JOURNAL OF REPRODUCTION AND FERTILITY

SUPPLEMENT 53

THE EPIDIDYMIS: CELLULAR AND MOLECULAR ASPECTS

Proceedings of the Boden Conference on
The Epididymis: Cellular and Molecular Aspects

held at
Ranelagh House,
Robertson
NSW, Australia
February 1998

Edited by Russell C. Jones, Michael K. Holland
and Christine Doberska

Journal of **REPRODUCTION** *and fertility*
1998

First published 1998

ISSN 0449 3087
ISBN 0 906545 33 1

JOURNALS OF REPRODUCTION AND FERTILITY LTD

The Journals of Reproduction and Fertility Ltd produce the *Journal of Reproduction and Fertility* and *Reviews of Reproduction.*

The *Journal of Reproduction and Fertility* publishes novel and significant papers on the molecular biology, biochemistry and physiology of reproduction, including lactation, and early embryogenesis in man and other animals. The *Journal* is the official organ of the Society for the Study of Fertility.

The *Journal* also publishes Supplements which are distinct from the regular issues, are not associated with any particular volume and are known by their serial number and date.

Reviews of Reproduction publishes topical, concise, well-illustrated reviews, contributed by leading research workers, on basic mechanisms in reproductive biology and comments on recent developments in the field, new hypotheses and highlights of scientific meetings. Articles are commissioned by the Editorial Board in consultation with the International Advisory Panel, and are peer-reviewed by experts in the field.

Published by **The Journals of Reproduction and Fertility Ltd.**

Agents for distribution: **Portland Press, PO Box 32, Commerce Way, Whitehall Industrial Estate, Colchester, CO2 8HP, Essex, UK; Tel: 44(0)1206 796351; FAX: 44(0)1206 799331; e-mail: sales@portlandpress.co.uk**

Printed by **Cambridge University Press**

CONTENTS

SUMMING UP

Chair: B. P. Setchell and R. C. Jones

ACKNOWLEDGEMENTS

This volume is a report of the Boden Conference on *The Epididymis: Cellular and Molecular Aspects* which was held at Ranelagh House, Robertson, NSW, Australia, 24–28 February 1998. There were 63 participants from 15 countries, and nearly all of the major laboratories in the field were represented. The meeting was organized as a workshop with time allocated for the presentation and discussion of 22 invited talks and 37 submitted miniposters. Participants received the book of miniposters about a month before the meeting so that discussions of the miniposters were informed. The main contributions at the conference were refereed for publication as this supplement of the *Journal of Reproduction and Fertility*.

We are grateful to those who made the Boden Conference a success: the invited speakers for the quality of their presentations at the meeting, those who presented miniposters, those who contributed to discussions, and for the timely submission of the manuscripts contained in this supplement. We are also grateful to colleagues in the US and Europe who provided generous support and advice towards organizing the conference and this monograph: J. M. Bedford, T. G. Cooper, B. T. Hinton, H. D. M. Moore, M-C. Orgebin-Crist and P. Y. D. Wong.

The conference was sponsored by The Australian Academy of Science, The Australian Society for Reproductive Biology, Cook Australasia Pty Ltd, the CRC for the Conservation and Management of Marsupials, The International Society for Andrology, The Journals of Reproduction & Fertility Ltd, Organon (Australia) Pty Ltd, the Research Management Committee of The University of Newcastle, Schering Research Foundation, Serono Australia Pty Ltd and the Vertebrate Biocontrol CRC. The Australian Academy of Science provided the seeding support from a fund established by the late Dr Alec Boden FAA.

The Organizing Committee of the meeting greatly appreciated the attendance at the meeting of Dr Christine Doberska, Managing Editor of the *Journal of Reproduction and Fertility*. Her professional approach and efforts ensured that most manuscripts were discussed with authors during the meeting and that agreement was reached among editors, reviewers and authors on necessary revisions.

Organizing Committee:
D. M. de Kretser
M. K. Holland
A. M. Jequier
R. C. Jones
B. P. Setchell

PREFACE

A publication on the epididymis is timely for a number of reasons. Most importantly, there is a developing interest in applying modern molecular techniques to study the epididymis. Work during the 1950s–1970s, by Lennart Nicander and others, on the structural differentiation of the epididymis is being revisited at the molecular level and shows regionalization, and is improving our understanding of the molecular regulation of regional gene expression by luminal and systemic factors. Its significance in regard to differentiation has recently been highlighted by Sonnenberg-Reithmacher and co-workers who showed that the primary defect after the targeted deletion of the c-ros tyrosine kinase receptor is failure to develop an initial segment of the epididymis. This causes sterility without an effect on sperm production. Molecular methods are also helping to determine the roles of some of the 150–200 proteins present in the epididymal lumen, and should provide a basis for interpreting the function and regulation of the epididymis. It is only possible to identify 6–10 processes that would involve luminal proteins in the epididymis, so it is not obvious why so many proteins are present. The role of oestrogens in epididymal function is currently controversial. R. A. Hess and co-workers report that fluid reabsorption by the ductuli efferentes is inhibited in the oestrogen receptor knockout mouse, whereas J. Clulow and co-workers report that the reabsorptive function of the ductuli efferentes is inhibited by oestrogen therapy. There is also a developing interest in the immunology of the epididymis (and the rest of the male reproductive tract) to control infections and sexually transmitted diseases, and to achieve immunocontraception in males. Finally, now that modern technologies achieve fertilization with spermatozoa that have not been exposed to the epididymis there is a need to pursue the findings of M-C. Orgebin-Crist, in the 1960s, which indicated that the passage of spermatozoa through the epididymis improved their chances of inducing normal egg development.

Work on humans over the last decade has questioned whether the epididymis is really necessary, as sperm aspirated from the ductuli efferentes of blocked tracts can sometimes fertilize *in vitro*, and one patient has produced fertile spermatozoa after anastomosis of the vas deferens to the rete testis. These findings may indicate that humans are different from other mammals in their requirement for post-testicular sperm maturation as it has not been possible to achieve fertilization with spermatozoa recovered from the rete testis of any other species of mammal. Further, it is questioned whether spermatozoa that have not passed through proximal regions of the epididymis are as potent as spermatozoa that have passed through all of the duct. That is, for example, would semen that was only exposed to part of the epididymis achieve as many pregnancies as semen exposed to the whole epididymis if samples of both were mixed and inseminated into females? It is also questioned whether males with an impairment affecting sperm storage in the epididymis could successfully compete with intact males when there is competition between males that may involve multiple matings of females?

The controversy over the importance of the epididymis emphasizes that presently '...there is little sense of the biological significance of epididymal functions in the context of conception as a whole...' (J. M. Bedford, personal communication). Obviously, the epididymis has evolved to cope with the constraints imposed on spermatozoa by the processes involved in internal fertilization. However, it may also enhance a male's prospects of achieving paternity in a competitive mating system. Clearly, the accumulation and storage of spermatozoa by the epididymis is advantageous in the competition between males to achieve paternity. However, it is not known whether the epididymis also plays a role in improving the potency of an individual's sperm in achieving fertilization.

The main objective of this publication has been to provide statements of current work on the epididymis. Consequently, most reports are on sperm maturation even though sperm storage is a very important function of the mammalian epididymis. The paucity of interest on sperm storage is unfortunate as there are important practical applications for knowledge of how the epididymis can maintain sperm viability for weeks–months. The emphasis on sperm maturation will probably change when more is known of the function of the epididymal proteins. Currently, the distinction is blurred between proteins that have a storage or protective role and those that have a maturation role. Some proteins that have been identified may have protective roles (for example against reactive oxygen species, enzymatic action and the immune system), but some of the protection may be to control sperm maturation processes involving enzymatic modification of sperm proteins, and redox regulation of maturation by reactive oxygen species. On the other hand, redox regulation may be involved in regulating or suppressing sperm motility and metabolism in the epididymis.

A concern that developed in editing this volume was the considerable variation between workers in their reference to specific regions of the epididymis. References based on anatomy are interpreted in different ways by different workers. References to the segments proposed by Glover and Nicander in 1971 also lead to ambiguities as it is not possible to apply the classification to all mammalian species. Reference to the 'initial segment' may also be ambiguous as Fawcett and Hoffer in 1979 showed that there is more than one initial segment. The only unambiguous way to identify specific regions is to refer to the appropriate report that relates the structural differentiation of the duct mucosa to the anatomy of the epididymis. A qualification of this suggestion is the need to recognize that there is an inaccuracy in the diagram of the rat epididymis by Reid and Cleland (1957) which was corrected by Nicander and co-workers in 1983.

The Boden Conference was recognized as the second international conference on the epididymis, the first being a one day meeting in Hong Kong in 1992. The longer meeting, the convivial atmosphere of the venue and the timeliness of the meeting contributed towards its success. There was an excellent exchange of ideas, and significant contacts were established as a prelude to the conference and during the conference. An important outcome of the conference was an agreement to continue the series of international conferences on the epididymis, and B. T. Hinton and T. T. Turner have undertaken to organize the third meeting in the USA in 2002.

Russell C Jones
Chairman
Organizing Committee

PARTICIPANTS AT THE BODEN CONFERENCE ON THE EPIDIDYMIS: CELLULAR AND MOLECULAR ASPECTS

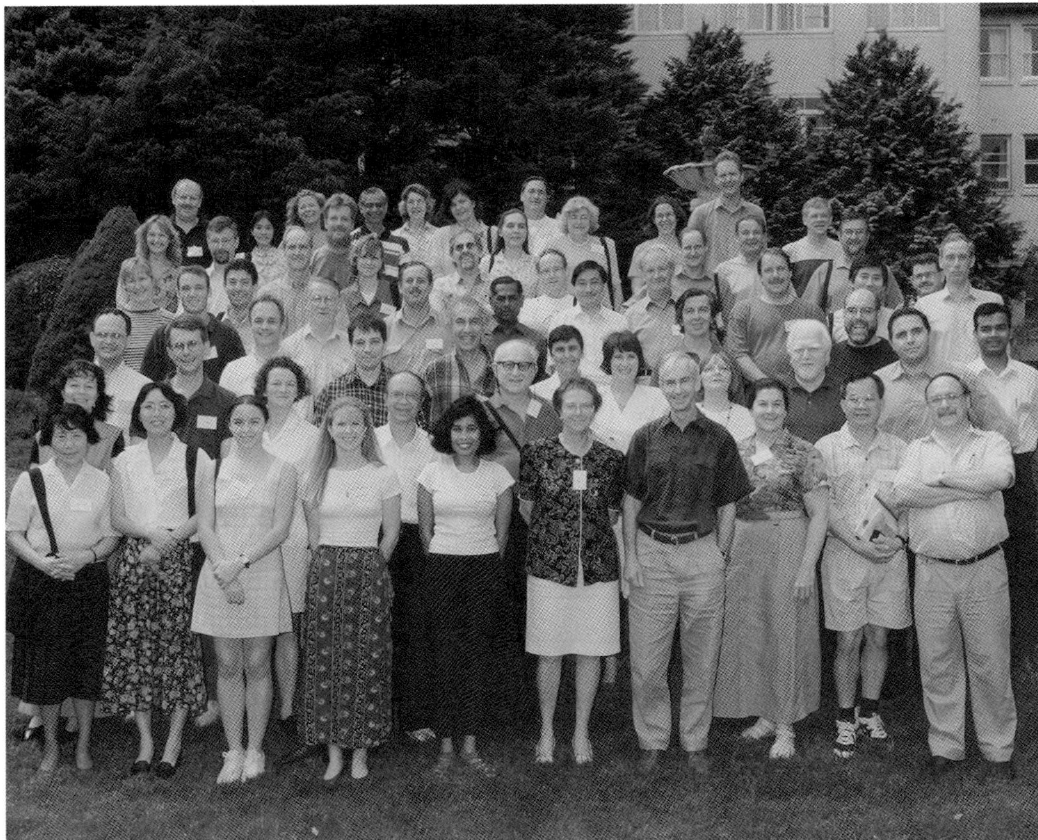

Starting from the front, from left to right: **Row 1**: L-L. Zhang, S. Y. Man, B. A. Lewis, N. G. Newcombe, D. C. Peiris, M-C. Orgebin-Crist, R. C. Jones, E. Smithwick, M. Lin, M. K. Holland. **Row 2**: F. Dacheux, T. T. Turner, C. Osterhoff, C. Pholpramool, L. M. Lewins, M. H. Fourie, C. A. Doberska. **Row 3**: R. A. Hess, J. A. Aitken, J. Drevet, D. M. de Kretser, L. G. Young, B. Robaire, P. Patrizio, L. Samayawardhena. **Row 4**: C. Kirchhoff, B. Nixon, P. Vernet, B. P. Setchell, P. M. Summers, M. A. Akbarsha, P. Y. D. Wong, R. Schoysman, H. D. M. Moore, R. Sullivan, N. U. L. Kvist, N. Okamura, D. J. Kay, R. Jones. **Row 5**: J. Frayne, J-L. Dacheux, B. T. Hinton, D. Bomgardner, R. Ivell, O. Fröhlich, T. G. Cooper, A. R. Jones, L. Hall, W. G. Breed. **Row 6**: K. W. Beagley, C-H. Yeung, Y. B. Kvist, J. Clulow, D. R. P. Tulsiani, M. Setchell, E. Töpfer-Pedersen, P. Seiler, P. Young, A. M. Jequier, E. Ekstedt, R. I. McLachlan. J. D. Kirby, Y. K. Kirby and S. J. Jones are not present.

Journal of Reproduction and Fertility Supplement **53**, 1–14

Fluid and electrolyte reabsorption in the ductuli efferentes testis

J. Clulow, R. C. Jones, L. A. Hansen and S. Y. Man

Department of Biological Sciences, University of Newcastle, NSW 2308, Australia

The efferent ducts of mammals are a series of ducts that are arranged in parallel and reabsorb most of the fluid released with spermatozoa from the testis. This function is essential for spermatogenesis, and for sperm maturation and storage in the epididymis. There is evidence for the involvement of three major transport processes in the bulk reabsorption of water and low molecular weight solutes from the ducts: active solute transport, passive (presumably paracellular) diffusion and fluid phase endocytosis. A small back-flux into the ducts via anion secretion also appears to occur. Control of fluid reabsorption by the efferent ducts is emerging as a complex process with multiple components. Reabsorption is flow dependent which provides local control of reabsorption with a rapid response to changes in luminal conditions. Sex steroids (oestrogen as well as androgen), but not mineralocorticosteroids, are involved in the chronic control of reabsorption in the ducts. Control of epithelial transport in the efferent ducts appears to be mediated by cAMP and probably other signal transduction systems.

Introduction

The efferent ducts of mammals (Jones and Jurd, 1987; Ilio and Hess, 1994) transport fluid and spermatozoa from the rete testis to the ductus epididymidis. Their primary function is the reabsorption of most of the testicular fluid released with spermatozoa. A growing body of evidence (Ilio and Hess, 1994; Eddy *et al.*, 1996; Hess *et al.*, 1997a) indicates that this function of the efferent ducts is essential for spermatogenesis and for the completion of sperm maturation and storage of spermatozoa in the epididymis. However, the mechanisms of fluid reabsorption by the efferent ducts, particularly of micro-solutes (electrolytes and low molecular weight organic compounds) and water, which make up the bulk of the reabsorbed fluid, are poorly understood. In addition, there is still a limited understanding of how epithelial transport is regulated to achieve the appropriate concentration of spermatozoa and luminal flow rate in fluid entering the ductus epididymidis. This review considers the current state of knowledge of fluid reabsorption by the efferent ducts (concentrating on water and micro-solutes), and proposes a model of fluid reabsorption that identifies the key features that need to be considered in future research aimed at understanding the central role of the efferent ducts in the function of the male extratesticular sperm ducts. The reader is referred to other reviews for a consideration of general aspects of efferent duct structure and function (Robaire and Hermo, 1998; Ilio and Hess, 1994) and of the reabsorption of macromolecules (Hermo *et al.*, 1988) by endocytosis.

Testicular Fluid Output and Reabsorption in the Efferent Ducts

When considering the reabsorption of testicular fluid, it is important to distinguish between the role of the efferent ducts and the caput epididymidis. Understandably, many earlier studies and reviews (see discussion in Clulow *et al.*, 1994) confounded reabsorption in these two regions of the male ducts. The reason for this was partly a failure to recognize the special role of the efferent ducts, but also technical difficulties in sampling fluids in the efferent ducts, and the initial segment of the epididymis where long stereocilia contaminate micropuncture samples (Jones *et al.*, 1987). It is now clear that a substantial change in the rate of fluid reabsorption represents a radical shift in function from the efferent ducts to the ductus epididymidis. In comparison to the efferent ducts, the ductus epididymidis, including the initial segments, carries out little net fluid reabsorption (Tables 1 and 2, see discussion Clulow *et al.*, 1994). Estimates of the proportion of testicular fluid output that is reabsorbed by the efferent ducts, which are not confounded by including the caput epididymidis, are available for a limited number of species, including the boar (90%; Crabo, 1965), bull (90%; Crabo, 1965), echidna (74%; Djakiew and Jones, 1983), tammar wallaby (87%; Jones and Clulow, 1987), elephant (96%; Jones, 1980) and rat (96%, Clulow *et al.*, 1994). For the rat, estimates of testicular fluid output are in the range of 30–50 µl h^{-1} (Tuck *et al.*, 1970; Free and Jaffe, 1979; Clulow *et al.*, 1994), and the flow rate reduces to only about 2 µl h^{-1} in fluid entering the ductus epididymidis. This flow rate under normal physiological conditions is remarkably stable (Clulow *et al.*, 1994; Man *et al.*, 1997).

Techniques for Studying Fluid Reabsorption in the Efferent Ducts

The efferent ducts are derived from the tubules of the mesonephric kidney (Du Bois,1969). Two regions of the ductuli can be recognized in mammals. In rats, for example, the initial zone consists of five to seven fairly straight ducts running parallel to one another. Distally, they form the coni vasculosi where the ducts are more sinuous and anastomose with one another eventually reducing to a single, common efferent duct (Jones and Jurd, 1987; Ilio and Hess, 1994). The structure of the ducts is similar to that of renal tubules and has led to renal techniques and transport models being applied to the ducts (Clulow *et al.*, 1994, 1996; Man *et al.*, 1997). Techniques used include sampling of the luminal contents by micropuncture (Clulow *et al.*, 1994), and microperfusion of individual ducts *in vivo* (Clulow *et al.*, 1996) and *in vitro* (Montorzi and Labiano, 1970). A modified renal microperfusion technique, the 'split droplet', has not been applied to the efferent ducts, but has considerable potential (one study that reported the application of split droplets to the rat efferent ducts (Holbrugger, 1980) was later confirmed to have been performed on the initial segment of the epididymis (Holbrugger, 1982)). Hess *et al.* (1997a) reported an *in vitro* technique in which the change in diameter of a ligated mouse duct was used to measure fluid reabsorption.

In our laboratory, two distinctly different *in vivo* techniques have been developed for the study of fluid transport by the efferent ducts of the anaesthetized rat (Clulow *et al.*, 1994; Clulow *et al.*, 1996). The first technique is micropuncture of the efferent ducts in conjunction with microcannulation of the proximal ductus epididymidis (zone 1a: Reid and Cleland, 1957; Fig. 1). The micropuncture sites include the proximal end of the initial zone of the efferent ducts (which samples rete testis fluid), the distal end of the initial zone, and the coni vasculosi. This procedure is used to sample luminal contents and to measure the rate of fluid entry from the rete testis into the ducts and the rate of efflux from the terminal end of the ducts into the ductus epididymidis, as well as rates of reabsorption in different regions and in the whole efferent ducts. Essentially, this procedure provides a measure of net fluid reabsorption by the efferent ducts in the intact animal. An additional procedure developed at the same time (Clulow *et al.*, 1994) used a micro-capillary pipette, rather than centrifugation, to sieve spermatozoa from plasma in micropuncture samples, reducing the probability of leakage of sperm cytoplasmic contents during separation.

The second technique is microperfusion of single efferent ducts *in vivo* (Fig. 2). This procedure involves the double cannulation and microperfusion of a single efferent duct in the initial zone. The proximal cannula is used to perfuse solutions at controlled rates through the duct, the modified perfusate (collectate) being accumulated in the distal collection cannula. A major difference between *in vivo* perfusion of the efferent ducts and the ductus epididymidis (Wong and Yeung, 1978) and renal tubules (Park and Maack, 1984) is that inulin cannot be used as a marker of fluid (volume) reabsorption in the efferent ducts because of its high permeability across the epithelium (Fig. 5). Furthermore, a limitation of the microperfusion technique is that it treats the epithelium as a single compartment, and does not differentiate between the roles of ciliated and non-ciliated cells in water

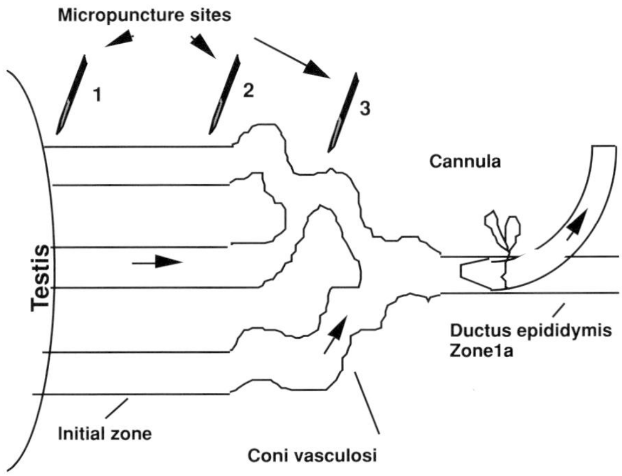

Fig. 1. Micropuncture and cannulation sites in the efferent ducts (initial zone and coni vasculosi) and ductus epididymis of the rat. Reproduced with permission from Clulow *et al.* (1994).

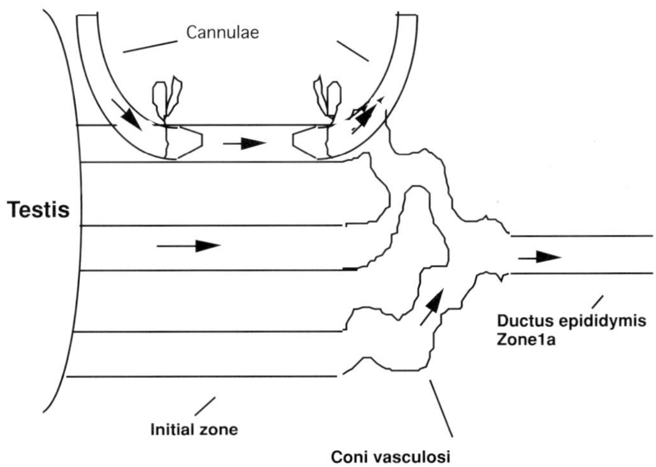

Fig. 2. System for microperfusion of the rat efferent ducts *in vivo*. Reproduced with permission from Clulow *et al.* (1996)

and electrolyte transport. Ciliated cells, while not the major cell type in the efferent ducts, are nevertheless, common, and their frequency increases from the proximal to the distal regions (Jones and Jurd, 1987; Wang *et al.*, 1994). They are distributed randomly among the principal cells, singly, or in clumps of from two to five cells (Wang *et al.*, 1994).

The Efferent Ducts as a Transporting Epithelium

Numerous structural studies (see discussions by Jones and Jurd, 1987; Wang *et al.*, 1994; Ilio and Hess, 1994) have demonstrated that the epithelial cells of the efferent ducts have structural features indicative of transporting epithelia. These features include high densities of mitochondria, well-developed microvilli and endocytotic apparatus and, importantly, tight junctional complexes typical of 'leaky' epithelia (Suzuki and Nagano, 1978; Lopez *et al.*, 1997). Table 1 shows estimates of fluid

Table 1. Estimates of net fluid fluxes across the mucosa of various transporting epithelia

Epithelium	Flux ($\mu l\ cm^{-2}\ h^{-1}$)	Epithelium	Flux ($\mu l\ cm^{-2}\ h^{-1}$)
Rat cauda epididymidis[1]	0.1	Dog ileum[2]	17.0
Frog skin[2]	1.1	Guinea-pig gall bladder[2]	23.0
Human ileum[2]	3.0	Rabbit ileum[2]	27.0
Turtle urinary bladder[2]	5.2	Rabbit gall bladder[2]	50.0
Human jejunum[2]	6.9	Dog gall bladder[2]	60.0
Fowl cloaca[2]	8.4	Quail efferent ducts[3]	100.4
Necturus gall bladder[2]	8.6	Rat proximal kidney tubule[4]	90.0–190.0
Rat efferent ducts[1]	17.2		

[1]Table 2; [2]House, 1974 p. 429; [3]Clulow and Jones, 1988; [4]Wang *et al.*, 1994

transport (net reabsorption) by the efferent ducts for the only species for which estimates are available and for several other transporting epithelia. It shows that the efferent ducts of rats have a moderately high rate of net reabsorption, although that rate is only about 10% of the estimate for the proximal renal tubule, which is the most active mammalian transporting epithelium. The rate of fluid reabsorption by the efferent ducts of the Japanese quail is very high, indicating that an avian model animal would be useful for studying fluid reabsorption by the efferent ducts.

There are insufficient experimental data to provide a reasonably complete, integrated model for epithelial transport in the efferent ducts. However, there is sufficient evidence to support a partial model (Figs 3, 4). The key components of transport are considered below: (i) active solute transport (ii) passive (diffusive) permeability (iii) fluid phase endocytosis and (iv) secretion.

Active solute transport: the sodium pump

As with other transporting epithelia, the sodium gradient across the plasma membrane generated by the active sodium pump (Na^+–K^+-ATPase) would appear to be the main source of energy driving primary and secondary active solute transport across the duct epithelium. Substantial Na^+–K^+-ATPase activity, located in the basolateral membranes, has been demonstrated in the efferent ducts (Byers and Graham, 1990; Ilio and Hess, 1992, 1994). Addition of the sodium pump inhibitors, vanadate and ouabain, together to perfusates of a rat efferent duct reduces reabsorption by up to 70% (L. A. Hansen, J. Clulow and R. C. Jones, unpublished). In addition, removal of Na^+ from the lumen during microperfusion abolishes fluid reabsorption (L. A. Hansen, J. Clulow and R. C. Jones, unpublished). Table 2 shows a comparison of the relationship between Na^+ and fluid transport and the activity of the sodium pump in the efferent ducts and the cauda epididymidis of the rat. Although Na^+–K^+-ATPase activity in the efferent ducts is less than in the cauda epididymidis, both net Na^+ and fluid transport by the ducts are two orders of magnitude greater than in the cauda epididymidis. In addition, the rate of Na^+ transport in the efferent ducts is much closer to the theoretical maximum for the sodium pump (3 Na^+ per ATP hydrolysed; Jørgensen, 1980; Burckhardt and Greger, 1992) than in the epididymis. These differences between the efferent ducts and the ductus epididymidis are indicative of the different functions of the two regions of the male tract: bulk fluid flow in the efferent ducts with high Na^+ and fluid fluxes, without the generation of substantial trans-epithelial gradients; and low Na^+ and fluid transport in the ductus epididymidis, where the sodium pump contributes to the generation of substantial luminal gradients rather than to substantial transepithelial transport. Nevertheless, a portion of Na^+ transport in the efferent ducts may be by passive, paracellular conductance, see below, suggesting that, even in the efferent ducts, the sodium pump may not be as fully utilized for epithelial transport as might be concluded from Table 2, unlike the proximal kidney tubule where Na^+ transport is greater than can be accounted for by the sodium pump capacity (Burckhardt and Greger, 1992).

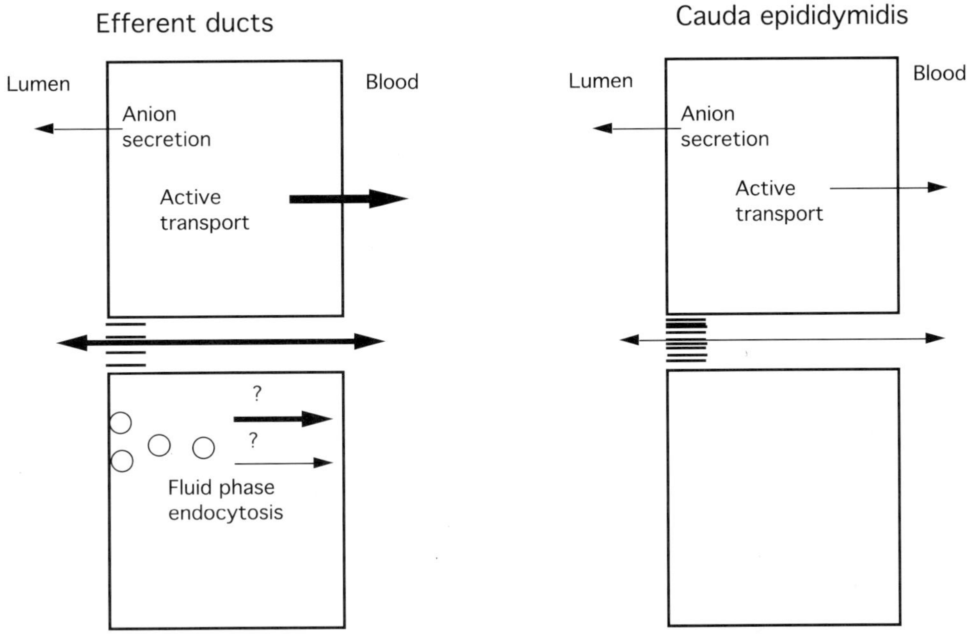

Fig. 3. Generalized model of epithelial transport in the efferent ducts and cauda epididymidis of the rat. Arrows indicate relative magnitude of fluxes.

Na^+-dependent transport in the efferent ducts appears to be mediated to a large extent by the Na^+–H^+ exchanger; addition of 1.0–7.5 mmol amiloride ml^{-1} to luminal perfusates during microperfusion *in vivo* reduces fluid reabsorption in a dose-dependent manner by up to 70% (L. A. Hansen, J. Clulow and R. C. Jones, submitted). There is also evidence of considerable carbonic anhydrase activity in the efferent ducts (Cohen *et al.*, 1976; Goyal *et al.*, 1980; Ekstedt and Ridderstråle, 1992), and unpublished data (N. Newcombe, J. Clulow, S. Y. Man and R. C. Jones) for the rat which indicates that bicarbonate reabsorption by the efferent ducts is extensive. It is probable that, as in the proximal kidney tubule, Na^+–H^+ exchange and carbonic anhydrase are associated in the reabsorption of bicarbonate (Burckhardt and Greger, 1992).

Evidence for the role of a high diffusional permeability in the efferent ducts

Although a number of studies and reviews (see discussion in Jones and Jurd, 1987; Ilio and Hess, 1994) have discussed the relative contribution of fluid phase endocytosis and active solute transport to reabsorption by the efferent ducts, the possible contribution of passive permeability has received little attention. On the basis of two sources of evidence, it is suggested that high diffusional permeability (to both water and low molecular weight solutes) is one of the most important features of epithelial transport in the efferent ducts. First, micropuncture studies of the efferent ducts (Clulow *et al.*, 1994) indicate that during the reabsorption of fluid in the initial zone and part of the coni vasculosi, the concentration of electrolytes in the lumen changes with a trend towards equilibration with concentrations in blood plasma. This trend towards equilibrium involves increases in the concentration of some electrolytes (for example Na^+) and decreases in others for example K^+, Cl^- (Table 3), and the equilibration of blood and luminal osmolality. This equilibrium occurs even though a high rate of water and electrolyte reabsorption occurs at the same time (Table 3). The second source of evidence is that when the initial zone is perfused with different fluids (for example Krebs Ringer bicarbonate and native rete testis fluid), there is a trend towards the equilibration of

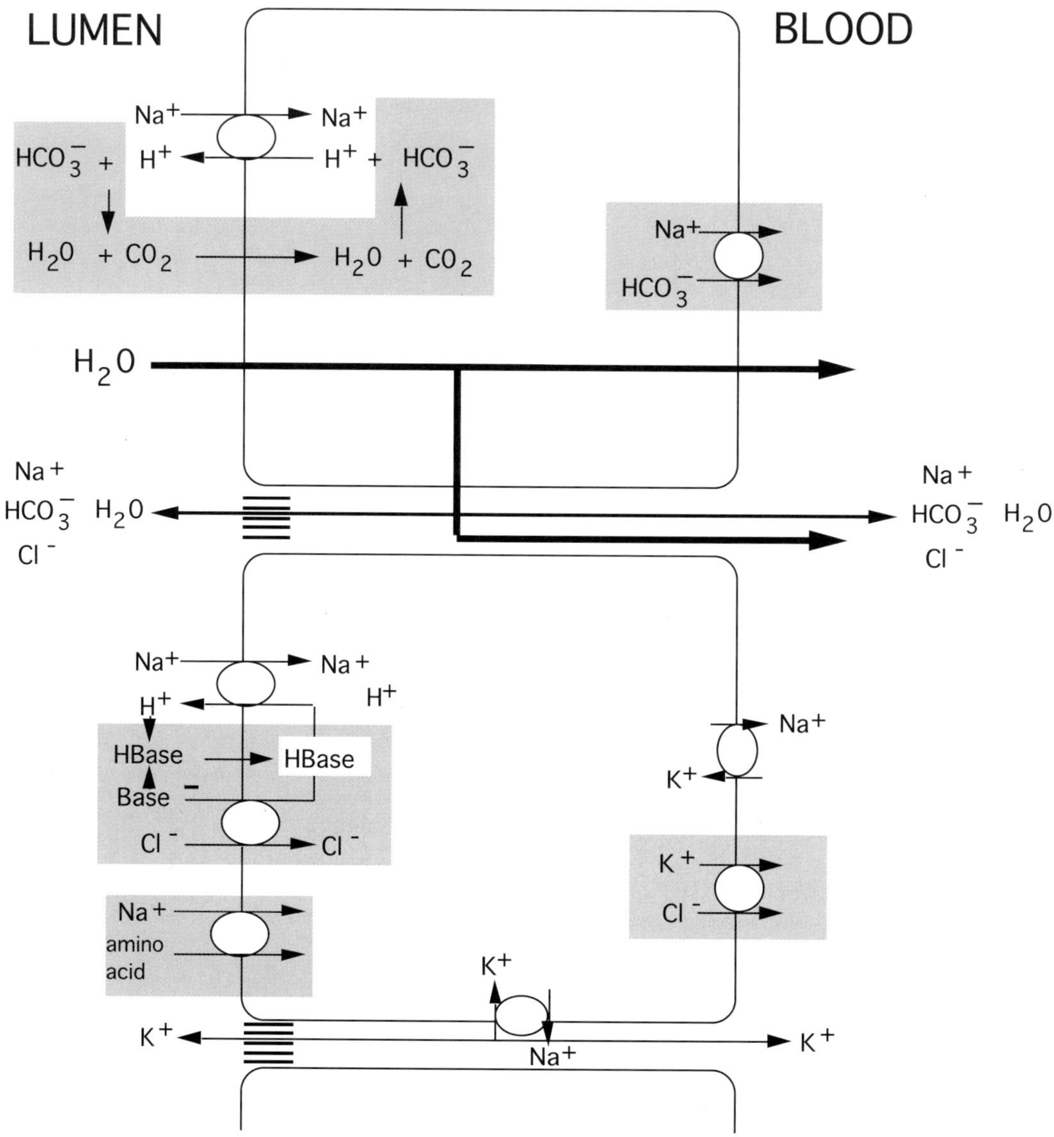

Fig. 4. Model of epithelial transport of water and electrolytes in the efferent ducts of the rat. Hypothetical pathways are stippled.

osmolality and luminal electrolytes between the lumen and the blood (Clulow *et al.*, 1996) even when the perfusion rate is varied considerably. Other unpublished data (L. A. Hansen, J. Clulow and R. C. Jones) indicates that the equilibration of osmolality occurs even when a solution containing only isotonic mannitol is perfused through the ducts causing considerable efflux of mannitol from the ducts and influx of Na^+, K^+ and Cl^- into the ducts.

The route for the passive diffusion of substances across the efferent duct epithelium has not been determined, although most probably paracellular water and solute fluxes through the intercellular spaces are important contributors. Wang *et al.* (1994) showed that there is an increased convolution (folding) of the lateral cell membrane, and hence of the volume of the lateral intercellular spaces, from the apical to the basal poles of the non-ciliated cells in the rat. Such an expansion of the

Table 2. Estimates of Na^+–K^+-ATPase (Na^+ pump) activity, and net Na^+ and fluid fluxes *in situ* in the initial zone of the efferent ducts and cauda epididymidis of the rat

Parameter	Efferent ducts	Cauda epididymidis	Efferent ducts: cauda epididymidis[g]
Fluid flux (μl cm^{-2} h^{-1})[a]	17.2[h]	0.1[i,j,k]	172
Na^+ flux (nmol cm^{-2} h^{-1})[b]	1756[h,m]	5.5[i,j,k,l]	319
Na^+–K^+-ATPase activity (nmol P_i mm^{-1} h^{-1})	7.60[n]	26.1[n]	0.29
Na^+–K^+-ATPase activity (nmol P_i cm^{-2} h^{-1})[b]	1407[m,n]	1855[i,n]	0.76
Maximum capacity Na^+ pump[c] (nmol Na^+ cm^{-2} h^{-1})[b]	4221[m,n]	5565[l,n]	0.76
Na^+ transport per ATP[d] (mol Na^+ per mol ATP)	1.248[h,m,n]	0.003[i,j,k,l,n]	416
Na^+ transport (% max Na^+ pump capacity)[e]	41.6[h,m,n]	0.1[i,j,k,l,n]	416
Fluid flux per ATP (nl $nmolP_i^{-1}$)[f]	5.86[h,m,n]	0.04[i,k,j,n]	155

Surface areas calculated treating the ducts as straight-sided cylinders: [a]per cm^{-2} of luminal surface area; [b]per cm^{-2} of basal surface area; [c]Activity of Na^+–K^+-ATPase (nmol P_i cm^{-2} h^{-1}) × 3; [d]Molar ratio of net Na^+ transport per mol of ATP hydrolysed by Na pump; [e]Molar ratio of net Na^+ transport to maximum capacity of Na^+ pump × 100; [f]Ratio of fluid flux (nl cm^{-2} h^{-1}) to activity of Na^+–K^+-ATPase (nl P_i cm^{-2} h^{-1}); [g]Ratio of efferent duct value to cauda epididymidis value in same row. Values calculated or taken from: [h]Clulow *et al.*, 1994; [i]Djakiew and Jones, 1982; [j]Hinton and Setchell, 1980; [k]Tuck *et al.*, 1970; [l]Levine and Marsh, 1971; [m]Jones and Jurd, 1987; [n]S. Y. Man, J. Clulow and R. C. Jones, unpublished.

intercellular space should decrease resistance to flow and favour both active solute and passive diffusional transport across the epithelium. Other findings that are consistent with a high paracellular permeability in the efferent ducts are the demonstration by Suzuki and Nagano (1978) that the tight junctions are less developed than in other regions of the sperm ducts, and the report by Chan *et al.* (1995a) of a low transepithelial resistance in cultured efferent duct cells. Nevertheless, the presence of water and ion channels (Brown *et al.*, 1993; Chan *et al.*, 1995a) in the efferent duct epithelium may also contribute substantial passive transcellular movement.

Potassium: a possible marker for modelling diffusional permeability in the efferent ducts

Potassium undergoes the greatest relative change in concentration of any electrolyte during passage through the efferent ducts. Its behaviour both in the intact system (Table 3) and during microperfusion *in vivo* (Table 4) indicates it is equilibrating as a simple diffusional solute. In this respect, a model of K^+ transport generated by Weinstein (1988) for the proximal kidney tubule (see the discussion of this model in Giebisch *et al.*, 1991) integrates active K^+ uptake by the epithelial cells from the serosal side and passive K^+ flux through the intercellular spaces. In this model (which predicts an equilibrium [K^+] in the lumen within 1 mmol l^{-1} of blood plasma), Na^+–K^+-ATPase actively removes K^+ from the intercellular space, while a diffusional flux of K^+ occurs between the intercellular space and the lumen (across the tight junction) and the intercellular space and the vascular compartment. Unpublished data (L. A. Hansen, J. Clulow and R. C. Jones) suggests such an equilibration occurs in the efferent ducts of the rat: when the rat ducts are perfused with pure mannitol and other K^+-free solutions, concentrations of K^+ in the lumen equilibrate close to that in blood plasma.

Thus, the limited data that are available support a model of the efferent ducts as a leaky epithelium with a highly permeable paracellular pathway which allows solutes to readily enter or

Table 3. Concentration of solutes and osmolality in blood and luminal fluids of the efferent ducts of the rat.

Parameter	Blood plasma	Rete testis	Coni vasculosi	Proximal[a] ductus epididymidis	Caput epididymidis
Na^+ (mmol l^{-1})	151 ± 2	137 ± 3[b]	144 ± 3*	137 ± 2[b]*	104
Cl^- (mmol l^{-1})	107 ± 1	130 ± 3[b]	113 ± 3*	117 ± 3[b]	25
K^+ (mmol l^{-1})	4.9 ± 0.2	13.3 ± 0.7[b]	5.7 ± 0.3*	11.6 ± 0.5[b]*	20.5
Mg^{2+} (mmol l^{-1})	3.0 ± 0.2	1.5 ± 0.3[b]	2.7 ± 0.3*	1.7 ± 0.2[b]*	2.0
Ca^{2+} (mmol l^{-1})	2.6 ± 0.1	0.9 ± 0.3[b]	2.2 ± 0.3*	1.3 ± 0.2[b]*	0.9
Phosphorus (mmol l^{-1})	4.1 ± 0.3	1.2 ± 0.3[b]	3.2 ± 0.4*	4.5 ± 0.6*	59.0
Sulphur (mmol l^{-1})	29.6 ± 0.9	0.9 ± 0.1[b]	5.5 ± 2.0[b]*	2.4 ± 0.5[b]*	13.8
Protein (µg µl^{-1})	60.3 ± 1.6	0.6 ± 0.1[b]	1.7 ± 0.6[b]*	3.4 ± 0.4[b]*	22.4
Osmolality (mosm kg^{-1})	305 ± 3	307 ± 3	303 ± 3	301 ± 2	315
% fluid reabsorbed[c]			71 %	86 %	

[a]Zone 1a (Reid and Cleland, 1957) see Fig. 1. Data from Clulow *et al.* (1994), except for the caput epididymidis which is from Levine and Marsh (1971); Jenkins *et al.* (1980); Turner *et al.* (1984); [b]indicates mean values significantly different from blood ($P < 0.05$), *indicates mean values significantly different from mean for adjacent proximal site ($P < 0.05$). Data for caput epididymidis not tested. Note: protein is only solute not equilibrated between efferent duct fluid (coni vasculosi) and blood (elemental sulphur incorporated in protein).[c]Percentage fluid reabsorbed between site and adjacent proximal site.

Table 4. Potassium concentration in blood plasma and in samples of native rete testis fluid and Krebs Ringer–bicarbonate, before (perfusate) and after (collectate) microperfusion of a single efferent duct at five different rates (means ± SEM, n = 5–10).

Parameter	Krebs Ringer-bicarbonate	Native rete testis fluid
Blood plasma	5.2 ± 0.4	4.7 ± 0.4**
Perfusate	5.2 ± 0.3	17.2 ± 0.4***
Collectate from perfusion at:		
0.025 µl min^{-1}	4.9 ± 0.4	5.4
0.05 µl min^{-1}	3.6 ± 0.3	5.2 ± 0.5
0.1 µl min^{-1}	4.0 ± 0.3	5.7 ± 0.5
0.2 µl min^{-1}	4.3 ± 0.6	7.6 ± 1.1
0.4 µl min^{-1}	5.5 ± 0.6	9.8 ± 0.9

Values for blood plasma or perfusate [K^+] are significantly different from collectates where: **$P < 0.01$, ***$P < 0.001$. Data indicate that a high luminal [K^+] and perfusion load saturates the capacity of the ducts to absorb K^+, otherwise an equilibrium between blood and luminal [K^+] is achieved. From Clulow *et al.* (1996).

leave the ducts (contributing to the efficiency of bulk fluid reabsorption), and prevents the establishment of major concentration gradients of organic compounds that occur (Hinton and Setchell, 1980; Hinton *et al.*, 1979, 1980) in the ductus epididymidis.

Fluid phase reabsorption

The occurrence of endocytosis as a mechanism for the reabsorption of proteins by both fluid and adsorptive endocytosis in the efferent ducts is well established. Tracer studies have shown progression of endocytosed protein from the apical membrane to tertiary lysosomes (Hermo *et al.*, 1988), and most of the protein released from the testis is reabsorbed by endocytosis in the efferent ducts. In rats, for example, 80 % of the protein released from the rete testis (29 µg h^{-1}) is reabsorbed (Clulow *et al.*, 1994). A more problematic question, however, is the contribution of fluid phase

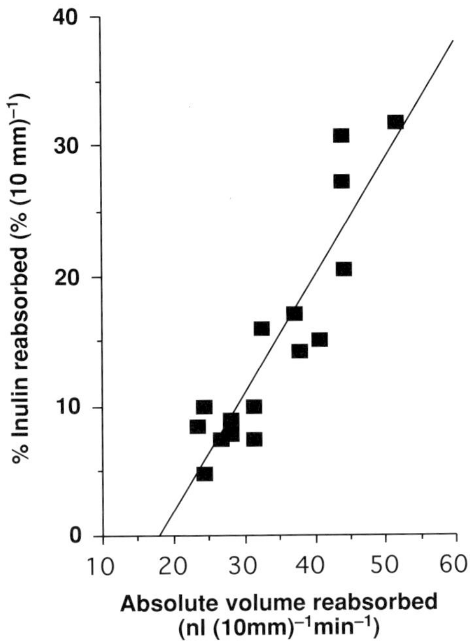

Fig. 5. Percentage inulin reabsorbed from Krebs Ringer Bicarbonate microperfusates of rat efferent ducts against absolute volume reabsorbed.

endocytosis to the uptake of fluid and electrolytes from the lumen of the ducts. Although there has been some discussion in the literature (Jones and Jurd, 1987; Ilio and Hess, 1994) concerning the relative contribution of active solute versus fluid phase endocytosis, there is a lack of experimental evidence to resolve the issue at this stage. Unpublished data (Fig. 5) from our laboratory indicate that up to 30 % of inulin (a fluid volume marker) added to the perfusate may be reabsorbed from microperfused rat efferent ducts. At least part of the inulin reabsorption is likely to be by fluid phase endocytosis. Reabsorption of inulin appears to be flow dependent, suggesting some interaction with other flow rate dependent aspects of reabsorption such as Na^+ transport.

Secretion versus reabsorption in the efferent ducts

The net movement of water and electrolytes during transport through the efferent ducts is overwhelmingly in favour of reabsorption. In rats, more than 95 % of the water, Na^+, K^+ and Cl^- (Clulow *et al.*, 1994), and HCO_3^- (N. Newcombe, J. Clulow, S. Y. Man and R. C. Jones, unpublished) is reabsorbed. Nevertheless, a considerable body of work by Wong and co-workers (Wong *et al.*, 1992; Chan *et al.* 1995a,b) indicates that the epithelium of the efferent ducts and the ductus epididymidis are capable of anion secretion (Cl^- and $HCO3^-$) via apical channels; Cl^- entry from the serosal surface occurs via a Na^+:K^+: $2Cl^-$ symport. This anion secretion is mediated by a number of hormonal and neurohormonal compounds, which in turn act by second messenger systems to stimulate anion secretion (Chan *et al.*, 1995b). In particular, a rise in intracellular cAMP and Ca^{2+} has been implicated in increasing anion secretion above basal values (Chan *et al.*, 1995b). In the ductus epididymidis (where the rate of Na^+ dependent fluid reabsorption is low; Table 2), anion secretion is considered to be an important counterbalance to reabsorption, preventing obstruction of the lumen by excessive fluid reabsorption (Wong *et al.*, 1992). However, it is less certain that it plays a significant role in the efferent ducts, where anion and fluid transport massively favour reabsorption over secretion.

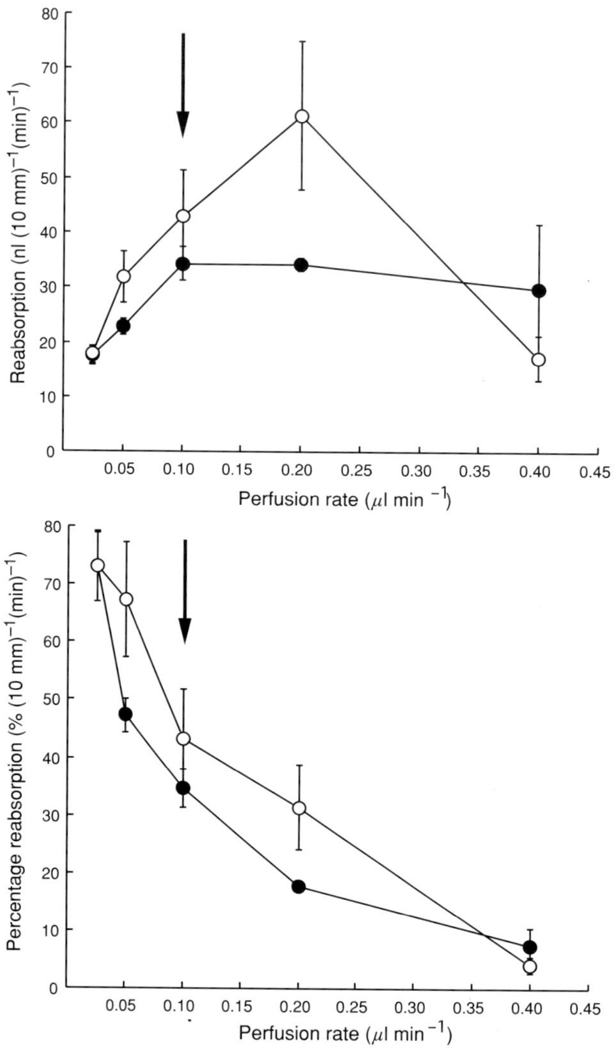

Fig. 6. Reabsorption of fluid ((●) Krebs Ringer bicarbonate and (○) rete testis fluid) against perfusion rate for single ducts from the initial zone of the efferent ducts of the rat perfused *in vivo*. Values are means ± SEM, $n = 5$. (a) Reabsorption (nl min^{-1}) normalized per 10 mm duct length. (b) Percentage reabsorption of perfusate (% min^{-1}), normalized per 10 mm duct length. Arrow indicates estimated initial perfusion rate in situ. Reproduced with permission from Clulow *et al.* (1996).

Control of Reabsorption

The control of fluid reabsorption in the efferent ducts is poorly understood, although the subject is now generating considerable interest with recent evidence from oestrogen receptor knockout (ERKO) mice that oestrogen is required for fluid reabsorption within the efferent ducts (Eddy *et al.*, 1996; Hess *et al.*, 1997a). The concept of the control of reabsorption is very important, as reabsorption must be precisely regulated if a large volume of fluid from the testis is to be reduced to a small volume of fluid entering the efferent ducts at a constant rate with only minimal deviation from the

Table 5. Testicular fluid and sperm output, and fluid flow from the efferent ducts of the rat following treatment with sex steroids and their antagonists.

Treatment	Seminal vesicles (g)	Testicular fluid output (μl h^{-1})*	Daily sperm production (no. d$^{-1}\times10^6$)	$[Sperm]_{RT}$ (no. μl$^{-1}\times10^4$)	$[Sperm]_{1a}$ (no. μl$^{-1}\times10^5$)	$Flow_{1a}$ (μl h^{-1})
Untreated	1.9 ± 0.2 (13)	47 (28–87)	27.3 ± 2.9 (16)	2.4 ± 0.4 (19)	6.0 ± 0.50 (15)	1.8 ± 0.1 (16)
Testosterone	2.7 ± 0.1 (17)[c]	50 (27–107)	28.1 ± 3.6 (5)	2.3 ± 0.5 (5)	8.5 ± 0.70 (5)	1.4 ± 0.3 (5)
Flutamide	1.5 ± 0.1 (9)[a]	33 (16–68)	19.0 ± 3.0 (5)	2.4 ± 0.5 (5)	6.4 ± 1.28 (5)	1.3 + 0.1 (5)[a]
Oestradiol	1.2 ± 0.1 (7)[c]	57 (21–137)	16.0 ± 4.0 (5)[a]	1.2 ± 0.2 (8)[a]	1.8 ± 0.70 (5)[c]	4.6 ± 0.9 (5)[c]
Tamoxifen	1.5 ± 0.1 (6)	45 (24–82)	27.2 ± 4.6 (5)	2.5 ± 0.3 (5)	8.1 ± 0.99 (5)	1.4 ± 0.1 (5)[a]

*Values in brackets show 95% confidence limits. $[Sperm]_{RT}$ = sperm concentration in rete testis fluid; $Flow_{1a}$, $[Sperm]_{1a}$ = flow rate and sperm concentration, respectively, of fluid leaving the efferent ducts i.e. entering the ductus epididymidis. Values are means ± SEM. Number of animal replicates are shown in parentheses. [a]($P < 0.05$) and [c]($P < 0.001$) indicate significant differences between means for untreated and treated rats within the same column. Data from Hansen *et al.* (1997).

mean flow rate (see above). Emerging evidence suggests that there are multiple mechanisms controlling fluid reabsorption by the efferent ducts, as in the kidney (Ilio and Hess, 1994; Clulow *et al.*, 1996; Hess *et al.*, 1997a; Hansen *et al.*, 1997). Given the complex interactions that would be expected of multiple control systems, understanding how reabsorption in the efferent ducts is so precisely regulated will be challenging. On the basis of a study of microperfused rat efferent ducts, Clulow *et al.* (1996) reported that reabsorption is flow dependent (Fig. 6) paralleling the same process that has been demonstrated in the proximal renal tubule. It appears to be at least partly, if not entirely, mediated through the Na^+–H^+ exchanger (L. A. Hansen, J. Clulow and R. C. Jones, unpublished) and provides an acute response to changes in luminal flow rate within minutes. Other control mechanisms seem to exert a more chronic effect on reabsorption (Ilio and Hess, 1994; Hess *et al.*, 1997a; Hansen *et al.*, 1997).

Sex steroids as first messenger control systems

There is now strong evidence (Ilio and Hess, 1994; Eddy *et al.*, 1996; Hess *et al.*, 1997a; Hansen *et al.*, 1997) that sex steroids are of central importance in regulating fluid reabsorption in the efferent ducts, as can be seen by deviations from the normal rate of fluid release from the efferent ducts into the epididymis, when the sex steroid status of rats is altered by administrating oestrogens, androgens or their antagonists (Table 5). The efferent ducts are well endowed with both androgen (Cooke *et al.*, 1991a) and oestrogen receptors (Cooke *et al.*, 1991b; Hess, *et al.*, 1997b; Fisher *et al.*, 1997), a situation complicated even more by the recent identification of two types of oestrogen receptors in the male (Hess *et al.*, 1997b). Separating the relative contribution of androgens and oestrogens to the control of efferent duct fluid reabsorption is, however, likely to be challenging, and recent studies on the effects of oestrogen in rats and mice have provided apparently conflicting results (Hess *et al.*, 1997a; Hansen *et al.*, 1997).

In the ER intact rat, testosterone administration causes a small increase in fluid reabsorption, whereas oestradiol reduces fluid reabsorption substantially, causing a 2.5-fold increase in the flow rate from the terminal end of the efferent ducts (Hansen *et al.*, 1997; Table 5). This response is seen whether fluid reabsorption is measured by cannulation of the terminal end of the efferent ducts (Fig. 1), or by the completely separate technique of *in vivo* microperfusion (Fig. 2). In the same study, tamoxifen, an anti-oestrogen, increased fluid reabsorption, as did the pure anti-androgen, flutamide. Interpretation of the actions of these antagonists is complicated, however, as tamoxifen may also have oestrogenic or anti-androgenic effects, and flutamide, by increasing systemic androgen concentrations, may act as an androgen agonist (see discussion in Hansen *et al.*, 1997). In addition, in the experiments of Hansen *et al.* (1997) oestrogen may have acted as an anti-androgen, reducing fluid reabsorption by reducing systemic testosterone, or by binding to androgen receptors. Nevertheless, one possible interprertation of these data is that, in the ER intact rat, androgens upregulate and oestrogens downregulate fluid reabsorption. The data of Hansen *et al.* (1997) are consistent with the report of Ilio and Hess (1994) that castration reduces Na^+–K^+-ATPase activity in the rat efferent ducts, as does the administration of oestrogen to intact rats. Interestingly, Ilio and Hess (1994) also showed that in castrated rats, the administration of oestrogen partially blocked the action of testosterone therapy in restoring Na^+–K^+-ATPase activity, suggesting some antagonistic effect of oestrogen against testosterone. Further evidence for a possible suppressive effect of oestrogen on fluid reabsorption comes from the study of Meistrich *et al.* (1975), in which oestrogen administration caused a decrease in the time taken for spermatozoa to transit through the epididymis in ER intact mice, an effect that may have been due to reduced fluid reabsorption by the efferent ducts. This interpretation is also consistent with the observation of a low sperm concentration in samples from the cauda epididymidis of a tammar receiving exogenous oestrogen (R. C. Jones, unpublished).

Nevertheless, conflicting data and interpretations have recently been reported on the role of oestrogens in efferent duct fluid reabsorption by Hess *et al.* (1997a) in studies on ERKO and ER intact mice. These workers reported that fluid reabsorption *in vitro* in the efferent ducts of ERKO mice was completely absent and that in ER intact mice, the anti-oestrogen, ICI 182,780, reduced fluid reabsorption (a response opposite to the effect of tamoxifen in rats). These workers interpreted their data as indicating that oestrogen action is required for fluid reabsorption to occur in the efferent ducts. The apparent conflict between the results of the different studies are likely to be resolved by one of two models: either oestrogen is essential for basal levels of fluid reabsorption, but also downregulates reabsorption, or else both oestrogen and testosterone support fluid reabsorption (in which case the decreased fluid reabsorption in the report of Hansen *et al.* (1997) was due to oestrogen acting as an anti-androgen). Irrespective of the separate contributions of oestrogens and androgens, the evidence is now very strong that sex steroid activity is essential to the precise control of fluid reabsorption displayed by the efferent ducts. By contrast, removal of the adrenal glands has no effect on reabsorption by the efferent ducts, indicating that aldosterone and other mineralocorticosteroids are not involved in the control of Na^+ and fluid transport (Man *et al.*, 1997).

Second messenger systems in the efferent ducts

There is little information on the role of signal transduction systems in the control of fluid reabsorption by the efferent ducts. The most detailed studies relate to the role of cAMP which appears to be involved in the stimulation of anion secretion by the cultured epithelial cells (Chan *et al.*, 1995b). New data from S. Y. Man, J. Clulow and R. C. Jones (unpublished), which indicate that 0.5 mmol cAMP l^{-1} in luminal perfusates totally abolishes fluid reabsorption in rat efferent ducts, conflicts with this action of cAMP (indicating how complex the control of fluid transport in the efferent ducts may be). It is possible that the abolition of reabsorption by cAMP may be due to increased anion secretion. However, given the evidence (see above) that anion secretion is a minor component of transport in the efferent ducts, it is more likely that cAMP downregulates reabsorption by suppression of the Na^+–H^+ exchanger as has been reported in the proximal kidney tubule (Harris, 1992). More research is needed before the role of signal transduction is adequately understood.

Conclusion

The role of the efferent ducts in reabsorbing most of the rete testis fluid released with spermatozoa is essential for normal function in the male reproductive tract. Although more interest is now being shown in understanding the physiology of the ducts, the fundamental mechanisms whereby they reabsorb fluid remain poorly understood. The regulatory systems whereby reabsorption is finely tuned to deliver modified fluid and spermatozoa into the initial segment of the epididymis at a precisely controlled rate is even less understood. Future research needs to target the fundamental transport processes, and the way these processes interact and are integrated by luminal and circulating factors, and by signal transduction. In particular, the role of three processes, active solute transport, passive (paracellular) diffusion and fluid phase endocytosis need to be more fully explored. Regulation of reabsorption by androgens and oestrogens is also a crucial question for future study.

References

Brown D, Verbavatz JM, Valenti G, Lui B and Sabolic I (1993) Localization of the CHIP28 water channel in reabsorptive segments of the rat male reproductive tract *European Journal of Cell Biology* **61** 264–273

Burckhardt G and Greger R (1992) Principles of electrolyte transport across plasma membranes of renal tubular cells. In *Handbook of Physiology* Section 8 Renal Physiology Vol. 1. pp 639–657 Ed. EE Windhager, Oxford University Press, NY

Byers S and Graham R (1990) Distribution of sodium–potassium ATPase in the rat testis and epididymis *American Journal of Anatomy* **188** 31–43

Chan HC, Lai KB, Fu WO, Chung YW, Chan PSF and Wong PYD (1995a) Regional differences in bioelectrical properties and anion secretion in cultured epithelia from rat and human male excurrent ducts *Biology of Reproduction* **52** 192–198

Chan HC, Zhou WL, Fu WO, Ko WH and Wong PYD (1995b) Different regulatory pathways involved in ATP-stimulated chloride secretion in rat epididymal epithelium *Journal of Cellular Physiology* **164** 271–276

Clulow J and Jones RC (1988) Studies of fluid and spermatozoal transport in the extratesticular ducts of the Japanese quail *Journal of Anatomy* **157** 1–11

Clulow J, Jones RC and Hansen LA (1994) Micropuncture and cannulation studies of fluid composition and transport in the ductuli efferentes testis of the rat: comparisons with the homologous metanephric proximal tubule *Experimental Physiology* **79** 915–928

Clulow J, Jones RC and Hansen LA (1996) *In vivo* microperfusion of the ductuli efferentes testis of the rat: flow dependence of fluid reabsorption *Experimental Physiology* **81** 633–644

Cohen JP, Hoffer AP and Rosen S (1976) Carbonic anhydrase localization in the epididymis and testis of the rat: histochemical and biochemical analysis *Biology of Reproduction* **14** 339–346

Cooke PS, Young P and Cunha GR (1991a) Androgen receptor expression in developing male reproductive organs *Endocrinology* **128** 2867–2873

Cooke PS, Young P, Hess RA and Cunha GR (1991b) Estrogen receptor expression in developing epididymis, efferent ductules and other male reproductive organs *Endocrinology* **128** 2874–2879

Crabo B (1965) Studies on the composition of epididymal content in bulls and boars *Acta Veterinaria Scandinavica* **6** (Supplement 5) 1–94

Djakiew D and Jones RC (1982) Stereological analysis of the epididymis of the echidna, *Tachyglossus aculeatus*, and Wistar rat *Australian Journal of Zoology* **30** 865–875

Djakiew D and Jones RC (1983) Sperm maturation, fluid transport and secretion and absorption of protein in the epididymis of the echidna, *Tachyglossus aculeatus. Journal of Reproduction and Fertility* **68** 445–456

Du Bois AM (1969) The embryonic kidney. In *The Kidney: Morphology, Biochemistry, Physiology* Eds C Rouiller and AF Muller, Vol. 1 pp 1–59 Academic Press, New York

Eddy EM, Washburn TF, Bunch DO, Goulding EH, Gladen BC, Lubahn DB and Korach KS (1996) Targeted disruption of the estrogen receptor gene in male mice causes alteration of spermatogenesis and infertility *Endocrinology* **137** 4796–4805

Ekstedt E and Ridderstråle Y (1992) Carbonic anhydrase localization in the testis and epididymis of the rabbit *Acta Anatomica* **143** 258–264

Fisher JS, Millar MR, Majdic G, Saunders PTK, Fraser HM and Sharpe RM (1997) Immunolocalization of estrogen receptor-α within the testis and excurrent ducts of the rat and marmoset monkey from perinatal life to adulthood *Journal of Endocrinology* **153** 485–495

Free MJ and Jaffe RA (1979) Collection of rete testis fluid from rats without previous efferent duct ligation *Biology of Reproduction* **20** 269–278

Giebisch G, Malnic G and Berliner RW (1991) Renal transport and control of potassium excretion. In *The Kidney* (4th Edn) Eds B Brenner and F C Rector Vol. 1, pp 283–317 W.B. Saunders, Philadelphia

Goyal HO, Ferguson JG and Hrudka F (1980) Histochemical activity of carbonic anhydrase in testicular and excurrent ducts of immature, mature intact and androgen-deprived bulls *Biology of Reproduction* **22** 991–997

Hansen LA, Clulow J and Jones RC (1997) Perturbation of fluid reabsorption in the efferent ducts of the rat by testosterone propionate, 17β-oestradiol 3-benzoate, flutamide and tamoxifen *International Journal of Andrology* **20** 265–273

Harris PJ (1992) Regulation of proximal tubule function by angiotensin *Clinical and Experimental Pharmacology and Physiology* **19** 213–222

Hermo L, Spier N and Nadler NJ (1988) Role of apical tubules in endocytosis in nonciliated cells of the ductuli efferentes of the rat: a kinetic analysis *American Journal of Anatomy* **182** 107–119

Hess RA, Bunick D, Lee K-H, Bahr J, Taylor JA, Korach KS and Lubahn DB (1997a) A role for oestrogens in the male reproductive system *Nature* **390** 509–512

Hess RA, Gist DH, Bunick D, Lubahn DB, Farrell A, Bahr J, Cooke PS and Green GL (1997b) Estrogen receptor (α and β) expression in the excurrent ducts of the adult male rat reproductive tract *Journal of Andrology* **18** 602–611

Hinton BT and Setchell BP (1980) Concentrations of glycerophosphocholine, phosphocholine and free inorganic phosphate in the luminal fluid of the rat testis and epididymis *Journal of Reproduction and Fertility* **58** 401–406

Hohlbrugger G (1980) A micropuncture study of transepithelial water reabsorption in the rat ductuli efferentes *Fertility and Sterility* **34** 50–54

Hohlbrugger G, Schweisfurth H and Dahlheim H (1982) Angiotensin I converting enzyme in rat testis, epididymis and vas deferens under different conditions *Journal of Reproduction and Fertility* **65** 97–103

House CR (1974) *Water transport in Cells and Tissues* p 429 Edward Arnold, London

Ilio KY and Hess RA (1992) Localization and activity of Na^{+}–K^{+}-

ATPase in the ductuli efferentes of the rat *The Anatomical Record* **234** 190–200

Ilio KY and Hess RA (1994) Structure and function of the ductuli efferentes: a review *Microscopy Research and Technique* **29** 432–467

Jenkins AD, Lechene CP and Howards SS (1980) Concentrations of seven elements in the intraluminal fluids of the rat seminiferous tubules, rete testis, and epididymis *Biology of Reproduction* **23** 981–987

Jones RC (1980) Luminal composition and maturation of spermatozoa in the genital ducts of the African elephant, *Loxodonta africana. Journal of Reproduction and Fertility* **60** 87–93

Jones RC and Clulow J (1987) Regulation of the elemental composition of the epididymal fluids in the tammar, *Macropus eugenii. Journal of Reproduction and Fertility* **81** 583–590

Jones RC and Jurd KM (1987) Structural differentiation and fluid reabsorption in the ductuli efferentes testis of the rat *Australian Journal of Biological Sciences* **40** 79–90

Jones RC, Clulow J, Stone GM and Setchell BP (1987) The role of the initial segments of the epididymis in sperm maturation in mammals. In *New Horizons in Sperm Cell Research* pp 63–74 Ed. H Mohri. Japan Scientific Society Press and Gordon and Breach Scientific, Tokyo

Jørgensen PL (1980) Sodium and potassium ion pump in kidney tubules *Physiological Reviews* **60** 864–917

Levine N and Marsh DJ (1971) Micropuncture studies of the electrochemical aspects of fluid and electrolyte transport in individual seminiferous tubules, the epididymis and the vas deferens in rats *Journal of Physiology* **213** 557–570

Lopez ML, Fuentes P, Retamal C and De Souza W (1997) Regional differentiation of the blood–epididymis barrier in the stallion *Journal of Submicroscopic Cytology and Pathology* **29** 353–363

Man SY, Clulow J, Hansen LA and Jones RC (1997) Adrenal independence of fluid and electrolyte reabsorption in the ductuli efferentes testis of the rat *Experimental Physiology* **82** 283–290

Meistrich ML, Hughes TJ and Bruce WR (1975) Alteration of epididymal sperm transport and maturation in mice by oestrogen and testosterone *Nature* **258** 145–147

Montorzi NM and Labiano SA (1970) Uptake of water, sodium and glucose by the ductuli efferentes of the hamster *"in vitro" Acta Physiologica Latinoamerica* **20** 135–139

Park CH and Maack T (1984) Albumin absorption and catabolism by isolated perfused proximal convoluted tubules of the rabbit *Journal of Clinical Investigation* **73** 767–777

Reid BL and Cleland KW (1957) The structure and function of the epididymis 1. The histology of the rat epididymis *Australian Journal of Zoology* **5** 223–246

Robaire B and Hermo L (1988) Efferent ducts, epididymis, and vas deferens: structure, functions and their regulation. In *The Physiology of Reproduction* Vol. 1. Ed. E Knobel and JD Neill. pp 999–1080 Raven Press, New York

Suzuki F and Nagano T (1978) Regional differentiation of cell junctions in the excurrent duct epithelium of the rat testis as revealed by freeze–fracture *Anatomical Record* **191** 503–519

Tuck RR, Setchell BP, Waites GMH and Young JA (1970) The composition of fluid collected by micropuncture and catheterization from the seminiferous tubules and rete testis of rats *Pflügers Archiv* **318** 225–243

Turner TT, Jones CE, Howards SS, Ewing LL, Zegeye B and Gunsalus GL (1984) On the androgen microenvironment of maturing spermatozoa *Endocrinology* **115** 1925–1932

Wang S, Jones RC and Clulow J (1994) Surface area of apical and basolateral plasmalemma of epithelial cells of the ductuli efferentes testis of the rat *Cell and Tissue Research* **276** 581–586

Weinstein AM (1988) Modeling the proximal tubule: complications of the paracellular pathway *American Journal of Physiology* **254** F297–F305

Wong PYD and Yeung CH (1978) Absorptive and secretory functions of the perfused rat cauda epididymidis *Journal of Physiology* **275** 13–26

Wong PYD, Huang SJ, Leung AYH, Fu WO, Chung YW, Zhou TS, Yip WWK and Chan WKL (1992) Physiology and pathophysiology of electrolyte transport in the epididymis. In *Spermatogenesis – Fertilization – Contraception: Molecular, Cellular and Endocrine Events in Male Reproduction* pp 319–344 Eds E Nieschlag and U-F Habenicht. Schering Foundation Workshop 4. Springer Verlag, Berlin

Journal of Reproduction and Fertility Supplement **53**, 15–22

The role of local angiotensins and prostaglandins in the control of anion secretion by the rat epididymis

P. S. Leung, H. C. Chan, Y. W. Chung, T. P. Wong and P. Y. D. Wong

Department of Physiology, Faculty of Medicine, the Chinese University of Hong Kong, Shatin, N.T., Hong Kong

Secretion of electrolytes and water by the epididymal epithelium is important in the formation of an optimal fluid environment for sperm maturation and storage. Recently, evidence has been obtained that anion/fluid secretion by the epididymis is subject to control by local humoral factors, among which the angiotensins play a significant role. This assertion is based on the morphological localization of various components of a local renin–angiotensin system (RAS) in the rat epididymis and the functional studies of angiotensins and their antagonists on anion secretion in cultured rat epididymal epithelia. More recent study has indicated that the effects of angiotensin II and other vasoactive peptides on anion secretion are mediated through an increase in prostaglandin formation. The pathway of synthesis involves the PLA_2-coupled receptor mediated breakdown of membrane phospholipids to arachidonic acid followed by conversion of arachidonic acid into the prostanoids by cyclooxygenases and other enzymes. The newly formed PGE_2 then diffuses out of the cells and acts on the EP2/4 receptors on the same or adjacent cells to increase intracellular cAMP. Accordingly, the pathways of activation by the paracrine factors all converge on the cystic fibrosis transmembrane conductance regulator (CFTR) as the final common effector in secretion. Studies on the biochemical pathways of paracrine control of fluid secretion may provide insight into the causes of epididymal irregularities in some forms of male infertility.

Introduction

It cannot be over-emphasized that the mammalian epididymis plays an indispensible role in reproduction. The epithelial cells lining the ductus epididymidis actively form a luminal fluid environment by secreting electrolytes and fluid (Wong, 1988). A cAMP-activated chloride channel (cystic fibrosis transmembrane conductance regulator, CFTR) on the apical membrane of the epithelial cells may play an integral role (Huang *et al.*, 1992; Chan *et al.*, 1994). The importance of this channel has been highlighted in the genetic disease, cystic fibrosis, in which, because of mutation of the CFTR gene (which encodes this channel), the CFTR protein cannot function as a cAMP-regulated Cl^- channel. Since this channel is also expressed by the fetal human epididymis (Harris *et al.*, 1991; Pollard *et al.*, 1991), it is believed that the disruption of fluid secretion by the Wolffian duct epithelial cells during fetal development underpins the obstruction and agenesis of the epididymis/vas in men with cystic fibrosis (Wong, 1998).

Secretion of anions and fluid by the epididymis is controlled by noradrenaline released from adrenergic nerves and by circulating catecholamines. These agents act through the β-adrenergic receptors to increase intracellular cAMP, which then activates the CFTR to allow Cl^- and HCO_3^- efflux. The cAMP-dependent anion channel activation is the rate limiting step in secretion (Leung and Wong, 1993). Previous work in our laboratory has shown that secretion is also controlled by humoral agents which include bradykinin (Cuthbert and Wong, 1986) endothelin (Wong *et al.*, 1989), calcitonin gene related peptide (Leung *et al.*, 1992), arginine vasopressin (Lai *et al.*, 1994), pituitary adenylate cyclase-activating polypeptide (Zhou *et al.*, 1997) and angiotensins (Wong *et al.*, 1990). In this paper, we present evidence of a local renin–angiotensin system (RAS), its physiological role and the biochemical pathways that lead to the stimulation of anion/fluid secretion by the epididymis.

Evidence for a Local RAS in the Rat Epididymis

The physiological role of a systemic renin–angiotensin system (RAS) in the regulation of blood pressure and fluid volume has been well documented (Peach, 1977). The circulating angiotensin II has diverse physiological functions which include vasoconstriction, aldosterone secretion and induction of drinking through the interaction with two pharmacologically defined receptor subtypes, type 1 (AT_1) and type 2 (AT_2) present throughout the body. AT_1 receptors have been shown to be G protein-coupled and may involve activation of phospholipase C (PLC), PLA_2, PLD or adenylate cyclase (Timmermans and Smith, 1996). However, the receptor–response coupling of AT_2 remains obscure. AT_1 receptors mediate most, if not all, of the known effects of angiotensin II, whereas the functions of AT_2 receptors are unknown (Bottari *et al.*, 1993). In recent years, a tissue or local RAS has been found in many mammalian tissues (Ganong, 1994) which contain not only the product, angiotensin II, but also the precursor, angiotensinogen and the enzymes necessary for the formation of angiotensin II, and their respective genes (Phillips *et al.*, 1993). The expression of these genes appears to be regulated by neurohumoral agents. The expression of mRNA encoding angiotensinogen in rat tissues, for instance, is found to be regulated by dexamethasone, oestrogen, testosterone and thyroxine (Campbell and Habener, 1986; Ellison *et al.*, 1989).

The presence of a tissue RAS in the rat epididymis has been implicated on the basis of the following evidence. First, angiotensin I, angiotensin II, renin and angiotensin converting enzyme are found in the epididymis (Wong and Uchendu, 1990, 1991). Second, exogenously applied angiotensin II stimulates anion secretion by the rat epididymis (Wong *et al.*, 1990). Third, angiotensin II has been localized in the basal cells of the epididymal epithelium (Zhao *et al.*, 1996). More recently, studies involving *in situ* hybridization, immunocytochemistry and western blot analysis have demonstrated expression of mRNA encoding angiotensinogen in the epithelial cells of the rat epididymis (Fig. 1). These results, taken together, lend support to the notion that the epididymis possesses all of the components necessary for the formation of angiotensin II, in keeping with the model of a tissue RAS suggested previously (Phillips *et al.*, 1993).

Studies of the Angiotensin Receptors

An indispensible step in executing a physiological function of a tissue RAS is the interaction of angiotensin II with specific receptors on the cell surface. The identification of angiotensin receptors in the epididymis is therefore an essential step in assessing the role of a RAS in the epididymis. An immunocytochemical approach has been used to detect specific angiotensin receptors in the rat epididymis. AT_1 and AT_2 receptors were demonstrated in the epididymis at different developmental stages (Leung *et al.*, 1977a). They are predominantly localized on the basal side of the cell membrane of the principal cells (Fig. 2). Electrophysiological investigation using the short-circuit current technique also demonstrated a marked stimulation of chloride secretion by basolateral application of angiotensin II compared with apical application (Wong *et al.*, 1990). Furthermore, the effect of angiotensin II is blocked by losartan, a specific AT_1 antagonist, but not by PD123177, a specific AT_2 antagonist, indicating that AT_1 receptors may play a role in the regulation of electrolyte and fluid secretion (Leung *et al.*, 1977b). As mentioned before, the source of the angiotensin II is the basal cells and its receptors are on the basal membrane of the principal cells. The close proximity of the basal cells to the principal cells supports the scenario that angiotensin II released from the basal cells

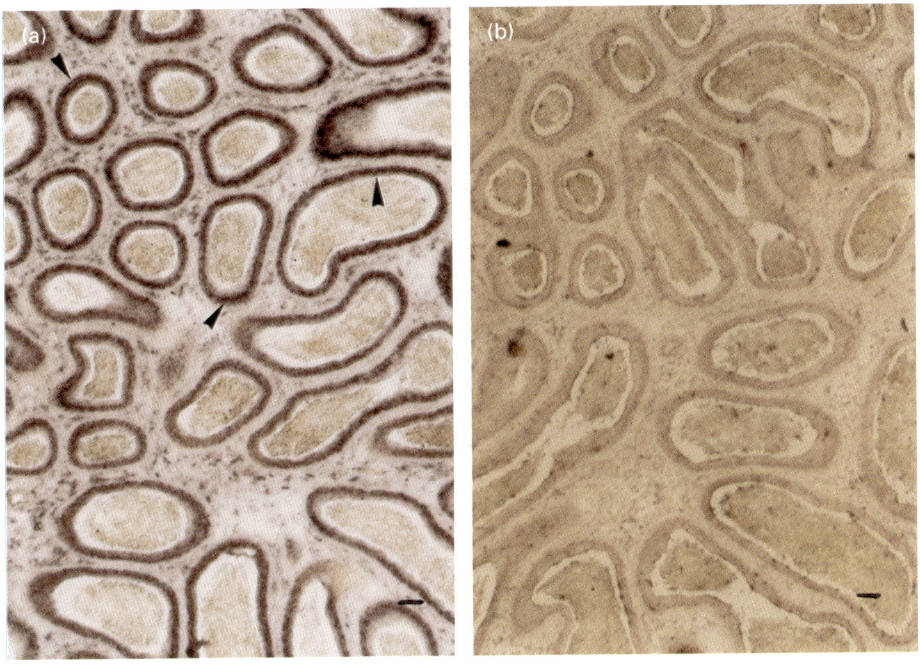

Fig. 1. *In situ* hybridization of mRNA encoding angiotensinogen in the rat epididymis. (a) Specific signal for mRNA encoding angiotensinogen was localized in the epithelial cells of the caput epididymidis (arrowheads) using antisense riboprobes. (b) Absence of mRNA signal for angiotensinogen using sense riboprobes. Scale bars represent 200 μm. A 600 bp angiotensinogen cDNA cloned in pBluescript was used to generate digoxigenin-labelled antisense and sense riboprobes using T3 and T7 polymerases, respectively. Sections from the rat caput epididymidis were fixed with freshly prepared 4% paraformaldehyde, followed by digestion with proteinase K (1 μg ml^{-1}). Sections were subsequently incubated overnight at 42°C in a humidified chamber with antisense or sense riboprobes (20 ng ml^{-1}) containing 50% formamide, 4 × saline sodium citrate (SSC), 0.25% mg yeast tRNA ml^{-1}, 0.25% mg salmon sperm DNA ml^{-1}, 100 mg dextran sulfate ml^{-1} and 1 × Denhardt's solution. Hybridized probes were detected with anti-digoxigenin antibody conjugated to alkaline phosphatase (1:500) and visualized by nitroblue tetrazolium chloride/ bromo-chloro-iodolyl-phosphate (NBT/BCIP) detection. Positive reaction gave a purple colour.

stimulates the adjacent principal cells to secrete anions or fluid. This arrangement is consistent with a paracrine role of a local RAS in the epididymis.

Stage-specific Expression of Angiotensin II Receptor Subtypes in the Rat Epididymis

Although angiotensin II acts in a paracrine fashion to regulate fluid secretion by the epididymis through AT_1 receptors (Leung *et al.*, 1977b), it is of interest to study gene expression of specific angiotensin II receptor subtypes at different developmental stages. Using semi-quantitative reverse transcription–polymerase chain reaction (RT–PCR) coupled with specific primers based on the corresponding angiotensin II receptor subtype genes for AT_{1a}, AT_{1b} and AT_2, we have demonstrated the differential expression of mRNAs for these receptor subtypes in the epididymides of mature and immature rats (Leung *et al.*, 1998). In the mature rat epididymis, mRNAs for AT_{1a} and AT_{1b} are predominantly expressed, but mRNA for AT_2 is not expressed. However, AT_{1a} and AT_2 mRNAs, but not AT_{1b} mRNA, are expressed in the immature rat epididymis. This finding suggests that AT_1 and AT_2 receptor subtypes are developmentally regulated. AT_1 receptors are involved in the regulation of

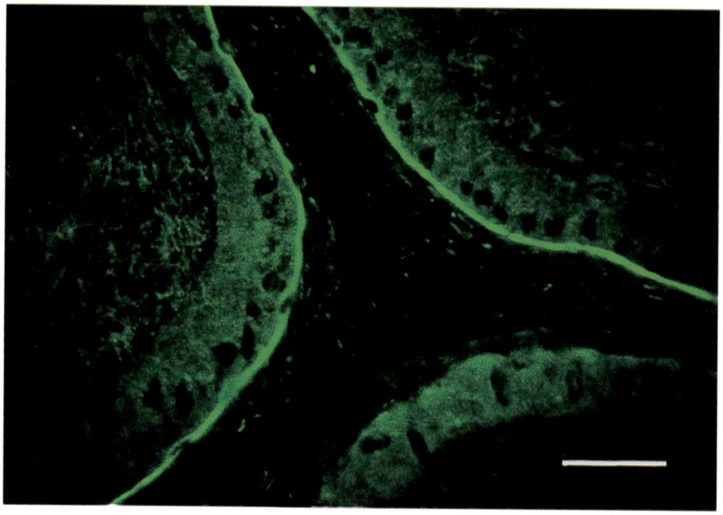

Fig. 2. Immunohistochemical localization of AT_1 receptors in the rat cauda epididymidis. Intense immunofluorescent staining was detected in the basal surface of the epithelial cells. Scale bar represents 200 µm. Reproduced from Leung *et al.* (1997a) with permission from the *Journal of Membrane Biology*.

anion secretion in the epididymis (AT_{1a} in immature and AT_{1a} and AT_{1b} in mature), whereas the AT_2 receptor subtype may play other roles in the epididymides of immature animals.

Effect of Castration on Gene Expression

Since it is well documented that the structural and functional integrity of the epididymis are controlled by androgens (Orgebin-Crist, 1973; Wong and Yeung, 1977, 1978; Toney and Danzo, 1989; Abou-Haila *et al.*, 1996) and by testicular factors flowing along the lumen of the efferent duct (Winer and Wolgemuth, 1995; Vernet *et al.*, 1997), it is of interest to determine whether the expression of the RAS components in the rat epididymis is affected by castration. We studied the expression of mRNAs for angiotensinogen and angiotensin II receptors in the epididymis of normal rats and in rats castrated for 21 days. The results show that castration greatly reduced the expression of the AT_1 receptor gene (Fig. 3). Currently, we are investigating whether the effects are due to withdrawal of androgens, the secretory products from the testis, or both. The dependence on other hormones is also being investigated.

Role of Prostaglandins in Mediating the Effects of Angiotensin II and Other Peptides

It is known that many vasoactive peptide hormones including angiotensins (Wong *et al.*, 1990), endothelin (Wong *et al.*, 1989), arginine vasopressin (AVP) (Lai *et al.*, 1994) and bradykinins (Cuthbert and Wong, 1986) stimulate secretion of chloride (and hence fluid) in the epididymis through an increase in prostanoid synthesis via the enzyme prostaglandin synthetase (PGS), as aspirin, piroxicam, indomethacine and L-745,337, which are inhibitors of the enzyme, abolish the responses to the peptides. Two forms of prostaglandin synthetase (cyclooxygenase, COX) are now known to be expressed by mammalian cells. COX-1, which is expressed by the platelets, kidney and gastrointestinal tract (Funk *et al.*, 1991; Kargman *et al.*, 1996), is thought to be involved in normal processes of homeostasis, whereas COX-2, which is stimulated by pro-inflammatory agents, is

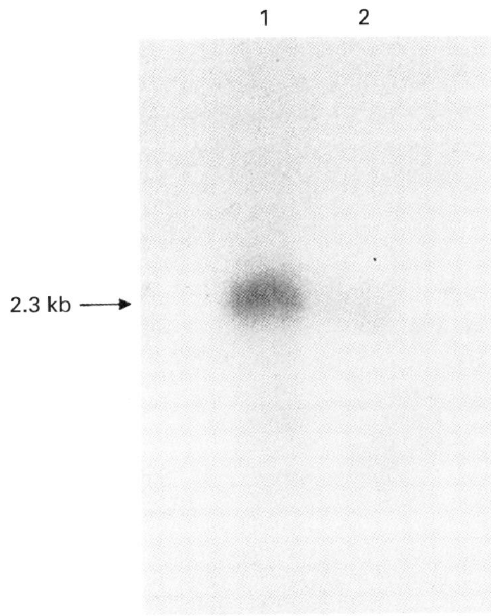

Fig. 3. Effect of castration on the expression of mRNA encoding the AT_1 receptor in the rat epididymis using northern blot analysis. Lane 1, a transcript of about 2.3 kb (arrow) corresponding to the mRNA encoding the AT_1 receptor was detected in the epididymis of normal rats. Lane 2, expression of mRNA encoding AT_1 was almost abolished in rats castrated for 21 days.

thought to mediate the oedematous, nociceptive and pyretic effects of inflammation (Harada *et al.*, 1996). We conducted experiments with inhibitors with presumed selectivity towards COX-1 or COX-2 at appropriate concentrations (Riendeau *et al.*, 1997) and found that the stimulatory effects of the vasoactive peptides on chloride secretion by the epididymis is likely to be mediated by COX-1. It is known that COX converts arachidonic acid (AA) to prostaglandin G_2 (PGG_2). This unstable intermediate is then converted to PGH_2 which is the common precursor of the prostanoids, the prostaglandins, thromboxanes and the prostacyclins. To determine which COX product is responsible for the Cl^- secretory response to the vasoactive peptides, we have studied the effects of externally applied PGE_2, PGD_2, $PGF_{2\alpha}$, U46619 and cicaprost, which are specific agonists for prostaglandin E, prostaglandin D, prostaglandin F, thromboxane and prostacyclin receptors, respectively, on chloride secretion by cultured rat epididymal epithelia (Coleman *et al.*, 1994). Among them only PGE_2 could mimic the effects of the hormones. The results therefore show that the active prostanoid is likely to be PGE_2 acting on the prostaglandin E (EP) receptors. Using specific EP receptor agonists, we showed that the physiological responses to the peptides and PGE_2 were reproduced by 11-deoxy PGE_1, a specific EP4 receptor agonist, but not by sulprostone, a specific EP1 receptor agonist. Since the former receptor is linked to the cAMP/PKA signal transduction pathway and the latter to the Ca^{2+}/IP_3 pathway respectively (Coleman *et al.*, 1994), this study indicates that the peptide hormones regulate electrolyte and fluid secretion by the epididymis via a common transport protein, the CFTR, which functions as a cAMP-activated Cl^- channel. According to the model depicted in Fig. 4, these peptides first interact with specific receptors on the basal surface of the principal cells leading to activation of PLA_2 with release of arachidonic acid (AA) from membrane phospholipids (PL). AA is converted to PGG_2 and PGH_2 by the cyclooxygenases (COX) and then to PGE_2 by a specific isomerase. The PGE_2 formed diffuses out of the cells and acts on the

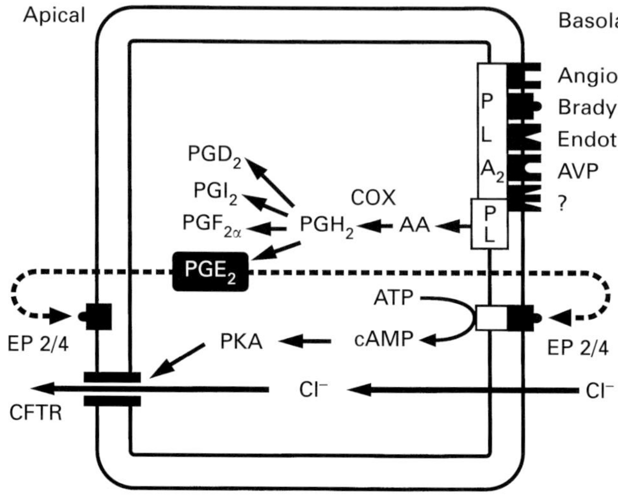

Fig. 4. Schematic diagram showing the role of prostaglandin E_2 (PGE_2) in mediating the effects of angiotensin II, bradykinin, endothelin and arginine vasopressin (AVP). These peptides interact with specific receptors on the basal surface of the principal cells leading to activation of phospholipase A_2 (PLA_2) with release of arachidonic acid (AA) from membrane phospholipids (PL). AA is converted to PGE_2 via cyclooxygenases (COX) and other enzymes. PGE_2 formed diffuses out of the cells and acts on the prostaglandin EP2/4 receptors on the basolateral and apical membranes of the principal cells to increase intracellular cAMP which then activates the apical cystic fibrosis transmembrane conductance regulator (CFTR) to effect secretion. In cystic fibrosis and congenital bilateral absence of the vas deferens (CBAVD), the CFTR protein is abnormal and this results in loss of paracrine hormone-mediated secretion.

prostaglandin EP2/4 receptors on the basolateral and apical membranes of the principal cells to increase intracellular cAMP which then activates the apical CFTR to effect secretion. Because the effects of the paracrine peptides all converge on the CFTR, this may explain why the epididymis is severely affected in cystic fibrosis or in congenital bilateral absence of the vas deferens (CBAVD) in which the CFTR gene is disrupted by gene mutation. Under these circumstances, although the Ca^{2+} pathway which terminates on a Cl^- channel distinct from CFTR is apparently unaffected in cystic fibrosis, it could not have maintained sufficient secretion to support normal epididymal function (Leung *et al.*, 1996).

Conclusion

New evidence from our laboratory has added to our understanding of the paracrine control of electrolyte and fluid transport in the epididymis. Using the rat epididymis as a model, we established that the mammalian epididymis expresses a full complement of a tissue RAS. The physiological role of the end product angiotensin II is to regulate electrolyte/fluid transport in the epididymis. The system is therefore important in the formation of a correct epididymal microenvironment for sperm maturation and storage. Both AT_1 and AT_2 receptors for angiotensin II are identified in the rat epididymis and their expressions appear to be developmentally regulated. The AT_1 receptor subtype is present in the epididymides of immature and mature rats, whereas AT_2 subtype is present only in immature rats. These results, together with the findings that the stimulation of anion secretion by angiotensin II is blocked by AT_1 antagonist and not by AT_2 antagonist suggest that the AT_1 receptor mediates the secretory response to angiotensins, whereas the AT_2 receptor mediates growth and differentiation or other functions of the immature epididymis. The recent finding that the AT_1 receptor gene is downregulated by castration may be taken to indicate that the epididymal RAS, in common with many epididymal functions, is regulated by androgens or testicular factors transported down along the lumen of the duct from the testis.

As with other peptide hormones, angiotensin II stimulates anion secretion by the epididymis through activation of membrane PLA_2, which leads to the production of arachidonic acid from membrane lipids. Arachidonic acid is converted *de novo* to prostaglandin E_2 by the enzyme prostaglandin synthetase, or the cyclooxygenase. The newly formed PGE_2 diffuses out from the cells and acts on prostaglandin E receptors, notably the EP2/4 subtypes, on the basolateral as well as the apical membranes, to increase intracellular cAMP which activates an apical Cl^- channel (CFTR) resulting in secretion of anions, and secondarily, water. In cystic fibrosis and in CBAVD, the gene encoding the CFTR protein is disrupted by gene mutation and this results in the loss of cAMP-driven secretion. Since the pathways of stimulation of secretion by the peptide hormones (paracrine factors) and adrenergic agents (adrenergic nerve) all converge on the CFTR as the final effector of secretion, it is expected that fluid secretion by the epididymis would be severely disrupted under these clinical conditions. This may explain why the epididymis is highly vulnerable to CFTR gene mutation. The anomaly of the RAS and the associated eicosanoid formation may be involved in the obstructive and inflammatory diseases of the epididymis and future research in this area is likely to be of considerable interest.

The authors are grateful to Professor R. Jones of the Department of Pharmacology, The Chinese University of Hong Kong for his invaluable advice on the study of eicosanoids. This work was supported by the Research Grants Council, Hong Kong and the International Consortium on Male Contraception, Population Council, New York.

References

Abou-Haila A, Tulsiani DR, Skudlarek MD and Orgebin-Crist MC (1996) Androgen regulation of molecular forms of beta-D-glucuronidase in the mouse epididymis: comparison with liver and kidney *Journal of Andrology* **17** 194–207

Bottari DP, de Gasparo M, Steckelings UM and Levens NR (1993) Angiotensin II receptor subtypes: characterization, signalling mechanisms and possible physiological implications *Frontiers in Neuroendocrinology* **14** 123–171

Campbell DJ and Habener JF (1986) Angiotensinogen gene is expressed and differentially regulated in multiple tissues of the rat *Journal of Clinical Investigation* **78** 31–39

Chan HC, Fu WO, Chung YW, Zhou TS and Wong PYD (1994) Adrenergic receptors on cultured rat epididymal cells: regulation of chloride conductances *Biology of Reproduction* **51** 1041–1045

Coleman RA, Smith WL and Narumiya S (1994) VIII. International Union of Pharmacology Classification of Prostanoid Receptors: properties, distribution, and structure of the receptors and their subtypes *Pharmacological Reviews* **46** 205–229

Cuthbert AW and Wong PYD (1986) Electrogenic anion secretion in cultured rat epididymal epithelium *Journal of Physiology* **378** 335–346

Ellison KE, Ingelfinger JR, Pivor M and Dzau VJ (1989) Androgen regulation of rat renal angiotensinogen messenger RNA expression *Journal of Clinical Investigation* **83** 1941–1945

Funk CD, Funk LB, Kennedy ME, Pong AS and Fitzgerald GA (1991) Human platelet/erythroleukemia cell prostaglandin G/H synthase: cDNA cloning, expression, and gene assignment *FASEB Journal* **5** 2304–2312

Ganong WF (1994) Reproduction and the renin–angiotensin system *Neuroscience and Biobehavioral Reviews* **19** 241–250

Harada Y, Hatanaka K, Kawamura M, Saito M, Ogino M, Majima M, Ohno T, Ogino K, Yamamoto K, Taketani Y, Yamamoto S and Katori M (1996) Role of prostaglandin H synthase-2 in prostaglandin E_2 formation in rat carrageenin-induced pleurisy *Prostaglandins* **51** 19–33

Harris A, Chalkley GC, Lankester SA and Coleman LS (1991) Expression of the cystic fibrosis gene in human development *Development* **113** 305–310

Huang SJ, Leung AYH, Fu WO, Chung YW, Zhou TS, Chan PSF and Wong PYD (1992) Electrophysiological studies of anion secretion in cultured human epididymal cells *Journal of Physiology* **455** 455–469

Kargman S, Charleson S, Cartwright M, Frank J, Riendeau D, Mancini J, Evans J and O'Neill G (1996) Prostaglandin G/H synthase-1 and -2 in rat, dog, monkey, and human gastrointestinal tract tissues: localization, enzyme activity and inhibition by NSAIDs *Gastroenterology* **111** 445–454

Lai KB, Fu WO, Ko WH, Chan HC and Wong PYD (1994) The effect of [Arg^8]-vasopressin on electrogenic chloride secretion in cultured rat epididymal epithelia *American Journal of Physiology* **267** C607–C616

Leung AYH and Wong PYD (1993) The epididymis as a chloride secreting organ *News in Physiological Sciences* **9** 31–35

Leung AYH, Leung PY, Cheng-Chew SB and Wong PYD (1992) The role of calcitonin gene-related peptide in the regulation of anion secretion by the rat and human epididymis *Journal of Endocrinology* **133** 259–268

Leung AYH, Wong PYD, Yankaskas JR and Bucher RC (1996) cAMP- but not Ca^{2+}-regulated Cl^- conductance is lacking in cystic fibrosis mice epididymides and seminal vesicles *American Journal of Physiology* **271** C188–C193

Leung PS, Chan HC, Fu LXM, Leung PY, Cheng, Chew SB and Wong PYD (1997 a) Angiotensin II receptors:

localization of type I and type II in rat epididymides of different developmental stages *Journal of Membrane Biology* **157** 97–104

Leung PS, Chan HC, Fu LXM, Zhou WL and Wong PYD (1997b) Angiotensin II receptors, AT_1 and AT_2 in the rat epididymis: immunocytochemical and electrophysiological studies *Biochimica et Biophysica Acta* **1357** 65–72

Leung PS, Yao XQ, Chan HC, Fu LXM and Wong PYD (1998) Differential gene expression of angiotensin II receptor subtypes in the epididymides of mature and immature rats *Life Sciences* **62** 461–468

Orgebin-Crist MC (1973) Maturation of spermatozoa in the rabbit epididymis: effect of castration and testosterone replacement *Journal of Experimental Zoology* **185** 301–310

Peach MJ (1977) Renin–angiotensin system: biochemistry and mechanisms of action *Physiological Reviews* **57** 313–370

Phillips MI, Speakman EA and Kimura B (1993) Levels of angiotensin and molecular biology of the tissue renin–angiotensin systems *Regulatory Peptides* **43** 1–20

Pollard CE, Harris A, Coleman L and Argent BE (1991) Chloride channels on epithelial cells from cultured human fetal epididymis *Journal of Membrane Biology* **124** 275–284

Riendeau D, Percival MD, Boyce S, Brideau C, Charleson S, Cromlish W, Ethier D, Evans J, Falgueyret J-P, Ford-Hutchinson AW, Gordon R, Grieg G, Gresser M, Guay J, Kargman S, Léger S, Mancini JA, O'Neill G, Ouellet M, Rodger IW, Thérien M, Wang Z, Webb JK, Wong E, Xu L, Young RN, Zamboni R, Prasit P and Chan C-C (1997) Biochemical and pharmacological profile of a tetrasubstituted furanone as a highly selective COX-2 inhibitor. *British Journal of Pharmacology* **121** 105–117

Timmermans PB and Smith RD (1996) The diversified pharmacology of angiotensin II-receptor blockade *Blood Pressure Supplement* **2** 53–61

Toney TW and Danzo BJ (1989) Estrogen and androgen regulation of protein synthesis by the immature rabbit epididymis *Endocrinology* **125** 231–242

Vernet P, Faure J, Dufaure JP and Drevet JR (1997) Tissue and developmental distribution, dependence upon testicular factors and attachment to spermatozoa of GPX5, a murine epididymis-specific glutathione peroxidase *Molecular Reproduction and Development* **47** 87–98

Winer MA and Wolgemuth DJ (1995) The segment-specific pattern of A-raf expression in the mouse epididymis is regulated by testicular factors *Endocrinology* **136** 2561–2572

Wong PYD (1988) Mechanism of adrenergic stimulation of anion secretion in cultured rat epididymal epithelium *American Journal of Physiology* **254** F121–F133

Wong PYD (1998) *CFTR* gene and male fertility *Molecular Human Reproduction* (in press)

Wong PYD and Uchendu CN (1990) The role of angiotensin-converting enzyme in the rat epididymis *Journal of Endocrinology* **125** 457–465

Wong PYD and Uchendu CN (1991) Studies on the renin–angiotensin system in primary monolayer cell cultures of the rat epididymis *Journal of Endocrinology* **131** 287–293

Wong PYD and Yeung CH (1977) Hormonal regulation of fluid reabsorption in isolated rat cauda epididymis *Endocrinology* **101** 1391–1397

Wong PYD and Yeung CH (1978) Absorptive and secretory functions of the perfused rat cauda epididymis *Journal of Physiology* **275** 13–26

Wong PYD, Fu WO and Huang SJ (1989) Endothelin stimulates short circuit current in cultured rat epididymal epithelium *British Journal of Pharmacology* **98** 1191–1196

Wong PYD, Fu WO, Huang SJ and Law WK (1990) Effect of angiotensins on electrogenic anion transport in monolayer cultures of rat epididymis *Journal of Endocrinology* **125** 449–456

Zhao W, Leung PY, Cheng Chew SB, Chan HC and Wong PYD (1996) Localization and distribution of angiotensin II in the rat epididymis *Journal of Endocrinology* **149** 217–222

Zhou WL, Leung PS, Wong TP, Dun NJ, Wong PYD and Chan HC (1997) Local regulation of epididymal anion secretion by pituitary adenylate cyclase-activating polypeptide *Journal of Endocrinology* **154** 389–395

Journal of Reproduction and Fertility Supplement **53**, 23–31

Sperm maturation *in vitro*: co-culture of spermatozoa and epididymal epithelium

H. D. M. Moore[1,2], L. A. Samayawardhena[1] and I. A. Brewis[1,2]

[1]*Department of Molecular Biology & Biotechnology; and*
[2]*Obstetrics & Gynaecology, University of Sheffield, Sheffield S10 2UH UK*

Sperm maturation involves an intimate interaction between spermatozoa and the epididymal epithelium. Aspects of this relationship can be examined by co-incubating epididymal spermatozoa with epididymal epithelium *in vitro*. Plaques of epididymal epithelium from a variety of species (for example rodents, dogs, humans) can be maintained in culture medium supplemented with growth factors and androgens. When co-incubated with these epithelial cultures, immature epididymal spermatozoa undergo maturation changes that lead to the acquisition of progressive motility, zona binding and, in some instances, fertilizing capacity *in vitro*. The use of such co-culture techniques for the understanding of sperm maturation *in vitro* and *in vivo* is reviewed with reference to recent experiments.

Introduction

Experimental approaches for investigating sperm maturation are rather limited. Micro-puncture and cannulation studies (see Setchell, *et al.*, 1994) give important information about the epididymal luminal milieu but sampling the narrow epididymal tubule, particularly in the proximal region of the duct can be difficult. Ethical considerations also restrict the type of studies carried out in man and laboratory animals. In an attempt to overcome some of these limitations, *in vitro* culture techniques have been developed. These methods cannot reproduce the conditions that occur *in situ* and are deficient in several aspects of epididymal physiology. Nevertheless, they provide valuable insights into sperm maturation events, and may eventually have a practical application in clinical medicine, for developing new methods of contraception, and for assessing the effects of toxicants on fertility. Here, some of the progress made with sperm maturation *in vitro* is reviewed and recent experiments from our laboratory are described. Reviews of epididymal sperm maturation are provided elsewhere (Cooper, 1986; Moore, 1990, Bedford and Hoskins, 1990; Turner, 1995; Moore and Akhondi, 1996; Moore, 1996).

Treatment of Epididymal Spermatozoa with Epididymal Secretory Preparations and Other Substances *In Vitro*

There is a complex series of interactions between epididymal secretions and spermatozoa as they migrate along the epididymis (see for example, Vreeburg *et al.*, 1992; Tulsiani *et al.*, 1993), so it is surprising that even the simple incubation of immature epididymal spermatozoa *in vitro* with epididymal protein extracts or other substances has met with some success. The inherent ageing of immature epididymal spermatozoa *in vitro* will not alone promote fertilizing capacity and the degree of sperm maturation that has been achieved by simple incubations or more complex co-culture methods (see below) depends to a large extent on the initial maturity of the spermatozoa being treated. For example, in perhaps the first unequivocal demonstration of sperm maturation *in vitro*, Orgebin-Crist and Jahad (1979) added crude cytoplasmic extracts of sperm-free rabbit epididymis from the distal corpus epididymidis to rabbit spermatozoa recovered from the proximal corpus epididymidis that had been previously incubated *in vitro* for 24 h. This procedure significantly increased the fertilizing capacity of the epididymal spermatozoa. In rabbits, the fertilizing capacity of spermatozoa increases substantially as they move from the proximal to the distal corpus epididymidis, and thus factors in the epididymal extract were presumed to have induced this final maturation process. Similar procedures in hamsters have shown that epididymal extracts incubated with immature spermatozoa can enhance the fertilizing capacity *in vivo* and *in vitro* (Gonzalez-Echeverria *et al.*, 1984). In this case, the extracts were charcoal filtered to remove androgens or other steroids that might have had a direct effect. When spermatozoa are retrieved from the more proximal regions of the epididymis of laboratory animals, simple incubations *in vitro* are insufficient for the development of full fertilizing capacity. However, alterations in the motility patterns of immature spermatozoa have been observed by adding various epididymal preparations or specific substances known to be present within the epididymis. For example, the concentration of L-carnitine in epididymal fluid increases considerably in the corpus epididymidis and when added *in vitro* to rat spermatozoa recovered from the caput epididymidis will increase their progressive motility. Furthermore, the epididymal secretory proteins, forward motility protein (FMP; Acott, *et al.*, 1983) and acidic epididymal glycoprotein (AEG; Pholpramool *et al.*, 1983) have been shown to alter the motility pattern of immature spermatozoa *in vitro*. Whether these substances specifically influence the development of sperm motility or are merely beneficial for sperm viability has not been resolved. In hamsters, the stiffening of the flagellar beat of immature spermatozoa leads to progessive motility and can be induced by sulphydryl oxidation agents *in vitro* (Cornwall *et al.*, 1986). This observation is consistent with the general increase in the number of disulphide bonds in spermatozoa as they mature (Bedford and Hoskins, 1990) and hence incubation conditions that permit or promote sulphydryl oxidation may act by enhancing sperm maturation in a non-specific way.

Alterations in the phosphorylation of sperm proteins also accompany epididymal maturation as shown, for example, in hamsters (Devi *et al*, 1997). Since the phosphorylation of a 95 kDa receptor tyrosine kinase is an important feature of induction of the acrosome reaction by the zona at fertilization in rodents and humans (Leyton and Saling, 1989; Burks *et al.*, 1995), we examined protein phosphorylation in hamster epididymal spermatozoa in response to soluble zona. The results of a typical experiment are shown in Fig. 1. Spermatozoa derived from the distal corpus to distal cauda epididymidis displayed a significant increase in tyrosine phosphorylation of 90 and 110 kDa components in response to zona, which is consistent with the result of Nixon *et al.* (1996). Spermatozoa from the caput and proximal corpus epididymides expressed similar tyrosine phosphorylated components but they did not respond to zona. Surprisingly in these experiments, spermatozoa retrieved from the distal cauda epididymidis showed the greatest increase in zona-dependent tyrosine phosphorylation even though spermatozoa from the proximal cauda epididymidis are also capable of fertilization. This finding suggests that storage in the epididymis may alter the sensitivity of spermatozoa to respond to a specific ligand under particular conditions *in vitro*. Such a maturation and storage process may also involve the removal or unmasking of determinants from the surface of the spermatozoon. An example of this is the induction of physiological acrosome reactions (by solubilized zona) in mouse spermatozoa when they are washed after incubation under capacitating conditions (Biegler *et al.*, 1994).

Epididymal Epithelial Cell Cultures

Initially, the culture of epididymal epithelium from laboratory animals or humans involved techniques using isolated fragments of tubules (Orgebin-Crist and Jahad, 1979; Tezon and Blaquier, 1981). Such protocols proved successful in terms of secretory activity and sperm maturation, but usually these primary organ cultures could be maintained for only a few days and access to the tubule lumen was limited. Nevertheless, such experiments indicated that androgen was needed in the medium (Vazquez *et al.*, 1986) and usually both testosterone and dihydrotestosterone are now added

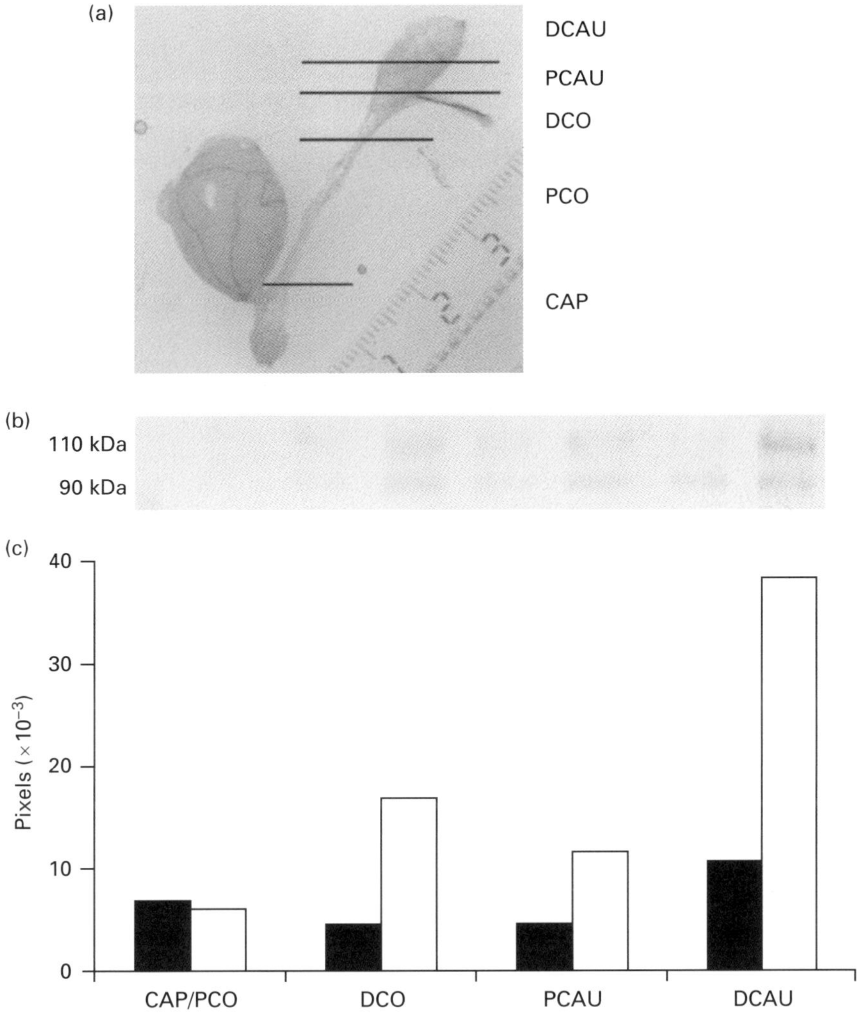

Fig. 1. Hamster spermatozoa (1×10^6 per lane) derived from regions of the epididymis (a) displayed an increase in tyrosine phosphorylation of 90 and 110 kDa proteins in response to soluble zona proteins (10ZP) as determined by immunoblotting (b). Only spermatozoa from the distal corpus and proximal/distal cauda epididymides displayed a significant response (c) as presented by semi-quantitative measurement of band intensity (pixel points).

to epididymal cultures to maintain epithelial function (Orgebin-Crist *et al.*, 1975). These androgens bind to corresponding receptors present in the epithelium but a more complex mixture of steroids may be beneficial for epithelial function. More recently, it has been shown that α-oestrogen receptors are present in the efferent ducts and initial segment of the rat epididymal epithelium and may regulate fluid resorption (Hess *et al.*, 1997a,b). β-Oestrogen receptor mRNA is also present throughout the male tract. Thus it is likely that a combination of androgens and oestrogens may be necessary to maintain full epididymal function.

More sophisticated epididymal organ cultures have been established (Klinefelter and Hamilton, 1985) by perifusion of lengths of rat caput epididymal tubule in the presence of high concentrations of carnitine. In the first 3 days of culture, spermatozoa become progressively motile on dilution, implying that certain aspects of maturation have occurred. Unfortunately, more defined cell culture procedures that reduce the epididymal epithelium to a purified single cell suspension of principal cells (Kierszenbaum *et al.*, 1981; Joshi, 1985) disrupt epithelial architecture and this results in rapid de-differentiation and loss of function in culture. In this respect, fibroblasts present in the myoid layer of the epididymal tubule have been shown to maintain epithelial secretory activity (Carballada and Saling, 1997). Hence, most of the current methods for the primary culture of epididymal epithelium use washed fragments or plaques of epithelium prepared by repetitive collagenase digestion (Moore *et al.*, 1990). This protocol (Fig. 2) generates plaques of epididymal epithelium from rodent (Moore and Hartman, 1986; Bongso and Trounson, 1996; Carballada and Saling, 1997), dog (Pera *et al.*, 1996) or human tissue (Moore *et al.*, 1992; Akhondi *et al.*, 1997) that evert overnight in culture and form contiguous spheres of epithelium with the apical surface facing outwards. Principal cells remain polarized and continue to secrete proteins for many days and sometimes weeks in the presence of androgens (Akhondi *et al.*, 1997) and for preparations of human epididymis, at least, there is little fibroblast overgrowth while the epithelial cells are functional. Various techniques have been adopted to support normal epithelial cell function including the use of semi-permeable support and extracellular matrix to produce polarized monolayers (Byers *et al.*, 1986; Cooper *et al.*, 1990; Klinefelter, 1992; Raczek *et al.*, 1994 and 1995). In the case of human tissue, a major obstacle to successful epithelial culture is the large amount of connective tissue around the epididymal tubule which often prevents adequate fragmentation. Tissue samples from vasectomy volunteers or from patients with testicular cancer to whom no anti-androgen treatment has been

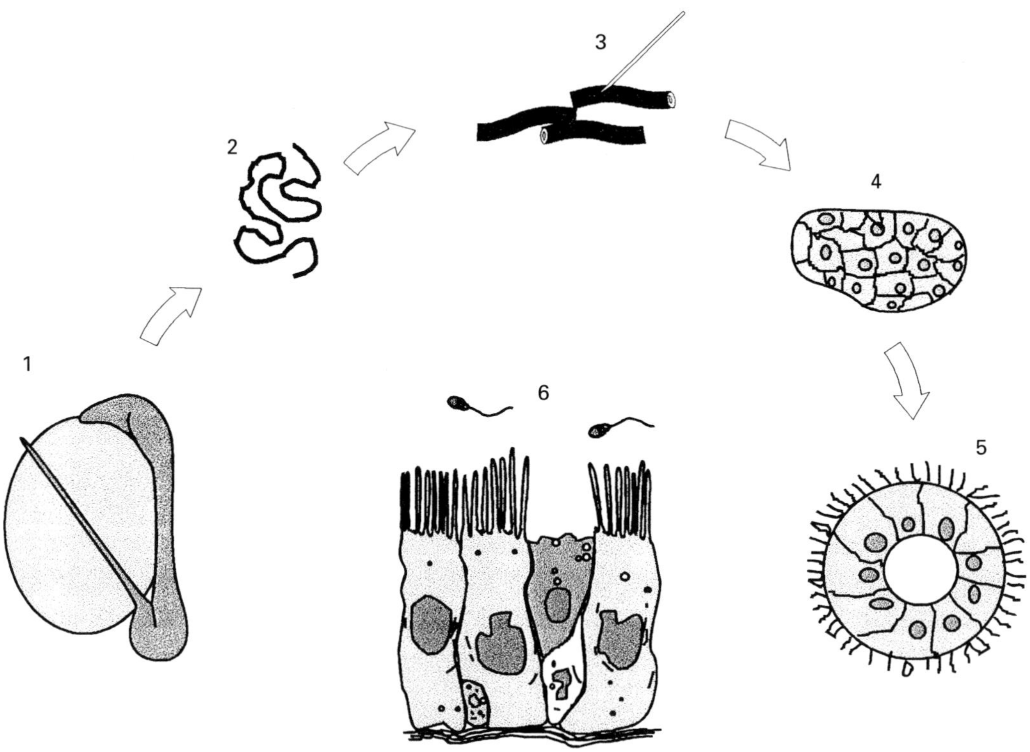

Fig. 2. A diagram of the protocol for generating functional epididymal epithelial cultures. (1) Epididymal tissue is recovered from the distal caput epididymidis to the proximal cauda epididymidis, sliced into small pieces and placed in principal cell medium (PCM). (2) After washing free of spermatozoa, the tissue is agitated with collagenase (0.1% w/v) to digest connective elements and produce fragments of tubules. (3) Under the dissecting microscope, tubules are split with a needle and washed again in PCM. (4) Plaques of epithelium are placed in PCM. (5) Overnight the plaques evert and form spheres of epithelium with microvilli facing outwards. (6) Epithelial spheres are transferred to new Petri dishes or are placed on filters coated with extracellular matrix components. Epididymal spermatozoa are co-incubated with these cultures and undergo maturation changes.

given produce much better cultures than samples from men given anti-androgen or oestrogen (sex change patients) therapy. These treatments may disrupt the androgen and oestrogen receptors of epididymal principal cells (Moore *et al.*, 1992).

Co-culture Systems

Although it has not been possible to achieve fertilization with sperm collected from the rete testis of laboratory animals, some of the later stages of maturation have been achieved by co-culture of spermatozoa that have already traversed part of the epididymis. But, currently it is not possible to bring about all the changes to spermatozoa required for acquisition of full fertility by co-culture. An example is the *in vitro* development of the fertilizing ability of hamster epididymal spermatozoa after co-culture with epithelium from the proximal cauda epididymidis (Moore *et al.*, 1986). Spermatozoa retrieved from the distal corpus epididymidis have a weak progressive motility, poor zona binding and hence low fertilizing ability *in vitro*. When co-incubated for 6 h with epithelial cell cultures from the cauda epididymidis, these spermatozoa bind avidly to hamster oocytes but their fertilizing capacity remains low because motility is not enhanced sufficiently. However, when spermatozoa were retained within the distal corpus epididymidis between ligatures around the duct and then co-cultured, spermatozoa exhibited good motility due to an ageing effect but had low fertility until co-incubated with epithelial cultures. When spermatozoa from the caput epididymidis were incubated with epithelial cultures from the corpus epididymidis, motility was enhanced for 24 h, but other aspects of maturation such as zona-binding could not be improved (Smith *et al.*, 1986). Recently, we have been able to show that changes in the motility of epididymal hamster spermatozoa from the cauda epididymidis are related to the age of the epididymal epithelium in culture (Fig. 3). Spermatozoa co-cultured with epithelium maintained for 5 and 7 days exhibit a significant improvement in motility with respect to straight-line velocity and the proportion of motile cells after incubation for 6 and 12 h compared with shorter or longer epithelial cultures

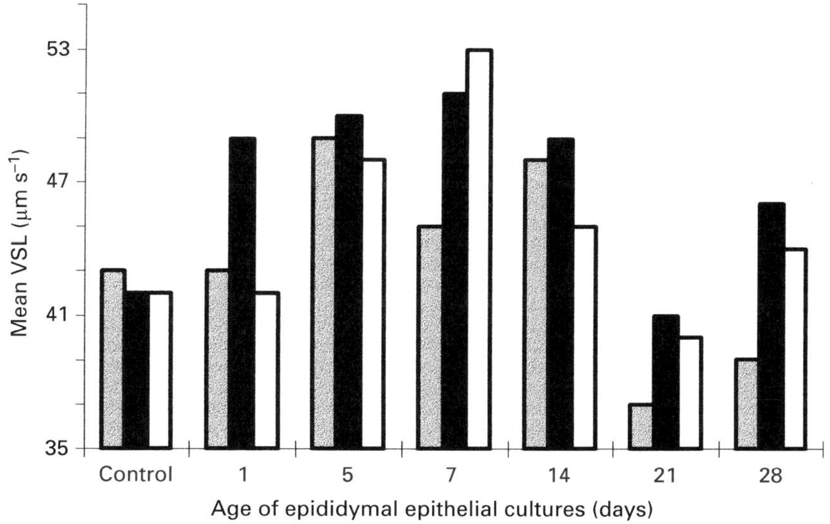

Fig. 3. Mean change in the straight-line velocity (VSL, μm s^{-1}) of hamster spermatozoa co-incubated (for ▨ 2 h; ■ 4 h; and □ 6 h) with epididymal epithelial cultures derived from the caput and corpus epididymides on various days previously. Over a 6 h co-incubation, progressive motility of spermatozoa increased most consistently when incubated with epididymal cultures 5 and 7 days old (significantly different from other values $P < 0.005$). $n = 10$ SEM = < 5% of each value. This corresponded to optimal expression of androgen receptors after the initial formation of the cultures (about day 3).

(Samayawardhena and Moore, 1998). The beneficial effects of epithelium at this time are related to when androgen receptors of epithelial cells are maximally expressed in culture and hence epididymal secretory function is maximal.

Human Sperm Maturation and Storage in Co-culture

Promising results have also been obtained with a co-culture system involving human tissue (Akhondi *et al.*, 1997). Primary cell cultures of distal caput or corpus epithelial cell preparations can be maintained for up to 12 weeks without substantial overgrowth of fibroblasts, as determined with monoclonal antibodies to cytokeratin. With co-incubations carried out at 37°C and medium replenished every other day, approximately 50% of spermatozoa were motile after 8 days and, in one case at least, a few spermatozoa survived for up to 17 days with progressive motility. Because of the scrotal position of the epididymis, it would be expected that co-cultures would be sensitive to body temperature of 37°C. Although epididymal function *in vitro* does seem to be temperature-sensitive in some species (Pera *et al.*, 1996; Carballada and Saling, 1997), it did not seem crucial in the human co-culture system in which the spermatozoa and epithelial cells were resilient to body temperature under the appropriate conditions. In this respect, the condition of human post-vasectomy ejaculates closely parallels *in vitro* sperm survival in co-culture. Spermatozoa retained in the vas deferens distal to the vas ligation will be stored close to core body temperature. A progressive decline in sperm viability occurs with a complete loss of motility in 84% of semen samples by 13 days after vasectomy (Bedford and Zelikosky, 1979) and 100% of samples by 15 days after vasectomy (Jouannet and David, 1978). Richardson *et al.* (1984) constructed a regression equation for this decline in the viability of post-vasectomy spermatozoa and found that a complete loss of sperm motility was calculated to occur at about 16 days. This corresponds closely to the 17 days maximum survival of spermatozoa in co-incubations with epididymal epithelial culture, suggesting that this is the inherent maximum survival time of human spermatozoa. The ability of spermatozoa to penetrate zona-free hamster eggs was still apparent in some individuals 8 days after vasectomy (Richardson *et al.*, 1984) indicating that at this stage a reasonable proportion of cells were functionally competent. This time period also corresponds to the proportion (50%) of spermatozoa displaying progressive motility during co-incubations. These spermatozoa retained intact acrosomal membranes and were often associated with the apical surface of epididymal principal cells in culture. Spermatozoa separated from the epithelial cultures by filters that allowed passage of macromolecules, or were incubated solely in conditioned medium, had a significantly shorter survival time. Hence, *in vitro* at least, an intimate sperm–epithelial interaction may be important for sperm survival and possibly maturation. This could be due to the need for membrane exchange of GPI anchored moieties (Kirchhoff and Hale, 1996) and the labile nature of epididymal secretions. Co-incubation with cultures other than epididymal epithelial cells were unsuccessful in promoting sperm maturation (Moore *et al.*, 1992), although in some cases they did enhance sperm motility and viability (Akhondi *et al.*, 1997). Human oviductal cells in culture have a beneficial effect on washed ejaculated human spermatozoa in terms of viability, synergistic induction of capacitation and induction of hyperactivated motility (Kervancioglu *et al.*, 1995; Chian and Sirard, 1995; Pacey *et al.*, 1995) and these effects seem to be more specific than with other epithelial cell lines (Vero cells; Kervancioglu *et al.*, 1995).

Epididymal Epithelial Factors *In Vitro*

Exactly how epididymal epithelium maintains sperm viability *in vitro* still remains unclear and several factors may be involved. In the hamster co-culture system, a 34 kDa glycoprotein secretion of principal cells of the proximal corpus epididymidis was identified *in vivo* or *in vitro* (Smith *et al.*, 1986). During co-culture conditions this epitope was transferred onto the post-acrosomal and annulus region of spermatozoa concomitant with their acquisition of progressive motility. More recently, we have shown that this glycoprotein is also expressed by rat epididymal cells in culture and binds to spermatozoa (Moore and Akhondi, 1996). Klinefelter and colleagues (1992) also reported on a 34–36 kDa group of proteins expressed by rat epithelial cells in culture which bind to spermatozoa. Treatment with ethane dimethane sulphonate (EDS) inhibited sperm maturation and diminished secretion of the 34–36 kDa (and 36–38 kDa) proteins to almost undetectable values. A 44 kDa secretory protein also binds to rat spermatozoa during co-culture and has been implicated in the maintenance of sperm viability and fertilizing capacity. A similar protein is expressed by human epididymal epithelial cells, specifically binding to washed human ejaculated spermatozoa which then maintain viability for a prolonged period of co-incubation (Moore and Akhondi, 1996). In the rat, this protein is the protease inhibitor α_1 anti-trypsin (Akhondi and Moore, unpublished). A major mRNA of the human epithelium also encodes a protease inhibitor (Kirchhoff *et al.*, 1991). Previous co-culture investigations using immature human epididymal spermatozoa have identified proteins with molecular masses of 20–22 kDa, 38–40 kDa and 66–69 kDa as being important for maturation (Tezon *et al.*, 1985; Moore *et al.*, 1992).

In addition, the epididymis may prevent oxidative stress in spermatozoa. In the rat, at least, it has been shown that gamma glutamyl transpeptidase is present in the lumen particularly in the proximal region (Hinton *et al.*, 1991). This enzyme regulates the concentration of glutathione, which is a potent antioxidant that can protect against free oxygen radicals that might otherwise attack sperm membranes. Whether such enzymes do in fact act in this way or are present under culture conditions remains to be determined.

Conclusion

The epididymal epithelial–sperm co-culture system is still far removed from the conditions prevailing in the epididymis. Spermatozoa are motile, and in far lower concentration ($\times 10^5$) than in the lumen of the tubule ($\times 10^8$). But an important aspect of co-culture experiments is that close interactions between spermatozoa and epithelial cells can be examined in detail. The observation that spermatozoa may undergo maturation changes and display prolonged survival when androgen-dependent epithelial cells are present indicates that conditions mimic to some extent processes *in situ* and therefore may yield important information related to epididymal sperm maturation and storage.

The technical assistance of Mark Morgan is much appreciated. The work was supported by The Medical Research Council.

References

Acott TS, Katz DF and Hoskins DD (1983) Movement characteristics of bovine epididymal spermatozoa. Effects of forward motility protein and epididymal maturation *Biology of Reproduction* **29** 389–399

Akhondi MA, Chapple C and Moore HDM (1997) Prolonged survival of human spermatozoa when co-incubated with epididymal cell cultures *Human Reproduction* **12** 514–522

Bedford JM and Hoskins DD (1990) The mammalian spermatozoon: morphology, biochemistry and physiology. In *Marshall's Physiology of Reproduction* (4th *Edn*) Vol. 2 pp 379–568 Ed. GE Lamming, Churchill Livingston, London

Bedford JM and Zelikosky G (1979) Viability of spermatozoa in the human ejaculate after vasectomy *Fertility and Sterility* **32** 460–463

Beigler BE, Aarons DJ, George BC and Poirier GR (1994) Induction of physiological acrosome reactions in caput epididymal spermatozoa of mice *Journal of Reproduction and Fertility* **100** 219–224

Bongso A and Trounson A (1996) Evaluation of motility, fertilising ability and embryonic development of murine epididymal sperm after coculture with epididymal epithelium *Human Reproduction* **11** 1451–1456

Burks DJ, Carballada R, Moore HDM and Saling PM (1995) A tyrosine kinase from human sperm interacts with the zona pellucida at fertilization *Science* **269** 83–86

Byers SW, Hadley MA, Djakiew D and Dym M (1986) Growth and characterisation of polarised monolayers of epididymal epithelial cells and Sertoli cells in dual environment culture chambers *Journal of Andrology* **7** 59–68

Carballada R and Saling PM (1997) Regulation of mouse epididymal epithelium *in vitro* by androgens, temperature and fibroblasts *Journal of Reproduction and Fertility* **110** 171–181

Chian R-G and Sirard MA (1995) Fertilizing ability of bovine spermatozoa cocultured with oviduct epithelial cells *Biology of Reproduction* **52** 156–162

Cooper TG (1986) *The Epididymis, Sperm Maturation And Fertilisation* Springer-Verlag, Heidelberg

Cooper TG, Yeung CH, Meyer R and Schulze H (1990) Maintenance of human epididymal epithelial cell function in monolayer culture *Journal of Reproduction and Fertility* **90** 81–91

Cornwall GA, Smyth TB, Vindnigh D, Harter C, Robinson J and Chang TSK (1986) Induction and enhancement of progressive motility in hamster caput epididymal spermatozoa *Biology of Reproduction* **35** 1065–1074

Devi KU, Ahmad MB and Shivaji S (1997) A maturation-related differential phosphorylation of the plasma membrane proteins of the epididymal spermatozoa of the hamster by endogenous protein kinases *Molecular Reproduction and Development* **47** 341–350

Gonzalez-Echeverria F, Cuasicu PS, Piazza A, Pineiro L and Blaquier JA (1984) Addition of an androgen-free epididymal protein extract increases the ability of immature hamster spermatozoa to fertilize *in vivo* and *in vitro*. *Journal of Reproduction and Fertility* **71** 433–437

Hess RA, Gist DH, Bunick D, Lubahn DB, Farell A, Bahr J, Cooke PS and Greene GL (1997a) Estrogen receptor (alpha and beta) expression in the excurrent ducts of the adult male rat reproductive tract *Journal of Andrology* **18** 602–611

Hess RA, Bunick D, Lee K-H, Bahr J, Taylor JA, Korach KS and Lubahn DB (1997b) A role for oestrogens in the male reproductive system *Nature* **390** 509–512

Hinton BT, Palladino MA, Mattmueller DR, Bard D and Good K (1991) Expression and activity of gamma glutamyl transpeptidase in the rat epididymis *Molecular Reproduction and Development* **28** 40–46

Joshi MS (1985) Isolation and cell culture of the epithelial cells of cauda epididymidis of the bull *Biology of Reproduction* **33** 187–200

Jouannet P and David G (1978) Evolution of the properties of semen immediately following vasectomy *Fertility and Sterility* **29** 435–441

Kervancioglu ME, Djahanbakhch O and Aitken RJ (1995) Epithelial cell coculture and the induction of sperm capacitation *Fertility and Sterility* **61** 1103–1108

Kierszenbaum AL, Lea AO, Petrusz P, French FS and Tres LL (1981) Isolation, culture and immunocytochemistry characterization of epididymal epithelial cells from pubertal and adult rats *Proceedings of the National Academy of Sciences USA* **78** 1675–1679

Kirchhoff C and Hale G (1996) Cell to cell transfer of glycosylphosphatidylinositol-anchored membrane proteins during sperm maturation *Molecular Human Reproduction* **2** 177–184

Kirchhoff C, Habben I, Ivell R and Krull N (1991) A major human epididymis-specific cDNA encodes a protein with sequence homology to extracellular proteinase inhibitors *Biology of Reproduction* **45** 350–357

Klinefelter GR (1992) A novel system for the co-culture of epididymal epithelial cells and sperm from adult rats *Journal of Tissue Culture Methods* **14** 195–200

Klinefelter GR and Hamilton DW (1985) Synthesis and secretion of proteins by perifused caput epididymal tubules and association of secreted proteins with spermatozoa *Biology of Reproduction* **33** 1017–1027

Leyton L and Saling P (1989) 95 kd sperm proteins bind ZP3 and serve as tyrosine kinase substrates in response to zona binding *Cell* **57** 1123–1130

Moore HDM (1990) The epididymis In *Scientific Foundations of Urology* pp 399–410 Eds GD Chisholm and WD Fair. Heimann Medical, Oxford

Moore HDM (1996) The influence of the epididymis on human and animal sperm maturation and storage *Human Reproduction* **11** 103–110

Moore HDM and Akhondi MA (1996) *In vitro* maturation of mammalian spermatozoa *Reviews of Reproduction* **1** 54–60

Moore HDM and Hartman TD (1986) *In-vitro* development of the fertilizing ability of hamster epididymal spermatozoa after co-culture with epithelium from the proximal cauda epididymidis *Journal of Reproduction and Fertility* **78** 347–352

Moore HDM, Hartman TD and Smith CA (1986) *In vitro* culture of hamster epididymal epithelium and induction of sperm motility *Journal of Reproduction and Fertility* **78** 327–336

Moore HDM, Curry M and Pryor JP (1990) *In vitro* culture of epididymal epithelium for the study of mammalian sperm maturation In *In Vitro Approaches to Mammalian Gamete Maturation and Embryonic Development* pp1–9 Eds A Lauria and F Gandolfi, Serovet, Rome

Moore, HDM, Curry MR, Penfold LM and Pryor JP (1992) The culture of human epididymal epithelium and *in vitro* maturation of epididymal spermatozoa *Fertility and Sterility* **58** 776–783

Nixon VL, Brewis IA and Moore HDM (1996) Induction of protein tyrosine phosphorylation in hamster spermatozoa is associated with capacitation state and zona induction of the acrosome reaction *Journal of Reproduction and Fertility Abstract Series* **18** Abstract 30

Orgebin-Crist M-C and Jahad N (1979) The maturation of rabbit epididymal spermatozoa in organ culture: stimulation by epididymal cytosolic extracts *Biology of Reproduction* **21** 511–516

Orgebin-Crist MC, Danzo BJ and Davies J (1975) Endocrine control of the development and maintenance of sperm fertilizing ability in the epididymis. In *Handbook of Physiology, Endocrinology V, section 7, Male Reproductive Tract* pp 319–337 Eds R Greep and D Hamilton. American Physiological Society, Washington

Pacey AA, Hill CJ, Scudamore IW, Warren MA, Barratt CLR and Cooke ID (1995) The interaction *in vitro* of human spermatozoa with epithelial cells from the human uterine (Fallopian) tube *Human Reproduction* **10** 360–366

Pera I Ivell R and Kirchoff C (1996) Body temperature (37°C) specifically down regulates the messenger ribonucleic acid for the major sperm surface antigen CD52 in epididymal cell culture *Endocrinology* **137** 4451–4459

Pholpramool C, Lea OA, Burrow PV, Dott HM and Setchell BP (1983) The effects of acidic epididymal glycoprotein (AEG) and some other proteins on the motility of rat epididymal spermatozoa *International Journal of Andrology* **6** 240–248

Raczek S, Yeung CH, Wagenfeld A, Hertle L, Schulze H and Cooper TG (1994) Epithelial monolayers from human epididymal and efferent duct tubules; testosterone metabolism and effects of culture conditions on cell height and confluence *Epithelium Cell Biology* **3** 126–136

Raczek S, Yeung CH, Hasilik A, Robenek H, Hertle L, Schulze H and Cooper TG (1995) Immunocytochemical localisation of some lysosomal hydrolases, their presence in luminal fluid and their direction secretion by epididymal cells in culture *Cell and Tissue Research* **280** 415–425

Richardson DW, Aitken RJ and Loudon NB (1984) The functional competence of human spermatozoa recovered after vasectomy *Journal of Reproduction and Fertility* **70** 575–579

Samayawardhena LA and Moore HDM (1998) Motility characteristics of hamster epididymal spermatozoa co-incubated with epididymal epithelial cultures *in vitro. Proceedings of the Boden Conference on the Epididymis* P6

Setchell BP, Maddocks S and Brook DE (1994) Anatomy, vasculature, innervation and fluids of the male reproductive tract. In *Physiology of Reproduction* (2nd Edn) pp1063–1176, Eds E Knobil and JD Neill. Raven Press, New York

Smith CA, Hartman TD and Moore HDM (1986) A determinant of Mr 34,000 expressed by hamster epididymal epithelium binds specifically to spermatozoa in co-culture *Journal of Reproduction and Fertility* **78** 337–345

Tezon JG and Blaquier JA (1981) The organ culture of human epididymal tubules and their response to androgens *Molecular and Cellular Endocrinology* **3** 233–242

Tezon JG, Ramella E, Cameo MS, Vasquez MH and Blaquier JA (1985) Identification of androgen-induced proteins in human epididymis *Biology of Reproduction* **32** 584–590

Tulsiani DRP, Skudlarek MD, Holland MK and Orgebin-Crist M-C (1993) Glycosylation of rat sperm plasma membrane during epididymal maturation *Biology of Reproduction* **48** 417–428

Turner TT (1995) On the epididymis and its role in the development of the fertile ejaculate *Journal of Andrology* **16** 292–298

Vazquez MH, de Lariminat MA and Blaquier JA (1986) Effect of androgen on androgen receptors in cultured human epididymis *Journal of Endocrinology* **111** 343–348

Vreeburg JMT, Holland MK and Orgebin-Crist M-C (1992) Binding of epididymal proteins to rat spermatozoa *in vivo. Biology of Reproduction* **47** 588–597

Journal of Reproduction and Fertility Supplement **53**, 33–45

The dog as a model system to study epididymal gene expression

R. Ivell, I. Pera, K. Ellerbrock, A. Beiglböck, K. Gebhardt, C. Osterhoff and C. Kirchhoff

IHF Institute for Hormone and Fertility Research, University of Hamburg, Grandweg 64, 22529 Hamburg, Germany

Advances in understanding the role of the epididymis in human sperm maturation and fertility are dependent upon the availability of appropriate model systems in which to examine regulatory mechanisms and functions in a controllable fashion. Of a number of mammalian species studied by us and others, we suggest that the dog epididymis offers an excellent compromise in terms of the similarity of the specific genes expressed to those in the human, their mode of regulation, and the availability of tissues suitable for cell culture studies. We have developed a set of important tools in the form of epididymis-specific canine cDNA clones and cell culture methods, with which to examine the functioning of the epididymal epithelial cells *in vitro*, as well as the expression of specific genes *in vivo*, under normal and pathological conditions (e.g. cryptorchidism). Using this model system, we have elaborated the regional patterns of gene expression *in vivo* for several of the major secretory protein genes of the canine epididymis, and we have examined the importance of androgens and temperature on gene expression *in vitro*.

Introduction

The mammalian epididymis represents a specialization of the male reproductive tract (efferent duct/ vas deferens) the function of which, although not well-defined, correlates with the acquisition by testicular spermatozoa of the ability to fertilize oocytes *in vivo* and *in vitro*, a change which appears to involve interactions between spermatozoa and proteins secreted by the epididymis. In order to understand epididymal function better, an animal model is required, with which to analyse epididymal gene expression, its regulation and functions.

In earlier studies we have identified a number of cDNA clones from a human epididymal cDNA library that appear to be expressed specifically in the epididymis, by comparison with human testis, brain or liver (Kirchhoff *et al.*, 1990, 1991, 1993, 1996; Osterhoff *et al.*, 1994, 1997). These specific products were numbered sequentially HE(human epididymis)1–HE6, and mainly represent small secretory glycoproteins, although HE6 encodes a novel G-protein coupled membrane receptor (Osterhoff *et al.*, 1997). These cDNA clones have been used as representative probes for human epididymal function, to analyse RNA from the epididymides of a number of different mammalian species by northern blot hybridization (Kirchhoff *et al.*, 1990, 1996; Uhlenbruck *et al.*, 1993). Even at low stringency, rodents indicated the presence of only two homologues (HE1, HE6; subsequently a functional homologue of HE5/CD52 has also been detected; Kirchhoff, 1994, 1996), whereas bulls, sheep and cats have an additional gene product (HE4; Kirchhoff *et al.*, 1990). The most homology was found with porcine epididymal RNA (additionally HE3; Kirchhoff *et al.*, 1994). One species that appeared to offer a good compromise between tissue availability and number of human homologues expressed (four of six) proved to be the dog. In most large European cities there is a high incidence of routine male castration of dogs for contraceptive purposes, or for what are defined as behavioural disturbances (aggression, promiscuity), in which the scrotal contents are removed to reduce circulating androgens. Such animals are in general endocrinologically normal and exhibit normal spermatogenesis. Thus we have available a frequent source of ethically unproblematic epididymal tissue obtained from local veterinary practices, which is suitable both for studies on *in vivo* gene expression or for the establishment and study of epididymal cells in culture. The aim of the present review is to describe in detail the canine epididymis and our current understanding of the regulation of epididymal gene expression based on the dog model.

Morphology and Development of the Canine Epididymis

The mammalian epididymis can be divided into three regions, caput, corpus and cauda (Glover and Nicander, 1971; Hamilton, 1990), based on a combination of gross morphology and histology, with the caput including the efferent ducts from the testis and being situated cranially on the testis, and the corpus and cauda being more or less closely apposed to the tunica albuginea of the testis. The cauda epididymidis is subjected to maximal scrotal cooling. Unlike the epididymis in some mammalian species, in the dog the corpus region does not become reduced to a narrow isthmus separating caput from cauda, but is a substantial component of the epididymis. This is reflected by the relationship of the relative wet weights of the different regions (dissected according to Glover and Nicander, 1971) calculated from a range of different breeds of dog (caput 22.4 ± 2.8 %, corpus 34.8 ± 6.1 %, cauda 42.8 ± 7.8 %; based on data in Ellerbrock *et al.*, 1994). The male reproductive organs in the dog vary in size following a positive allometry (Woodall and Johnstone, 1988). The size of the epididymis can vary greatly from one breed of dog to another: in a Chihuahua it may weigh only 0.3 g wet weight, whereas in a large dog such as a Deutsche Dogge, it may weigh up to 10 g (Woodall and Johnstone, 1988; Ellerbrock *et al.*, 1994). Given this variation in size, one should be aware of the possibility that this is reflecting a difference in the pattern of circulating and local growth factors, and hence that there may also be breed-specific differences in epididymal gene expression. However, in one comparison between breeds using northern hybridization of a constant amount of total epididymal RNA, expression of the CE1, CE4 and CE5 gene transcripts (the canine homologues of HE1, HE4 and HE5, respectively) showed no variation in relative quantity (Ellerbrock *et al.*, 1994).

Detailed studies of the histology and ultrastructure of the dog epididymis (Hammar, 1897; Chandler *et al.*, 1981; Orsi, 1983) emphasize a very similar cellular structure to that described for other species.

The epididymis, like the vas deferens and the vesicular glands (seminal vesicles), is a derivative of the embryonic mesonephric duct. However, carnivores lack any organ corresponding to the vesicular gland or seminal vesicle and the bulbourethral gland. The male accessory glands in the dog comprise, therefore, besides the vas deferens and the epididymis, only the prostate, which is a derivative of the urogenital sinus. It is therefore to be expected that in the dog possibly some of the functions normally associated with the vesicular glands in other species are taken over by the other organs of the male tract, including the epididymis. Recently, it was shown that transplanting embryonic canine epididymal tissue to the mouse kidney capsule led to a graft structure more similar to a vesicular gland than to an epididymis (Chan and Wong, 1996), suggesting that in developmental terms these organs are more similar indeed than their gross morphology would suggest.

Little is known of the early development of the epididymis in the dog. However, there are several studies assessing postnatal development, and in particular testicular and epididymal descent and cryptorchidism. Cryptorchidism or hemicryptorchidism is not uncommon amongst dogs (Pendergrass and Hayes, 1975), and provides an interesting pathological situation in which to investigate the effects particularly of abdominal, as opposed to scrotal, temperature on epididymal differentiation and gene expression. In one of the few studies on the postnatal development of the canine epididymis, it was shown that oestradiol treatment *in vivo*, acting via oestrogen receptors, led to a relatively undifferentiated epididymal epithelium, to a gross enlargement of the organ and an increase particularly of the connective tissue compartment (Connell and Donjacour, 1985).

Tissue-specific Gene Expression in the Canine Epididymis

The cells of the epididymal epithelium in the dog are furnished with a large Golgi apparatus, and evidence of considerable apocrine secretion. Although such secretions will include small molecules and electrolytes, a large portion will be made up of tissue-specific proteins. Since ejaculated canine semen has a comparable sperm density to that in other species with vaginal insemination (about 10^8 ml^{-1} with an ejaculate volume of 3–30 ml) we can assume that there are similar requirements of the epididymis with regard to sperm storage and maturation, and in particular to the numbers of spermatozoa passing through the epididymis at any one time.

Concerning the composition of epididymal fluid in the dog, Brooks (1990) collated an excellent review on the composition of the fluid secretions from different regions of the male tract across a wide variety of species, including the dog. Essentially, in terms of electrolyte balance, pH, carnitine, glycerophosphocholine and phosphocholine, and most other measured parameters, including enzymes and steroids, the dog epididymis is no different from most other species, including man (Mennella and Jones, 1977; Jones, 1978; Brooks, 1990). An exception is the complete lack of fructose in canine seminal fluid, which is believed to be due to the lack of the vesicular gland (Brooks, 1990). Taken together, these data imply that the physiological milieu that the dog epididymis provides for spermatozoa in transit is essentially no different from that of other species, including man.

In tissue sections, most spermatozoa, as might be expected, are seen within the lumen of the cauda epididymidis. Thus, if the majority of epididymal secretory products are involved in some way in interactions with spermatozoa in transit, they are likely to be (i) specialized proteins, i.e. tissue-specific, and (ii) frequent gene products. In studies on gene expression in the human epididymis, differential screening of a human epididymal cDNA library has yielded six different gene products (HE1–HE6) with a high degree of tissue-specificity and with frequencies in the range of 0.01–0.50 %. Similar findings, although for different gene products, have been obtained for mice and rats.

The dog epididymis was originally chosen as a model system because we had been able to show by northern blot hybridization the presence of canine homologues for the human epididymal genes HE1, HE4 and HE5. Screening of a canine epididymal cDNA library using the human cDNAs as probes produced full-length canine homologues of these gene transcripts (now named CE1, CE4 and CE5, for canine epididymal protein 1, 4 and 5, respectively), with frequencies of 3.3, 0.7 and 2.6 %. Although these appear to be nearly an order of magnitude more abundant than their human homologues, this is not unexpected given the age of the human donors, and the comparatively poor quality of human ejaculated spermatozoa. Northern blot hybridization of RNA from several different canine tissues (Fig. 1) showed that the CE1 and CE5 genes were expressed in a highly tissue-specific fashion, as had also been shown for humans. CE4 was maximally expressed in the epididymis but, at least in the dog, also appears to be expressed in some other tissues with a marked mucosal component, such as uterus and lung, and also weakly in the liver (Fig. 1).

Given these results, it was decided to apply a similar differential cloning approach to the dog epididymis, as was used to identify epididymis-specific human cDNA clones. In the human study, cDNA clones were identified because they were present in the epididymis but not in the testis, used here as negative control. The focus in this study had been specifically on post-testicular maturation events. Subsequent hybridization studies in the human, however, showed that there was little difference between using testis or another tissue as negative control; the epididymal-specific genes tended to be highly specific just to the epididymis and to very few other tissues. Therefore, in the dog project, cDNA clones were sought that were expressed in the epididymis but not in the liver. In this way, it was anticipated that the majority of common, specifically expressed genes not related to general metabolic or householding functions should be identified.

Although preliminary studies were carried out using the new procedure of differential display RT–PCR to identify tissue-specific gene transcripts, this was found to be quite unsuitable for this application. The reasons for this were (i) many of the interesting and specific epididymal transcripts are short (< 1 kb), and therefore there is only a small probability that random primers for the reverse transcription or PCR reactions will prime within such short transcripts, and an even lower

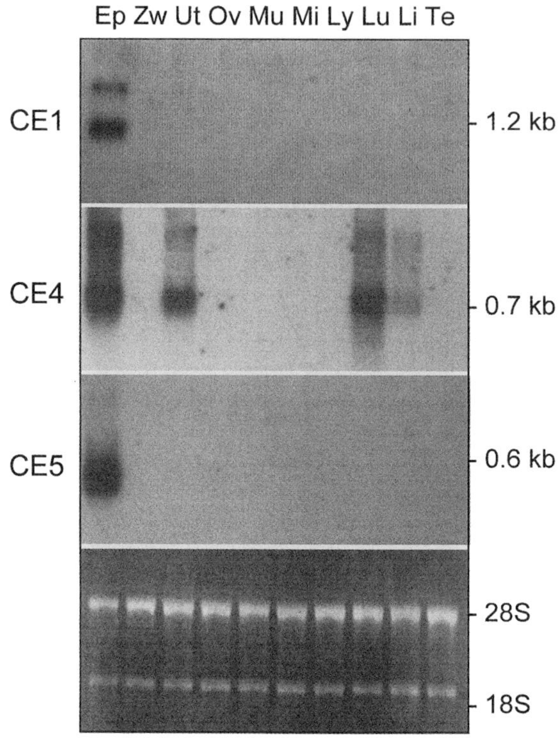

Fig. 1. Northern blot hybridization of total RNA from various canine tissues, using as probes the full-length cDNA clones CE1, CE4 and CE5, as indicated, labelled with ^{32}P by random primer extension. 10 mg RNA were loaded per slot as follows: Ep, epididymis; Zw, diaphragm; Ut, uterus; Ov, ovary; Mu, skeletal muscle; Mi, spleen; Ly, lymph nodes; Lu, lung; Li, liver; Te, testis.

probability that PCR products in the desired size range of 100–500 bp will be generated, and (ii) subsequent testing showed that the selection of 26 random primers generally used for differential display RT–PCR were incapable of hybridizing within the sequences of the known differentially expressed genes CE1, CE4 and CE5, even with a high degree of sequence corruption. It was therefore decided to apply a rigorous differential screening protocol similar to that used for the screening of the human epididymal cDNA library. This method applies complex cDNA probes derived by reverse transcription of poly(A)-enriched RNA prepared from the positive (epididymis) and negative (liver) tissues in the presence of oligo(dT) as primer and [α-^{32}P]dCTP as radiolabel. These probes are hybridized to duplicate membrane replicas of non-confluent bacteriophage plaques of the dog epididymal cDNA library. The major limitation of this procedure is that although the bacteriophage target cDNA is in excess, positively hybridizing signals will only be evident for transcripts present at a relatively high frequency within the complex radiolabelled cDNA probe. Nevertheless, our experience shows that transcripts with a frequency as low as 0.01 % can be detected with this method, which is within the range we expect for gene products of importance for specific epididymal function.

7700 cDNA clones of a canine epididymal cDNA library were screened using this approach. Approximately 400 cDNA clones were classified as positive (epididymis-specific). Since many of these are likely to represent the common genes CE1, CE4 and CE5, the replica membranes were hybridized once more against a mixed probe specific for these three gene transcripts. After this step

175 positive cDNA clones remained unaccounted for, and hence might represent novel epididymis-specific gene transcripts. These were arrayed and subjected to a secondary screening using complex cDNA probes derived from testis and from lung RNA to eliminate possible remaining false positives. 99 cDNA clones remained epididymis-positive after this step. 95 of these were subjected to partial DNA sequencing (four proved unsequenceable), revealing that these represented a total of 78 different genes, of which database searching showed that only 18 represented known sequences (for any species). Of the remaining 60 novel cDNA clones, a number of these have now been used as probes in northern blot hybridization of poly(A)-enriched canine RNA from the epididymis, lung and testis. So far, seven of these show epididymis-specific northern hybridization signals and are currently the subject of more detailled characterization. However, since the remaining cDNA clones appear to be represented as single copies only in the screened cDNA library, it is likely that their expression frequency is only very low (i.e. ≤ 0.01 %), and hence probably below the detection limit for northern blot hybridization using total RNA. Subsequent hybridization of the original cDNA library using several of the purified novel cDNA clones as probes implies that the efficiency of detection of such clones in the original differential screening using the complex epididymal cDNA probe is only about 50 %. Thus, about half the differentially expressed cDNA clones may remain undetected, possibly because of ineffective hybridization or because of overlap or overcrowding of cDNA clones on the original membrane replicas. Nevertheless, we are confident that using this procedure we have identified the majority of tissue-specifically expressed gene transcripts in the canine epididymis, with an expression frequency greater than 0.05 %, as well as a large number of novel and interesting cDNA clones whose level of expression is below this frequency.

Canine Epididymal Genes

CE1

CE1 is the canine equivalent of the human HE1 gene (Ellerbrock *et al.*, 1994; Kirchhoff *et al.*, 1996), and with an estimated frequency of 3.3 % is probably the most abundant of the gene transcripts expressed in the epididymis. The ca. 1.3 kb transcript has been fully sequenced (Ellerbrock *et al.*, 1994) and encodes a secreted glycoprotein of 149 amino acids, with an anticipated molecular mass of ca. 15–20 kDa, although western blotting of the human protein suggests a molecular mass in the range 20–27 kDa probably because of extensive glycosylation. Immunohistochemistry using an antibody raised against the bovine HE1 homologue (Fig. 2) shows marked specific staining in the epithelial cells of the canine epididymis, and also in the tubular lumen. *In situ* hybridization in sections of dog epididymis indicates that CE1 is expressed throughout the epididymis, except for the efferent ducts, and with weaker signals in the cauda than in caput and corpus epididymis (Fig. 3; Pera *et al.*, 1994). Although the HE1 protein is a major constituent of epididymal and seminal fluid it does not appear to be present on the surface of ejaculated spermatozoa (Kirchhoff *et al.*, 1996). Indeed, homology to peptide fragments of a protein from ram epididymal fluid suggests that CE1 and its homologues may be responsible for cholesterol transfer within the epididymal lumen (Baker *et al.*, 1993).

CE4

Like CE1, the CE4 gene transcripts (ca. 0.7 kb) are highly conserved across species and encode a small secretory polypeptide (Ellerbrock *et al.*, 1994). *In situ* hybridization in the dog epididymis localizes the relatively low abundance CE4 gene transcripts to most parts of the caput, corpus and cauda epididymides (Fig. 3), although with weakest signals in the central corpus, and stronger signals in the caput and proximal cauda epididymidis (Pera *et al.*, 1994). This 125 amino acid CE4 protein (molecular mass ca. 12–15 kDa) has a single site for *N*-glycosylation, and belongs to the cysteine-rich family of whey acidic proteins, of which several members are described as extracellular protease inhibitors (Kirchhoff *et al.* 1991). Antibodies raised against the human HE4 protein react

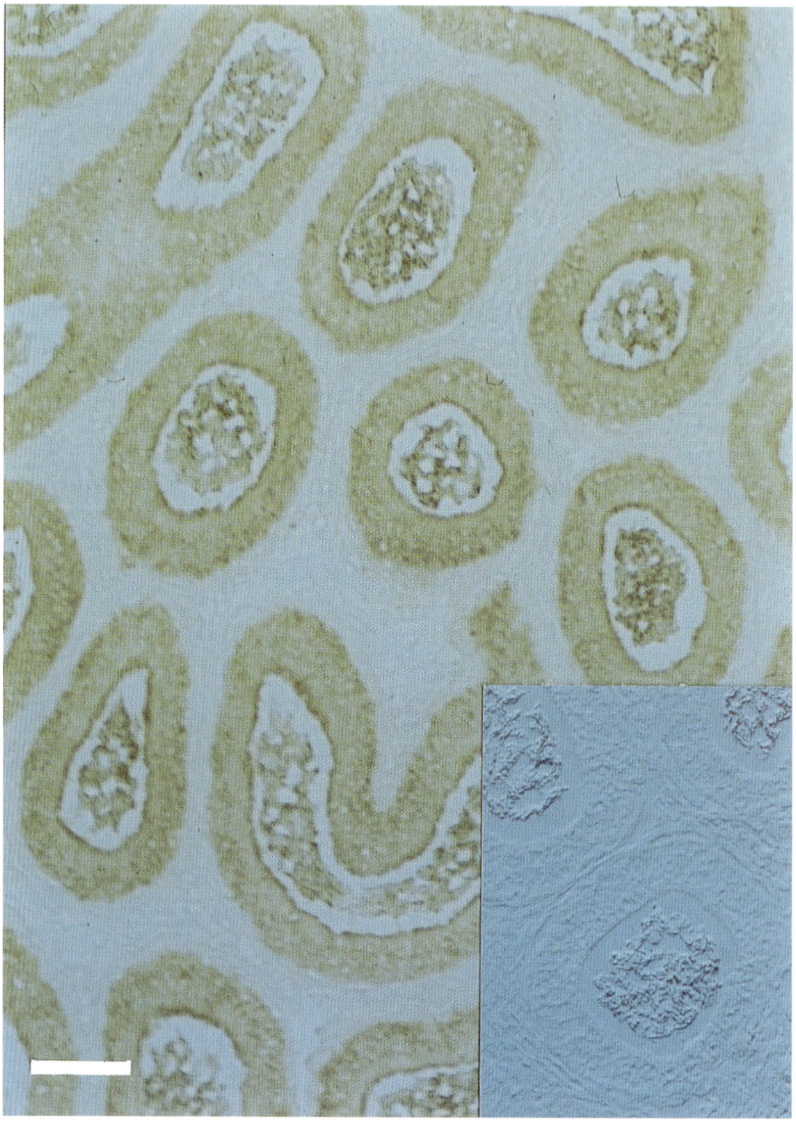

Fig. 2. Immunohistochemistry for CE1 epitopes in cryostat sections of canine epididymis. A rabbit antiserum raised against the bovine HE1 homologue (Larsen *et al.*, 1997) was applied at a dilution of 1:200, and visualized (brown chromogen) using the Envision system (Dako, Hamburg). Normal non-immune rabbit serum was used at the same dilution as negative control in place of the primary antiserum (insert). Scale bar represents 100 µm.

specifically with the epithelial cells in human (Osterhoff *et al.*, 1995), porcine and bovine epididymis (Uhlenbruck *et al.*, 1993), as well as with freshly ejaculated human spermatozoa. However, the interaction between the HE4 protein and the sperm surface appears to be only transitory, the protein appearing to disengage from the spermatozoa in fresh medium (Osterhoff *et al.*, 1995). Thus at least in the human the HE4 protein appears to have several properties reminiscent of a so-called decapacitation factor (Brooks, 1990).

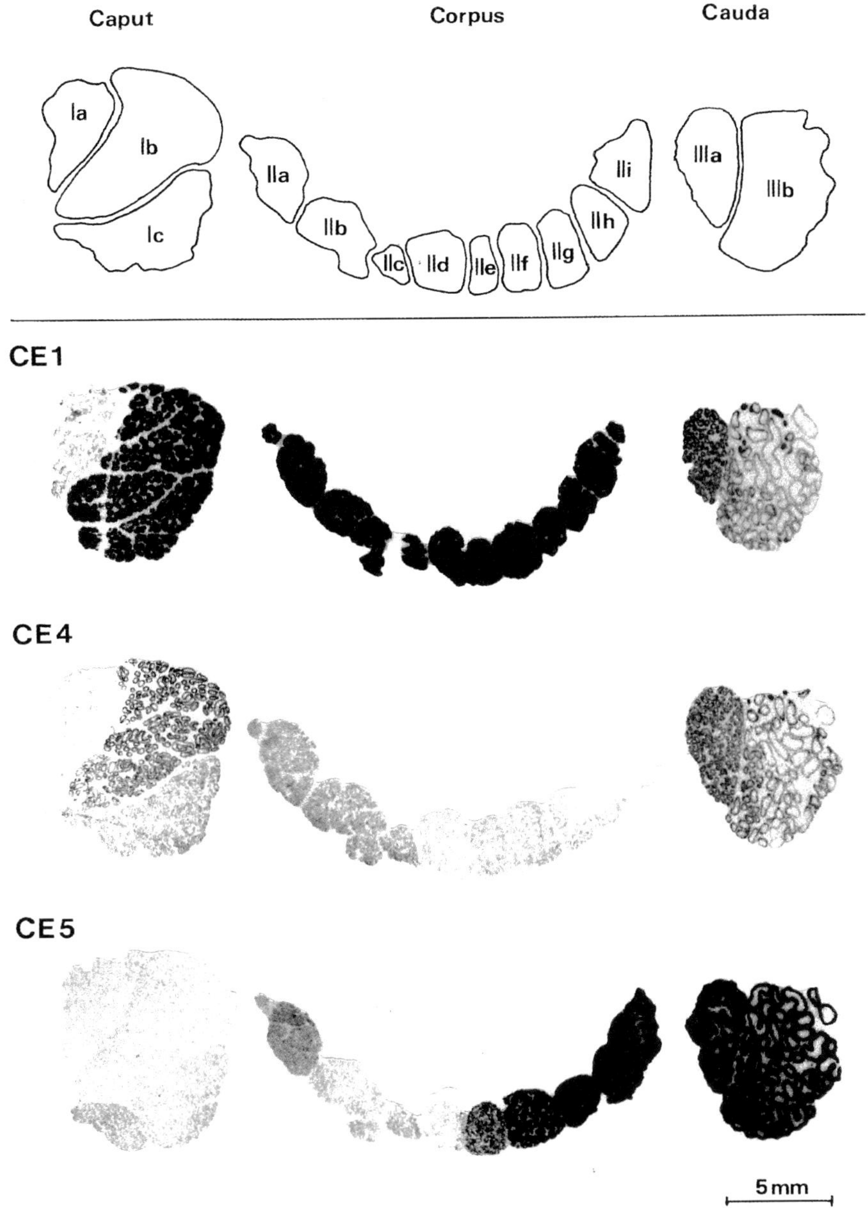

Fig. 3. *In situ* hybridization for CE1, CE4 and CE5 gene transcripts in longitudinal cryosections of an intact canine epididymis (caput, corpus and cauda were mounted separately, but all processed simultaneously). Roman numerals signify arbitrary subdivisions defined by connective tissue septa within the caput, corpus and cauda regions. As probes specific ^{32}P-labelled cRNAs prepared by *in vitro* transcription were applied and specific hybridization signals (black coloration) visualized by autoradiography using Kodak X-Omat film. For details, see Pera *et al.*, 1994. (Reproduced with permission from Pera *et al.*, 1994)

CE5

CE5 is the canine homologue of the human HE5 gene product (Ellerbrock *et al.*, 1994), which has been shown to be identical in its primary polypeptide structure to the lymphocyte antigen CD52 (Kirchhoff *et al.*, 1993; Kirchhoff and Hale, 1996). This small secretory glycopeptide, which is encoded by a small 0.6 kb mRNA, is additionally furnished with a C-terminal signal sequence indicating the post-translational addition of a glycosyl-phosphatidylinositidyl (GPI) anchor. Extensive immunological and flow-cytometric studies in humans show that this small epididymal glycopeptide is secreted in large amounts into the epididymal lumen and becomes inserted into the sperm membrane via its GPI anchor. The mechanisms by which this occurs are unclear, but may involve direct contact between the sperm membrane and the seminosome products of epididymal apocrine secretion (Kirchhoff and Hale, 1996; Aumüller *et al.*, 1997; Yeung *et al.*, 1997). Unlike the preceding epididymal genes, the CE5 gene is expressed almost exclusively in the distal epididymis, mainly within the distal corpus and cauda epididymides (Fig. 4; Pera *et al.*, 1994), which is similar to the expression of HE5 gene in humans, and of the functional CD52 homologues in rodents (Kirchhoff, 1994, 1996; Pera *et al.*, 1997).

CE6

The CE6 gene product in the dog epididymis has only been partially characterized as an RT–PCR product, derived from canine epididymal mRNA using internal oligonucleotide primers based on the human HE6 sequence (Osterhoff *et al.*, 1997). In humans a low abundance (ca. 0.01 %), ca. 5kb transcript encodes a novel member of the G-protein-coupled, 7-transmembrane-domain family of cell surface receptors. The encoded protein, HE6, is unusual in being not closely related to other members of the peptide receptor superfamily, and may represent the first member of a new subfamily. It has a large (ca. 620 amino acid) extracellular N-terminus which appears to be highly glycosylated, with structural features similar to mucins. The intracellular C-terminus is relatively long (ca. 130 amino acids) and contains several putative sites for specific phosphorylation (Osterhoff *et al.*, 1997). An analysis of a number of different tissues from the human and rat suggests that this gene product is very specifically expressed in the epididymal epithelium. It will be therefore of very great interest to determine the nature of the ligand, if any, that could interact with this receptor protein.

CE7

CE7 is a recently identified (Beiglböck *et al.*, 1998) canine epididymal gene transcript (ca. 1.5 kb) that encodes a polypeptide with high homology to the secretory glutathione peroxidase-like protein, GPX5, identified in the epididymides of mouse, rat, pig and macaque monkey (Faure *et al.*, 1991; Perry *et al.*, 1992; Vernet *et al.*, 1997). Although evidently related to the glutathione peroxidase family of enzymes, GPX5 is very specifically expressed only in the epididymis and lacks the selenocysteine considered to be an intrinsic part of the enzymatic active site. The mouse homologue appears to be secreted by the epithelium into the epididymal lumen where it appears to bind to the sperm surface (Vernet *et al.*, 1997). *In situ* hybridization in the canine epididymis and northern blot hybridization to epididymal fragments show that the CE7 mRNA is predominantly expressed in the caput epididymidis; the hybridization signal intensity decreases in the corpus epididymidis and is virtually absent in the cauda epididymidis and in the vas deferens (Pera, 1997; Beiglböck *et al.*, 1998).

CE8–CE13

As a result of the most recent differential screening procedures (see above), we have obtained partial cDNA clones for a further six canine genes, CE8 to CE13, expressed in the epididymis. Database searching of partial sequence information shows that all of these transcripts represent novel genes for any species. The preliminary northern blot hybridization analyses suggest that most are represented by relatively short gene transcripts: CE8, 0.7 kb; CE9, 1.1 kb; CE10, 0.65 kb; CE11, 2.5 kb; CE12, 1.3 kb; CE13, 3.5 kb).

Regionalization of Gene Expression within the Epididymis

The epididymis is a linear and vectorial organ. This is reflected in its morphology (see above) and the pattern of specific gene expression, both of which reflect a temporal succession of functions, vis-à-vis the spermatozoa in transit. From the point of view of spermatozoa leaving the testis, the functions occurring in the caput epididymidis must precede those in the corpus and cauda epididymides, correlating therefore with the acquisition by the spermatozoa of oocyte fertilizing ability. Looking at the dynamics of sperm transport through the epididymis, although absolute velocities are difficult to calculate because of the changes in fluid uptake and secretion, in general spermatozoa pass rapidly through the caput and corpus epididymides and are retained for storage within the distal cauda epididymis. This is reflected morphologically by the relative diameters of the epididymal lumen in the different regions, and is confirmed in tissue sections by the observation of spermatozoa predominantly in the cauda epididymidis.

Looking at specific gene expression, we find very similar patterns of mRNA distribution in the canine epididymis to those in the human; some genes are expressed predominantly in the caput epididymis, such as CE7 or HE2, others such as CE4 and CE1 are more generally expressed, but especially in the caput and corpus epididymides, and finally there are genes, such as CE5, with a mainly distal, caudal mode of expression (Krull *et al.*, 1993; Pera *et al.*, 1994; Beiglböck *et al.*, 1998). Since all of these genes represent common, secreted proteins, we can then assume that CE7 is required to act first on the spermatozoa, then the others interact, and finally, and particularly during storage, a molecule like CE5 will be expressed. This is particularly remarkable in that CE5 is expressed at a very high concentration, and is furnished with a GPI-anchor with which it can intercalate over the entire sperm cell membrane. Furthermore, its extracellular domain is considerably glycosylated, such that the CE5 molecule is likely to comprise most of the sperm glycocalyx during storage in the cauda epididymidis, and may serve to mask other sperm antigens from interaction with luminal proteins or antibodies.

The regionally specific patterns of epididymal gene expression, which have also been observed in the patterns of sperm function (Bedford and Hoskins, 1990), lectin binding (for example Yanagimachi, 1994) and in enzyme-histochemical reactions (for example Calvo *et al.*, 1995), reflect specific regional differences in epididymal cell metabolism and in particular in the expression of nuclear transcription factors. Although it is known that certain transcription factors are expressed in the canine epididymis, for example the nuclear receptors for oestradiol, androgens and progesterone (Younis *et al.*, 1979), there is no evidence as yet for a regional distribution of these factors. Of considerable interest, however, is the observation from the *in situ* hybridization (Fig. 4) that, within the epididymis, genes may be expressed homogeneously within a particular small domain defined by connective tissue septa, but that from one domain to the next the level may be quite different albeit also homogeneous within that next domain. The connective tissue epididymal septa appear thus to define homogeneous functional units, as has been suggested for the seminiferous tubules in the human testis (Ergün *et al.*, 1997). Whether such functional units are controlled by blood supply or innervation is unknown, but this implies an important aspect of epididymal metabolism which would appear to be independent of the events occurring within the epididymal lumen.

Primary Cultures of Canine Epididymal Epithelial Cells to Study the Regulation of Epididymal Gene Expression

By using small explants of intact canine epididymal tissue to seed culture medium, it is possible to generate confluent epididymal epithelial cell cultures of high purity (Ellerbrock *et al.*, 1994; Pera *et *al.*, 1996). It would appear that under these conditions only the epithelial cells grow out from the initial fragments to form a continuous monolayer of flattened polygonal cells. Cytokeratin was used as a marker for epithelial cells, and the monolayers were shown to be more than 90 % epithelial cells. In a medium containing selenium, transferrin and vitamins A and E as supplements, together with 10 % fetal calf serum, the epithelial cell cultures would remain stable for at least 7 days. Culture growth involved mainly the epithelial cells, and was both by cell migration and proliferation as shown by bromodeoxyuridine staining (Pera *et al.*, 1996).

An important feature of the canine epididymal cell culture is that the epididymis-specific gene transcripts appear to be maintained to a certain degree during culture up to 7 days, although the expression of some genes appears to be more stable than others. Furthermore, all cells appear to retain expression of the androgen receptor over this period (Pera *et al.*, 1996). In earlier experiments we could show by *in situ* hybridization that all of the epididymal epithelial cells were able to express the CE1 mRNA (Ellerbrock *et al.*, 1994), thus extracting total RNA from whole cultures reflects the metabolism of the majority of the cells in culture. In a subsequent series of experiments (Pera, 1997; Pera *et al.*, 1996) the effects of testosterone, growth factors (nerve growth factor, NGF; epidermal growth factor EGF; and transforming growth factor β,$TGFß_1$), serum addition and temperature were tested over various time intervals, and the epididymal mRNAs CE1, CE4 and CE5 measured by northern blot hybridization. For both CE1 and CE4, there was little evidence for an influence of any of these factors. The CE4 mRNA appeared to be more stably expressed in culture than was CE1, which showed a steady decline in hybridization intensity with time in culture. However, there was a major effect of temperature on CE5 (CD52) mRNA. Cultures grown at scrotal temperature (33 °C) still showed significant CE5 mRNA after 5 days, compared with cultures grown at abdominal temperature (37 °C), in which at 5 days CE5 mRNA was no longer detectable (Pera *et al.*, 1996). Preliminary experiments with transcription inhibitors suggested that this was a gene-specific effect of temperature on mRNA stability, rather than on transcription *per se*, although more extensive experimentation is necessary to verify this. Moreover, it has to be a direct effect of temperature on the epididymal cells rather than an effect mediated by the testis.

These experiments highlight two very interesting points. First, although the accessory glands of the male reproductive tract have generally been considered to be androgen dependent, this appears difficult to demonstrate for the expression of certain epididymis-specific genes in the somewhat artificial conditions of epididymal cell culture. Second, abdominal, as opposed to scrotal, temperature does not have a big effect on cultured epididymal epithelial cells in general; however, it has a major effect on the expression of at least one important and specific epididymal gene, CE5 (CD52).

This effect of temperature is particularly relevant in consideration of the negative effects of cryptorchidism on sperm function. Whereas high temperature through development is known to have a major effect on spermatogenesis, less is known about temperature effects on the epididymis, and yet from its location in the coolest part of the scrotum, the epididymis is *a priori* probably more susceptible to increased temperature. In preliminary studies on hemicryptorchid canine epididymides, in which the scrotal organ could be used as control, it was shown that endogenous CE5 mRNA was substantially reduced in the abdominal epididymis, compared with that in the scrotum (Pera *et al.*, 1996), although the relative distribution of the specific mRNA between caput, corpus and cauda epididymides remained similar. This was different from the situation for CE7 (GPX5; Beiglböck *et al.*, 1998). Although there was a massive reduction in the overall CE7 mRNA in the abdominal epididymis, this was due specifically to a loss of expression in the caput epididymidis; the levels of CE7 mRNA in the corpus and cauda epididymidis appeared to be virtually unaffected, or even increased. In contrast to these two genes, CE1 and CE4 mRNA appeared only slightly reduced in the cryptorchid epididymis (Pera, 1997; Beiglböck *et al.*, 1998). Although the cryptorchid situation is complex, involving developmental aspects and reduction of androgen concentrations as well as direct temperature effects, these observations suggest that temperature *per se* may have a marked direct impact not only on the specific gene expression, but also on the relationships between the different regions of the epididymis. A similar observation was made for genes expressed in a hemicryptorchid porcine epididymis (Uhlenbruck *et al.*, 1993). For the porcine equivalents of CE1 and CE4 mRNAs, there was also a shift in the regional pattern of expression within the abdominal epididymis compared with the scrotal organ.

Future Prospects and Limitations

The dog epididymis appears to fulfil many of the criteria required of a good model for the study of human epididymal function and sperm maturation. Tissue is generally readily available in an ethically acceptable manner from local veterinary practices, where dogs are being routinely castrated for non-endocrinological complaints. Although dogs are genetically very variable, leading to marked variation in organ size, preliminary studies suggest that this aspect does not impair its suitability as a model system. On the other hand, breed-specific incidence of infertility-related pathology (for example cryptorchidism) could make the genetic variability rather an asset in the study of this species. The dog appears to be quite human-like in terms of the epididymis-specific genes being expressed, and their regional distribution within the epididymis, implying a similarity in physiology and function. Thus studies on specific gene regulation should have direct relevance to human physiology. Finally, the ease and stability of the canine epididymal cell culture, as well as the size of the organs available, mean that for *in vitro* experiments of this type, including coculture, an optimal system is available.

However, there are disadvantages in the use of the dog for male reproductive research. First, there is only limited basic andrological information, including pharmacological studies, although fortunately the use of the dog as a model of prostatic hyperplasia has led to numerous studies on the use of different anti-androgens. Little is known of spermatogenesis and functional parameters of the male gamete, both before and after post-testicular maturation events. Finally, although *in vitro* fertilization is possible, the female biology of carnivores is such that routine functional tests of sperm–oocyte interaction and fertilization are still problematic.

Although we have been considering the dog as a model of human epididymal function, it should not be forgotten that there is a major international requirement for novel contraceptive development with regard to overpopulation in the wild of another member of the family Canidae, the European fox (Bradley, 1994). An understanding of canine epididymal function could have major implications in the development of appropriate immunocontraceptive strategies for the fox based on post-testicular sperm antigens. Indirectly, a successful application of an immunocontraceptive agent, even in the fox, would also be important in any development of such strategies in humans.

The authors are particularly grateful to the German Federal Ministry of Science and Technology (BMBF; project 01 KY 9502), as well as the German Research Council (DFG; project Ki317/5-1) for supporting aspects of the work reported here. They would also like to thank the Ernst Schering Research Foundation for a fellowship in support of K. Ellerbrock.

References

Aumüller G, Renneberg H, Schiemann PJ, Wilhelm B, Seitz J, Konrad L and Wennemuth G (1997) The role of apocrine released proteins in the post-testicular regulation of human sperm function *Advances in Experimental Medicine and Biology* **424** 193–220

Baker CS, Magargee SF and Hammerstedt RH (1993) Cholesterol transfer proteins from ram cauda epididymal and seminal plasma *Biology of Reproduction* **48** (Supplement 1) P111

Bedford JM and Hoskins DD (1990) The mammalian spermatozoon: morphology, biochemistry and physiology. In *Marshall's Physiology of Reproduction, Volume 2, Reproduction in the Male* pp 379–568 Ed. GE Lamming. Churchill Livingstone, Edinburgh

Beiglböck A, Pera I, Ellerbrock K and Kirchhoff C (1998) Canine epididymis-specific mRNA encodes secretory glutathione peroxidase-like protein *Journal of Reproduction and Fertility* **112** 357–367

Bradley MP (1994) Experimental strategies for the development of an immunocontraceptive vaccine for the European red fox, *Vulpes vulpes*. *Reproduction, Fertility and Development* **6** 307–317

Brooks DE (1990) Biochemistry of the male accessory glands. In *Marshall's Physiology of Reproduction, Volume 2, Reproduction in the Male*, pp 569–690. Ed. GE Lamming. Churchill Livingstone, Edinburgh

Calvo A, Pastor LM, Horn R and Pallares J (1995) Histochemical study of glycoconjugates in the epididymis of the hamster (*Mesocricetus auratus*) *Histochemical Journal* **27** 670–680

Chan TW and Wong YC (1996) Induction of seminal vesicle morphogenesis from dog epididymal epithelium *Anatomy and Embryology, Berlin* **194** 391–398

Chandler JA, Sinowatz F and Pierrepoint CG (1981) The ultrastructure of dog epididymis *Urological Research* **9** 33–44

Connell CJ and Donjacour A (1985) A morphological study of the epididymides of control and estradiol-treated prepubertal dogs *Biology of Reproduction* **33** 951–969

Ellerbrock K, Pera I, Hartung S and Ivell R (1994) Gene expression in the dog epididymis: a model for human epididymal function *International Journal of Andrology* **17** 314–323

Ergün S, Kilic N, Harneit S, Paust HJ, Ungefroren H, Mukhopadhyay A, Davidoff M and Holstein AF (1997) Microcirculation and the vascular control of the testis *Advances in Experimental Medicine and Biology* **424** 163–180

Faure J, Ghyselinck NB, Jiminez C and Dufaure JP (1991) Specific distribution of messenger ribonucleic acids for 24-kilodalton proteins in the mouse epididymis as revealed by *in situ* hybridization: developmental expression and regulation in the adult *Biology of Reproduction* **44** 13–22

Glover TD and Nicander L (1971) Some aspects of structure and function in the mammalian epididymis *Journal of Reproduction and Fertility Supplement* **13** 39–50

Hamilton DW (1990) Anatomy of mammalian male accessory reproductive organs. In *Marshall's Physiology of Reproduction, Volume 2, Reproduction in the Male,* pp 691–746 Ed. GE Lamming. Churchill Livingstone, Edinburgh

Hammar JA (1897) Über Sekretionserscheinungen im Nebenhoden des Hundes *Archive für Anatomie und Entwicklungsgeschichte, Supplement* **1** 1–42

Jones R (1978) Comparative biochemistry of mammalian epididymal plasma *Comparative Biochemistry and Physiology* **61B** 365–370

Kirchhoff C (1994) A major messenger ribonucleic acid of the rodent epididymis encodes a small glycosdyl-phosphatidylinositol-anchored lymphocyte surface antigen *Biology of Reproduction* **50** 896–902

Kirchhoff C (1996) CD52 is the 'major maturation-associated' sperm membrane antigen *Molecular Human Reproduction* **2** 9–17

Kirchhoff C and Hale G (1996) Cell-to-cell transfer of glycosylphosphatidylinositol-anchored membrane proteins during sperm maturation *Molecular Human Reproduction* **2** 177–184

Kirchhoff C, Osterhoff C, Habben and Ivell R (1990) Cloning and analysis of mRNAs expressed specifically in the human epididymis *International Journal of Andrology* **13** 155–167

Kirchhoff C, Habben I, Ivell R and Krull N (1991) A major human epididymis-specific cDNA encodes a protein with sequence homology to extracellular proteinase inhibitors *Biology of Reproduction* **45** 350–357

Kirchhoff C, Krull N, Pera I and Ivell R (1993) A major mRNA of the human epididymal principal cells, HE5, encodes the leucocyte differentiation CDw52 antigen peptide backbone *Molecular Reproduction and Development* **34** 8–15

Kirchhoff C, Pera I, Rust W and Ivell R (1994) A major human epididymis-specific gene product, HE3, is the first representative of a novel gene family *Molecular Reproduction and Development* **37** 130–137

Kirchhoff C, Osterhoff C and Young L (1996) Molecular cloning and characterization of HE1, a major secretory protein of the human epididymis *Biology of Reproduction* **54** 847–856

Krull N, Ivell R, Osterhoff C and Kirchhoff C (1993) Region-specific variation of gene expression in the human epididymis as revealed by *in situ* hybridization with tissue-specific cDNAs *Molecular Reproduction and Development* **34** 16–24

Larsen LB, Ravn P, Boisen A, Berglund L and Petersen TE (1997) Primary structure of EPV20, a secretory glycoprotein containing a previously uncharacterized type of domain *European Journal of Biochemistry* **243** 437–441

Mennella MRF and Jones R (1977) The activity of some nucleolytic enzymes in semen and in the secretions of the male reproductive tract *Andrologia* **9** 15–22

Orsi AM (1983) Regional histology of the epididymis of the dog. A light microscope study *Anatomische Anzeige, Jena* **153** 441–445

Osterhoff C, Kirchhoff C, Krull N and Ivell R (1994) Molecular cloning and characterization of a novel human sperm antigen (HE2) specifically expressed in the proximal epididymis *Biology of Reproduction* **50** 516–525

Osterhoff C, Kirchhoff C and Ivell R (1995) Fate of two novel human sperm antigens HE4 and HE5 during *in vitro* capacitation. In *Human Sperm Acrosome Reaction. Colloque INSERM,* Vol. 236 pp 393–394 Eds P Fénichel and J Parinaud. John Libbey Eurotext, Paris

Osterhoff C, Ivell R and Kirchhoff C (1997) Cloning of a human epididymis-specific mRNA, HE6, encoding a novel member of the seven transmembrane-domain receptor superfamily *DNA and Cell Biology* **16** 379–389

Pendergrass TW and Hayes HM (1975) Cryptorchidism and related defects in dogs: epidemiological comparisons with man *Teratology* **12** 51–56

Pera I (1997) *Regulation der Genexpression der 'Principal Cells' des Nebenhodens von Säugertieren* PhD Thesis, University of Hamburg

Pera I, Ivell R and Kirchhoff C (1994) Regional variation of specific gene expression in the dog epididymis as revealed by *in situ* transcript hybridization *International Journal of Andrology* **17** 324–330

Pera I, Ivell R and Kirchhoff C (1996) Body temperature (37°C) specifically down-regulates the messenger ribonucleic acid for the major sperm surface antigen CD52 in epididymal cell culture *Endocrinology* **137** 4451–4459

Pera I, Derr P, Yeung CH, Cooper TG and Kirchhoff C (1997) Regionalized expression of CD52 in rat epididymis is related to mRNA poly(A) tail length *Molecular Reproduction and Development* **48** 433–441

Perry AC, Jones R, Niang LS, Jackson RM and Hall L (1992) Genetic evidence for an androgen-regulated epididymal secretory glutathione peroxidase whose transcript does not contain a selenocysteine codon *Biochemical Journal* **285** 863–870

Russell LD, Ettlin RA, Sinha Hikim AP and Clegg ED (1990) *Histological and Histopathological Evaluation of the Testis* Cache River Press, Vienna, IL

Uhlenbruck F, Sinowatz F, Amselgruber W, Kirchhoff C and Ivell R (1993) Tissue-specific genes as an indicator of epididymis-specific functional status in the boar, bull and stallion *International Journal of Andrology* **16** 53–61

Vernet P, Faure J, Dufaure JP and Drevet JR (1997) Tissue and developmental distribution, dependence upon testicular factors and attachment to spermatozoa of GPX5, a murine epididymis-specific glutathione peroxidase *Molecular Reproduction and Development* **47** 87–98

Woodall PF and Johnstone IP (1988) Dimensions and allometry of testes, epididymides and spermatozoa in the domestic dog (*Canis familiaris*) *Journal of Reproduction and Fertility* **82** 603–609

Yanagimachi R (1994) Mammalian fertilization. In *The Physiology of Reproduction* pp 189–317 Ed. Knobil E and Neill JD. Raven Press, New York

Yeung CH, Schröter S, Wagenfeld A, Kirchhoff C, Kliesch S, Poser D, Weinbauer GF, Nieschlag E and Cooper TG (1997) Interaction of the human epididymal protein CD52 (HE5) with epididymal spermatozoa from men and cynomolgus monkeys *Molecular Reproduction and Development* **48** 267–275

Younes MA, Evans BA, Chaisiri N, Valotaire Y and Pierrepoint CG (1979) Steroid receptors in the canine epididymis *Journal of Reproduction and Fertility* **56** 45–52

Journal of Reproduction and Fertility Supplement **53**, 47–57

Testicular regulation of epididymal gene expression

B. T. Hinton, Z. J. Lan, D. B. Rudolph, J. C. Labus and R. J. Lye

Department of Cell Biology, University of Virginia Health Sciences Center, Charlottesville, Virginia 22908, USA

Normal epididymal function is regulated by androgens and testicular factors. Our studies have been directed towards identifying testicular factors that regulate the function of the initial segment and the mechanisms by which this is achieved. The initial segment appears to be critical for normal sperm maturation in view of recent gene knock-out studies. Previous and ongoing studies from this and other laboratories have shown that the expression of several genes including proenkephalin, cystatin-related epididymal specific (CRES), 5α-reductase and γ-glutamyl transpeptidase (GGT) within the initial segment is highly dependent upon the presence of testicular factors. A lumicrine mechanism of regulation of these genes is proposed. The regulation of gamma-glutamyl transpeptidase (GGT) is described as a model enzyme for studying the role and identification of testicular factors. GGT appears to play an important role in the protection of spermatozoa from oxidative stress. Multiple GGT mRNAs (II–IV) are expressed within the epididymis, but GGT mRNA IV is the only form that is highly expressed in the initial segment, especially within zone 1A, and is regulated by testicular factors. Testicular factors control this transcript by regulating both its rate of transcription and its stability. Evidence is presented to suggest that basic fibroblast growth factor (bFGF) is a candidate testicular factor that regulates GGT activity in the epididymis. Basic FGF may regulate gene expression in the epididymis via the ras–raf–MAPK second messenger pathway and by members of the *Ets* transcription family.

Introduction

It is well established that a functional epididymis is dependent upon androgens produced by the testis. However, it has become clear from the initial studies of Danzo *et al.* (1977) and later studies by several investigators that the testis may support epididymal function by other mechanisms. In this instance, there is substantial evidence to show that factors originating in the testis are secreted into the seminiferous tubule and are then transported into the rete testis, through the efferent ducts and into the epididymal lumen, to regulate epididymal function. This is neither an endocrine nor an autocrine type of regulation, although it could be considered paracrine in nature. In collaboration with Drs Terry T. Turner and Charles J. Flickinger , the term 'lumicrine' has been coined to define the regulation of cells via factors secreted or produced by another group of cells through a luminal or ductal system. Previous observations support the concept that a factor can be secreted in one part of a luminal system and influence another cell type downstream. For example, studies by Skinner and Rowson (1967, 1968) demonstrated that the ampulla of the vas deferens remained underdeveloped after unilateral vasectomy. These investigators (Skinner and Rowson, 1968) also showed that it was the loss of testosterone, presumably originating in the testis, from the lumen that resulted in the failure of the ampulla to develop after vasectomy. With the discovery of synthesis and secretion of androgen-binding protein (ABP) by the testis (French and Ritzen, 1973a,b; Danzo, 1974; Ritzen and French, 1974; Cameo and Blaquier, 1976), several investigators suggested that ABP and androgens (testosterone, dihydrotestosterone or both hormones) were responsible for the maintenance of a normal proximal epididymis (Danzo *et al.*, 1977; Fawcett and Hoffer, 1979; Nicander *et al.*, 1983; see review by Robaire and Viger, 1995). However, proteinaceous factors other than ABP may regulate epididymal protein synthesis and secretion (Brooks, 1979; Brooks, 1983; Sujarit *et al.*, 1990; Holland *et al.*, 1992; Lan *et al.*, 1998).

This paper will review the evidence for the regulation of epididymal function by a lumicrine mechanism, and present results from our laboratory and from others about the identity of such factors.

Evidence That Testicular Factors Affect Epididymal Function

It is well known that the morphology of the rat initial segment (zones 1A, B and C; Reid and Cleland, 1957) region is altered after ligation of the efferent ducts (Danzo *et al.*, 1977; Fawcett and Hoffer, 1979; Nicander *et al.*, 1983; Abe *et al.*, 1984), so it is not surprising that the expression of proteins and genes in this epididymal region is also altered. Although general protein synthesis and secretion by the initial segment and proximal caput is affected by loss of testicular factors (Jones *et al.*, 1980; Brooks, 1983, 1987; Holland and Orgebin-Crist, 1988), the expression of several specific mRNAs and proteins within the initial segment has been shown to depend upon the presence of testicular factors. These include proenkephalin (Garrett *et al.*, 1990), retinoic acid binding protein (Zwain *et al.*, 1992), CRES gene (Cystatin Related Epididymal Specific; Cornwall *et al.*, 1992), 5α-reductase (Robaire *et al.*, 1977; Robaire, 1979; Viger and Robaire, 1994), gamma-glutamyl transpeptidase (GGT) mRNA IV (Palladino and Hinton, 1994), A-raf (Winer and Wolgemuth , 1995), glutathione peroxidase (GPX5; Rigaudiere *et al.*, 1992; Vernet *et al.*, 1997), polyomavirus enhancer activator 3 (PEA3; Lan *et al.*, 1997) and ADAM 7 (A Disintegrin And Metalloprotease 7; Cornwall and Hsia, 1997).

It is of interest that expression of GGT mRNA IV, and of mRNA encoding PEA3, 5 alpha-reductase (type 1) and proenkephalin is high in zone 1A (Reid and Cleland, 1957) of the rat initial segment, and that all are profoundly affected by loss of testicular factors. Cell death or apoptosis, necrotic cells and cytoplasmic regression are also observed in this region after efferent duct ligation (Nicander *et al.*, 1983). Although cell death was observed in zones 1B and 1C, the severity was considerably less compared with that in zone 1A (Nicander *et al.*, 1983). The difference in cell death between initial segment regions may be due to the greater frequency of mitosis in cells located in zone 1A compared with cells in the distal initial segment (Nicander *et al.*, 1983). Hence, the function(s) of zone 1A of the initial segment appears to be highly dependent upon factor(s) of testicular origin.

It is apparent that the initial segment is important for sperm maturation because a c-ros tyrosine kinase receptor knock-out results in an underdeveloped initial segment and male infertility (Sonnenberg-Riethmacher *et al.*, 1996).

What Are The Testicular Factors That Regulate Epididymal Function?

Presumably, rete testis fluid contains one or more putative factors originating in the testis that regulate epididymal function. Rete testis fluid contains two major components, spermatozoa and fluid, and either one or both can be considered as regulators of epididymal gene expression.

Hypothesis 1: testicular spermatozoa regulate epididymal function

Spermatozoa make up approximately 1% of the volume of rete testis fluid and are concentrated to about 20% of fluid within the efferent ducts (Clulow *et al.*, 1994, 1996). There are 3×10^7 spermatozoa ml^{-1} rete testis fluid (see Setchell, 1978). It is possible that this number of spermatozoa entering the initial segment would influence epididymal cells by either acting as a ligand or carrying a factor into the epididymis.

Evidence to suggest that spermatozoa regulate epididymal gene expression comes from the work of Garrett *et al.* (1990). In this study, expression of mRNA encoding proenkephalin was assessed in the initial segment of rats after treatment with the drug busulfan to cause a transient loss of early developing germ cells. Results showed that during the time of sperm depletion in the proximal epididymis, there was a decline in expression of proenkephalin mRNA, and its expression returned to normal values after the re-appearance of spermatozoa. These authors provided three possible interpretations of their findings. The first interpretation is that spermatozoa can regulate gene expression in the initial segment by direct contact with the principal cells. A more obvious possibility is that spermatozoa act as a carrier of testicular factor(s), although direct contact of spermatozoa with the apical surface of the epididymal cells cannot be ruled out. The second possibility is that the cytoplasmic droplet is absorbed by the principal cells of the proximal epididymis and factors within the droplet regulate gene expression. The third interpretation is that the developing germ cells induce Sertoli cells to produce a factor that passes into the lumen. This hypothesis seems the most plausible as many of the products synthesized and secreted by Sertoli cells are highly dependent upon the presence of germ cells. An alternative interpretation of this study is that busulfan itself can directly affect expression of the proenkephalin gene or that busulfan has a direct affect on production of testicular factor by Sertoli cells. In support of this suggestion, Brooks (1979) showed that busulfan treatment can directly affect epididymal weight, epididymal ABP concentration and pyruvate carboxylase activity.

The role of testicular spermatozoa in regulating epididymal gene expression or epididymal function could be examined by isolating and microperfusing testicular spermatozoa into the epididymal duct after ligation of the efferent ducts for different periods. Gene expression, protein synthesis or the activity of a protein could be measured after microperfusion and compared with control values. The possibility that spermatozoa themselves can regulate epididymal gene expression is intriguing and warrants further investigation.

Hypothesis 2: soluble component(s) of rete testis fluid can regulate epididymal gene expression

The composition of rete testis fluid differs from that of blood plasma (see review by Hinton and Setchell, 1995). It contains numerous ions and organic solutes including inositol and amino acids, in addition to steroids (Turner *et al.*, 1984; see also Setchell and Brooks, 1988). The total protein concentration is quite low, approximately 1 mg ml^{-1} for many species (Setchell, 1978). Albumin, androgen-binding protein (ABP), α_2-macroglobulin, clusterin (SGP-2), growth factors (Brown *et al.*, 1981; Feig *et al.*, 1980; Buch *et al.*, 1988; see review by Skinner, 1995) as well as enzymes including esterase, malate dehydrogenase, aspartate aminotransferase, galactosyltransferase and acid phosphatase (Suominen and Setchell, 1972; Koskimies and Kormano, 1973; Hamilton, 1980), contribute to the protein content of rete testis fluid. Ions, organic solutes, steroids and protein components of rete testis fluid are all candidate factors that may control epididymal gene expression.

The most obvious protein candidate, and the protein that has been studied most extensively, is androgen-binding protein (ABP). Several investigators originally suggested that ABP is the testicular factor that regulates functions of the proximal regions of the epididymis (Danzo *et al.*, 1977; Fawcett and Hoffer, 1979; Nicander *et al.*, 1983). Although the precise role of ABP is not yet known, the hypothesis presented by Robaire and Viger (1995) seems plausible. These investigators suggested that ABP is synthesized by Sertoli cells under the influence of testosterone secreted by Leydig cells. ABP is secreted into the seminiferous tubule and enters the initial segment of the epididymis. ABP with bound androgen is taken up by the principal cells where it can regulate epididymal nuclear 5α-reductase (microsomal 5α-reductase is presumably regulated by circulating androgens). This mechanism would provide high concentrations of dihydrotestosterone, the active androgen, to mediate androgen action in this epididymal region. Studies by Turner *et al.* (1995) also showed that sex-hormone binding globulin (an ABP analogue) stimulated protein synthesis and secretion by the caput epithelium after introduction of ABP into the caput lumen. These studies support the hypothesis that testicular ABP plays a role in proximal epididymal function.

Evidence to suggest that additional testicular factors are needed for normal proximal epididymal function comes from the studies of Brooks (1979) and Lan *et al.* (1998). Brooks (1979) showed that even in the absence of androgen-binding protein in the proximal epididymis, the activity of some glycolytic enzymes remained unchanged as did the weight of the tissue. The experiments performed by Lan *et al.* (1998) are described below.

Rete testis fluid appears to contain potential negative regulators. For example, Brooks (1983) showed that two proteins not synthesized in the initial segment of normal rats were synthesized and secreted after orchidectomy. If testosterone was administered after orchidectomy, these proteins were still synthesized and secreted. Hence, a factor(s) from the testis is probably responsible for the downregulation of these proteins. Upon closer inspection of the two proteins, it appears that these may be the subunits of clusterin (SGP-2). Holland *et al.* (1992) also showed the appearance of a 40 kDa protein in the mouse proximal epididymis after efferent duct ligation. Whether the 40 kDa identified by Holland *et al.* (1990) is also one of the subunits of clusterin remains to be clarified because Cyr and Robaire (1992) showed that the expression of clusterin mRNA was not regulated by testicular factors.

Studies by our laboratory (Lan and Hinton, unpublished observations) have shown that several nuclear and cytoplasmic proteins isolated from the initial segment are phosphorylated after efferent duct ligation (Fig. 1). This finding supports the idea that testicular factors may regulate cytoplasmic and nuclear phosphatases in the initial segment. Hence, under normal conditions some cytoplasmic and nuclear proteins in the initial segment are in a dephosphorylated state. The finding that testicular factors regulate the phosphorylation state of initial segment proteins may have important implications in view of our discussion below concerning second messenger pathways, and the possible involvement of testicular factors in the regulation of apoptosis in the initial segment (Nicander *et al.*, 1983; Turner and Riley, personal communication).

Hypothesis 3: genes within the initial segment are regulated by changes in blood flow or innervation caused by efferent duct ligation

The hypothesis that testicular factors regulate the expression of genes and proteins in the initial segment can be tested by performing an efferent duct ligation and measuring the amount of mRNA or protein and comparing the values with those of non-ligated controls. Data obtained from such a set of experiments are often interpreted to mean that a factor(s) of testicular origin is responsible for any changes measured. However, the data may be interpreted in another manner. Brown and Waites (1972) showed that after efferent duct ligation for 7 days, blood flow to the proximal epididymis of rats and rabbits was reduced. Since blood flow to an organ is critical for its normal function, the effects of efferent duct ligation on protein and gene expression may be due to a reduction in blood flow to the initial segment. However, blood flow to the initial segment was not reduced after efferent duct ligation for 1 day, so that any changes in expression of proteins and genes during this time would support the idea that it is due to a loss of a testicular factor(s) rather than to changes in blood flow.

An efferent duct ligation may compromise innervation to the initial segment which may result in changes in epithelial function. Although experiments to test this hypothesis have not been performed, it has been shown, for example, that loss of sympathetic innervation to the cauda epididymidis of rats results in alteration of luminal fluid proteins (Ricker *et al.*, 1996). It is recognized that the efferent ducts and the initial segment may not have extensive autonomic innervation, but loss of any type of innervation to the efferent ducts may result in changes of function of epithelial cells in this region. Further experiments are needed to test this hypothesis.

Regulation of Epididymal Gamma-Glutamyl Transpeptidase (GGT) as a Model Enzyme For Studying the Role and Identification of Testicular Factors

Introduction

Gamma-glutamyl transpeptidase (GGT: EC 2.3.2.2) is a key enzyme in the metabolism of the tripeptide glutathione (GSH: γ-Glu-Cys-Gly), an important antioxidant (see Hinton *et al.*, 1996 for

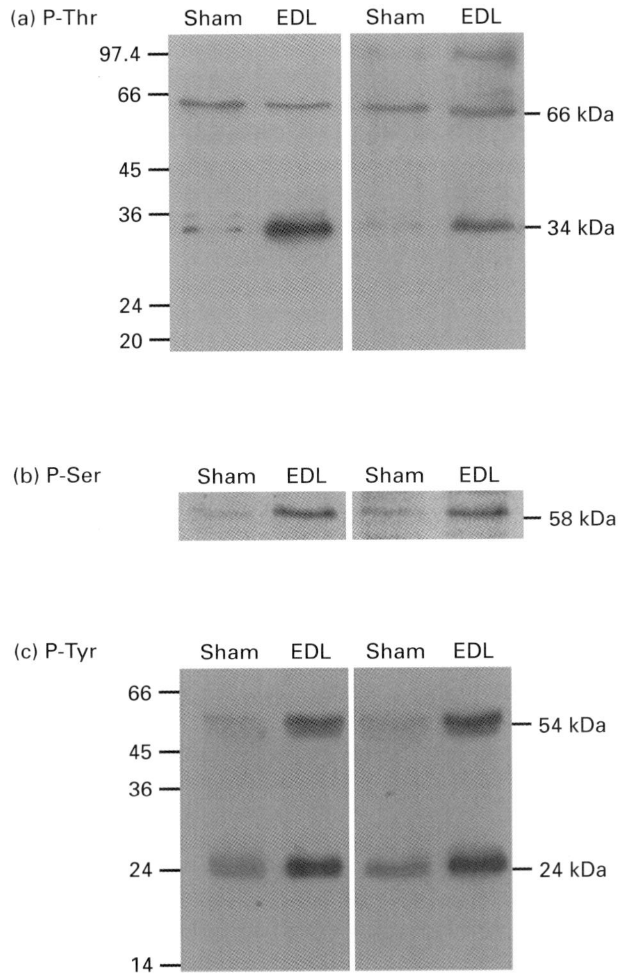

Fig. 1. Western blot analysis of initial segment nuclear extracts (a, b; 50 μg protein per lane) and whole cell extracts (c; 80 μg protein per lane) from sham-operated rats (Sham) and rats that had previously undergone an efferent duct ligation (EDL) for 3 days. The proteins were separated by polyacrylamide gel electrophoresis, transferred to cellulose acetate and probed with monoclonal antibodies to phosphothreonine (P-Thr), phosphoserine (P-Ser) and phosphotyrosine (P-Tyr). Molecular weight markers are shown on the left hand side. Data shown are from two animals per group. Note that in (a), a protein of apparent molecular mass 34 kDa showed a stronger antibody signal in tissue removed from animals that had undergone an EDL compared with sham tissue. Similar results are seen in (b) for a 58 kDa protein, and in (c) for 54 and 24 kDa proteins. These data indicate that each of these proteins is in a dephosphorylated state under normal physiological conditions. In (a), the phosphorylation state of the 66 kDa protein was not altered following EDL (Lan and Hinton, unpublished observations). The identity of these proteins is not known.

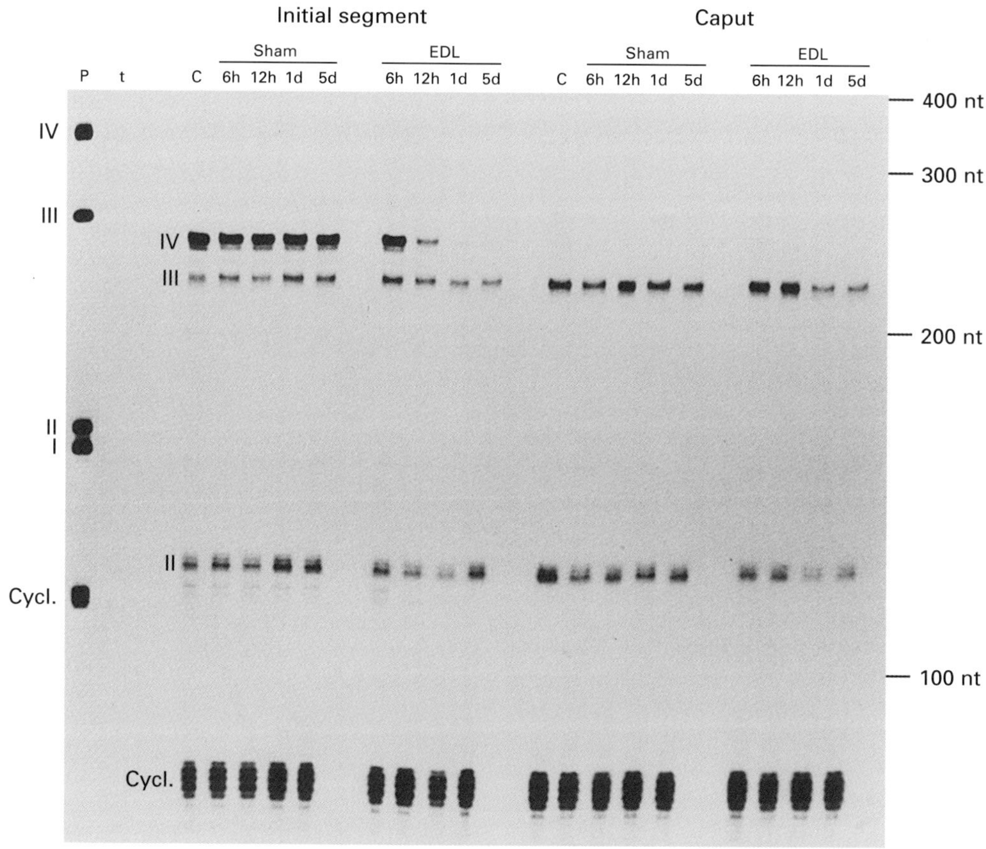

Fig. 2. Ribonuclease protection analyses of total RNA from the initial segment and caput regions of the rat epididymis after unilateral efferent duct ligation (EDL). Ten micrograms of total RNA isolated from the initial segment and caput of sham-operated control rats and rats after unilateral EDL for 6 h, 12 h, 1 day and 5 days were subjected to ribonuclease protection analyses with four GGT 5′ untranslated region-specific cRNA probes and the cyclophilin antisense transcript. An 18 h exposure with an intensifying screen is shown. P, undigested GGT probes and cyclophilin (Cycl) probe; C, 10 μg total RNA from control unoperated rats; t, tRNA control hybridization. Note that expression of GGT mRNA IV only declines following loss of testicular factors after 12 h EDL. The decline is due to both changes in stability and transcription rate (see Rudolph and Hinton, 1997). Reproduced by kind permission from Palladino and Hinton (1994) and The Endocrine Society.

review). Upon oxidation of GSH to the dimer (GSSG), GGT rapidly cleaves the gamma bond between glutamate and cysteine; it is the only known enzyme that can perform this reaction. The remaining dipeptide, Cys-Gly, is then cleaved by a dipeptidase to yield cysteine and glycine. GGT and dipeptidase are generally located on the epithelial brush border of tissues involved in secretion and absorption, for example kidney, small intestine, pancreas and epididymis. Hence, upon metabolism of GSSG into its constituent amino acids, each amino acid is then transported into the respective cell type for the resynthesis of reduced glutathione.

Our previous studies have shown that three forms of GGT mRNAs (II, III and IV) are expressed in the rat epididymis in a region-dependent manner (Palladino *et al.*, 1994), and each mRNA appears to be under the control of a different promoter. The expression of GGT mRNAs is highest in the proximal epididymal regions which coincides with highest enzyme activity and protein content as measured by biochemical assays and western blot analysis, respectively (Hinton *et al.*, 1991; Lan *et al.*,

1998). Expression of GGT mRNAs II and III is quite low in the caput compared with the very high expression of GGT mRNA IV within the initial segment (Palladino *et al.*, 1994). Expression of GGT mRNA IV in the initial segment depends upon the presence of testicular factors (Palladino and Hinton, 1994; Fig. 2). The expression of GGT mRNA IV in the initial segment declined to approximately 50% of control values after efferent duct ligation for 24 h.

Testicular factors maintain rate and stability of GGT mRNA IV transcription

It is well known that the amount of RNA observed on a northern blot analysis or RNase protection assay represents the steady-state level of that particular transcript. The steady-state expression of a transcript is a balance between the rate of transcription and its decay (see Nielsen and Shapiro, 1990). Therefore, the decline of GGT mRNA IV expression after loss of testicular factors could be due to either a decline in the rate of transcription or a decrease in stability. Our studies have shown that the rate of transcription of GGT mRNA IV declines to approximately 70% of control values within 12 h of loss of testicular factors. Loss of testicular factors also results in an initial rapid decay of GGT mRNA IV with a half-life of less than 1 h followed by a slower decay with an approximate half-life of 8 h. Secondary-structure models indicate that there are two families (α and β) of folding patterns for the 5′ untranslated region (UTR) of GGT mRNA IV in epididymal cells. Analysis revealed that one 5′ UTR folding pattern (α-family) was more thermodynamically stable than the other (β-family). It is suspected that the rapid decay of GGT mRNA IV observed during the first hour of loss of testicular factors is due to the decay of mRNAs in the β-family. The subsequent decay with a half-life of 8 h may be due to the decay of mRNAs in the α-family. The mechanisms by which this is achieved remain unclear but may involve differential binding of a stabilizing complex to each configuration or to differences in susceptibility of the mRNAs to cellular nucleases. Therefore, testicular factors maintain transcription rates and stabilize GGT mRNA IV under normal physiological conditions (Rudolph and Hinton, 1997).

A member of the Ets transcription family, PEA3, regulates expression of GGT mRNA IV

In an effort to search for testicular factor(s) that regulate the expression of GGT mRNA in the initial segment, the promoter region of this transcript was analysed using the Genetics Computer Group (Madison, WI) sequence analysis computer software package. Several conserved polyomavirus enhancer activator 3 (PEA3) binding motifs were found. PEA3 is a member of the *Ets* (E26 transformation specific) transcription family that has DNA binding activity to the motif 5′-AGGAAG-3′ (Martin *et al.*, 1988; Xin *et al.*, 1992). The protein contains acidic and glutamate-rich regions, *Ets*-binding domain, and has a molecular weight of 62 kDa. PEA3 is expressed in several tissues including mouse brain and epididymis as well as several cell lines (Xin *et al.*, 1992). Studies have shown that PEA3 binds to the promoter region of a number of different genes including human synapsin II (Petersohn *et al.*, 1995) and collagenase (Gutman and Wasylyk, 1990; Gum *et al.*, 1996). DNA binding and transcriptional activity of PEA3 is regulated by serum, growth factors, non-nuclear oncogenes and tumour promoters (Wasylyk *et al.*, 1989; Gutman and Wasylyk, 1990; Gum *et al.*, 1996).

PEA3 mRNA is highly expressed in the initial segment of the rat epididymis, coincident with GGT mRNA IV expression (Lan *et al.*, 1997). *In situ* hybridization analysis revealed that PEA3 mRNA and GGT mRNA IV are primarily localized to zone 1A and B (Reid and Cleland, 1957) of the initial segment (Rudolph and Hinton, unpublished observations) and immunocytochemical analysis shows that PEA3 is localized to the nucleus (Suarez-Quian, Lan and Hinton, unpublished observations). Expression of PEA3 mRNA was also shown to be reduced to approximately 40% of the control level after efferent duct ligation for 12 h (Lan *et al.*, 1997). Hence, the expression of PEA3 mRNA in the initial segment depends upon the presence of testicular factors. Western blot analysis showed that PEA3 protein is present in initial segment nuclear protein extracts. Electrophoretic mobility shift assays showed that this nuclear extract specifically bound to a PEA3 DNA binding motif, and southwestern analysis demonstrated that the DNA–protein complex contained PEA3. Studies are underway to examine the regulation of transactivation of GGT mRNA IV by PEA3. Evidence suggests that other members of the *Ets* transcription family are also present in nuclear extracts of the initial segment, and may also play a role in transactivation of genes in this region (Lan *et al.*, 1997). A recent study by Drevet *et al.* (1998) has shown that PEA3 may be an inhibitor of transcription of the epididymal glutathione peroxidase 5 (gpx5) gene. Activation of GGT mRNA IV promoter by PEA3 was also inhibited or not observed when either COS-1 or NRK-52E cell lines were used, respectively (Lan and Hinton, unpublished observations). However, our studies using initial segment primary cultures have shown that PEA3 or another member of the *ets* family is needed for the formation of the pre-initiation transcriptional complex but that PEA3 may also modulate promoter activity (Lan and Hinton, unpublished observations).

Basic FGF is a testicular factor that regulates GGT protein content and enzyme activity

Previous studies have shown that the collagenase gene is regulated by both PEA3 and growth factors (Gum *et al.*, 1996). In addition, the testis synthesizes and secretes growth factors (see review by Skinner, 1993). In the light of these findings, a hypothesis was formulated. It was proposed that growth factors originating in the testis would regulate expression of PEA3 mRNA which in turn would regulate expression of GGT mRNA for the maintenance of normal GGT enzyme activity. A series of experiments was performed to test this hypothesis. GGT enzyme activity and protein content were measured in the initial segment after efferent duct ligation (EDL) for 3 days. Results from these experiments showed a 30–40% decrease in activity and protein content compared with controls. Initial segment pieces from animals that had undergone an EDL were then incubated in rete testis fluid or a number of candidate molecules to determine whether GGT enzyme activity and protein content returned to control values. Results showed that a protein-like molecule of greater than 10 kDa that is not ABP in rat rete testis fluid returned GGT enzyme activity and protein content in the initial segment to control values. Neither steroids nor EGF had an effect but phorbol ester and bFGF were effective in returning GGT enzyme activity and protein content to control values. Western blot analysis showed that bFGF is present in rete testis fluid as well as in epididymal fluid (Lan *et al.*, 1998) and that bFGF receptor mRNA is present in the initial segment (Lan and Hinton, unpublished observations).

Basic FGF may regulate GGT activity by the ras-raf–MAPK pathway

It is proposed that bFGF is one of the testicular factors that regulate epididymal function. Specifically, it is suggested that bFGF regulates GGT activity via a second messenger pathway, probably via the ras-raf-MAPK pathway (A-raf mRNA is present in the initial segment; Winer and Wolgemuth, 1995), that activates PEA3 expression (O'Neill *et al.*, 1994; Wasylyk *et al.*, 1989), which in turn regulates GGT mRNA expression and enzyme activity (Fig. 3). Basic FGF may also have a direct effect on GGT protein content and enzyme activity. In view of the importance of this hormone in the development and differentiation of the epididymis, it is anticipated that bFGF regulates other genes and plays a major role in epididymal function (Alarid *et al.*, 1991).

Conclusion

In summary, the studies described in this review provide evidence that epididymal function is regulated and maintained by a lumicrine mechanism, and therefore supports hypothesis 2 as previously described. However, the data presented here do not eliminate the possibility of alternative regulatory mechanisms as described in hypotheses 1 and 3. Regulation of gene expression within the epididymis appears to be complex. Many hormones and binding proteins of testicular origin are presented to the epididymis via the vascular supply and the efferent ducts to

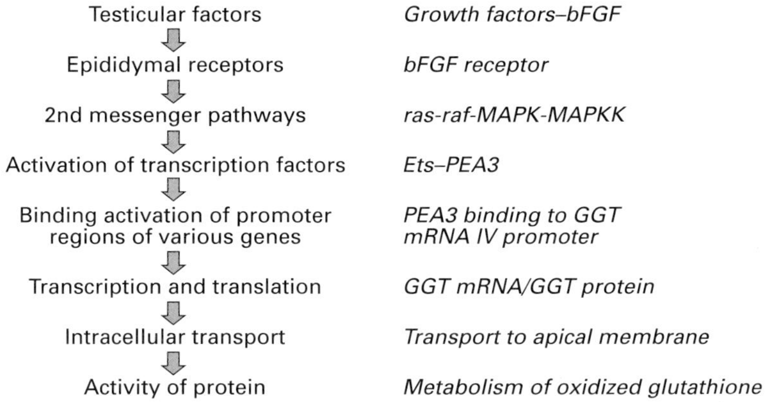

Fig. 3. Schematic representation of our working hypothesis showing how epididymal function can be maintained and regulated by a lumicrine mechanism. The left hand side outlines a general pathway by which protein activity in the epididymis is maintained by testicular factors. The right hand side shows putative candidates that may be involved in this pathway in zone 1A (Reid and Cleland, 1957) of the initial segment. It is suggested that to maintain normal epididymal function in this region of the epididymis, basic fibroblast growth factor (bFGF) is secreted by the testis into the lumen of the seminiferous tubule and then passes out of the testis through the rete testis and efferent ducts and into the lumen of the initial segment. Basic FGF then binds to its receptor located on the apical surface of the epithelial cells whereupon it activates a signal transduction pathway. It is hypothesized that the second messenger pathway involves the activation of ras, A-raf and MAPK. Transcription factors such as members of the E26 transformation specific transcription (Ets) family, polyomavirus enhancer activator (PEA3), are then activated, bind to the promoter region of GGT mRNA IV and modulate promoter activity. GGT mRNA IV is transcribed, the protein translated and transported to the apical cell surface. The protein is oriented in the apical surface membrane such that the catalytic site faces into the lumen. Under these conditions, enzyme activity is normal.

ensure normal epididymal function. Some of these hormones and binding proteins may activate gene expression through second messenger pathways and involve unique transcriptional factors. It is important to dissect the pathways involved in gene regulation in the proximal epididymis in view of the importance of this region in sperm maturation.

Studies presented in this paper were supported by NIH grants HD 32979 (BTH), training grant T-30-DKO7642 (DBR) and P-30 HD28934 Center for Cellular and Molecular Studies in Reproduction, from The Rockefeller Foundation and the Ernst Schering Research Foundation. The authors would like to thank Dr. Charles Flickinger for critical reading of the manuscript.

References

Abe K, Takano H and Ito T (1984) Interruption of the luminal flow in the epididymal duct of the corpus epididymidis in the mouse, with special reference to differentiation of the epididymal epithelium *Archives Histologica Japonica* **47** 137–147

Alarid ET, Cunha GR, Young P and Nicoll CS (1991) Evidence for an organ- and sex-specific role of basic fibroblast growth factor in the development of the fetal mammalian reproductive tract *Endocrinology* **129** 2148–2154

Brooks DE (1979) Influence of testicular secretions on tissue weight and on metabolic and enzyme activities in the epididymis of the rat *Journal of Endocrinology* **82** 305–313

Brooks DE (1983) Effect of androgens on protein synthesis and secretion in various regions of the rat epididymis, as analysed by two-dimensional gel electrophoresis *Molecular Cellular Endocrinology* **29** 255–270

Brooks DE (1987) Developmental expression and androgenic regulation of the mRNA for major secretory proteins of the rat *Molecular Cellular Endocrinology* **53** 59–66

Brown KD, Henville A and Setchell BP (1981) Rete testis fluid contains a growth factor for cultured fibroblasts *Journal of Physiology* **310** 79P

Brown PDC and Waites GMH (1972) Regional blood flow in the epididymis of the rat and rabbit: effect of efferent duct ligation and orchidectomy *Journal of Reproduction and Fertility* **28** 221–233

Buch JP, Lamb DL, Lipschultz LI and Smith RG (1988) Partial characterization of a unique growth factor secreted by human Sertoli cells *Fertility and Sterility* **49** 658–665

Cameo MS and Blaquier JA (1976) Androgen specific proteins in rat epididymis *Journal of Endocrinology* **69** 47–55

Clulow J, Jones RC and Hansen LA (1994) Micropuncture and cannulation studies of fluid composition and transport in the ductuli efferentes testis of the rat: comparisons with the homologous metanephric proximal tubule *Experimental Physiology* **79** 915–928

Clulow J, Hansen LA and Jones RC (1996) *In vivo* microperfusion of the ductuli efferentes testis of the rat: flow dependence of fluid reabsorption *Experimental Physiology* **81** 633–644

Cornwall GA and Hsia N (1997) ADAM 7, a member of the ADAM (A Disintegrin and Metalloprotease) gene family is specifically expressed in the mouse anterior pituitary and epididymis *Endocrinology* **138** 4262–4270

Cornwall GA, Orgebin-Crist M-C and Hann SR (1992) The CRES gene: a unique testis regulated gene related to the cystatin family is highly restricted in its expression to the proximal region of the mouse epididymis *Molecular Endocrinology* **6** 1653–1664

Cyr DG and Robaire B (1992) Regulation of sulfated glycoprotein-2 (clusterin) messenger ribonucleic acid in the rat epididymis *Endocrinology* **130** 2160–2166

Danzo BJ, Eller BC and Orgebin-Crist M-C (1974) Studies on the site of origin of the androgen binding protein present in epididymal cytosol from mature intact rabbits *Steroids* **24** 107–122

Danzo BJ , Cooper TG and Orgebin-Crist M-C (1977) Androgen binding protein (ABP) in fluids collected from the rete testis and cauda epididymidis of sexually mature and immature rabbits and observations on morphological changes in the epididymis following ligation of the ductuli efferentes *Biology of Reproduction* **17** 64–77

Fawcett DW and Hoffer AP (1979) Failure of exogenous androgen to prevent regression of the initial segments of the rat epididymis after efferent duct ligation or orchiectomy *Biology of Reproduction* **20** 162–181

Feig LA, Bellve AR, Erickson NH and Klagsbrun M (1980) Sertoli cells contain a mitogenic polypeptide *Proceedings of the National Academy of Sciences USA* **77** 4774–4778

French FS and Ritzen EM (1973a) Androgen binding protein in efferent duct fluid of rat testis *Journal of Reproduction and Fertility* **32** 479–483

French FS and Ritzen EM (1973b) A high affinity androgen binding protein (ABP) in rat testis: evidence for secretion into efferent duct fluid and absorption by epididymis *Endocrinology* **93** 88–95

Garrett JE, Garrett SH and Douglass J (1990) A spermatozoa-associated factor regulates proenkephalin gene expression in the rat epididymis *Molecular Endocrinology* **4** 108–118

Gum R, Lengyel E, Juarez J, Chen JH, Sato H, Seiki M and Boyd D (1996) Stimulation of 92 kDa gelatinase B promoter activity by ras is mitogen-activated protein kinase I and requires multiple transcription factor binding sites including closely spaced PEA / ets and AP-1 sequences *Journal of Biological Chemistry* **271** 10672–10680

Gutman A and Wasylyk B (1990) The collagenase gene promoter contains a TPA and oncogene-responsive unit encompassing the PEA3 and AP-1 binding sites *European Molecular Biology Organisation Journal* **9** 2241–2246

Hamilton DW (1980) UDP-galatactose: *N*-acetylglucosamine galactosyltransferase in fluids from the rat rete testis and epididymis *Biology of Reproduction* **23** 377–385

Hinton BT and Setchell BP (1995) Fluid secretion and movement. In *The Sertoli Cell* pp 249–267 Ed. LD Russell and MD Griswold. Cache River Press, Florida

Hinton BT, Palladino MA, Mattmueller DR, Bard D and Good K (1991) Expression and activity of gamma-glutamyl transpeptidase in the rat epididymis *Molecular Reproduction and Development* **28** 40–46

Hinton BT, Palladino MA, Rudolph DB, Lan ZJ and Labus JC (1996) The role of the epididymis in the protection of spermatozoa. In *Current Topics in Developmental Biology* Vol. 33 pp 61–102 Ed. RA Pederson and GP Schatten. Academic Press, New York

Holland MK and Orgebin-Crist M-C (1988) Characterization and hormonal regulation of protein synthesis by the murine epididymis *Biology of Reproduction* **38** 487–496

Holland MK, Vreeburg JTM and Orgebin-Crist M-C (1992) Testicular regulation of epididymal protein secretion *Journal of Andrology* **13** 266–273

Jones R, Brown CR, von Glos KI and Parker MG (1980) Hormonal regulation of protein synthesis in the rat epididymis: characterization of androgen-dependent and testicular fluid dependent proteins *Biochemical Journal* **188** 667–676

Koskimies AI and Kormano M (1973) Proteins in fluids from the seminiferous tubules and rete testis in the rat *Journal of Reproduction and Fertility* **34** 433–444

Lan Z-J, Palladino MA, Rudolph DB, Labus JC and Hinton BT (1997) Identification, expression and regulation of the transcription factor polyomavirus enhancer activator 3, and its putative role in regulating the expression of gamma-glutamyl transpeptidase mRNA-IV in the rat epididymis *Biology of Reproduction* **57** 186–193

Lan Z-J, Labus JC and Hinton BT (1998) Regulation of gamma-glutamyl transpeptidase catalytic activity and protein level in the initial segment of the rat epididymis by testicular factors: role of basic fibroblast growth factor *Biology of Reproduction* **58** 197–206

Martin ME, Piette J, Yaniv M, Tang WJ and Folk WR (1988) Activation of the polyomavirus enhancer by a murine activator protein 1 (AP1) homolog and two contiguous proteins *Proceedings of the National Academy of Sciences USA* **85** 5839–5844

Nicander L, Osman DI, Ploen L, Bugge HP and Kvisgaard KN (1983) Early effects of efferent ductule ligation on the proximal segment of the rat epididymis *International Journal of Andrology* **6** 91–102

Nielsen DA and Shapiro DJ (1990) Insights into hormonal control of messenger RNA stability *Molecular Endocrinology* **4** 953–957

Palladino MA and Hinton BT (1994) Expression of multiple gamma-glutamyl transpeptidase messenger ribonucleic acid transcripts in the adult rat epididymis is differentially regulated by androgens and testicular factors in a region-specific manner *Endocrinology* **135** 1146–1156

Palladino MA, Laperche Y and Hinton BT (1994) Multiple forms of gamma-glutamyl transpeptidase messenger ribonucleic acid are expressed in the adult rat testis and epididymis *Biology of Reproduction* **50** 320–328

Petersohn D, Schoh S, Brinkmann DR and Thiel G (1995) The human synapsin II gene 8 promoter – possible role for the transcription factors Zif 268/EGR-1, polyomavirus enhancer activator 3, and AP2 *Journal of Biological Chemistry* **269** 17152–17159

Reid BL and Cleland KW (1957) The structure and function of the epididymis: histology of the rat epididymis *Australian Journal of Zoology* **5** 223–246

Ricker DD, Chamness SL, Hinton BT and Chang TSK (1996) Changes in luminal fluid protein composition in the rat cauda epididymidis following partial sympathetic denervation *Journal of Andrology* **17** 117–126

Rigaudiere N, Ghyselinck NB, Faure J and Dufaure JP (1992) Regulation of the epididymal glutathione peroxidase-like protein in the mouse: dependence upon androgens and testicular factors *Molecular Cellular Endocrinology* **89** 67–77

Ritzen EM and French FS (1974) Demonstration of an androgen binding protein (ABP) in rabbit testis: secretion in efferent duct fluid and passage into the epididymis *Journal of Steroid Biochemistry* **5** 151–154

Robaire B (1979) Effects of unilateral orchidectomy on rat epididymal Δ^4-5α-reductase and 3α hydroxysteroid dehydrogenase *Canadian Journal of Physiology and Pharmacology* **57** 998–1003

Robaire B and Viger RS (1995) Regulation of epididymal epithelial cell functions *Biology of Reproduction* **52** 226–236

Robaire B, Ewing LL, Zirkin BR and Irby DC (1977) Steroid Δ^4-5α-reductase and 3α-hydroxysteroid dehydrogenase in the rat epididymis *Endocrinology* **101** 1379–1390

Rudolph DB and Hinton BT (1997) Stability and transcriptional regulation of gamma-glutamyl transpeptidase mRNA expression in the initial segment of the rat epididymis *Journal of Andrology* **18** 501–512

Setchell BP (1978) *The Mammalian Testis* Paul Elek, London

Setchell BP and Brooks DE (1988) Anatomy, vasculature, innervation, and fluids of the male reproductive tract. In *The Physiology of Reproduction* pp 753–836 Ed. E Knobil and JD Neill Raven Press, New York

Skinner JD and Rowson LEA (1967) Effect of unilateral cryptorchidism on sexual development in the pubescent male animal *Journal of Reproduction and Fertility* **14** 349–350

Skinner JD and Rowson LEA (1968) Some effects of unilateral cryptorchidism and vasectomy on sexual development of the pubescent ram and bull *Journal of Reproduction and Fertility* **42** 311–321

Skinner MK (1995) Secretion of growth factors and other regulatory factors. In *The Sertoli Cell* pp 237–247 Ed. LD Russell and MD Griswold. Cache River Press, Florida

Sonnenberg-Riethmacher E, Walter B, Riethmacher D, Godecke S and Birchmeier C (1996) The c-ros tyrosine receptor controls regionalization and differentiation of epithelial cells in the epididymis *Genes and Development* **10** 1184–1193

Sujarit S, Jones RC, Setchell BP, Chaturapnich G, Lin M and Clulow J (1990) Stimulation of protein secretion in the initial segment of the rat epididymis by fluid from the ram rete testis *Journal of Reproduction and Fertility* **88** 315–321

Suominen J and Setchell BP (1972) Enzymes and trypsin inhibitor in the rete testis fluid of rams and boars *Journal of Reproduction and Fertility* **30** 235–245

Turner TT, Jones CE, Howards SS, Ewing LL, Zegeye B and Gunsalus GL (1984) On the androgen microenvironment of maturing spermatozoa *Endocrinology* **115** 1925–1932

Turner TT, Miller DW and Avery EA (1995) Protein synthesis and secretion by the rat caput epididymidis *in vivo*: influence of the luminal microenvironment *Biology of Reproduction* **52** 1012–1019

Vernet P, Faure J, Dufaure J-P and Drevet JR (1997) Tissue and developmental distribution, dependence upon testicular factors and attachment to spermatozoa of GPX, a murine epididymis-specific glutathione peroxidase *Molecular Reproduction and Development* **47** 87–98

Viger RS and Robaire B (1994) Immunocytochemical localization of 4-ene steroid 5α-reductase type 1 along the rat epididymis during postnatal development *Endocrinology* **134** 2298–2306

Winer MA and Wolgemuth DJ (1995) The segment-specific pattern of A-raf expression in the mouse epididymis is regulated by testicular factors *Endocrinology* **136** 2561–2572

Xin JH, Cowie A, Lachance P and Hassell JA (1992) Molecular cloning and characterization of PEA3, a new member of the Ets oncogene family that is differentially expressed in mouse embryonic cells *Genes and Development* **6** 481–496

Zwain IH, Grima J and Cheng CY (1992) Rat epididymal retinoic acid-binding protein: development of a radio-immunoassay, its tissue distribution, and its changes in selected androgen-dependent organs after orchiectomy *Endocrinology* **131** 1511–1526

Journal of Reproduction and Fertility Supplement **53**, 59–65

Structure and putative function of a murine epididymal retinoic acid-binding protein (mE-RABP)

J-J. Lareyre[1], M-G. Mattéi[2], S. Kasper[3,5,6], M. E. Newcomer[4,6], D. E. Ong[4,6], R. J. Matusik[3,5,6], and M-C. Orgebin-Crist[1,3,6*]

Departments of [1]Obstetrics and Gynecology, [3]Cell Biology, [4]Biochemistry, [5]Urologic Surgery, and [6]Center for Reproductive Biology Research, Vanderbilt University, School of Medicine, Medical Center North, Room D2303, Nashville, TN, 37232-2633, USA; and [2]INSERM U406, Faculté de médecine de la Timone, Boulevard Jean Moulin, 13385, Marseille Cedex 5, France

Vitamin A is required to maintain the epididymal epithelium. In this report, the characterization and putative functions of a murine epididymal retinoic acid-binding protein (mE-RABP) that is secreted into the lumen from the mid-/distal caput epididymidis are discussed. The amino acid sequence analysis of the mE-RABP preprotein shows that mE-RABP is the mouse orthologue of the rat epididymal secretory protein I (ESPI). These proteins belong to the lipocalin superfamily and bind to active retinoids but not to retinol. Therefore, we propose that mE-RABP may function as an extracellular retinoid carrier-protein involved in the paracrine regulation of epididymal function by retinoids.

Introduction

Epididymal function is primarily under androgen control (Orgebin-Crist, 1996, for review), but unidentified testicular factors (Douglass *et al.*, 1991), oestrogen (Toney and Danzo, 1988; Hess *et al.*, 1997), growth factors (Lan *et al.*, 1998) and retinoic acid (Astraudo *et al.*, 1995) have also been implicated. Vitamin A is essential for the development and maintenance of many epithelial tissues including the epididymis (Mason, 1939). Retinoids exert their action by binding to nuclear receptors that function as ligand-activated transcription factors. Overexpression of a dominant negative retinoic acid receptor α (RARα) receptor in transgenic mice promotes the loss of organization of the columnar epithelium lining the cauda epididymidis followed by its transformation into a squamous-like epithelium which results in infertility (Costa *et al.*, 1997). Likewise, the double RARα and retinoid X receptor (RXR) knock-out mutant mice display not only aspermatogenesis but also vacuolization of the epididymal epithelium (Mendelsohn *et al.*, 1994). These studies emphasize the important role of retinoids in maintaining the epididymal epithelium.

In this report, we describe the characterization of a mouse epididymal retinoic acid-binding protein (mE-RABP) that may be involved in the retinoid signalling pathway.

Characterization of the mE-RABP Protein

A mouse epididymal secretory protein of 18.5 kDa has been described (MEP10: Rankin *et al.*, 1992b) and this has subsequently been renamed mE-RABP. This protein is synthesized by the principal cells of the mid- and distal caput epididymidis, and is secreted into the lumen. The mE-RABP protein is

* Correspondence: Center for Reproductive Biology Research, Vanderbilt University, School of Medicine, Medical Center North, Room D2303, Nashville, TN, 37232–2633, USA

```
mE-RABP                             MESIMLFTLLGLCVGLAAGTEAAVVKDFDVNKFLGFWYEIALAS
Proteins B/C                        MENIMPFALLGLCVGLAAGTEGAVVKDFDISKFLGFWYEIAFAS
LESPIV                             MIAVLLLVFGMTPDYIFPVSADIPVVPNFDAQKTVGKWHPIGMAS

mE-RABP      KMGAYGLAHKEEK-MGAMVVELKENLLALTTTYYNEGHCVLEKVAATQVD--GSAKYKVTRI
Proteins B/C KMGTPGLAHKEEK-MGAMVVELKENLLALTTTYYSEDHCVLEKVTATEGD--GPAKFQVTRL
LESPIV       KLPEVPEYEQKISPMDHMV-ELTDGDMKLTANY-MDGVCKEATAMLKHTDKPGVFKFT----

mE-RABP      SGEKEVVVVATDYMTYTVIDITSLVAGAVHRAMKLYSRSLDNNGEALNN-FQKIALKHGFSE
Proteins B/C SGKKEVVVEATDYLTYAIIDITSLVAGAVHRTMKLYSRSLDDNGEALYN-FRKITSDHGFSE
LESPIV       -G-GEIRMMDIDYEKYLIMYMKKSTFE----AMYLSARGSD-VGDDIKEKFKKLVLEQNFPE

mE-RABP      TDIHILKHDLTCVNALQSGQI
Proteins B/C TDLYILKHDLTCVKVLQSAAESRP
LESPIV       AHIKYFNAEQ-CTPTAA
```

Fig. 1. The primary amino acid sequences of murine epididymal retinoic acid-binding protein (mE-RABP), rat proteins B/C (Brooks *et al.*, 1986), and lizard epididymal secretory protein IV (Morel *et al.*, 1991) are aligned (Matrix: BLOSUM62). The conserved amino acids between mE-RABP and the other lipocalin proteins are shaded. Signal peptide cleavages are indicated by broken arrows. N-terminal microsequences of purified proteins are shown in bold letters. Boxed regions indicate the conserved motifs G-X-W and T-D-Y and the two cysteine residues that are believed to be important for the three-dimensional structure.

partially reabsorbed by clear cells located in the distal corpus and proximal cauda epididymidis (Vierula *et al.*, 1995); it does not bind tightly to spermatozoa since it can be easily dissociated under low-salt conditions (Rankin *et al.*, 1992a). N-terminal amino acid sequence analysis determined a high homology (86%) with two rat epididymal secretory proteins B/C (Brooks *et al.*, 1986) resulting from an alternative cleavage of a single precursor. These proteins B/C, also known as ESPI (Girotti *et al.*, 1992), were later identified as epididymal retinoic acid-binding proteins EBP1/EBP2 (Ong and Chytil, 1988) (Fig. 1). Like EBP1/EBP2, mE-RABP binds active retinoids (9-*cis* and all *trans* retinoic acid), but not retinol (Rankin *et al.*, 1992b).

EBP1 has been crystallized (Newcomer and Ong, 1990) and its X-ray structure determined (Newcomer, 1993). The rat EBP1 is a globular protein of the approximate dimension 40Å × 50Å × 35Å. The center of the protein contains a deep binding pocket 15Å across at the entrance and 20Å deep. The basic structural framework of the molecule is an eight stranded up-and-down β sheet which twists into a barrel. One end of the barrel is closed by a single turn of an α helix. The front end of the barrel is open and provides entrance to the binding site. The topology of E-RABP is similar to that of members belonging to the lipocalin superfamily (human plasma retinol binding protein (Newcomer *et al.*, 1984), human β-lactoglobulin (Papiz *et al.*, 1986), insecticyanin (Holden *et al.*, 1987), bilin-binding protein (Huber *et al.*, 1987), mouse major urinary protein and rat $\alpha_2\mu$-globulin (Bocskei *et al.*, 1992), and bovine odorant-binding protein (Bianchet *et al.*, 1996; Tegoni *et al.*, 1996)). The predicted amino acid sequence of rat E-RABP further implies that E-RABP belongs to the lipocalin superfamily (Brooks, 1987a).

Degenerate oligonucleotides corresponding to the N-terminal amino acid sequence of the major and minor forms of mE-RABP were used to obtain the cDNA encoding mE-RABP (Lareyre *et al.*, 1998a). The predicted amino acid sequence showed a 75% identity (90% homology) with rat proteins B/C (Brooks *et al.*, 1986). The tertiary structure of mE-RABP was modelled using the amino acid sequence (Brooks *et al.*, 1986) and structure (Newcomer, 1993) of the rat protein (Lareyre *et al.*, 1998a). Although sequence differences occur between the rat and the mouse protein in surface amino acids, only three changes were found in the binding pocket. These changes do not affect the space required to bind retinoic acid. The predicted amino acid sequence homology, the ligand-binding specificity, and three-dimensional structure confirm that mE-RABP is the mouse orthologue of the rat epididymal secretory protein and is a member of the lipocalin superfamily.

Another androgen-dependent lipocalin related to mE-RABP (26.5% identity, 48% homology) was

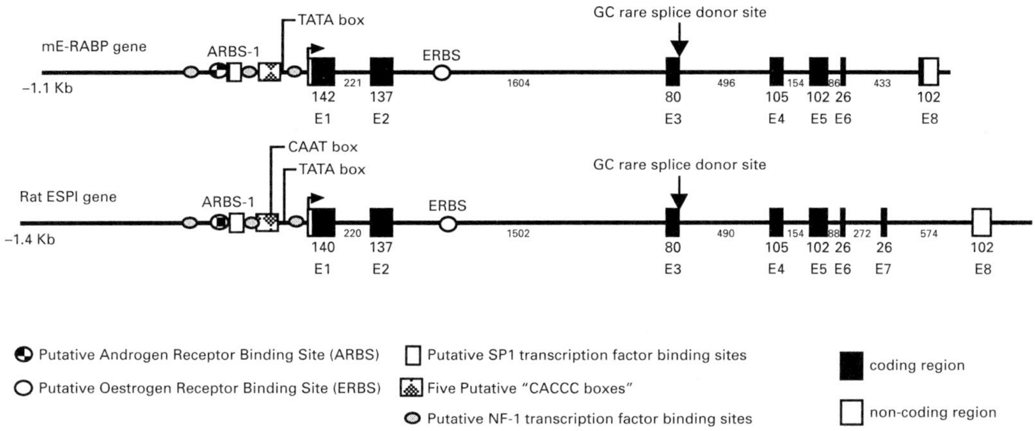

Fig. 2. The genomic organization of the murine epididymal retinoic acid-binding protein (mE-RABP) gene is compared with that of the rat ESPI gene (Girotti *et al.*, 1992). The exon/intron boundaries of the exons E2, E3, E4 and E6 encoding important structural domains (motifs G-X-W and T-D-Y and two cystein residues) are compared and found highly conserved. The location of conserved putative regulatory elements on mE-RABP and epididymal secretory protein I (ESPI) genes is illustrated.

described in lizard epididymal fluid (Morel *et al.*, 1991, 1993) (Fig. 1). The antibody raised against mE-RABP recognized an antigen in the human caput epididymidis (Lareyre, unpublished data). This suggests that a retinoic acid-binding protein belonging to the lipocalin superfamily has been conserved during evolution.

Genomic Organization and Chromosomal Localization of the mE-RABP Gene

The mE-RABP protein is encoded by a single copy gene (Fig. 2). Its structure is similar, but not identical, to that of the rat ESPI gene since exon 7 of the rat gene is absent (Fig. 2). In addition, no CAAT box is present in the mouse gene. However, the comparison of the nucleotide sequence between these two genes shows that all the exon/intron boundaries are conserved as well as several putative regulatory elements (Lareyre *et al.*, 1998b).

Fluorescent *in situ* hybridization studies map the mE-RABP gene to the proximal region [A3-B] of mouse chromosome 2 (Lareyre *et al.*, 1998b). This region is analogous to those on human chromosome 10 [10p] and 9 [9q] (Fig. 3). Other genes encoding related lipocalins, such as prostaglandin D synthase or C8 gamma subunit, are also localized within the same proximal region of murine chromosome 2 (Fig. 3). Since these genes have a genomic organization similar to the mE-RABP gene, we believe that these genes are evolutionarily related and may have evolved from a duplication of a single ancestral gene within the [A3-B] region of the murine chromosome 2.

A mutation resulting in a urogenital syndrome was also reported in the region [A3-B] of the mouse chromosome 2 (Lane and Birkenmeier, 1993). A similar human syndrome named Nail-patella-syndrome has also been mapped to human chromosome 9 (Nadeau *et al.*, 1992).

Further studies will be required to determine whether mE-RABP is involved in the differentiation process of the mouse epididymis.

Region-specific Expression and Hormonal Regulation of the mE-RABP Gene

Although the epididymis consists of a single convoluted duct composed of one major cell type, it displays a high degree of region-specific expression of a large number of genes (Orgebin-Crist 1996, for review). *In situ* hybridization experiments determined that mE-RABP mRNA expression was restricted to the caput epididymidis (Lareyre *et al.*, 1998b). Although mE-RABP and rat proteins B/C

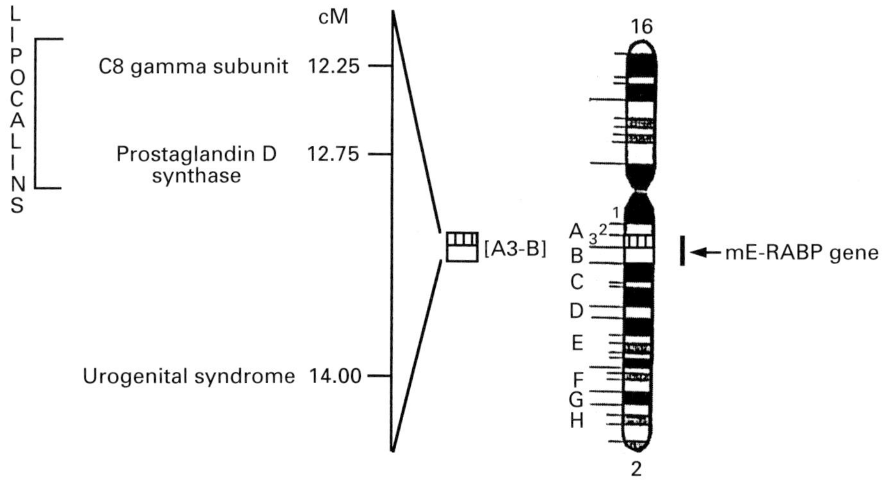

Fig. 3. The chromosomal location of the murine epididymal retinoic acid-binding protein (mE-RABP) gene in the region [A3-B] of the mouse chromosome 2 is shown on the idiogram of the G-banded (2;16) Robertsonian translocation. The physical map indicates that other genes encoding lipocalins such as the C8 gamma subunit and the prostaglandin D synthase genes are located in this region. The urogenital syndrome is also mapped in this area (Lane and Birkenmeier, 1993).

are homologous, the mRNA expression patterns are different. In the rat, proteins B/C mRNA is expressed uniformly in the efferent ducts and all the caput epididymidis including the initial segment (Garrett *et al.*, 1991). In the mouse, mE-RABP mRNA is expressed in a gradient pattern from the mid- to the distal caput epididymidis, but is undetectable in the efferent ducts and in the initial segment (Lareyre *et al.*, 1998a). Although it is difficult to compare the segments of the caput epididymidis from different species, it appears that the regulation of region-specific expression of E-RABP may be different in the mouse and rat epididymis.

To identify *cis*-DNA regulatory element(s) involved in the tissue-specific expression of the mE-RABP gene, we have studied the expression of a transgene containing 5 kb of the 5′ flanking region driving the CAT reporter gene (Lareyre *et al.*, 1997). Transgene expression is restricted to the caput epididymidis, demonstrating that important *cis*-DNA regulatory element(s) required for epididymis- and region-specific gene expression are located within the 5 kb upstream from the mE-RABP gene promoter.

Androgens are required for epididymal sperm maturation (Dyson and Orgebin-Crist, 1973; Orgebin-Crist and Tichenor, 1973). Previous studies have shown that castration of adult mice results in the loss of the mE-RABP expression (Holland and Orgebin-Crist, 1988). Northern blot analyses showed that castration, but not efferent duct ligation, led to a rapid decrease in mE-RABP mRNA expression (0.7% of control, 10 days after castration). Moreover, testosterone propionate or dihydrotestosterone injections to castrated mice restored mE-RABP mRNA expression. The restoration of the overall region-specific pattern of expression was similar to that seen in the intact mice. Therefore, these results suggest that the regulation of mE-RABP gene expression is primarily dependent on circulating androgens.

Androgens bind to a nuclear receptor that belongs to the ligand-activated transcription factor superfamily (Lubahn *et al.*, 1988). The binding of the androgen receptor to *cis*-acting DNA regulatory elements named androgen response elements (AREs) results in the modulation of the target gene transcription (Beato, 1989). Preliminary studies have shown the presence of a functional androgen response region (ARR) within the mE-RABP gene promoter (Lareyre *et al.*, 1997). AREs identified to date bind to other steroid receptors *in vitro* (glucocorticoids, mineralocorticoids, progesterone receptors) when they are maintained in the context of the promoter region. The mE-RABP gene ARR is inducible only by androgens, but not by glucocorticoids (Lareyre *et al.*, 1997). Therefore, the mE-RABP gene ARR is a unique model to study, *in vitro*, molecular mechanisms that lead to a specific hormonal response. Thus, mE-RABP gene expression may be directly regulated by androgens at the transcriptional level *in vivo*. However, it cannot be excluded that androgens may also regulate the turnover of mE-RABP mRNA.

The expression of mE-RABP mRNA progressively reappeared between 15 and 60 days after castration without reaching the control level (20% of control) (Lareyre *et al.*, 1998b). In the prostate gland, an androgen-dependent mRNA encoding another lipocalin protein named probasin was observed to rebound to precastration values 12 days after castration (Sweetland *et al.*, 1988). However, to our knowledge, the rebound of an androgen-regulated gene has not been reported before in the epididymis. Moreover, expression of the gene encoding rat proteins B/C does not rebound after long-term castration (Brooks, 1987b) suggesting that the rebound of mE-RABP mRNA is unique to the mouse. It is unlikely that adrenal androgens are involved since the concentration of epididymal androgens remains low during long-term castration in the mouse (Rigaudiere *et al.*, 1992). This atypical behaviour suggests that other transcription factor(s) (repressor or activator) may cooperate with the androgen receptor to control mE-RABP gene expression at a transcriptional or post-transcriptional level.

Putative Function of the Epididymal Retinoic Acid-Binding Protein (E-RABP)

The lipocalins have been classified as extracellular transport proteins involved in the delivery of small lipophilic molecules (Flower, 1996). Since the amino acid sequence analysis and ability to bind retinoic acid place mE-RABP in the lipocalin superfamily, the most plausible function for mE-RABP is as a transport protein for retinoic acid within the epididymis.

Several hypothetical scenarios can be envisaged for the function of mE-RABP. In the first scenario, retinol is delivered to the caput epididymal cells bound to retinol binding protein (RBP). Within the cytoplasm, retinol is bound to cellular retinol binding protein type I (CRBPI) and converted to retinoic acid which is subsequently bound by E-RABP. The retinoic acid/E–RABP complex may then be secreted into the lumen from the caput and delivered to spermatozoa or to epididymal cells downstream from the caput. However, delivery to the spermatozoa appears unlikely since no significant increase in sperm retinoic acid content occurs between spermatozoa from the caput and cauda epididymidis (Pappas *et al.*, 1993). The latter possibility may be more plausible, since the integrity of the cauda epithelium is dependent on retinoids (Costa *et al.*, 1997) , but expression of CRBPI is low in the cauda epididymidis (Porter *et al.*, 1985). The luminal mE-RABP may deliver retinoids to the epithelial cells of the cauda epididymidis.

Another scenario is that mE-RABP is secreted into the lumen of the caput and captures retinoids released from spermatozoa. This may regulate the retinoids in spermatozoa before they reach the oocyte. In *Xenopus laevis* eggs, an early and temporary expression of RAR and RXR mRNAs is observed upon fertilization (Blumberg *et al.*, 1992). It is not known whether this occurs in rodents but it implies that retinoids may regulate early stages of development immediately after fertilization.

In addition, mE-RABP may also deliver sperm-derived retinoic acid to epithelial cells to relay to the cells a sperm-derived signal (retinoic acid) that would affect gene transcription. Such a model has been proposed for the regulation of proenkephalin gene expression in the rat caput epididymidis by an unidentified sperm-associated factor (Garrett *et al.*, 1990).

In conclusion, E-RABP may play a key role in the sperm maturation process or in the paracrine regulation of epididymal function by retinoids.

This work was supported by NIH grants HD03820, HD05797 and HD25206 and by 'La Ligue contre le Cancer'.

References

Astraudo C, Lefevre A, Boue F, Durr F and Finaz C (1995) *In vivo* regulation of rat epididymal proteins by retinoids: analysis by two-dimensional electrophoresis *Archives of Andrology* **35** 247–259

Beato M (1989) Gene regulation by steroid hormones *Cell* **56** 335–344

Bianchet MA, Bains G, Pelosi P, Pevsner J, Snyder SH, Monaco HL and Amzel LM (1996) The three-dimensional structure of bovine odorant binding protein and its mechanism of odor recognition *Nature Structural Biology* **3** 934–939

Blumberg B, Mangelsdorf DJ, Dyck JA, Bittner DA, Evans RM and De Robertis EM (1992) Multiple retinoid-responsive receptors in a single cell: families of retinoid "X" receptors and retinoic acid receptors in the *Xenopus* egg *Proceedings of the National Academy of Sciences USA* **89** 2321–2325

Bocskei Z, Groom CR, Flower DR, Wright CE, Phillips SE, Cavaggioni A, Findlay JB and North AC (1992) Pheromone binding to two rodent urinary proteins revealed by X-ray crystallography *Nature* **360** 186–188

Brooks DE (1987a) The major androgen-regulated secretory proteins of the rat epididymis bear sequence homology with members of the alpha 2μ-globulin superfamily *Biochemistry International* **14** 235–240

Brooks DE (1987b) Developmental expression and androgenic regulation of the mRNA for major secretory proteins of the rat epididymis *Molecular and Cellular Endocrinology* **53** 59–66

Brooks DE, Means AR, Wright EJ, Singh SP and Tiver KK (1986) Molecular cloning of the cDNA for two major androgen-dependent secretory proteins of 18.5 kilodaltons synthesized by the rat epididymis *Journal of Biological Chemistry* **261** 4956–4961

Costa SL, Boekelheide K, Vanderhyden BC, Seth R and McBurney MW (1997) Male infertility caused by epididymal dysfunction in transgenic mice expressing a dominant negative mutation of retinoic acid receptor alpha *Biology of Reproduction* **56** 985–990

Douglass J, Garrett SH and Garrett JE (1991) Differential patterns of regulated gene expression in the adult rat epididymis *Annals of the New York Academy of Sciences* **637** 384–398

Dyson AL and Orgebin-Crist MC (1973) Effect of hypophysectomy, castration and androgen replacement upon the fertilizing ability of rat epididymal spermatozoa *Endocrinology* **93** 391–402

Flower DR (1996) The lipocalin protein family: structure and function *Biochemical Journal* **318** 1–14

Garrett SH, Garrett JE and Douglass J (1990) A spermatozoa-associated factor regulated proenkephalin gene expression in the rat epididymis *Molecular Endocrinology* **4** 108–118

Garrett SH, Garrett JE and Douglass J (1991) *In situ* histochemical analysis of region-specific gene expression in the adult rat epididymis *Molecular Reproduction and Development* **30** 1–17

Girotti M, Jones R, Emery DC, Chia W and Hall L (1992) Structure and expression of the rat epididymal secretory protein I gene. An androgen-regulated member of the lipocalin superfamily with a rare splice donor site *Biochemical Journal* **281** 203–210

Hess RA, Bunick D, Lee KH, Bahr J, Taylor JA, Korach KS and Lubahn DB (1997) A role for oestrogens in the male reproductive system *Nature* **390** 509–512

Holden HM, Rypniewski WR, Law JH and Rayment I (1987) The molecular structure of insecticyanin from the tobacco hornworm *Manduca sexta* L. at 2.6 A resolution *EMBO Journal* **6** 1565–70

Holland MK and Orgebin-Crist MC (1988) Characterization and hormonal regulation of protein synthesis by the murine epididymis *Biology of Reproduction* **38** 487–496

Huber R, Schneider M, Mayr I, Muller R, Deutzmann R, Suter F, Zuber H, Falk H and Kayser H (1987) Molecular structure of the bilin binding protein (BBP) from *Pieris brassicae* after refinement at 2. 0 A resolution *Journal of Molecular Biology* **198** 499–513

Lan ZJ, Labus JC and Hinton BT (1998) Regulation of gamma-glutamyl transpeptidase catalytic activity and protein level in the initial segment of the rat epididymis by testicular factors: role of basic fibroblast growth factor *Biology of Reproduction* **58** 197–206

Lane PW and Birkenmeier CS (1993) Urogenital syndrome (us): a developmental mutation on chromosome 2 of the mouse *Mammalian Genome* **4** 481–484

Lareyre JJ, Kasper S, Ong DE, Matusik RJ and Orgebin-Crist MC (1997) The 5′ flanking region of mE-RABP gene targets transgene expression in the epididymis *Molecular Biology of the Cell* **8** (Supplement)1888 (Abstract)

Lareyre JJ, Mattei M-G, Kasper S, Ong DE, Matusik RJ and Orgebin-Crist M-C (1998a) Genomic organization and chromosomal localization of the murine Epididymal Retinoic Acid Binding Protein (mE-RABP) gene *Molecular Reproduction and Development* **50** 387–395

Lareyre JJ, Zheng W-L, Zhao G-Q, Kasper S, Newcomer ME, Matusik RJ, Ong DE and Orgebin-Crist M-C (1998b) Molecular cloning and hormonal regulation of a murine epididymal retinoic acid-binding protein mRNA *Endocrinology* **139** 2971–2981

Lubahn DB, Joseph DR, Sar M, Tan J, Higgs HN, Larson RE, French FS and Wilson EM (1988) The human androgen receptor: complementary deoxyribonucleic acid cloning, sequence analysis and gene expression in prostate *Molecular Endocrinology* **2** 1265–1275

Mason KE (1939) Relation of the vitamins to the sex glands. *Sex and Internal Secretions* (2nd Edn) pp 153–239 Eds E Allen, CH Danforth and EA Doisy. Williams & Wilkins, Baltimore

Mendelsohn C, Lohnes D, Decimo D, Lufkin T, LeMeur M, Chambon P and Mark M (1994) Function of the retinoic acid receptors (RARs) during development (II). Multiple abnormalities at various stages of organogenesis in RAR double mutants *Development* **120** 2749–2771

Morel L, Depeiges A and Dufaure JP (1991) Molecular cloning and characterization of a cDNA encoding for the mature form of a specific androgen dependent epididymal protein *Cellular and Molecular Biology* **37** 757–764

Morel L, Dufaure JP and Depeiges A (1993) LESP, an androgen-regulated lizard epididymal secretory protein family identified as a new member of the lipocalin superfamily *Journal of Biological Chemistry* **268** 10274–10281

Nadeau JH, Davisson MT, Doolittle DP, Grant P, Hillyard AL, Kosowsky MR and Roderick TH (1992) Comparative map for mice and humans *Mammalian Genome* **3** 480–536

Newcomer ME (1993) Structure of the epididymal retinoic acid binding protein at 2. 1 A resolution *Structure* **1** 7–18

Newcomer ME and Ong DE (1990) Purification and crystallization of a retinoic acid-binding protein from rat epididymis. Identity with the major androgen-dependent epididymal proteins *Journal of Biological Chemistry* **265** 12876–12879

Newcomer ME, Jones TA, Aqvist J, Sundelin J, Eriksson U, Rask L and Peterson PA (1984) The three-dimensional structure of retinol-binding protein *EMBO Journal* **3** 1451–1454

Ong DE and Chytil F (1988) Presence of novel retinoic acid-binding proteins in the lumen of rat epididymis *Archives of Biochemistry and Biophysics* **267** 474–478

Orgebin-Crist MC (1996) Androgens and epididymal function. In *Pharmacology, Biology, and Clinical Applications of Androgens* pp 27–38 Eds D Bhasin, HL Gabelnick, Spieler JM, Swerdloff RS, Wang C. Wiley-Liss, Inc., New York

Orgebin-Crist MC and Tichenor PL (1973) Effect of testosterone on sperm maturation *in vitro*. *Nature* **245** 328–329

Papiz MZ, Sawyer L, Eliopoulos EE, North AC, Findlay JB,

Sivaprasadarao R, Jones TA, Newcomer ME and Kraulis PJ (1986) The structure of beta-lactoglobulin and its similarity to plasma retinol-binding protein *Nature* **324** 383–385

Pappas RS, Newcomer ME and Ong DE (1993) Endogenous retinoids in rat epididymal tissue and rat and human spermatozoa *Biology of Reproduction* **48** 235–247

Porter SB, Ong DE, Chytil F and Orgebin-Crist MC (1985) Localization of cellular retinol-binding protein and cellular retinoic acid-binding protein in the rat testis and epididymis *Journal of Andrology* **6** 197–212

Rankin TL, Tsuruta KJ, Holland MK, Griswold MD and Orgebin-Crist MC (1992a) Isolation, immunolocalization, and sperm-association of three proteins of 18, 25, and 29 kilodaltons secreted by the mouse epididymis *Biology of Reproduction* **46** 747–766

Rankin TL, Ong DE and Orgebin-Crist MC (1992b) The 18-kDa mouse epididymal protein (MEP 10) binds retinoic acid *Biology of Reproduction* **46** 767–771

Rigaudiere N, Ghyselinck NB, Faure J and Dufaure JP (1992) Regulation of the epididymal glutathione peroxidase-like protein in the mouse: dependence upon androgens and testicular factors *Molecular and Cellular Endocrinology* **89** 67–77

Sweetland R, Sheppard PC, Dodd JG and Matusik RJ (1988) Post-castration rebound of an androgen regulated prostatic gene *Molecular and Cellular Biochemistry* **84** 3–15

Tegoni M, Ramoni R, Bignetti E, Spinelli S and Cambillau C (1996) Domain swapping creates a third putative combining site in bovine odorant binding protein dimer *Nature Structural Biology* **3** 863–867

Toney TW and Danzo BJ (1988) Developmental changes in and hormonal regulation of estrogen and androgen receptors present in the rabbit epididymis *Biology of Reproduction* **39** 818–828

Vierula ME, Rankin TL and Orgebin-Crist MC (1995) Electron microscopic immunolocalization of the 18 and 29 kilodalton secretory proteins in the mouse epididymis: evidence for differential uptake by clear cells *Microscopy Research and Technique* **30** 24–36

Journal of Reproduction and Fertility Supplement **53**, 67–72

Expression of CRISP proteins in the male equine genital tract

A. Schambony, O. Hess, M. Gentzel and E. Töpfer-Petersen*

Tierärztliche Hochschule Hannover, Institut für Reproduktionsmedizin, Bünteweg 15, D-30559 Hannover, Germany

Cysteine rich secretory proteins (CRISPs) have been detected immunochemically in the equine male genital tract. CRISPs are secretory products of the epididymis, the ampulla and the seminal vesicle. A particular feature of the horse is the abundance of CRISPs in seminal plasma. CRISPs can also be detected in extracts of testicular, epididymal and ejaculated spermatozoa in increasing amounts. Unlike other seminal plasma proteins, they cannot be removed completely from spermatozoa by high salt treatment. The remaining CRISP antigens are localized on the midpiece, and the postacrosomal and equatorial region of the sperm head. Tissue distribution and localization of CRISPs on equine spermatozoa point to a role of these proteins in epididymal sperm maturation and equine reproduction.

Introduction

Interactions of the sperm surface with the secretory products of the epididymis appear to be essential features of the post-testicular maturation process that enables spermatozoa to fertilize the ovum. Two of the proteins associating with the sperm membrane during their passage through the epididymal tract, the rat proteins D and E, were the first described members of the emerging cysteine-rich secretory protein (CRISP) family (Cameo and Blaquier, 1976). Biochemical and functional studies on rat proteins DE indicate that these proteins play an essential role in the gamete fusion process. The appearance of DE binding sites during oogenesis has been correlated with the acquisition of fusibility of the rat oocyte (Cohen *et al.*, 1996). These DE receptors can be saturated with purified protein leading to a complete inhibition of gamete fusion. Sperm–egg fusion is prevented by preincubation of spermatozoa with antibodies directed against the proteins DE (Rochwerger *et al.*, 1992); in contrast, the binding of spermatozoa to the oocyte is not inhibited.

The structurally related members of the CRISP protein family are characterized by 16 conserved cysteine residues (Haendler *et al.*, 1993; Eberspaecher *et al.*, 1995) and occur in many species from plants to mammals.

In the horse one of the major seminal plasma proteins is a member of the CRISP family (Calvete *et al.*, 1994). The accessibility of reasonable amounts of equine CRISP-3 provides a tool for biochemical and functional studies on equine CRISP proteins and their role in the reproductive system.

Materials and Methods

All chemicals used were purchased from Applichem, Merck, or Roth if not indicated otherwise and were of analytical grade or better.

A polyclonal antiserum was raised in chicken using HPLC-purified stallion seminal plasma protein 3 (CRISP-3) (Schambony *et al.*, 1997). This antiserum was used to detect CRISP proteins on

*Correspondence

Table 1. Tissue distribution of equine cysteine-rich secretory proteins (CRISP)

Tissue type	Immunohistology	Sperm extracts
Testis	–	+
Caput epididymidis	+	–
Corpus epididymidis	+	+
Cauda epididymidis	+	+
Ampulla	+	n.d.
Seminal vesicle	+	n.d.
Prostate gland	–	n.d.
Bulbourethal gland	–	n.d.
Salivary gland	n.d.	n.d.

n.d. – not determined
Liver, spleen, and muscle were used as control tissues; CRISPs were not detected immunochemically in these tissues.

tissue sections, Western blots and in indirect immunofluorescence. All assays were carried out following standard protocols. A biotinylated goat–anti-chicken IgY (Vector) and streptavidine horseradish peroxidase conjugate (Calbiochem) were used in immunohistology and Western blots with the substrates diaminobenzidine (DAB, Sigma) and 4-chloronaphtol (Biorad), respectively. For indirect immunofluorescence a goat–anti-chicken-IgY-Cy 3 probe (Dianova) was used.

Tissue samples were obtained from a 5-year-old healthy stallion and fixed in 4% formalin immediately after dissection, dehydrated using increasing ethanol concentrations and embedded in paraffin wax. Ultrathin sections were mounted on slides, rehydrated and probed as described above.

Spermatozoa were sampled from testis and caput, corpus and cauda epididymides with slight agitation in PBS and washed twice with PBS before protein extraction. Sperm proteins were solubilized using 1% (w/v) octylglycopyranoside, 1 mmol PMSF l^{-1}, 10 mmol benzamidine l^{-1} in PBS, and separated from cellular debris by centrifugation for 10 min at 13 000 *g*. The extracted proteins were separated by SDS–PAGE (Laemmli, 1970), blotted onto a PVDF membrane and CRISPs were detected immunochemically.

Semen samples were collected from healthy stallions of Hannover breed, 6–12 years old, using an artificial vagina. Spermatozoa were washed three times with PBS and twice with phosphate-buffered 0.5 mol NaCl l^{-1}(pH 7.4) and resuspended in PBS. Smear preparations of spermatozoa were air dried, fixed in methanol and used for indirect immunofluorescence.

Results and Discussion

One of the major equine seminal plasma proteins has proved to be a member of the CRISP protein family (Calvete *et al.*, 1994; A. Schambony *et al.*, in press). The abundant secretion of CRISPs by the accesory sexual glands is a unique feature of the horse, although the physiological function of these large amounts of CRISPs in stallion seminal plasma is not clear. The tissue distribution of CRISPs in the equine male genital tract and whether CRISPs associate with stallion spermatozoa were investigated. The expression and location of equine CRISP proteins were studied by immunochemical methods.

The expression of CRISP proteins in the tissues of the stallion genital tract was studied using immunohistochemical techniques and a polyclonal antiserum. CRISP proteins were not detected in the testis, but throughout the epididymis, in the ampulla and the seminal vesicle (Table 1). The CRISP antigen is present in the secretory epithelial cells and the ciliary border coating the lumen of caput, corpus and cauda epididymides (Fig.1 a–c). The antigen is also present on spermatozoa in the lumen of the epididymis (Fig. 1b). This observation could be confirmed by Western blotting of sperm

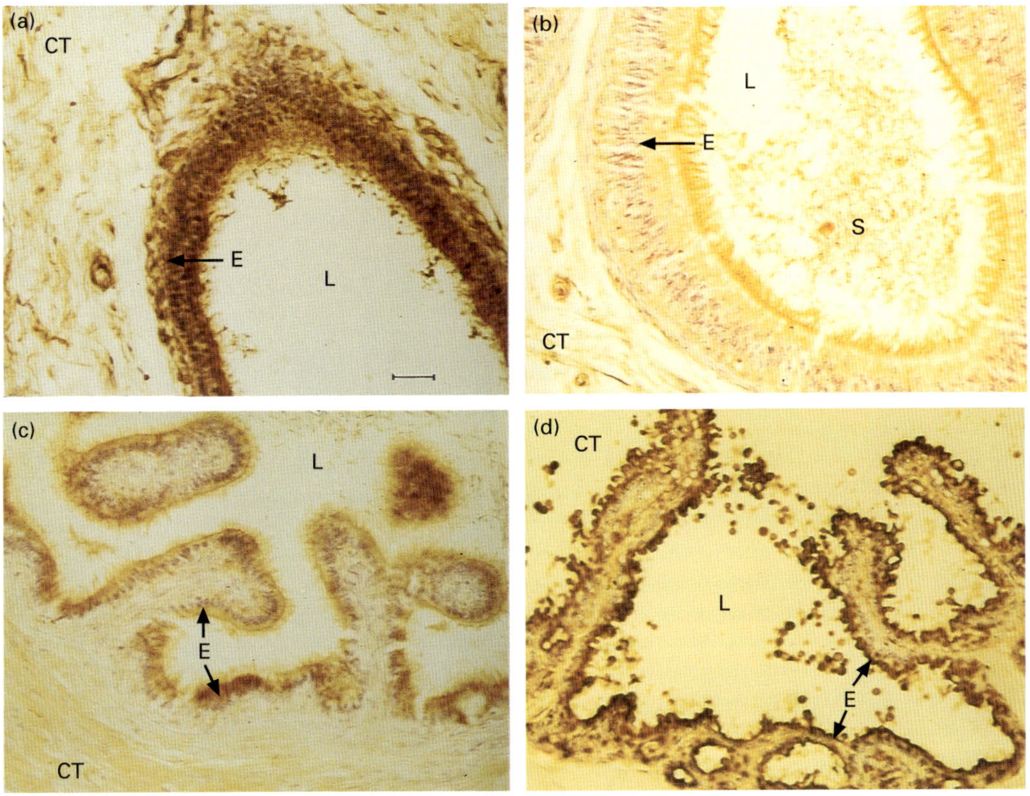

Fig. 1. Immunohistological detection of cysteine-rich secretory protein (CRISP) antigens in equine (a) caput, (b) corpus and (c) cauda epididymides and (d) ampulla. The distribution of CRISP antigens was visualized using a secondary antibody conjugated to horseradish peroxidase and diaminobenzidine (DAB) as substrate resulting in a brown precipitate. CRISPs are present throughout the epididymis (a–c) in epithelial cells (E) and in the ciliary border of the epithelium, but not in the surrounding connective tissue (CT). An association with epididymal spermatozoa (S) is observed in the lumen (L) of corpus (b) and cauda (c) epididymides. In the ampulla (d) strong staining of epithelial cells (E), intracellularly and particularly on the surfaces directed toward the lumen (L) is visible. Scale bar represents 20 μm.

extracts. CRISP antigens are present on spermatozoa isolated from corpus and cauda epididymides. In addition, a faint signal was obtained with testicular sperm extracts, although CRISP antigens were not detected in testis tissue by immunohistochemistry. This could be due to the higher sensitivity of western blotting, allowing the detection even of small amounts of CRISPs.

The expression of CRISPs in the epididymis and the association with spermatozoa is in agreement with the distribution of CRISPs reported for other species (Cameo and Blaquier, 1976; Haendler *et al.*, 1993; Eberspaecher *et al.*, 1995) and point to a role of CRISPs in equine reproduction. Nevertheless these findings do not explain the abundant presence of CRISP-3 in the stallion seminal plasma.

Immunohistology yielded strong staining of CRISP antigens in tissue sections of the ampulla, showing their presence in and on the surface of the epithelial cells (Fig. 1d). Sections of the seminal vesicle showed weak expression of CRISPs, while no CRISP antigens were observed in sections of prostate and bulbourethral glands (Table 1). These results suggest that the ampulla could be the source of the dominant seminal plasma CRISP-3. These findings were confirmed by amplification of CRISP messenger RNA in reverse transcription (RT)–PCR (A. Schambony *et al.*, in press).

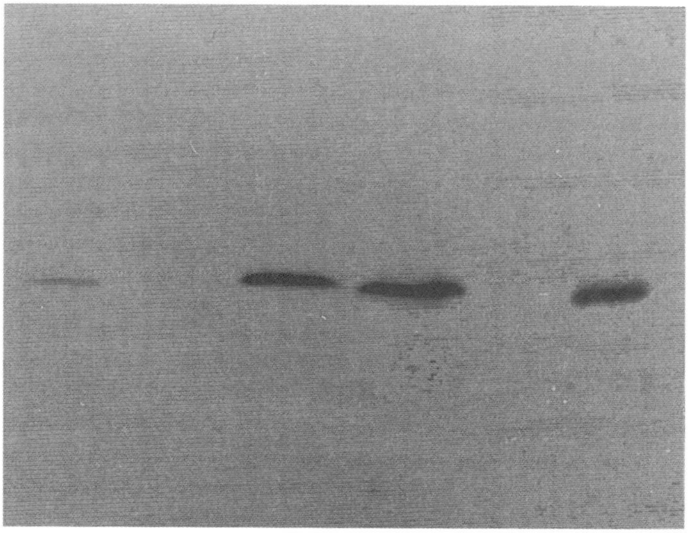

Fig. 2. Western blot of sperm extracts isolated from stallion testis (1), caput (2), corpus (3) and cauda (4) epididymides. Purified cysteine-rich secretory protein 3 (CRISP-3) (5) was used as a positive control. Sperm proteins were extracted using octylglycopyranoside, separated in SDS–PAGE, immobilized on PVDF membrane and probed with polyclonal anti-CRISP 3 antiserum. Small amounts of CRISP antigens can be detected in extracts of testicular spermatozoa (1). No signal was obtained in extracts of caput epididymal spermatozoa (2), while a strong staining of a 25 kDa band is observed in sperm extracts from corpus (3) and cauda (4) epididymides.

As CRISPs seem to associate with spermatozoa during their passage through the epididymis, we were interested in the location of CRISPs on stallion spermatozoa and the quality of the association. Ejaculates were washed three times with PBS and twice with high salt buffer (0.5 mol NaCl l^{-1}) to remove loosely bound proteins before staining. By indirect immunofluorescence microscopy CRISP antigen is visible on the postacrosomal and equatorial region of the sperm head and on the midpiece of salt-washed spermatozoa (Fig. 3), indicating that CRISPs associate tightly with the sperm membrane. Furthermore CRISPs are present in those regions of the sperm head involved in sperm–egg binding and fusion, pointing to a possible role of CRISPs in gamete interaction as reported for rat CRISPs, proteins D and E (Rochwerger *et al.*, 1992; Cohen *et al.*, 1996). Preliminary results indicate that the amount of CRISP antigen still present on spermatozoa after several washings with phosphate buffered 0.5 mol NaCl l^{-1} solution is directly correlated with the fertility of the stallion (Schambony *et al.* 1997) giving further evidence for an important role of CRISPs in equine reproduction.

Conclusion

We were able to demonstrate transcription and expression of CRISP proteins in the stallion genital tract and association to spermatozoa. CRISP antigens are located at those regions of the sperm head that participate in gamete interaction, the postacrosomal and equatorial segment. The CRISP proteins tightly bound to spermatozoa cannot be removed by harsh washing conditions and,

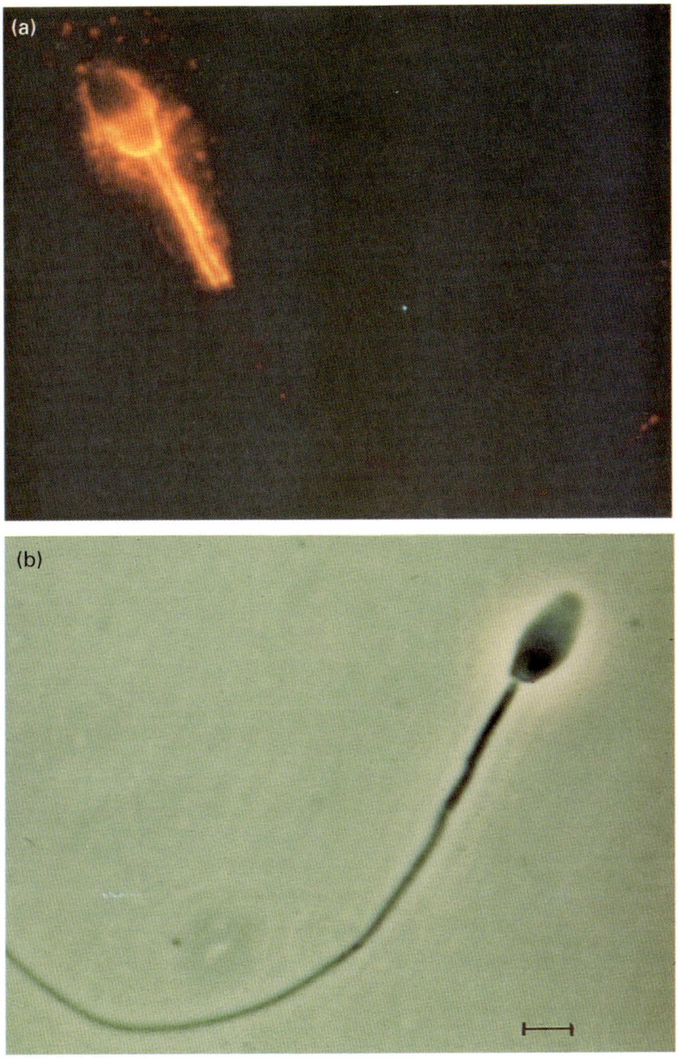

Fig. 3. Localization of cysteine-rich secretory protein (CRISP) antigens on washed stallion spermatozoa: (a) indirect immunofluorescence; (b) bright field. CRISP antigens are localized on the midpiece, the postacrosomal and the equatorial region of the sperm head of high salt treated spermatozoa representing the amount of CRISPs tightly associated to the sperm membrane. Scale bar represents 1 μm.

furthermore, the amount of sperm bound CRISPs could be correlated with the fertility of the stallion in preliminary studies. Our findings point to an important role of CRISP proteins in equine reproduction, and the accessibility of the equine CRISP-3 provides a powerful tool for investigating the physiological function of CRISPs in equine fertilization.

This work was financed by grants GRK 158/2-96 from Deutsche Forschungsgemeinschaft, Graduiertenkolleg, Zell- und Molekularbiologie in der Tiermedizin", Bonn, Germany, and BMBF 01 KY 95033 from Bundesministerium für Bildung und Forschung, Bonn, Germany

References

Calvete JJ, Nessau S, Mann, K, Sanz L, Sieme H, Klug E and Töpfer-Petersen E (1994) Isolation and biochemical characterization of stallion seminal plasma proteins *Reproduction in Domestic Animals* **29** 411–426

Cameo MS and Blaquier JA (1976) Androgen controlled specific proteins in rat epididymis. *Journal of. Endocrinology* **69** 47–55

Cohen DJ, Munuce MJ and Cuasnicù PS (1996) Mammalian sperm–egg fusion: the development of rat oolemma fusibility during oogenesis involves the appearance of binding sites for sperm protein "DE" *Biology of Reproduction* **55** 200–206

Eberspaecher U, Roosterman D, Krätzschmar J, Haendler B, Habenicht U-F, Becker A, Quensel C, Petri T, Schleuning WD and Donner P (1995) Mouse androgen-dependent epididymal glycoprotein CRISP-1 (DE/AEG): isolation, biochemical characterization and expression in recombinant form. *Molecular Reproduction and Development* **42** 157–172

Haendler B, Krätzschmar J, Theuring F and Schleuning W-D (1993) Transcripts for cysteine-rich secretory protein-1 (CRISP-1; DE/AEG) and the novel related CRISP-3 are expressed under androgen control in the mouse salivary gland *Endocrinology* **133** 192–198

Laemmli UK (1970) Cleavage of the structural proteins during the assembly of the head of bacteriophage T4 *Nature* **227** 680–685

Rochwerger L, Cohen DJ and Cuasnicù PS (1992) Mammalian sperm–egg fusion: the rat egg has complementary sites for a sperm protein that mediates gamete fusion *Developmental Biology* **153** 83–90

Schambony A, Hess O, Calvete JJ, Neumann U and Töpfer-Petersen E (1997) Horse seminal plasma protein 3: isolation, biochemical characterization, immunohistological localization and sperm coating characteristics *Reproduction in Domestic Animals* **32** 46

Schambony A, Gentzel M, Wolfes H, Raida M, Neumann U and Töpfer-Peterson E Equine CRIPS-3: primary structure and expression in the male genital tract *Biochemica et Biophysica Acta* (in press)

Journal of Reproduction and Fertility Supplement **53**, 73–84

Plasma membrane structure and remodelling during sperm maturation in the epididymis

Roy Jones

The Babraham Institute, Babraham, Cambridge CB2 4AT, UK

All mammalian spermatozoa are surrounded by a limiting plasma membrane that mediates many of the early events during fertilization. The membrane is derived originally from spermatogonia/spermatocytes in the testis but is then modified considerably during spermiogenesis, epididymal maturation and capacitation. It is characterized by an unusually high proportion of polyunsaturated phospholipids that give it special physical characteristics and compartmentalization of many of its component proteins and lipids into discrete domains on the head and tail. During passage of spermatozoa through the epididymis remodelling of the plasma membrane is commensurate with acquisition of motility and fertilizing capacity. Remodelling processes include uptake of secreted epididymal glycoproteins, removal or utilization of specific phospholipids from the inner leaflet of the bilayer, processing of existing or acquired glycoproteins by endoproteolysis and re-positioning of both protein and lipid components to different membrane domains. These modifications are carefully co-ordinated at different zones of the epididymis and indirectly affect intracellular membranes, organelles and even nucleoprotein. Maturation changes are described and appraised within the context of current concepts of membrane structure and fertilization.

Introduction

In common with all somatic cells, mammalian spermatozoa are surrounded by a limiting plasma membrane that maintains essential differences between the intracellular and extracellular environments. Within the spermatozoon, membranes also surround the acrosome, mitochondria and nucleus and serve to maintain gradients between the internal contents of each organelle and the limited amount of cytosol. Ultrastructurally, all these membranes conform to the classic bilayer arrangement yet they have different origins and different functions. The plasma membrane is ultimately derived from the spermatogonium but as spermatozoa differentiate in the testis and mature in the epididymis it is extensively remodelled by a variety of mechanisms that culminate in the development of fertilizing capacity. Thus, during spermiogenesis targeting and insertion of newly synthesized membrane components coupled with polarized migration is the basis for the establishment of separate membrane domains (acrosome, postacrosome, midpiece and principal piece; Cowan and Myles, 1993). This is followed by further modifications in the epididymis and later still, by changes during capacitation in the female tract. Precisely what remodelling means in quantitative terms is not at all clear. Most of the techniques that have been used to probe sperm membrane organization are qualitative and although they may indicate clear-cut differences between for example, testicular and cauda epididymidal spermatozoa, these differences may reflect between 5% and 50% of the total membrane. Even more uncertain are the underlying mechanisms that mediate these changes and how they are integrated with one another. Given that binding of spermatozoa to the zona pellucida and fusion with the oolemma involve surface membrane components in one way or another, a thorough knowledge of the biosynthesis and structure of the plasma membrane is clearly required. Defining differences between immature and mature spermatozoa is also important from a clinical perspective as a means of diagnosing the aetiology of

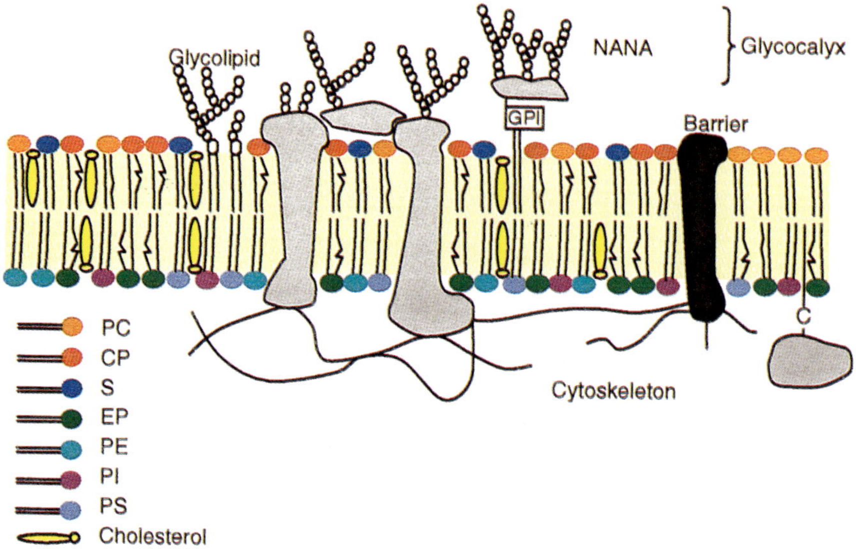

Fig. 1. Schematic drawing of the potential arrangement of lipid and protein components in the plasma membrane of a mammalian spermatozoon. The drawing is based on the original model by Singer and Nicolson (1972) and incorporates some current concepts of lipid and protein asymmetry. See text for details. CP, choline plasmalogen; EP, ethanolamine plasmalogen; PC, phosphatidylcholine; PE, phosphatidylethanolamine; PI, phosphatidylinositol; PS phosphatidylserine.

infertility in man and gaining insights into the key molecules that are crucial for fertilization. This review, therefore, will first of all appraise (briefly) current concepts of cell membrane structure with particular reference to spermatozoa and second, it will focus on mechanistic aspects of membrane remodelling that occur to spermatozoa as they pass through the epididymal duct.

Current Concepts of Plasma Membrane Structure and Function in Mammalian Cells

Lipids

The basic structure of a cell membrane is a bilayer arrangement of lipids that tend to form spontaneously in an aqueous environment (Singer and Nicolson, 1972; Fig. 1). Lipids constitute 50–60% of the mass of animal cell membranes; almost all of the remainder is protein. Quantitatively, this translates into about 10^9 lipid molecules in the plasma membrane of a typical cell the size of a leucocyte, although the degree of packing or density can vary to a surprising degree. The most abundant group is the phospholipids (PLs) of which phosphatidylcholine (PC), phosphatidylethanolamine (PE), phosphatidylserine (PS), sphingomyelin (SM) and phosphatidylinositol (PI) are the main constituents together with minor components such as phosphatidic acid (PA), lysphospholipids (LPC or LPE), cardiolipin (CL; found mainly in mitochondrial membranes), sterols (mostly cholesterol) and glycolipids. The last class contains complex carbohydrates attached to the polar head group and consequently vary substantially. In some specialized cells like spermatozoa, plasmalogen PLs are present in the form of choline plasmalogen (CP) or ethanolamine plasmalogen (EP) and together constitute 40–50% of the total PL. Plasmalogen PLs differ from diacyl PLs in having a fatty aldehyde substituted at the C2 atom via either a 1-alkyl or 1-alkenyl bond.

Besides heterogeneity in the nature of the polar head groups, PLs also differ according to the length and degree of unsaturation of attached acyl fatty acids which have a major influence on the properties of the membrane as a whole. Generally, the longer the acyl chain and the more *cis*-double bonds in it, the more distorted or 'kinked' their shape becomes, an arrangement that energetically favours a bilayer structure as opposed to a rigid micelle. Long-chain fatty acids are also more flexible and have higher 'fluidity' than saturated ones (see later).

A second feature of membrane PLs is that they are arranged asymmetrically in the bilayer, both laterally and transversely. Transverse asymmetry is due to the preferential accumulation of PE, PS and PI on the inner or cytoplasmic side of the bilayer whereas PC, SM and glycolipids are found predominantly on the outer or exoplasmic side. This arrangement is established during membrane biogenesis and is actively maintained by head-group specific PL translocases or flippases (Devaux, 1992). Lipid asymmetry seems to be widespread in cell membranes so that the detection of PS or PE in the exoplasmic face of the bilayer is one of the early signs of cellular apotosis. It is also of great functional relevance. Many transmembrane signalling systems, are dependent on specific PLs; for example, protein kinase C requires PS for activation and hence the complex is located on the cytoplasmic side of the plasma membrane (Devaux, 1992). Similarly, PI is the substrate for formation of polyphosphinositides that are important second messengers for triggering intracellular Ca^{2+} release. Conversely, glycolipids, which have diverse roles as receptor molecules for cell–cell recognition and interaction with the extracellular matrix are found mainly, if not exclusively, on the exoplasmic surface.

Unlike transverse movement or flip–flop, lateral diffusion of PLs within the plane of the bilayer is very rapid with typical diffusion coefficients of about 10^{-7} cm^2 s^{-1}. In more realistic terms, this means that for a bacterium 2 μm long a PL molecule could diffuse its entire length in about 1 s. PL diffusion is influenced greatly by fatty acyl chain length, degree of unsaturation and relative proportion of cholesterol. In general, PLs with short or unsaturated acyl chains form fluid phases, whereas long or saturated chains favour gel phases. Phase transition is temperature sensitive and usually very sharp (1 to 2 degrees) depending on the type of PL. Cholesterol also has a major effect on the phase state of PLs in membranes as it intercalates between fatty acyl chains in the hydrophobic interior of the bilayer and regulates their interactions with each other (Yeagle, 1985). Its effects are somewhat paradoxical depending on temperature and concentration; at high cholesterol:PL ratios (e.g. 1.0) and at 37°C it opposes fluidity, creates order and 'seals' membranes, whereas below phase transition temperatures cholesterol prevents acyl chains from binding to one another and therefore promotes fluidity. Thus, there is enormous scope for variation in the behaviour of lipid bilayers depending on the interplay between multiple controlling factors.

Despite their rapid diffusion, spatial segregation of PLs into specific domains on cell surfaces has been demonstrated on scales ranging from a few nanometers to micrometers. The most obvious examples are those associated with cellular structures such as tight junctions which provide a physical barrier to free diffusion between the apical and basolateral plasma membranes in the exoplasmic face of the bilayer. Another example of a macrolipid domain is the myelin sheath which has a composition very different from the plasma membrane of the myelin forming cell. On a smaller scale, there is the question of the formation and persistence of lipid microheterogeneities. This is still a contentious issue as it is not clear whether they are the results of lipid–lipid immiscibility, protein–lipid interactions or both (Edidin, 1992). The heterogeneous mixture of lipids in cell membranes also implies a wide-range of thermotropic phase transitions that, in theory, could promote a mosaic of fluid and gel phase lipids. The presence of these heterogeneities in time and space may be very small and contain only a few hundred PL molecules, for example the 'collar' lipids that form around certain transmembrane proteins. This preferential affinity of some proteins for specific PLs is found in caveoli and lipid 'rafts' within the plasma membrane (Harder and Simons, 1997). Caveoli (membrane invaginations free of clathrin) are enriched in cholesterol and glycospingolipids and have a proposed function in transcytosis. Lipid rafts containing selected proteins may also act as 'relay' stations for intracellular signalling events.

Proteins

Progress in elucidating the structure and function of proteins in cell membranes has been more rapid than with lipids, largely because of the relative ease with which they can be purified, sequenced and their function assessed by mutagenesis and null mutation or 'knock-out' experiments (Jennings, 1989). Although proteins make up about 40% of the total mass of the plasma membrane, being larger than lipids there are fewer of them – on average about one protein molecule for 50 lipid molecules. Proteins may occur singly or in the form of a large complex (for example pore proteins) and are major effectors of cell function. Their roles are diverse but structurally their association with the membrane falls into several well-defined categories. Transmembrane proteins span the entire bilayer owing to the presence of one or more short stretches of 20–30 hydrophobic amino acids arranged in the form of an alpha helix. These proteins are integral components of the membrane and require detergents for solubilization. An unusual subclass of these tightly bound proteins are those that do not have direct contact with the lipid bilayer but instead are anchored to it by covalently bound fatty acids, polyprenyl groups or glycosylphosphatidylinositol (GPI). In contrast, peripheral membrane proteins are weakly bound to the outside of the bilayer, usually by electrostatic interactions, and can be readily dissociated from it by extremes of pH, reducing agents or a high ionic strength medium. The presence of such 'coating' proteins on the surface membrane, therefore, depends on the nature of the environment to which the cell is exposed. A third class of proteins is restricted to the cytoplasmic face of the bilayer and the proteins are anchored either by a fatty acid (myristic or palmitic acid) or a prenyl group (farnesyl). Overall, the diverse nature of membrane-bound proteins and their different orientation to the lipid bilayer emphasises the asymmetry of the membrane.

One consequence of this asymmetry is that the outside of the membrane has a different charge to the inside (the outside is usually negative). An important contribution to charge is made by carbohydrates attached to either proteins (glycoprotein) or lipids (glycolipids), especially if the oligosaccharide chains terminate in sialic acids. Although oligosaccharides are made up of fewer than 15 different sugars, they are often branched and their potential arrangement is highly variable. Structurally, carbohydrate chains extend several microns from the surface of the membrane to form the so-called glycocalyx and currently are perceived as having two main functions: one is to keep other cells such as bacteria at a distance from the bilayer and prevent spontaneous membrane fusion and the other is to act as specific receptors for cell–cell recognition, for example rolling and binding of neutrophils to endothelial cells during inflammation. A third putative function that has only recently come to light is that the glycocalyx can hinder the lateral movement of proteins within the membrane, presumably via charge interactions since digestion with sialidases frequently increases diffusion coefficients.

Immediately below the lipid bilayer there is an extensive network of cytoskeletal fibres composed of specialized filamentous proteins such as actin and myosin (Pumplin and Bloch, 1993). Many transmembrane proteins are covalently attached to the cytoskeleton presumably because their orientation in the membrane is important for their function. Consequently their lateral mobility is much lower than that of unattached proteins. Paradoxically, however, the cytoskeleton participates in protein movement over large distances (5–10 microns) since processes such as capping, whereby antibody-induced patches are transported to one pole of the cell, are inhibited by agents that prevent actin polymerization–depolymerization reactions. The cytoskeleton is also involved in the positioning and maintenance of intramembraneous barriers between cells, such as those formed by tight junctions, that help to compartmentalize the plasma membrane functionally. Again the paradigm here is the polarized epithelial cell in which ion pumps and other molecules are sequestered onto the apical plasma membrane whereas receptors for intracellular matrix proteins are localized to the basal membrane. Passive diffusion of protein molecules through tight junctional barriers is actively impeded, at least on the exoplasmic face of the bilayer.

Modifications to the Plasma Membrane of Spermatozoa in the Epididymis

Remodelling of lipid components

The lipid composition of mammalian spermatozoa is well documented (for reviews see Hammerstedt *et al.*, 1979; Ladha, 1998). Three unusual features of sperm lipids are (i) the presence of large amounts of plasmalogen PLs, 30%–40% in some cases, (ii) the high content of polyunsaturated fatty acids, mostly 20:4, 22:5 and 22:6, and (iii) relatively low cholesterol: PL ratios ranging from 0.26 to 0.45 depending on the species. It has long been known that during passage of spermatozoa through the epididymis there is a decrease in the total cellular content of PLs of between 25% and 48% (see for example Scott *et al.*, 1967; Poulos *et al.*, 1973; Poulos *et al.*, 1975; Rana *et al.*, 1991). These values may seem large but they actually mask more impressive changes when individual classes of PL are compared. Three specific examples illustrate the point. In the ram PC decreases by 37%, PE by 45%, PI by 79%, PS by 78%, C by 35%, S by 17%, EP by 61% and CP by only 9% (Poulos *et al.*, 1975). In the bull PC decreases by 42%, PE by 66%, PS by 95%, C by 71%, S by 37%, EP by 73% and CP by only 16% (Poulos *et al.*, 1973). In the rat PC declines by 64%, PE by 71%, PI by 53%, PS by 82%, S by 16%, EP by 7% and CP by only 6% (Alveldano *et al.*, 1992). It is evident from these figures that the content of choline plasmalogen, already quantitatively the major PL in testicular spermatozoa, is remarkably consistent throughout maturation and that the changes are accounted for by other (minor) PLs. Thus, PL loss during sperm maturation is highly selective. An obvious problem with these data, however, is that whole cell compositional analysis may or may not reflect the situation in the plasma membrane. In part, this is due to the technical difficulties of purifying sperm plasma membranes for analysis. Attempts are noteworthy for their lack of quantitation (specific markers are rarely used and hence enrichment factors cannot be calculated), presumption of purity based of very subjective criteria (for example thickness of membrane) and disregard for the fact that some procedures (for example nitrogen cavitation) selectively demembranate sperm heads and not the tail. In addition, sperm membrane lipids can vary according to the diet of the animal and the method of semen collection (Evans and Setchell, 1979). However, even allowing for all these variables, a survey of the most reliable data indicates that lipids in the plasma membrane of cauda epididymidal spermatozoa are different in composition from those in testicular spermatozoa. In a careful study on maturing ram sperm membranes, Parks and Hammerstedt (1985) found a 46% and 48% decrease in total PL and cholesterol, respectively, with an increase in the sterol: PL ratio from 0.26 to 0.44. Choline PLs were relatively stable whereas the amounts of PE, PS and PI declined by more than 50%. Interestingly, the latter PLs are characteristically found on the cytoplasmic side of the plasma membrane. Palmitic acid (16:0) is the major PL-bound fatty acid present in immature spermatozoa, whereas in mature cells docosahexanoic acid (22:6) predominates, a finding consistent with the relative increase in the amount of CPs. Thus, it would seem from the available data that the loss of specific classes of PL from maturing spermatozoa as revealed by whole cell compositional analysis reflects to a reasonable extent the situation in the plasma membrane.

Two important questions that arise from these findings are (i), what mediates selective PL loss and (ii), what are the implications for the properties and behaviour of the plasma membrane? A long-standing idea pertaining to the first problem is that fatty acids derived from PLs provide the energy source for maturing spermatozoa since exogenous glucose is very low or absent in epididymal fluid (Mann, 1964). Compatible with this concept is the presence in epididymal fluid and spermatozoa of high concentrations of carnitine and acetylcarnitine that would facilitate the transfer of fatty acids into mitochondria for β-oxidation. Against this concept is the failure to detect any appreciable decrease in PL content in ejaculated ram spermatozoa during prolonged incubation *in vitro* and the absence in maturing epididymal spermatozoa of significant amounts of lysophosphatides resulting from phospholipase activity (Darin-Bennet *et al.*, 1973). The case for PLs as an energy source for spermatozoa in the epididymis, therefore, is not proven. Another possible explanation for PL loss is active lipid exchange proteins that would mediate transfer of PLs from spermatozoa to membrane bound vesicles in epididymal fluid. So far, such exchange proteins have not been reported and in any case, are likely to affect the PLs on the outside of the bilayer rather than those on the inner leaflet of the membrane. In this respect it is intriguing that PE, PI and PS are involved in many intracellular signalling processes in association with Ca^{2+} and may be utilized in these pathways as part of other remodelling events in preparation for example, for the acrosome reaction or acquisition of motility.

More far-reaching implications of selective changes to PLs during epididymal maturation of spermatozoa are to the biophysical properties of the bilayer and the behaviour of protein components within it. It is known from work on liposomes that the compositional criteria important

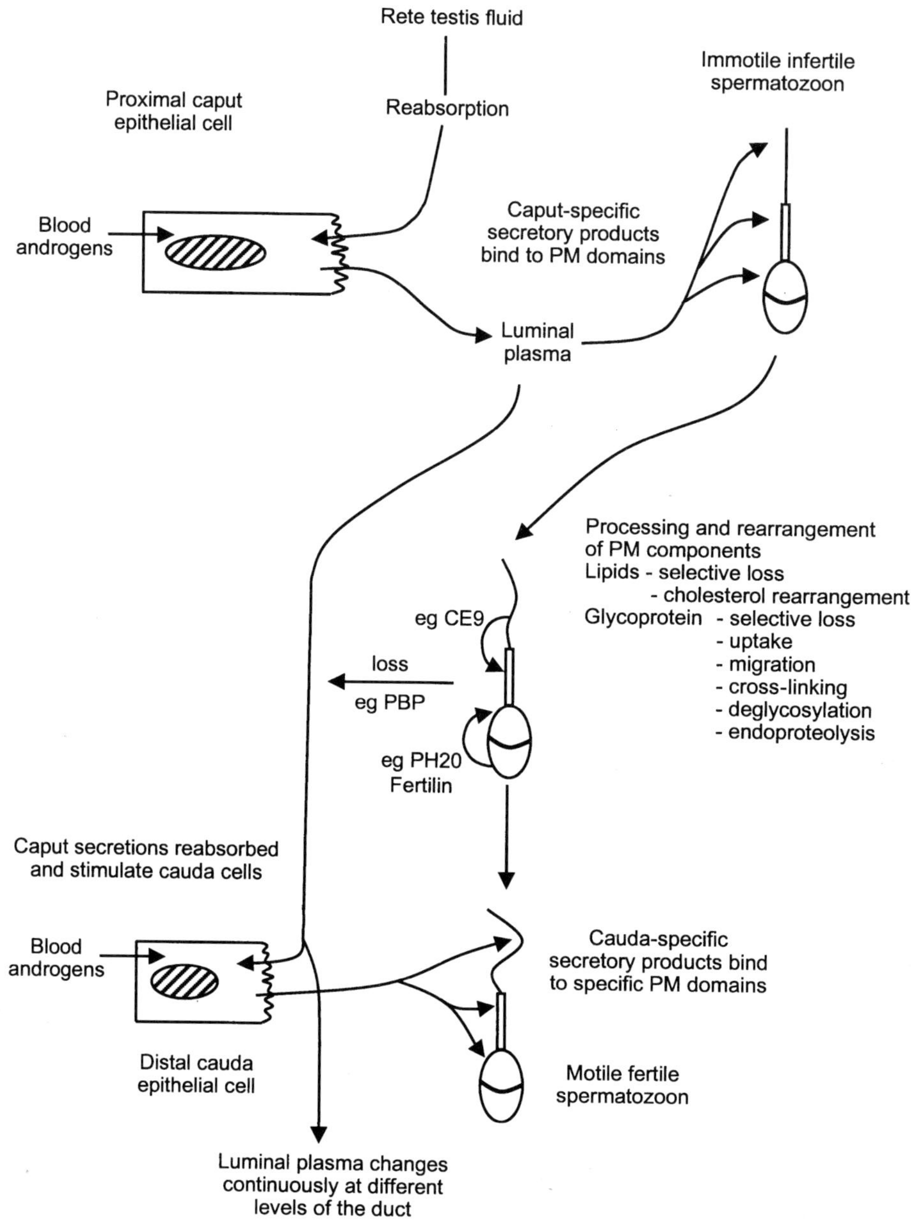

Fig. 2. Summary of processes involved in plasma membrane remodelling during maturation of spermatozoa in the mammalian epididymis. See text for details.

for fluidity are the ratios of cholesterol: PL, PE: PC and saturated:unsaturated fatty acids (reviewed by Ladha, 1998). As detailed above, during epididymal maturation the proportions of PE and saturated fatty acids decrease significantly while unsaturated fatty acids increase; this should, in theory, increase fluidity. However, in rams and goats at least, this is opposed by a relative increase in cholesterol (Rana *et al.*, 1991; Parks and Lynch, 1992). The resultant effects are very difficult to predict and point to the need for direct biophysical measurements of membrane behaviour during maturation. In human spermatozoa generalized polarization spectroscopy measurements with

Laurdan have detected only liquid crystalline (fluid) states in plasma membranes over a surprisingly large temperature range of 10°C–42°C with no evidence for gel phase lipids (Palleschi and Silvestroni, 1996). Fluorescence polarization, however, has demonstrated thermotropic phase transitions in whole spermatozoa and their plasma membrane vesicles during cooling, consistent with the view that there is lateral segregation of lipids within the membrane and co-existence of fluid and gel phases (Holt and North, 1986). However attractive this interpretation may be, it is still a contentious issue, as is the presence of transient hexagonal phase lipids within bilayer arrangements. Rana and Majumder (1990) measured a decrease in fluidity of goat sperm plasma membrane lipids during epididymal maturation by diphenylhexatriene polarization but the differences were small and could not be assigned to a particular region. Fluorescent recovery after photobleaching (FRAP), on the other hand, is a more informative procedure since it has the resolution to measure lateral diffusion of molecules in membrane domains a few microns in diameter. Wolf and Voglmayr (1984) measured diffusion of DiIC16 on testicular and ejaculated ram spermatozoa by FRAP analysis and found a small but significant increase in the diffusion coefficient during maturation on the acrosomal and postacrosomal domains but not on the tail. These data are somewhat questionable in the light of a recent finding that DiIC16 stains only dead or permeabilized spermatozoa which develop large immobile phases in their membrane lipids (Ladha *et al.*, 1997). Measurements of lipid dynamics in permeabilized cells, therefore, have to be viewed with considerable caution. Using a different lipid reporter probe, ODAF, and taking care to discriminate between live and dead cells, we have found that (i), lipid diffusion in live ram, mouse and bull testicular spermatozoa is significantly faster over the acrosome > postacrosome > midpiece > principal piece (Ladha *et al.*, 1997; Wolfe *et al.*, 1998); (ii) in ram spermatozoa (where membrane PLs decrease substantially during maturation) this pattern is maintained and exacerbated with an approximately threefold increase in diffusion coefficients over the sperm head but not the tail (James *et al.*, 1999). By contrast, in boar spermatozoa (where membrane PLs remain remarkably constant during maturation) diffusion coefficients for ODAF do not change significantly between testis and cauda epididymidis (James *et al.*, 1999). Thus, theoretical predictions about the effects of compositional changes on lipid diffusion have some experimental support although redistribution of specific PLs within the bilayer or their sequestration into different phases (fluid versus gel) may also be involved. In addition, the funcionality of putative diffusion barriers (posterior ring and annulus) within the membrane may change during maturation and have repercussions for antigen migration (see below).

Like somatic cells, sperm plasma membranes also show transverse lipid asymmetry. This can be demonstrated very clearly with a fluorescent tetracyclic polypeptide known as FL-Ro09-0198 that has specificity for ethanolamine PLs (Choung *et al.*, 1988). Fl-Ro09-0198 does not react with live, membrane-intact spermatozoa (ram, bull, boar, mouse; P. S. James, M. Umeda and R. Jones, unpublished). After permeabilization, however, the probe binds all over spermatozoa with the same pattern irrespective of the degree of maturation. This finding suggests that with respect to PE and EP, membrane remodelling in the epididymis does not perturb transverse lipid asymmetry. Similar experiments with Fl-Annexin V have been less successful, possibly because of the much smaller amounts of PS present in sperm membranes. In summary, therefore, the available data indicate that in most species the lipid content of sperm plasma membranes decreases significantly during epididymal maturation due to a loss of specific PLs, notably PE, EP, PS and PI, that is, PLs normally found on the inner leaflet of the bilayer. The mechanisms that mediate these changes are not understood but in theory the consequences for the biophysical behaviour of the plasma membrane are considerable. This may be due to complex compensatory mechanisms within the plasma membrane itself involving unsaturated fatty acids/cholesterol redistribution and/or the effects of proteins acquired from epididymal fluid.

Remodelling of protein components

Much attention has been directed over many years to comparing the proteins and glycoproteins in the plasma membrane of mature and immature spermatozoa on the premise that this may provide clues to the identity of the receptor molecules that mediate sperm–egg recognition. This view, however, has been confounded by the large number of differences between the two cell types and the associated problems of interpreting their significance. The opposite approach, of identifying molecules involved in fertilization by techniques such as antibody inhibition assays and zona binding and investigating their biogenesis in the epididymis and testis, has provided some novel clues to the subtlety of membrane remodelling processes during post-testicular sperm development.

Two widely used methods for investigating surface membrane proteins on cells are surface labelling with enzymes and 'mapping' by two-dimensional SDS-PAGE. Both techniques are only semi-quantitative at best yet valuable nonetheless. The first procedure labels specific groups on sugars or amino acids, such as terminal galactose/sialic or tyrosine residues, using large protein probes (that, in theory, should be membrane impermeable) like galactose oxidase and lactoperoxidase. There are substantial differences in these enzymes between testicular and cauda spermatozoa in rats, rams, monkeys and rabbits which together with possible artefacts in the techniques are well documented (Jones, 1989). Two-dimensional mapping of total membrane proteins and glycoproteins derived from caput and cauda spermatozoa has been reported for the rat and boar and has revealed many differences (as well as many similarities) between the two cell types (Olson and Hinton, 1985; Syntin *et al.*, 1996). The limitations of this approach are (i) the relative purity of the plasma membrane preparations (a technique that is appropriate to cauda spermatozoa may not be applicable to testicular spermatozoa); (ii) how representative the membrane preparations are of the whole cell; (iii) identifying the same protein on different maps due to subtle alterations in for example size or charge. Despite these drawbacks, however, membrane mapping studies in combination with surface probes like enzymes and antibodies have revealed many differences between testicular and caudal spermatozoa that are possible to relate to specific components secreted by the epididymis. Much data are now available on these secreted glycoproteins, their hormonal regulation and, in a limited number of cases, their sequences (see other reviews in this supplement). Rather than cataloguing all the epididymal glycoproteins that have been reported to interact with spermatozoa, the remainder of this review will concentrate on the mechanisms by which external proteins influence plasma membrane composition and behaviour.

Interactions between spermatozoa and epididymal secretory proteins

The most obvious and well documented pathway for membrane remodelling in the epididymis is uptake of glycoproteins directly from the luminal secretion. Many (about 50%) glycoproteins are synthesized and secreted in specific regions of the epididymis and bind to spermatozoa as they pass through that particular area. Two immediate questions that arise are the nature of the association of secreted glycoproteins with the plasma membrane (hydrophobic versus ionic) and the reasons why some glycoproteins bind to specific regions (for example acrosome only or tail only) whereas others are less discriminatory. Some secreted glycoproteins (it is not known what percentage) are only weakly bound by ionic bonds as they are readily dissociated by 1 M NaCl or pH >10.0. An example of this is HIS50 in the rat (Rifkin and Olson, 1985); this antigen is secreted specifically by the cauda epididymidis, localizes to the sperm acrosome and is easily solubilized by 0.4 M NaCl. A second example of a high salt and high pH dissociated protein is PBP the presence of which in luminal secretions throughout the epididymal duct is due to its 'leaching' from spermatozoa (Perry *et al.*, 1994).

The opposite scenario, in which a secreted epididymal glycoprotein binds very strongly to the sperm plasma membrane is shown by CDw52 antigen (also known as CAMPATH1, HE5 or SMemG; reviewed by Kirchhoff, 1996). CDw52 contains a GPI anchor and hence partitions into Triton X114, a characteristic feature of integral membrane proteins. On monkey and human spermatozoa it is localized on the tail and postacrosomal regions as they pass through the epididymis. CDw52 is present in epididymal secretions with an intact GPI anchor and it has been postulated that it is transferred to spermatozoa from membrane-bound vesicles or epididymosomes (cf prostasomes) by a mechanism similar to that found for cell–cell transfer between erythrocytes and endothelial cells (Kooyman *et al.*, 1995; Yeung *et al.*, 1997). Its transfer to the plasma membrane is related to the maturation status of the spermatozoon implying that its uptake is dependent on changes that precede its appearance in the luminal secretions (Yeung *et al.*, 1997).

Other potential mechanisms for binding soluble proteins strongly to the plasma membrane are, first, conformational changes in tertiary structure brought about by simple alterations in pH or concentrations of divalent cations that allow helically aligned hydrophobic residues to interact directly with lipids in the bilayer. This mechanism is well known from studies of viral fusion proteins (White, 1992) but has yet to be investigated in epididymal protein–sperm plasma membrane interactions. The second mechanism involves transglutaminase catalysed cross-linking of glutamine and lysine residues both within and between different proteins. In the presence of Ca^{2+}, transglutaminase has also been reported to covalently cross-link putrescine, spermidine and spermine to rat sperm membranes (Paonessa *et al.*, 1984). Since these polyamines are present in high concentrations in epididymal secretions and a uteroglobin-like protein has been detected in the epididymal epithelium of rabbits, there may be a parallel system for suppressing antigenicity of spermatozoa during maturation. This contention is supported by the presence of CD59 and CD55 (DAF) antigens on spermatozoa (Rooney *et al.*, 1993). The third mechanism is covalent attachment of fatty acids, (commonly myristic (14:0) or palmitic acids(16:)), to soluble proteins via an amide linkage on an N-terminal glycine followed by insertion into the lipid bilayer. Incorporation of radiolabelled palmitate into several membrane proteins has been reported in rat spermatozoa but it is not clear whether these proteins are lipid anchored (Srivastava and Olson, 1996). As with GPI anchors, an attractive feature of this mechanism is that preferential association of the fatty acid for a particular type of PL phase could localize the protein in a specific surface domain. Thus, the restricted distribution of at least some glycoproteins in the membrane would be determined and directed primarily by the disposition of lipids. The fourth mechanism, an extension of the third mechanism, is prenylation of soluble proteins by attachment of unsaturated hydrocarbon chains (for example farnesyl) via C-terminal cysteine residues to provide a hydrophobic 'tail' for membrane insertion. Prenylation and myristylation are anchoring mechanisms for attaching cytoplasmic proteins to the inner leaflet of the membrane and in this respect farnsyl transferase has been detected only within the cytoplasmic droplet (Olson *et al*, 1997). The fifth mechanism is 'protein-off–protein-on' exchange. An unusual type of membrane protein remodelling in the epididymis is replacement of testicular clusterin with an epididymal form of the same protein. Clusterin is ubiquitous in somatic tissues and has many functions including cell aggregation, cytolysis inhibition and lipoprotein transport. In the testis it is secreted by Sertoli cells as a heterodimeric glycoprotein and binds to spermatozoa in the seminiferous tubules. Testicular clusterin is removed from spermatozoa as they pass through the initial segment and is replaced by a lower molecular weight form secreted by the caput epididymidis (Sylvester *et al.*, 1991). The difference between the two forms seems to be in the degree of glycoslyation as the polypeptide chains are of similar size. The simplest interpretation of this phenomenon would be that epididymal clusterin displaces testicular clusterin by virtue of its higher affinity for the same receptor if it were not for the fact that they frequently have different cellular locations indicating that either the receptor changes its position during maturation in the epididymis or the proteins bind to different receptors and behave independently of each other.

Processing and realignment of plasma membrane components during sperm maturation

Processing and spatial re-alignment of plasma membrane components, whether originally present on testicular spermatozoa or newly acquired from epididymal secretions, are remodelling mechanisms that may be more widespread than is currently appreciated. Fertilin, PH20/2B1 and CE9 are membrane-bound glycoproteins on guinea-pig and rat spermatozoa that undergo site-specific endoproteolytic cleavage in the epididymis. In the case of fertilin, which is synthesized as a heterodimer during spermatogenesis, cleavage of the α-subunit takes place during spermiogenesis whereas the β-subunit cleavage is delayed until spermatozoa reach the distal caput epididymidis (Phelps *et al.*, 1990; Lum and Blobel, 1997). Both subunits are processed at a similar site which lies between the disintegrin and metalloproteinase domains and as a consequence, the size of the protein dimer decreases from about 190 kDa to about 80 kDa (values refer to guinea-pig fertilin). It is presumed that the N-terminal fragments thus released remain in a soluble form in the luminal fluid and either accumulate or are absorbed by epithelial cells lining the duct. Their ultimate fate, however, is not known. Similarly, CE9 glycoprotein on rat spermatozoa is cleaved near the N-terminus at Arg75; the smaller polypeptide is released from the larger subunit that contains the transmembrane domain (Petruszak *et al.*, 1991). In contrast, endoproteolytic cleavage of PH20/2B1 (sperm-specific forms of a membrane-bound hyaluronidase) at Arg312 takes place as spermatozoa pass through the caput epididymidis to produce a heterodimeric glycoprotein, the subunits of which are held together by disulphide bridges (Lathrop *et al.*, 1990; Jones *et al.*, 1996). All three glycoproteins have only one cleavage site, although there are numerous arginine residues throughout the protein sequence, implying that site-specific cleavage depends on the tertiary structure and presentation of the protein on the membrane surface. Endoproteolytic processing of 2B1 is not obligatory for hyaluronidase activity so any conformational changes that take place must be small or well removed from the active site of the enzyme. The source of the endoprotease that mediates this processing in the epididymis has not been established but preliminary experiments suggest that it is associated with spermatozoa. After thorough washing and culture of caput spermatozoa *in vitro* for 24 h, 2B1 glycoprotein still underwent cleavage at Arg312, although the α-subunit was about 5 kDa larger than the *in vivo* processed form, indicating that other changes must take place as well (Jones *et al.*, 1996). One obvious possibility is simultaneous deglycosylation as epididymal luminal fluid has long been known to contain high concentrations of exoglycosidases, especially α-mannosidase, β-D-galactosidase and *N*-acetylglucosaminidase (Tulsiani *et al.*, 1993). During culture for 24 h many spermatozoa degenerated and lost their acrosomes suggesting that acrosomal proteinases (acrosin?) may be responsible. In support of this hypothesis, Lum and Blobel (1997) found that guinea-pig fertilin-β could be endoproteolytically cleaved *in vitro* if caput spermatozoa were freeze–thawed beforehand. Together, this evidence suggests that the endoproteinase is intracellular but does not explain how it would be released *in vivo*.

A second feature of fertilin, PH20 and CE9 mentioned above is that their cellular location changes during epididymal maturation. For fertilin and PH20, a causal relationship between endoproteolysis and spatial reorganization is suggested by the finding that trypsinization of testicular spermatozoa *in vitro* mimics the repositioning of these antigens observed *in vivo* from their original location all over the sperm head to the postacrosomal region where they remain until maturation is complete (Phelps *et al.*, 1990). Rat sperm CE9 glycoprotein also changes its position from all over the tail of caput spermatozoa to the midpiece region of cauda spermatozoa, which may be caused by active migration in an anterior direction (Cesario and Bartles, 1994). In this case, however, trypsinization *in vitro* is unable to mimic the effect prompting speculation that anterior movement of CE9 *in vivo* is due to a change in the function of the annulus as an intramembranous barrier. If correct, then it implies that compartmentalization of plasma membrane components becomes compromised during maturation in a very specific way, as not all membrane components are free to diffuse between domains. Although 2B1 glycoprotein does not alter its domain position on the sperm tail during epididymal maturation, under capacitating conditions it actively migrates onto the acrosome where its hyaluronidase activity would facilitate penetration of spermatozoa through the cumulous oophorus (Jones *et al.*, 1990). Epididymal endoproteolysis may be an important prerequisite for this migration. Thus, processing and spatial realignment of plasma membrane antigens to a position where they become functionally active is an important aspect of epididymal maturation of spermatozoa irrespective of whether antigens are of testicular or epididymal origin.

Overall, therefore, the profile and distribution of protein antigens on the plasma membrane of spermatozoa changes continuously as they pass through the epididymal duct. The principal mechanisms responsible (summarized in Fig. 2) include uptake of glycoproteins directly from epididymal secretions (in some instances to specific regions of the sperm surface), processing (by endoproteolysis) of acquired or pre-existing glycoproteins and migration of antigens to new membrane domains. It is still not clear whether any of these epididymal antigens participate directly in the fertilization process or whether they have more subtle effects related to sperm survival in the cauda epididymidis, acquisition of motility and even capacitation in the female tract.

Conclusions

It is apparent from this overview of the sperm plasma membrane that although it conforms to a very large extent to the concepts pertaining to other cell membranes, there are many aspects of it that are unusual and unique. These include the high proportion of unsaturated alkyl-acyl and alkenyl-acyl phospholipids and the uptake of a variety of testis- and epididymal-specific glycoproteins. As a consequence it undergoes constant remodelling during epididymal maturation. Qualitatively, the differences between caput and cauda epididymidal spermatozoa appear large, although it is not clear precisely what this means in quantitative terms. Remodelling involves not only compositional changes brought about by uptake and removal of membrane proteins, but also processing and re-positioning of antigens to different membrane domains where they may assume novel functions as a consequence of a different microenvironment. It is of interest that several of the antigens that undergo the latter modifications (fertilin, PH20/2B1) are molecules that have a putative role in egg recognition and fusion. The evidence that the epididymis has an active role to play in membrane remodelling is substantial and indicates that it is carefully regulated at different levels of the duct. Lastly, it is likely that modifications to the sperm plasma membrane during maturation also have far-reaching effects on intracellular membranes and even to the nucleoprotein (for example remethylation of specific genes).

I am grateful to Dr Liz Howes for helpful comments on the manuscript and Mrs Linda Notton for preparation of the text figures.

References

Alveldano MI, Rotstein NP and Vermouth NT (1992) Lipid remodelling during epididymal maturation of rat spermatozoa *Biochemical Journal* **283** 235–241

Cesario MM and Bartles JR (1994) Compartmentalization, processing and redistribution of the plasma membrane protein CE9 on rodent spermatozoa *Journal of Cell Science* **197** 561–570

Choung S-Y, Kobayashi T, Takemoto K, Ishitsuka H and Inoue K (1988) Interaction of a cyclic peptide, Ro09-0198 with phosphatidylethanolamine in liposomal membranes *Biochimica et Biophysica Acta* **940** 180–187

Cowan AE and Myles DG (1993) Biogenesis of surface domains during spermiogenesis in the guinea pig *Developmental Biology* **155** 124–133

Darin-Bennet A, Poulos A and White IG (1973) A re-examination of the role of phospholipids as energy substrates during incubation of ram spermatozoa *Journal of Reproduction and Fertility* **34** 543–546

Devaux PF (1992) Protein involvement in trans-membrane lipid asymmetry *Annual Review of Biophysics and Biomolecular Structure* **21** 417–439

Edidin M (1992) Patches, posts and fences: proteins and plasma membrane domains *Trends in Cell Biology* **2** 376–380

Evans RW and Setchell BP (1979) Lipid changes during epididymal maturation in ram spermatozoa collected at different times of the year *Journal of Reproduction and Fertility* **57** 179–203

Hammerstedt RH, Keith AD, Hay S, Delucia N and Amann RP (1979) Changes in ram sperm membranes during epididymal transit *Archives of Biochemistry and Biophysics* **196** 7–12

Harder T and Simons K (1997) Caveolae, DIGS, and the dynamics of sphingolipid-cholesterol microdomains *Current Opinion in Cell Biology* **9** 534–542

Holt WV and North RD (1986) Thermotrophic phase transitions in the plasma membrane of ram spermatozoa *Journal of Reproduction and Fertility* **78** 447–457

James PS, Wolfe CA, Ladha S and Jones R (1999) Lipid diffusion in the plasma membrane of ram and boar spermatozoa during maturation in the epididymis measured by fluorescence recovery after photobleaching (FRAP) *Molecular Reproduction and Development* (in press)

Jennings ML (1989) Topography of membrane proteins *Annual Review of Biochemistry* **58** 999–1027

Jones R (1989) Membrane remodelling during sperm maturation in the epididymis *Oxford Reviews of Reproductive Biology* 285–337

Jones R, Shalgi R, Hoyland J and Phillips DM (1990) Topographical rearrangement of a plasma membrane antigen during capacitation of rat spermatozoa *in vitro*. *Developmental Biology* **139** 349–362

Jones R, Ma A, Hou S-T, Shalgi R and Hall L (1996) Testicular biosynthesis and epididymal endoproteolytic processing of rat sperm surface antigen 2B1 *Journal of Cell Science* **109** 2561–2570

Kirchoff C (1996) CD52 is the 'major maturation-associated' sperm membrane antigen *Molecular Human Reproduction* **2** 9–17

Kooyman DL, Byrne GW, McClellan S, Nielsen D, Tone M, Waldman H, Coffman TM, McCurry KR, Platt JL and Logan JS (1995) *In vivo* transfer of GPI-linked complement restriction factors from erythrocytes to the endothelium *Science* **269** 89–92

Ladha S (1998) Lipid heterogeneity and membrane fluidity in a highly polarized cell, the mammalian spermatozoon *Journal of Membrane Biology* **165** 1–10

Ladha S, James PS, Clark DC, Howes EA and Jones R (1997) Lateral mobility of plasma membrane lipids in bull spermatozoa: heterogeneity between surface domains and rigidification following cell death *Journal of Cell Science* **110** 1041–1050

Lathrop WF, Carmichael EP, Myles DG and Primakoff P (1990) cDNA cloning reveals the molecular structure of a sperm surface protein, PH.20, involved in sperm–egg adhesion and the wide distribution of its gene among mammals *Journal of Cell Biology* **111** 2939–2949

Lum L and Blobel CP (1997) Evidence for distinct serine protease activities with a potential role in processing the sperm protein fertilin *Developmental Biology* **191** 131–145

Mann T (1964) *Biochemistry of Semen and of the Male Reproductive Tract* Methuen, London

Olson GE and Hinton BT (1985) Regional differences in luminal fluid polypeptides of the rat testis and epididymis revealed by two-dimensional gel electrophoresis *Journal of Andrology* **6** 20–34

Olson GE, Nagdas SK and Winfrey VP (1997) Temporal expression and localization of protein farnesyltransferase during spermiogenesis and post-testicular sperm maturation in the hamster *Molecular Reproduction and Development* **48** 71–76

Palleschi S and Silvestroni L (1996) Laurdan fluorescence spectroscopy reveals a single liquid-crystalline lipid phase and lack of thermotropic phase transitions in the plasma membrane of living human sperm *Biochimica et Biophysica Acta* **279** 197–202

Paonessa G, Metafora S, Tajana G, Abrescia P, De Santis A, Gentile V and Porta R (1984) Transglutaminase-mediated modifications of the rat sperm surface *in vitro. Science* **226** 853–855

Parks JE and Hammerstedt RH (1985) Developmental changes in the lipids of ram epididymal spermatozoa plasma membrane *Biology of Reproduction* **32** 653–668

Parks JE and Lynch DV (1992) Lipid composition and thermotrophic phase behaviour of boar, bull, stallion, and rooster sperm membranes *Cryobiology* **29** 255–266

Perry ACF, Hall L, Bell AE and Jones R (1994) Sequence analysis of a mammalian phospholipid-binding protein from testis and epididymis and its distribution between spermatozoa and extracellular secretions *Biochemical Journal* **301** 235–242

Petruszak JAM, Nehme CL and Bartles JR (1991) Endoproteolytic cleavage in the extracellular domain of the integral plasma membrane protein precedes its redistribution from the posterior to the anterior tail of the rat spermatozoon during epididymal maturation *Journal of Cell Biology* **114** 917–927

Phelps B M, Koppel DE, Primakoff P and Myles DG (1990) Evidence that proteolysis of the surface is an initial step in the mechanism of formation of sperm cell surface domains *Journal of Cell Biology* **111** 1839–1847

Poulos A, Voglmayr JK and White IG (1973) Phospholipid changes in spermatozoa during passage through the genital tract of the bull *Biochimica et Biophysica Acta* **306** 194–202

Poulos A, Brown-Woodman PDC, White IG and Cox RI (1975) Changes in phospholipids of ram spermatozoa during migration through the epididymis and possible origin of prostaglandin $F_{2\alpha}$ in testicular and epididymal fluid *Biochimica et Biophysica Acta* **388** 12–18

Pumplin DW and Bloch RJ (1993) The membrane skeleton *Trends in Cell Biology* **3** 113–117

Rana APS and Majumder GC (1990) Changes in the fluidity of the goat sperm plasma membrane in transit from caput to cauda epididymis *Biochemistry International* **21** 797–803

Rana APS, Majumder GC, Misra S and Ghosh A (1991) Lipid changes of goat sperm plasma membrane during epididymal maturation *Biochimica et Biophysica Acta* **1061** 185–196

Rifkin JM and Olson GE (1985) Characterization of maturation-dependent extrinsic proteins of the rat sperm surface *Journal of Cell Biology* **100** 1582–1591

Rooney IA, Atkinson JP, Krul ES, Sconfeld G, Polakoski K, Saffity JE and Morgan BP (1993) Physiologic relevance of the membrane attack complex inhibitory protein CD59 in human seminal plasma: CD59 is present on extracellular organelles (prostasomes), binds cell membranes, and inhibits complement-mediated lysis *Journal of Experimental Medicine* **177** 1409–1420

Scott TW, Voglmayr JK and Setchell BP (1967) Lipid composition and metabolism and ejaculated ram spermatozoa *Biochemical Journal* **102** 456–461

Singer SJ and Nicolson GL (1972) The fluid mosaic model of the structure of cell membranes *Science* **175** 720–731

Srivastava A and Olson GE (1996) Studies on [^{3}H]palmitate-binding proteins of rat spermatozoa: a post-translational modification of membrane proteins by fatty acid acylation *Journal of Reproduction and Fertility* **108** 245–251

Sylvester S R, Morales C, Oko R and Griswold MD (1991) Localization of sulphated glycoprotein-2 (clusterin) on spermatozoa and in the reproductive tract of the male rat *Biology of Reproduction* **45** 195–207

Syntin P, Dacheux F, Druant X, Gatti JL, Okamura N and Docheux J-L (1996) Characterization and identification of proteins secreted in the various regions of the adult boar epididymis *Biology of Reproduction* **55** 956–974

Tulsiani DRP, Skudlarek MD, NagDas SK and Orgebin-Crist M-C (1993) Purification and characterization of rat epididymalfluid α-mannosidase: similarities to sperm plasma-membrane α-mannosidase *Biochemical Journal* **290** 427–436

White JM (1992) Membrane fusion *Science* **258** 917–924

Wolf DE and Voglmayr JK (1984) Diffusion and regionalization in membranes of maturing ram spermatozoa *Journal of Cell Biology* **98** 1678–1684

Wolfe CA, James PS, Mackie AR, Ladha S and Jones R (1998) Regionalized lipid diffusion in the plasma membrane of mammalian spermatozoa *Biology of Reproduction* **59** 1506–1514

Yeagle PL (1985) Cholesterol and the cell membrane *Biochimica et Biophysica Acta* **822** 267–278

Yeung CH, Schröter S, Wagenfield A, Kirchloff C, Kliesch S, Poser D, Weinbauer GF, Nieschlag E and Cooper TG (1997) Interaction of the human epididymal protein CD52 (HE5) with epididymal spermatozoa from men and cynomolgus monkeys *Molecular Reproduction and Development* **48** 267–275

Journal of Reproduction and Fertility Supplement **53**, 85–97

Role of luminal fluid glycosyltransferases and glycosidases in the modification of rat sperm plasma membrane glycoproteins during epididymal maturation

D. R. P. Tulsiani, M-C. Orgebin-Crist and M. D. Skudlarek

Center for Reproductive Biology Research and Department of Obstetrics and Gynecology, Vanderbilt University School of Medicine, Nashville, TN 37232–2633, USA

It is generally accepted that mammalian spermatozoa undergo biochemical and morphological changes during epididymal transit, collectively termed epididymal maturation. Although many details of the biochemical modification are not fully understood, lectin binding studies from several laboratories strongly suggest that glycan moieties of sperm plasma membrane glycoproteins are extensively modified as spermatozoa transit from the proximal to the distal epididymis. In the present article, we summarize our studies with two sets of glycan modifying enzymes, namely glycosyltransferases (synthetic enzymes) and glycosidases (hydrolytic enzymes) in rat spermatozoa collected from different regions of the epididymis, and similar enzyme activities present in the epididymal luminal fluid. Our data show that the activities of these enzyme are high in the epididymal luminal fluid (> 80% of the total enzyme activities was in the plasma). Evidence presented in this report also demonstrates that: (1) at least one sperm surface glycoprotein (apparent molecular mass of 86 kDa) is fucosylated *in vitro* when caput spermatozoa are incubated with GDP [^{14}C]fucose; and (2) a peanut agglutinin (PNA)-positive glycoprotein of 135–150 kDa present on plasma membrane of sperm from the caput (but not cauda) epididymidis is degalactosylated by digestion with purified luminal fluid β-D-galactosidase. Taken together, these results strongly suggest a role for glycoprotein modifying enzymes in the modification of sperm surface glycoproteins during epididymal maturation.

Introduction

Mammalian spermatozoa released from the seminiferous tubules and those present within the proximal regions of the epididymis are unable to bind to the zona pellucida (ZP), the extracellular coat that surrounds the oocyte, and fertilize the egg. They acquire progressive motility and fertilizing ability during passage through the epididymis. The maturation process in the epididymis involves several intracellular (Yanagimachi, 1994) and extracellular changes including modification of the sperm plasma membrane proteins by proteolysis (Blobel *et al.*, 1990; Tulsiani *et al.*, 1995a; Jones *et al.*, 1996) and glycan moieties of the sperm surface glycoproteins (Hammerstedt and Parks, 1987; Orgebin-Crist, 1987). Two sets of glycan modifying enzymes, namely glycosyltransferases, which add sugar residues from the nucleotide sugar (donor) to glycolipids and glycoproteins (Fig. 1), and glycosidases, which cleave sugar residues from the existing glycoconjugates (Tulsiani *et al.*, 1998), are present in the epididymal luminal fluid that surrounds spermatozoa (Skudlarek *et al.*, 1993; Tulsiani *et al.*, 1993) and are thought to have an important role. Although many details of these modifications are still not known, lectin binding studies provide evidence that glycan moieties of sperm plasma membrane glycoproteins undergo extensive modifications during epididymal transit. Thus, it has been suggested that glycosyltransferases, in conjunction with glycosidases, may be involved in the alteration of sperm plasma membrane glycoproteins.

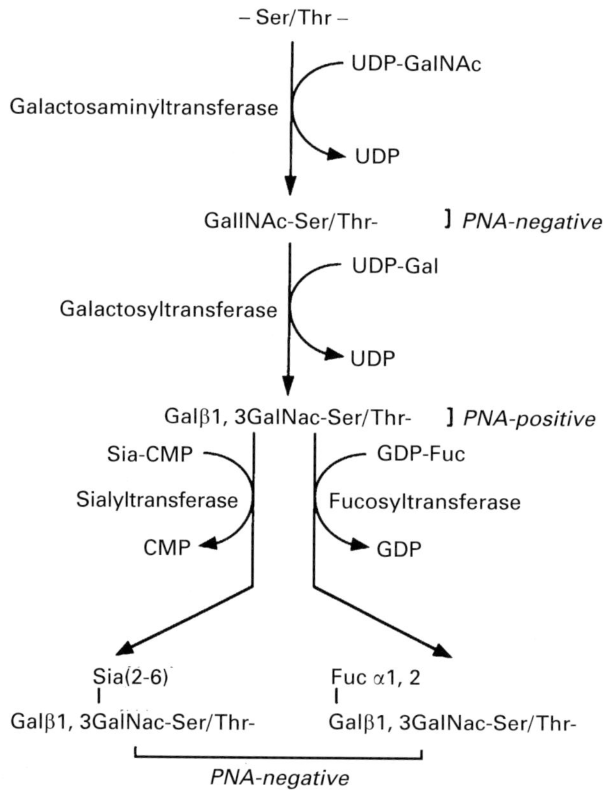

Fig. 1. Biosynthesis of *O*-linked glycoproteins. The *O*-linked glycosylation is catalysed by several glycosyltransferase activities in the lumen of the Golgi apparatus. Frequently, the *N*-acetylgalactosaminyl residue is first added to a specific serine/threonine site of the protein. Additional sugars are added by various glycosyltransferase activities to form a variety of *O*-linked oligosaccharides. The oligosaccharides that have affinity for peanut agglutinin (PNA) are identified. Whether epididymal luminal fluid glycosyltransferases function in a manner similar to the Golgi apparatus transferases is not yet known, nor is it known whether epididymal luminal fluid contains donor sugars (nucleotide sugars).

The purpose of the studies presented in this communication is to: (i) report several glycan modifying enzyme activities associated with spermatozoa from different regions of the epididymis and similar enzyme activities present in soluble form in the epididymal luminal fluid; (ii) present evidence that at least one glycosyltransferase (fucosyltransferase) is functional *in vitro*, and is capable of fucosylating an existing sperm plasma membrane glycoprotein of 86 kDa; and (iii) demonstrate that a peanut agglutinin (PNA)-positive glycoprotein of 135–150 kDa present on caput (but not cauda) sperm plasma membrane can be degalactosylated by digestion *in vitro* of the sperm plasma membrane with purified luminal fluid β-D-galactosidase. Taken together, the evidence suggests a potential role for the glycoprotein modifying enzymes in modification of sperm plasma membrane glycoproteins during epididymal maturation.

Table 1. Glycosyltransferase activities in spermatozoa from rat cauda epididymidis and luminal fluid[a]

Enzyme[b]	pH optimum	Total[c] units	Distribution (%)	
			Spermatozoa	Plasma
Galactosyltransferase	7.0	751 ± 70	11	89
Glucosaminyltransferase	6.8	50 ± 30	12	88
Fucosyltransferase	7.0	348 ± 50	19	81
Sialyltransferase	6.6	5.3 ± 0.6	8	92

[a]The rat distal cauda was flushed with PBS solution (pH 7.4) and the collected fluid was centrifuged at 500 *g* for 10 min. The pelleted spermatozoa were suspended in PBS. Aliquots were used for counting spermatozoa and enzyme assays. The supernatant was freed from the remaining spermatozoa and membranous components by high-speed centrifugation (105 000 *g* for 30 min) and the clear supernatant was used for enzyme assays. [b]All enzymes were assayed as described previously (Tulsiani *et al.*, 1990; Skudlarek *et al.*, 1991; Tulsiani *et al.*, 1993). [c]Values reported are the mean ± SD of 3–4 separate experiments (n = 4 rats per experiment).

Table 2. Glycosidase activities in spermatozoa from the rat cauda epididymidis and luminal fluid[a]

Enzyme[b]	pH optimum	Total[c] units	Distribution (%)	
			Spermatozoa	Plasma
[^{3}H]Gal-β-D-galactosidase	6.8	1710 ± 126	14	86
PNP-β-D-galactosidase	3.5	50 ± 0.6	10	90
PNP-β-D-glucuronidase	5.0	4 ± 0.3	14	86
PNP-α-D-mannosidase	4.4	72 ± 2.2	13	87
PNP-β-*N*-acetylglucosaminidase	4.6	20 ± 0.6	14	86

[a]The luminal contents were recovered from the distal cauda epididymidis by retrograde perfusion with PBS, and the collected fluid was centrifuged at 500 *g* for 10 min. The pelleted spermatozoa and the clear supernatant obtained by high-speed centrifugation (for details see Table 1) were used for enzyme assays. [b]All enzymes were assayed as described by Tulsiani *et al.* (1977); Tulsiani *et al.* (1990); and Skudlarek *et al.* (1993). [c]Values reported are the mean ± SD of 3–4 separate experiments (n = 4 rats per experiment).

Glycosyltransferase and Glycosidase Activities in the Rat Cauda Luminal Fluid and in Spermatozoa

In preliminary studies, we examined the distribution of several glycosyltransferase and glycosidase activities in the epididymal luminal fluid and spermatozoa. The luminal content from the distal cauda epididymidis was obtained by retrograde flushing of the vas deferens with PBS and after centrifugation, aliquots from the supernatant and sperm suspension were assayed for several glycosyltransferase and glycosidase activities at their optimal pH. Data presented in Tables 1 and 2, respectively, show that most of the glycosyltransferase (about 81–92 %) and glycosidase (approximately 90 %) activities in luminal fluid were present in soluble form in the plasma and only 10–19 % of the total enzyme activities were associated with the spermatozoa.

Sperm-associated Glycosyltransferase Activities

The rat epididymis, free of blood vessels and connective tissue and ducti efferenti, was dissected into five regions: proximal (1) and distal (2) caput, corpus (3) and proximal (4) and distal (5) cauda as described in Tulsiani *et al.* (1993). The five regions relate to the epididymal zones described by Reid and Cleland (1957): region 1, zones 1 and 2; region 2, zone 3 and the first half of zone 4; region 3, second half

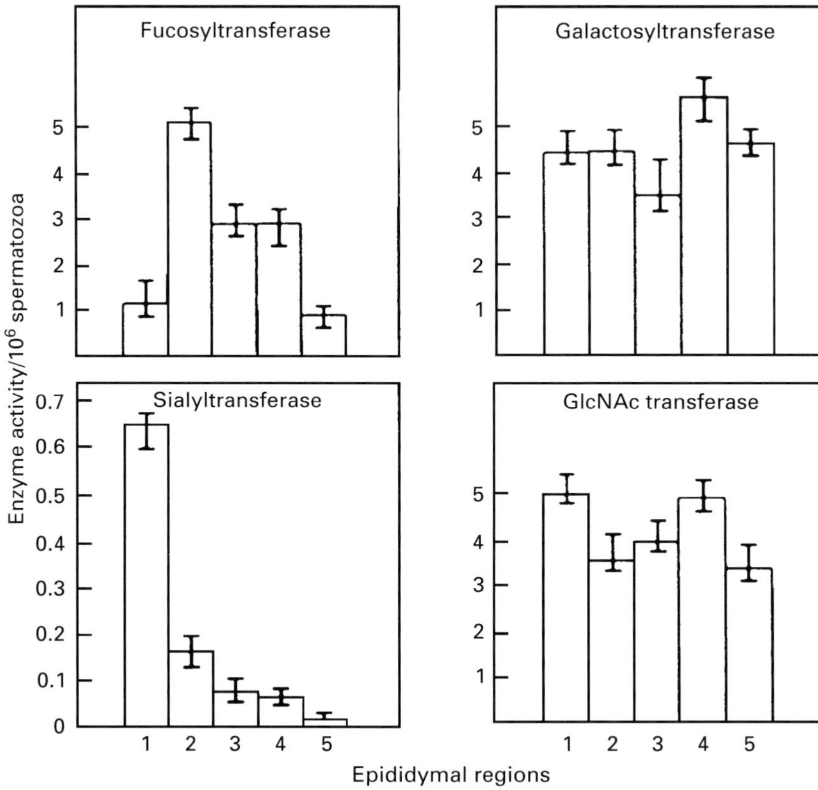

Fig. 2. Sperm-associated glycosyltransferase activities during epididymal maturation. Details of the preparation of rat spermatozoa and assay for enzyme activities are described by Tulsiani *et al.* (1993). Values reported are the mean of 3–4 separate animals, and the vertical bar shows the range in values. The epididymal regions are: (1) proximal caput; (2) distal caput; (3) corpus; (4) proximal cauda; (5) distal cauda. Reproduced with permission from Tulsiani *et al.* (1993).

of zone 4 and zone 5; region 4, zone 6A; and region 5, zone 6B. Each region was placed into a petri dish containing PBS (pH 7.4) and maintained at room temperature. The epididymal regions were minced and the mixture was gently shaken for 10–15 min to release spermatozoa. The cloudy supernatant was removed by aspiration, and centrifuged at 500 *g* for 10 min. The pelleted spermatozoa were gently suspended in PBS, and aliquots were used for counting spermatozoa by haemocytometer as well as for enzyme assay. Of the four glycosyltransferase activities assayed, only sialyltransferase and fucosyltransferase activities displayed maturation-dependent changes (Fig. 2). The former enzyme was several-fold higher in activity than on spermatozoa from the proximal caput, and the latter enzyme showed highest activity in the distal caput. There was a gradual decrease in the activities of these two transferases as the spermatozoa transits from the distal caput to the cauda epididymidis (Fig. 2).

Two lines of evidence strongly suggest that the observed decrease in the two transferase activities is not due to the loss of the cytoplasmic droplets (CDs) during isolation of spermatozoa (Tulsiani *et al.*, 1993). First, the CDs prepared from the caput and cauda spermatozoa showed similar transferase activities: second, the total transferase activities in the CDs were negligible compared with the activities of the enzyme in the spermatozoa (Tulsiani *et al.*, 1993). Taken together, these results allow us to conclude that the decrease in sialyltransferase and fucosyltransferase activities in cauda spermatozoa is not due to the loss of CDs.

It is important to remember that sperm cells are terminally differentiated with no known synthetic capability. Thus a possible explanation for the presence of high sialytransferase and fucosyltransferase activities in the proximal caput spermatozoa and distal caput spermatozoa, respectively, could be the binding of these enzymes from the epididymal luminal fluid to the sugar acceptor sites on the sperm surface glycoproteins and their release following sequential sialylation and fucosylation of these acceptor sites.

Incorporation of [^{14}C]Fucose into Caput Spermatozoa

Attempts were then made to obtain evidence for the presence of sugar acceptor sites on the caput spermatozoa. In these studies, we determined incorporation of radiolabelled fucose from donor sugar (GDP [^{14}C]fucose) into endogenous glycoproteins of the caput spermatozoa. Aliquots from the distal caput sperm suspension were added to the incubation mixture (100 µl) containing 50 mmol 3-[*N*-morpholino]propanesulfonic acid buffer l^{-1}, pH 7.0, 50 mmol NaCl l^{-1}, 5 mmol $MnCl_2$ l^{-1}, 5 mmol AMP l^{-1} and 1µCi of GDP[^{14}C]fucose, and the mixture was incubated at 37 °C for 6 h. After labelling *in vitro*, the spermatozoa were extensively washed to remove free GDP[^{14}C]fucose. Data showed a time-dependent incorporation of radioactive [^{14}C]fucose into caput spermatozoa but not into rat epididymal fluid glycoproteins or blood cells (Tulsiani *et al.*, 1993), suggesting the presence of endogenous [^{14}C]fucose acceptor sites on the caput spermatozoa.

The incorporation of [^{14}C]fucose into endogenous glycoproteins of distal caput spermatozoa increased with increasing concentration of the GDP[^{14}C]fucose or increasing number of the distal caput spermatozoa. By using optimal conditions of nucleotide sugar (1 µCi GDP[^{14}C]fucose), distal caput spermatozoa (5×10^6 cells) and incubation for 6 h at 37 °C, we were able to incorporate 16.1 pmole (about 5000 c.p.m.) of radiolabelled fucose into the endogenous components of the distal caput spermatozoa.

Characterization of [^{14}C]Fucose-labelled Sperm Surface Glycoproteins

The radiolabelled sperm suspension was mixed with an equal volume of double-strength Laemmli buffer (Laemmli, 1970), heated in a boiling water bath for 2–3 min and then centrifuged in a microfuge for 1–2 min. The [^{14}C]fucose-labelled glycopeptides in the supernatant were resolved by SDS-PAGE using denaturing gels consisting of 10–15% (w/v) linear gradients of acrylamide as described by Laemmli (1970), and the resolved components were revealed by autoradiography. When the gel was exposed for 25 days, a single band of 86 kDa was revealed (Fig. 3, lane A). However, longer exposure (47 days) revealed several additional (minor) bands (Fig. 3, lane B).

For identifying the [^{14}C]fucose-labelled glycan, the distal caput spermatozoa were fucosylated by incubation with GDP[^{14}C]fucose at 37 °C for 6 h as described above. The radiolabelled spermatozoa were extensively washed, followed by repeated extraction in 1% (w/v) SDS containing 40 mmol β-mercaptoethanol $l^{-1}$and heat treatment (100 °C for 5 min). The solubilized glycopeptide(s) were then treated with or without *N*-glycanase, an enzyme known to release all *N*-linked glycan moieties (Tarentino *et al.*, 1985). The enzyme treatment caused most of the radioactivity to be released into the ethanol soluble fraction (Tulsiani *et al.*, 1993), a result consistent with the suggestion that the *N*-linked glycan moiety(ies) on sperm glycoprotein is the site of fucosylation.

Glycosidase Activities in Rat Epididymal Luminal Fluid

As stated earlier, the luminal fluid is a rich source of glycosyltransferases as well as glycosidases. Although the former enzymes are optimally functional at the neutral pH (6.6–6.8) of the epididymal lumen, glycosidases are optimally active at acidic pH (3.5–5.0) when assayed using commercially available substrates, *p*-nitrophenyl glycosides or 4-methylumbelliferyl glycosides. To determine whether one of these acid glycosidases, namely β-D-galactosidase, could be functional in the

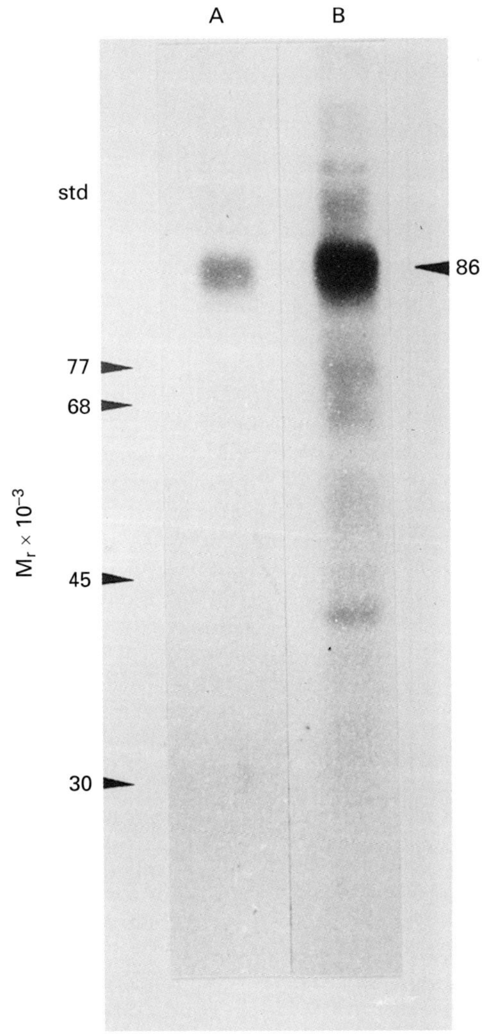

Fig. 3. Electrophoretic resolution of [^{14}C]fucose-labelled sperm proteins by SDS-PAGE. Distal caput spermatozoa (~ 5×10^6 cells) were incubated in a total volume of 0.1 ml containing 50 mmol 3-[*N*-morpholino] propanesulfonic acid buffer l^{-1}(pH 7.0), 50 mmol NaCl l^{-1}, 5 mmol AMP l^{-1} and 1 µCi GDP [^{14}C]fucose. After incubation at 37 °C for 6 h, the labelled spermatozoa were washed with 1 % phosphotungstic acid, 10 % trichloroacetic acid and ethanol–ether as described by Skudlarek *et al.* (1991). The washed spermatozoa were dissolved in 1 % (w/v) SDS containing 40 mmol β-mercaptoethanol $l^{-1}$and then in boiling water for 5 min, followed by centrifugation in a microfuge for 2 min. The supernatant containing approximately 2000 c.p.m. was resolved on a 10–15 % gradient gel under reducing conditions, and the resolved components were revealed by autoradiography. A: exposed for 25 days; B: exposed for 47 days. The positions of prestained standard marker proteins are shown on the left. Reproduced with permission from Tulsiani *et al.* (1993).

physiological pH of the epididymal lumen, we prepared and used a galactose-labelled glycoprotein substrate ([^{3}H]Gal-fetuin). Interestingly, these preliminary studies indicated that the luminal fluid β-D-galactosidase, which optimally cleaves PNP β-D-galactosidase at pH 3.5, shows maximum activity at pH 6.8 when glycoprotein ([^{3}H]Gal-fetuin) was used as a substrate (Skudlarek *et al.*, 1992; Tulsiani *et al.*, 1995). Competition studies indicated that the enzyme is capable of cleaving galactosyl residues present in a variety of linkages found in *O*- and *N*-linked glycan moieties of glycoproteins. Subsequent studies revealed that the luminal fluid β-D-galactosidase exists in two molecular forms, a 97 kDa form and an 84 kDa form (Skudlarek *et al.*, 1992). Despite the difference in their molecular masses, several lines of evidence indicated that the two molecular forms are chemically, catalytically and immunologically similar (Tulsiani *et al.*, 1995b). First, the two forms showed similar K_m values for the PNP β-D-galactoside and glycoprotein substrates. Second, both forms showed pH-dependent substrate preference, optimally cleaving the artificial (PNP-galactoside) substrate at acidic pH (3.5) and glycoprotein substrates at a significantly higher pH. Third, the *N*-terminal sequence analysis gave identical amino acid sequences for the two forms with a 63 % residue identity with the mouse β-D-galactosidase precursor. Fourth, de-*N*-glycosylation of the two forms generated a similar polypeptide of an apparent molecular mass of 70 kDa. Finally the two isoforms crossreacted with the anti-mouse liver β-D-galactosidase antibody. Despite these similarities, the two isoforms contained significantly different total carbohydrate content, and various amounts of high mannose/hybrid-type and complex-type glycans (Tulsiani *et al.*, 1995b). The differences in the *N*-linked glycan chains, as expected, had no detectable effect on the catalytic properties of the two isoforms.

Potential Role of the β-D-Galactosidases in Degalactosylation of Sperm Plasma Membrane Glycoproteins

As stated earlier, the sperm plasma membrane glycoproteins are extensively modified as spermatozoa travel from the caput to the cauda epididymidis. For instance the lectin PNA, which preferentially recognizes the terminal galactosyl residue of Galβ1,3GalNAc linkage found in *0*-linked glycoproteins, binds glycoproteins from rat caput but not from cauda sperm plasma membrane (Srivastava and Olson, 1991). The apparent loss of PNA affinity from the cauda sperm surface glycoprotein could either be due to masking of galactosyl residues, possibly by the addition of other sugar residues by the luminal fluid glycosyltransferases or cleavage of terminal galactosyl residues by the luminal fluid β-D-galactosidase. The availability of purified luminal fluid β-D-galactosidases has allowed us to examine the potential role of the enzymes in modification of PNA binding sperm surface glycoproteins present on the caput (but not cauda) sperm plasma membranes.

In the first set of experiments, the sperm plasma membrane-enriched fractions prepared from the caput and cauda spermatozoa by our published procedures (Tulsiani *et al.*, 1989) were resolved by the SDS-PAGE system of Laemmli carried out under reducing conditions (Laemmli, 1970). The resolved polypeptides were transferred by electrophoresis to a nitrocellulose membrane, and the glycopeptides containing a terminal galactosyl residue on disaccharide Galβ1,3Gal*N*Ac were identified by their ability to bind to peanut agglutinin (PNA) lectin. Data from these studies (Fig. 4) are in general agreement with an earlier report (Srivastava and Olson, 1991) and demonstrate that the PNA binds to several glycoproteins on the caput and cauda sperm plasma membranes. However, whereas a diffused glycopeptide band of an apparent molecular mass of 135–150 kDa could be seen in the caput sperm plasma membranes, the glycopeptide band was not present in the cauda sperm plasma membranes (Fig. 4). These results suggest that the diffused band present on the caput sperm plasma membrane may be modified during sperm maturation.

Next, we attempted to modify the caput sperm surface-specific glycoprotein by treatment of the caput sperm plasma membranes *in vitro* with the purified luminal fluid β-D-galactosidase (97 kDa isoform). In these studies, the salt-washed plasma membrane-rich fraction from rat caput spermatozoa was suspended in 100 mmol sodium cacodylate buffer l^{-1}, pH 6.6, and heat treated (80 °C for 1 h) to inactivate endogenous β-D-galactosidase and protease activities. Aliquots from the heat-treated membrane suspension containing 75 μg of membrane proteins were mixed with the

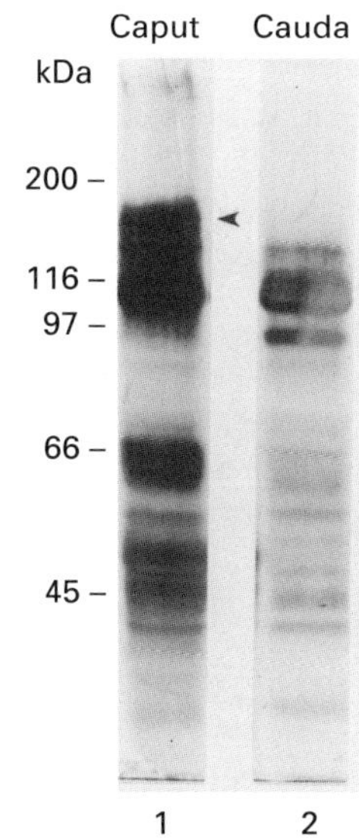

Fig. 4. Lectin (peanut agglutinin, PNA) blot analysis of caput and cauda sperm plasma membranes. Aliquots from the membrane suspension containing 50 μg membrane protein were subjected to electrophoresis on SDS-PAGE (7% acrylamide) under reducing conditions. After transfer to a nitrocellulose paper, the bands were revealed by probing with biotinylated-PNA as described by Tulsiani *et al.* (1995b). Lane 1: caput sperm plasma membrane; lane 2: cauda sperm plasma membrane. The prestained standard marker proteins are shown on the left. The PNA-positive glycoprotein of an apparent molecular mass 135–150 kDa present in the caput (but not cauda) sperm plasma membranes is indicated by the arrowhead. Reproduced with permission from Tulsiani *et al.* (1995b).

purified enzyme (4 units of 97 kDa form) and 10 μl toluene in a total volume of 100 μl and the mixture was incubated at 37 °C. Additional enzyme (4 units) was added after incubation for 4 h and 8 h, and the incubation was continued for 12 h. The reaction was stopped by heat treatment for 10 min and the samples analysed by SDS-PAGE (7% acrylamide gel) under reducing conditions, transferred to nitrocellulose sheets, and the glycoproteins detected by staining with biotinylated-PNA as described by Tulsiani *et al.* (1995b). There was a decrease in the PNA-positive glycoproteins with the time of β-D-galactosidase treatment (Fig. 5). The 135–150 kDa caput sperm plasma membrane-specific glycoprotein is the most sensitive to the β-D-galactosidase treatment, and virtually disappeared after treatment for 12 h. These results suggest a role for the luminal fluid β-D-galactosidase in modification of terminal galactosyl moieties on the sperm plasma membrane glycoproteins.

Potential Consequences of Biochemical Changes in Sperm Membrane Glycoproteins

Although there is extensive literature on epididymal maturation-associated remodelling of sperm plasma membranes (Jones, 1989) and alteration in the oligosaccharide portion of the sperm surface glycoproteins (Hammerstedt and Park, 1987; Orgebin-Crist, 1987; Yanagimachi, 1994), few studies have attempted to elucidate the mechanisms underlying these alterations. The presence of high concentrations of the glycoprotein-modifying enzymes in the epididymal lumen makes them primary candidates for these modifications. It is important to note that glycosyltransferases are synthetic enzymes and are usually associated with the Golgi apparatus where they modify *N*-linked and *O*-linked glycoproteins by transferring sugar residues from the nucleotide sugar (donor) to the sugar acceptor sites on glycan moieties. Since these enzymes are optimally active at neutral pH (Kornfeld and Kornfeld, 1985; Carraway and Hull, 1989), they will be functional at the physiological pH of the epididymal lumen which is thought to be 6.8 (Levine and Kelly, 1978). In contrast, glycosidases are hydrolytic enzymes and are usually present in a bag-like electron dense structure, the lysosome (de Duve, 1969), and are functional in the acidic environment of the lysosome. The hydrolytic enzymes are found in extracellular fluid, such as blood (Tulsiani *et al.*, 1977; Tulsiani and Touster, 1983) and luminal fluid (Skudlarek *et al.*, 1992; Tulsiani *et al.*, 1995b), and are optimally active at acidic pH when assayed with synthetic substrates. Their putative role when present in the physiologically neutral environment has not been elucidated.

It should be noted that only sialyltransferase and fucosyltransferase activities displayed maturation-dependent quantitative changes as spermatozoa transit from the proximal caput to the distal cauda (Fig. 2). A similar maturation-dependent decrease in the activity of sperm-associated fucosyltransferase (Ram *et al.*, 1989) and a lack of change in the activity of galactosyltransferase (Scully *et al.*, 1987) have been reported in mouse spermatozoa. The latter enzyme is thought to have a role in sperm–egg interaction by binding to glycan residues on the mouse ZP3 (Miller *et al.*, 1992). It has been suggested that the inability of immature caput spermatozoa to bind to the zona pellucida and fertilize an egg is due to the binding of galactosyltransferase inhibitor to the sperm surface enzyme and preventing it from recognizing the complementary glycan moieties (Macek and Shur, 1988).

Fucosyltransferase has been reported in the mouse germ cells, and is apparently involved in stage-specific fucosylation of the mouse pachytene spermatocytes and round spermatids (Gerton and Millette, 1986; Fenderson *et al.*, 1984; Cardullo *et al.*, 1989). These germ cells in culture incorporate [^{14}C]fucose into at least six common glycoproteins. In addition, eight sperm surface glycoproteins were reported to be fucosylated only in pachytene spermatocytes. These data suggest that a number of germ cell surface glycoproteins are fucosylated during spermatogenesis.

The studies *in vitro* presented here demonstrate that at least one more sperm surface glycoprotein can be fucosylated in the distal caput epididymidis. The fact that [^{14}C]fucose can be incorporated into spermatozoa *in vitro* suggests the presence of fucosyl acceptor components on these cells. Although the [^{14}C]fucose can be incorporated into the spermatozoa from all regions of the epididymis, the distal caput spermatozoa routinely showed highest labelling (Tulsiani *et al.*, 1993). The fact that radiolabelled fucose was incorporated into a major glycoprotein of apparent molecular mass of 86 kDa and several minor glycoproteins of the caput spermatozoa or sperm plasma membranes *in vitro*, and that *N*-linked glycan moiety(ies) on the 86 kDa glycoprotein is the site of fucosylation, allow us to suggest that the testicular spermatozoa are additionally fucosylated in the distal caput epididymidis.

In addition to the proposed role for the luminal fluid fucosyltransferase, β1,4 galactosyltransferase (UDP-galactose:*N*-acetylglucosamine galactosyltransferase) has a role in the galactosylation of sperm surface glycoprotein during epididymal maturation (Hamilton and Gould, 1982; Hamilton *et al.*, 1986). Ram and bull testicular spermatozoa carry low negative charge on entering the epididymis (Yanagimachi, 1994; Bedford, 1963; Holt, 1980; Hammerstedt *et al.*, 1982). However, the net negative charge increases as spermatozoa transit from the proximal to the distal epididymis. The increase in negative charge during epididymal maturation may be due to sialylation of sperm surface components (Holt, 1980). On the basis of sperm-associated sialyltransferase activities (Fig. 2), it is possible that the sialylation of rat sperm plasma membrane glycoproteins begins in the proximal caput epididymis. Additional studies are needed to confirm the precise site of sialylation.

In considering the fucosylation of sperm surface glycoproteins *in vitro*, it is important to comment on the availability of donor sugar (GDP-fucose) in the epididymal luminal fluid. For fucosylation, it is necessary to have fucosyltransferase, fucose acceptor site(s) on sperm surface glycoproteins, and the sugar donor. In this report, we have demonstrated the presence of sperm-associated enzyme and the fucose acceptor site(s). Whether epididymal luminal fluid contains GDP-fucose is not yet known.

As shown in Table 2, epididymal luminal fluid contains several glycosidases with catalytic and immunological properties similar to the hydrolytic enzymes present within lysosomes. These exo-enzymes catalyse hydrolytic cleavage of terminal sugar residues from the glycan portion of glycolipids and glycoproteins (Conzelman and Sandhoff, 1987). The hydrolytic enzymes are most often assayed using synthetic substrates (PNP-glycosides) which are optimally hydrolysed at acidic pH. Relatively few studies have compared the hydrolysis of the synthetic and natural (glycoproteins/glycan) substrates which suggests that the latter substrates are optimally cleaved at a slightly higher pH (Opheim and Touster, 1978; Tulsiani and Touster, 1978; and Tulsiani *et al.*, 1988). Thus, it was surprising to see a strikingly different pH-dependent substrate preference by purified luminal fluid β-D-galactosidase (pH optimum 3.5 with PNP-galactoside versus pH optimum 6.8 with [^{3}H]Gal-fetuin). It is important to mention that epididymal luminal fluid β-D-galactosidase undergoes pH-dependent association–dissociation (Tulsiani *et al.*, 1995b). In the epididymal lumen where pH is 6.6–6.8 (Levine and Kelly, 1978), the enzyme probably occurs in dissociated (monomeric and dimeric) forms. Thus, it is reasonable to suggest that the β-D-galactosidase undergoes pH-dependent conformational changes under conditions *in vivo*, and is mainly active towards the glycoprotein substrates.

We studied the action of luminal fluid β-D-galactosidase on sperm glycoproteins by first confirming an earlier report (Srivastava and Olson, 1991) suggesting that the caput sperm plasma membranes have a PNA-positive glycoprotein which is not present on the cauda sperm plasma membranes. Since the modification of the carbohydrate moieties during epididymal transit may be important for developing functionally mature spermatozoa, it was important to determine whether the PNA-positive caput sperm plasma membrane glycoproteins can be degalactosylated by digestion *in vitro* with purified luminal fluid β-D-galactosidase. Indeed, the enzyme treatment resulted in a gradual and preferential disappearance (degalactosylation) of the 135–150 kDa PNA-positive band (Fig. 5).

We do not know whether the fucosylation of 86 kDa glycoprotein or degalactosylation of 135–150 kDa glycoproteins in the caput spermatozoa are important for sperm function. It will be important to characterize these glycoproteins chemically, examine their localization, and functional role in sperm–egg interaction/fusion. Nonetheless, these studies demonstrate potential roles of luminal fluid fucosyltransferase and β-D-galactosidase in the modification of sperm surface glycoproteins during sperm maturation.

Finally, it is important to mention that the maturation-associated alterations of sperm plasma membrane are not limited to the effects of glycan modifying enzymes alone. In recent years, there have been reports that several sperm surface molecules are modified by proteolytic processing. For example, rat sperm plasma membrane mannosidase is synthesized in the testis in an enzymatically inactive or less active precursor form of 135 kDa which is proteolytically processed to an enzymatically active mature form of 115 kDa during development in the testis and maturation in the epididymis (Tulsiani *et al.*, 1995a). Similarly, guinea-pig sperm plasma membrane proteins PH 20 and PH 30 (Phelps *et al.*, 1991), mouse sperm antigen M42 (Lakoski *et al.*, 1988), rat sperm glycoprotein CE9 (Pertruszak *et al.*, 1991), and antigen 2B1 (Jones *et al.*, 1996) undergo proteolysis during sperm maturation. In addition to the modification of sperm plasma membrane proteins/glycoproteins, spermatozoa undergo intra-acrosomal modifications of several acrosomal enzymes including β-D-galactosidase (Skudlarek *et al.*, 1993), α-L fucosidase (Hancock *et al.*, 1993), acrosin (Nagdas *et al.*, 1992) and acrogranin (Anakwe and Gerton, 1990). Thus it seems likely that processing of sperm surface molecules and intra-acrosomal components is important in development of functionally mature spermatozoa.

Conclusion

Spermatozoa are produced by a complex set of morphological and biochemical differentiation events from proliferating diploid germ cells to haploid cells in the testes. Mammalian spermatozoa, as they leave the testis, are unable to fertilize an egg. They undergo modifications during epididymal

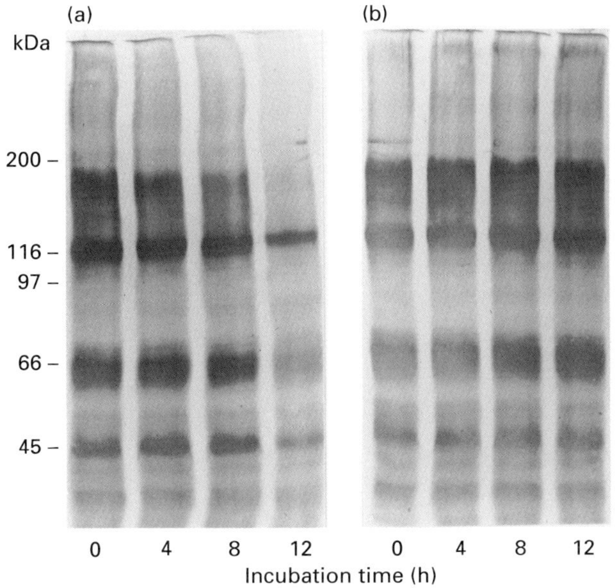

Fig. 5. Degalactosylation of caput sperm plasma membrane glycoproteins with the purified luminal fluid β-D-galactosidase. Rat caput sperm plasma membranes in 100 mmol sodium cacodylate buffer l^{-1} were heat treated (80 °C for 1 h) to inactivate any protease activities. Aliquots from the mixture containing 50 µg membrane proteins were mixed with (a) or without (b) purified β-D-galactosidase as described by Tulsiani *et al.* (1995b). At the indicated time intervals, the reaction was stopped by heat treatment, and the samples were processed by SDS-PAGE (under reducing conditions). The resolved polypeptides were transferred to a nitrocellulose sheet and the bands revealed by lectin (peanut agglutinin, PNA) blot. The position of standard marker proteins is shown on the left. Note a decrease in caput specific PNA-positive glycoproteins and disappearance of the 135–150 kDa band after treatment for 12 h with β-galactosidase. Reproduced with permission from Tulsiani *et al.* (1995b).

maturation. This article presents our *in vitro* studies in support of a putative role for the glycan modifying enzymes, glycosyltransferases and glycosidases, in the modification of sperm surface glycoproteins during epididymal maturation. From the discussion in this review, it is obvious that the maturation process reflects multiple extracellular (sperm surface) and intra-acrosomal modifications. Understanding the *in vivo* significance of these modifications during development of functionally mature spermatozoa awaits new approaches and development of sensitive methods for detection of nucleotide sugars in the luminal fluid and carbohydrate residues on sperm plasma membrane glycoproteins. An understanding of the maturation-associated modifications will allow new strategies for regulation of fertility.

The authors acknowledge the contribution of M. Holland and Y. Araki in some phases of these studies. We are indebted to Ms. Lynne Black for editorial assistance. Supported in part by grants HD 25869, HD 34041, HD 03820 and HD 05797 from the National Institute of Child Health and Human Development.

References

Anakwe OO and Gerton GL (1990) Acrosome biogenesis begins during meiosis: evidence from the synthesis and distribution of an acrosomal glycoprotein, acrogranin, during guinea pig spermatogenesis *Biology of Reproduction* **42** 317–328

Bedford JM (1963) Changes in electrophoretic properties of rabbit spermatozoa during passage through epididymis *Nature* **200** 1178–1180

Blobel CP, Myles DG, Primakoff P and White JM (1990) Proteolytic processing of a protein involved in sperm–egg fusion correlates with acquisition of fertilization competence *Journal of Cell Biology* **111** 69–78

Cardullo RA, Armant DR and Millette CF (1989) Characterization of fucosyltransferase activity during mouse spermatogenesis: evidence for a cell surface fucosyltransferase *Biochemistry* **28** 1611–1617

Carraway KL and Hull SR (1989) *O*-glycosylation pathway for mucin-type glycoproteins *Bioassay* **10** 117–121

Conzelman E and Sandhoff K (1987) Glycolipid and glycoprotein degradation *Advances in Enzymology and Related Areas of Molecular Biology* **60** 215–235

deDuve C (1963) The lysosome *Scientific American* **208** 64–72

Fenderson BA, O'Brien DA, Millette CF and Eddy EM (1984) Stage-specific expression of three cell surface antigens during murine spermatogenesis detected with monoclonal antibody *Developmental Biology* **103** 117–128

Gerton GL and Millette CL (1986) Stage-specific synthesis and fucosylation of plasma membrane proteins by mouse pachytene spermatocytes and round spermatids in culture *Biology of Reproduction* **35** 1025–1035

Hamilton DW and Gould RP (1982) Preliminary observation on enzymatic galactosylation of glycoproteins on the surface rat caput epididymal spermatozoa *International Journal of Andrology* **5** 73–80

Hamilton DW, Wenstrom JC and Baker JB (1986) Membrane glycoprotein from spermatozoa: partial characterization of an integral Mr = 24000 molecule from rat spermatozoa that is glycosylated during epididymal maturation *Biology of Reproduction* **34** 925–936

Hammerstedt RH and Park JE (1987) Changes in sperm surface associated with epididymal transit *Journal of Reproduction and Fertility* **34** 133–149

Hammerstedt RH, Hay CR and Amann RP (1982) Modification of ram sperm membranes during epididymal transit *Biology of Reproduction* **27** 745–754

Hancock LW, Raab LS and Aronson NN, Jr (1993) Synthesis and processing of rat sperm associated α-fucosidase *Biology of Reproduction* **48** 1228–1238

Holt WY (1980) Surface-bound sialic acid on ram and bull spermatozoa: deposition during epididymal transit and stability during washing *Biology of Reproduction* **23** 847–857

Jones R (1989) Membrane remodeling during sperm maturation in the epididymis *Oxford Reviews of Reproductive Biology* 285–337

Jones R, Ma A, Hous ST, Shalgi R, and Hall L (1996) Testicular biosynthesis and epididymal endoproteolytic processing of rat sperm surface antigen 2B1 *Journal of Cell Science* **109** 2561–2570

Kornfeld S and Kornfeld R (1985) Assembly of asparagine-linked oligosaccharides *Annual Reviews of Biochemistry* **54** 631–664

Laemmli UK (1970) Cleavage of structural proteins during the assembly of the head of bacteriophage T_4 *Nature* **227** 680–685

Lakoski KA, Carron CP, Cabot CL and Saling PM (1988) Epididymal maturation and the acrosome reaction in mouse sperm: response to zona pellucida develops coincident with modification of M42 antigen *Biology of Reproduction* **38** 221–233

Levine N and Kelly H (1978) Measurement of pH in the rat epididymis *in vivo*. *Journal of Reproduction and Fertility* **52** 333–335

Macek MD and Shur BD (1988) Protein–carbohydrate complementarity in mammalian gamete recognition *Gamete Research* **20** 93–109

Miller DJ, Macek MD and Shur BD (1992) Complementarity between sperm surface β 1,4–galactosyltransferase and egg-coat ZP3 mediates sperm–egg binding *Nature* **357** 589–592

Nagdas SK, Skudlarek MD, Orgebin-Crist M-C and Tulsiani DRP (1992) Biochemical alteration in proacrosin–acrosin system during epididymal maturation of the rat spermatozoa *Journal of Andrology* **13** 36–43

Opheim DJ and Touster O (1978) Lysosomal α-D-mannosidase of rat liver: purification and comparison with Golgi and cytosolic α-D-mannosidases *Journal of Biological Chemistry* **253** 1017–1023

Orgebin-Crist M-C (1987) Post-testicular development of mammalian spermatozoa. In *Morphological Basis of Human Reproduction Function Acta Medicine* pp 115–174. Plenum Press, New York

Patruszak JAM, Nehme CL and Bartles JR (1991) Endoproteolytic cleavage in the extracellular domain of the integral plasma membrane protein CE9 precedes its redistribution from the posterior to the anterior tail of the rat spermatozoa during epididymal maturation *Journal of Cell Biology* **114** 917–927

Phelps BM, Koppel DE, Primakoff P and Myles DG (1991) Evidence that proteolysis of the surface is an initial step in the mechanisms of formation of sperm surface domains *Journal of Cell Biology* **111** 1839–1847

Ram PA, Cardullo RA and Millette CF (1989) Expression and topographical localization of cell surface fucosyl-transferase activity during epididymal sperm maturation in the mouse *Gamete Research* **22** 321–332

Reid BL and Cleland KW (1957) The structure and function of the epididymis. 1. The histology of the rat epididymis *Australian Journal of Zoology* **5** 223–246

Skudlarek MD, Orgebin-Crist M-C and Tulsiani DRP (1991) Asparagine-linked glycoprotein biosynthesis in rat epididymis: presence of a mannosidase II-like enzyme *Biochemical Journal* **277** 213–221

Skudlarek MD, Tulsiani DRP and Orgebin Crist M-C (1992) Rat epididymal luminal fluid acid β-D-galactosidase optimally hydrolyses glycoprotein substrate at neutral pH *Biochemical Journal* **286** 907–914

Skudlarek MD, Tulsiani DRP, Nagdas SK and Orgebin-Crist M-C (1993) β-D-Galactosidase of rat spermatozoa: subcellular distribution, substrate specificity and molecular changes during epididymal maturation *Biology of Reproduction* **49** 204–213

Scully NF, Shapher JH and Shur BD (1988) Spatial and temporal expression of cell surface galactosyltransferase during mouse spermatogenesis and epididymal maturation *Developmental Biology* **124** 111–124

Srivastava A and Olson GE (1991) Glycoprotein changes in the rat sperm plasma membrane during maturation in the epididymis *Molecular Reproduction and Development* **29** 357–364

Tarentino AL, Gomez CM and Plummer TH, Jr (1985) Deglycosylation of asparagine-linked glycans by peptide: *N*-glycosidase F *Biochemistry* **24** 4665–4671

Tulsiani DRP and Touster O (1983) Swainsonine, a potent mannosidase inhibitor, elevates rat liver and brain lysosomal α-D-mannosidase, decreases Golgi α-D-mannosidase II, and increases the plasma levels of several acid hydrolases *Archives of Biochemistry and Biophysics* **224** 594–600

Tulsiani DRP and Touster O (1987) Substrate specificities of rat kidney lysosomal and cytosolic α-D-mannosidase and effects of swainsonine suggests a role of the cytosolic enzyme in glycoprotein catabolism *Journal of Biological Chemistry* **262** 6506–6514

Tulsiani DRP, Buschiazzo HO, Tolbert B and Touster O (1977) Changes in plasma hydrolase activities in hereditary and streptozotocin-induced diabetes *Archives of Biochemistry and Biophysics* **181** 216–227

Tulsiani DRP, Coleman VD and Touster O (1988) Rat epididymal α-D-mannosidase: purification, carbohydrate composition, substrate specificity, and antibody production *Archives of Biochemistry and Biophysics* **267** 60–68

Tulsiani DRP, Skudlarek MD and Orgebin-Crist M-C (1989) Novel α-D-mannosidase of rat sperm plasma membranes: characterization and potential role in sperm–egg interaction *Journal of Cell Biology* **109** 1257–1267

Tulsiani DRP, Skudlarek MD and Orgebin-Crist M-C (1990) Human sperm plasma membranes possess α-D-mannosidase activity but no galactosyltransferase activity *Biology of Reproduction* **42** 843–858

Tulsiani DRP, Skudlarek MD, Holland MK and Orgebin-Crist M-C (1993) Glycosylation of rat sperm plasma membranes during epididymal maturation *Biology of Reproduction* **48** 417–428

Tulsiani DRP, Nagas SK, Skudlarek MD and Orgebin-Crist M-C (1995a) Rat sperm plasma membrane mannosidase: localization and evidence for proteolytic processing during epididymal maturation *Developmental Biology* **167** 584–595

Tulsiani DRP, Skudlarek MD, Araki Y and Orgebin-Crist M-C (1995b) Purification and characterization of two forms of β-D-galactosidase from rat epididymal luminal fluid: evidence for their role in the modification of sperm plasma membrane glycoprotein(s) *Biochemical Journal* **305** 41–50

Tulsiani DRP, Abou-Haila A, Loeser CR and Pereira BMJ (1998) The biological and functional significance of the sperm acrosome and acrosomal enzymes in mammalian fertilization *Experimental Cell Research* **240** 151–164

Yanagimachi R (1994) Mammalian fertilization. In *The Physiology of Reproduction* pp 189–317 Eds E Knobil and JD Neill. Raven Press, New York

Journal of Reproduction and Fertility Supplement **53**, 99–107

Role of epididymal secretory proteins in sperm maturation with particular reference to the boar

J-L. Dacheux[1], X. Druart[1], S. Fouchecourt[1], P. Syntin[1], J-L. Gatti[1], N. Okamura[2] and F. Dacheux[1]

[1]*URA 1291 INRA-CNRS, Institut National de la Recherche Agronomique, Station de Physiologie de la Reproduction des Mammifères Domestiques, 37380 Monnaie, France; and*
[2]*Institute of Basic Medical Sciences, University of Tsukuba, Tsukuba, Ibaraki, 305, Japan*

This review considers the role of proteins secreted by the epididymis on post-testicular sperm maturation and storage. Two-dimensional gels show that 150 to 200 proteins are secreted into the epididymal lumen. Most are secreted in relatively small amounts; in rams, for example, fewer than ten contribute 90% of the total secretion and only two contribute 52% of the total protein secreted. Most of the proteins are confined to specific regions of the epididymis. The changing pattern of protein secretion along the epididymis corresponds to change in surface protein on spermatozoa, but no epididymal proteins have been identified that appear to be directly involved in modifying the sperm membrane. Most of the major proteins that have been identified seem to be playing a homeostatic role in maintaining the epididymal milieu for spermatozoa.

Introduction

Mammalian spermatozoa are the result of extensive cellular differentiation of spherical spermatids to become highly polarized and fully motile cells. Complex biochemical, physiological and morphological events take place in the testis during spermiogenesis and also during transit through the epididymis, where spermatozoa develop the capacity to fertilize eggs. Control of these cellular events involves numerous interactions between somatic cells and germ cells but the process is still poorly understood. Events in the testis are under the genomic regulation of the gamete, but when DNA begins to condense in the elongated spermatids, the transcription process in the germinal DNA decreases and then stops. The external milieu of the gamete is, therefore, believed to play an essential role during the subsequent differentiation stages both in the testis and the epididymis. Consequently, the functional integrity of the epididymal epithelium which maintains the epididymal milieu is essential for the production of fertile spermatozoa .

The nature of the interactions in the testis and in the epididymis are not fully understood. Some interactions, such as supply of energy substrates, external ionic environment for correct membrane potential, oxygen availability and elimination of metabolic residues of germ cells are linked to the preservation of the vital functions of the gametes. More specific interactions such as the development of a mature plasma membrane are involved in the induction or control of gamete differentiation. Among the various factors that are potentially involved, protein components are suspected of having an important role in the interactions between gametes and somatic cells. Although much information is available on epididymal secreted proteins in mammals, their role and importance in sperm physiology needs to be established more fully, particularly the role they play in membrane modifications involved in sperm maturation and fertilizing ability, and sperm survival during epididymal storage.

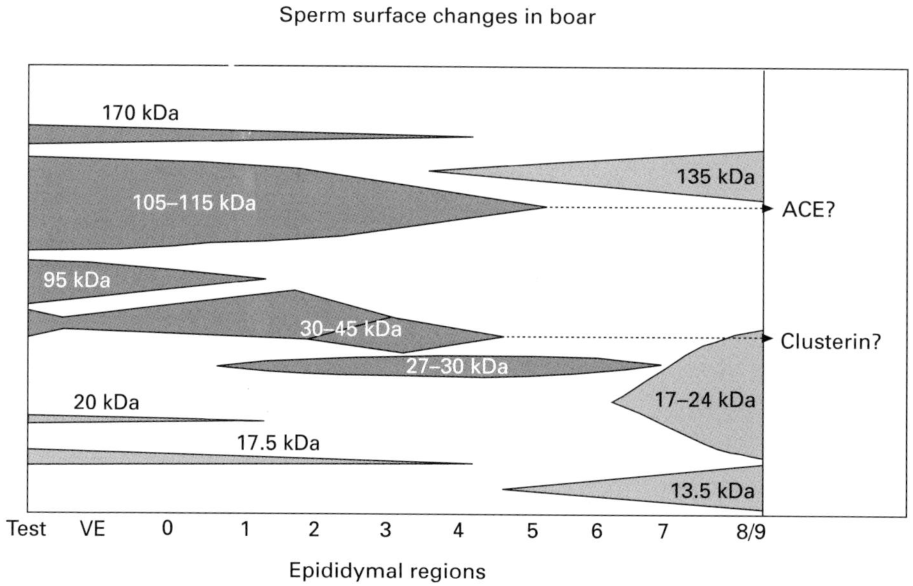

Fig.1. Distribution of major radiolabelled surface proteins of boar spermatozoa taken from different regions of the epididymis. Intensities of labelling have been estimated after one-dimensional electrophoresis separation (adapted from Dacheux *et al.*, 1989). Test, testis; VE, efferent ducts ; 0–8/9, epididymal regions; 0–4, caput epididymidis; 5–6, corpus epididymidis; 7–8/9, cauda epididymidis. ACE: angiotensin-converting enzyme.

Epididymal Sperm Maturation: Final Stages of Spermatogenesis

During epididymal transit, the sperm plasma membrane undergoes intense changes both in protein composition and in the distribution of specific protein. Considerable information is available concerning sperm surface changes during epididymal maturation. In all species that have been studied, specific surface proteins present on testicular spermatozoa are removed or modified during transit through the epididymis. This has been well illustrated by studies using radiolabelling to determine surface changes of the whole sperm population. In boars, most changes occur in the proximal region of the epididymis (Fig. 1). However, different testicular sperm proteins are modified in different regions of the epididymis. For example, in the ram and boar epididymis, a 95 kDa protein is no longer detected when spermatozoa enter in the proximal caput epididymidis, whereas a 105–115 kDa testicular sperm protein is not detected on the surface only when the spermatozoa reach the distal caput epididymis (Dacheux *et al.*, 1989; Dacheux and Voglmayr, 1983).

The sequential disappearance of testicular proteins on the sperm surface is thus a specific process that depends on the epididymal region but also on the sensitivity of the sperm membrane protein to be processed by specific proteases. Several testicular sperm surface proteins have been characterized and identified. For some, their disappearance from the sperm surface is clearly related to a specific endoproteolytic mechanism during epididymal transit. In guinea-pigs two sperm surface glycoproteins, PH20 and PH30, undergo several proteolytic cleavages. PH20 is first reduced from 66 kDa to 64 kDa and then cleaved into two fragments of 41 kDa and 27 kDa (Phelps *et al.*, 1990; Primakoff *et al.*, 1988; Jones *et al.*, 1996). PH30, consisting of two dimeric complexes, of 88 and 48 kDa, is also processed in the epididymis into two subunits of 48 and 28 kDa (Blobel *et al.*, 1990). In rats, a 40–48 kDa membrane protein (CE9) is cleaved into a 23–33 kDa epididymal form (Petruszak *et al.*, 1991) and a 135 kDa testicular plasma membrane promannosidase is converted into a 115 kDa enzymatically active form during sperm maturation (Tulsiani *et al.*, 1995).

For most of these proteins, part of the molecule remains in or on the membrane, but for others, such as the 105 kDa protein in boars, rams and horses, endoproteolysis liberates the protein from the surface (Gatti *et al.*, 1998).

As several surface proteins disappear from spermatozoa during epididymal transit or are being processed, several new antigens can be identified on the spermatozoa . Some of these associations are transitory, but several, mostly with a low molecular weight, are still present in the distal part of the epididymis. These new components originate from epididymal secretions. Much information about similarity between sperm membrane proteins and epididymal secretions is available for several species (Shabonowitz and Killian, 1987; Dacheux *et al.*, 1989; Chatterjee *et al.*, 1989; Cornwall *et al.*, 1990; Robitaille *et al.*, 1991). However, protein identities and the degree of similarity between the sperm surface component and the epididymal protein has rarely been established. The first has recently been described in rats, in which a sperm plasma membrane component has been found to be identical to an epididymal fluid-secreted protein (protein E) which belongs to the CRISP family of proteins (Cysteine-Rich Secretory protein) (Xu *et al.*, 1997).

The changes in the protein composition of the sperm membrane are often associated with the movement of the proteins into the different domains of the sperm surface that are established during spermatogenesis (Jones, 1989). This movement of surface proteins between domains occurs as the sperm travel through the epididymis. This phenomenon occurs for most of the surface components that are processed post-testicularly and also for some new surface components originating from epididymal fluid, such as a 135 kDa antigen relocated in the equatorial segment of boar spermatozoa (Okamura *et al.*, 1995a).

The relationship between sperm membrane maturation and the physiological changes in the spermatozoa are still not fully established. The presence or absence of definite antigens has often been correlated with a sperm property such as recognition and binding to the zona pellucida and perivitelline membrane of the oocyte or with initiation of sperm movement. However all molecular mechanisms have not been established.

The factors that control post-testicular sperm differentiation are linked to the presence of a specific environment in the epididymal milieu. To our knowledge, maturation of testicular spermatozoa has never been achieved under conditions *in vitro*. Epididymal sperm maturation appears to be the result of a pattern of sequential events that occurs only in consecutive epididymal regions.

Epididymal Secretory Proteins: Spatial Specificity

Among the different metabolic activities of the epididymal epithelium, the synthesis and secretion of proteins are probably the most important (Brooks, 1981). During the last ten years, a considerable amount of information has become available about the proteins secreted by the epididymis. The number of proteins secreted as estimated by electrophoresis is about several hundred for all mammalian species. Furthermore, for most of these compounds, several isoforms are secreted according to the epididymal region (Olson and Hinton, 1985; Syntin *et al.*, 1996). Two-dimensional electrophoresis patterns of secreted epididymal proteins provide a relatively complex map (Fig. 2). Most of the proteins are secreted in specific regions of the epididymis. The anterior region is the most active as estimated by the incorporation of radioactive methionine into the secreted proteins in all of the species studied (Del-Rio, 1979; Chaturapanich *et al.*, 1992; Jones and Clulow, 1994; Syntin *et al.*, 1996). In rams, boars and horses, protein secretion in this anterior part represents about 80% of the total protein secreted by the epididymis (Syntin *et al.*, 1996).

Several proteins are secreted in relatively large amounts and they represent most of the proteins secreted. In rams, among the one hundred proteins that have been identified by electrophoresis, fewer than 15 represent 90% of the total protein secreted, and two represent 52% of the protein secreted (Druart *et al.*, 1998). Similar results have been obtained in other species such as boars (Fig. 3).

Some secreted epididymal proteins have been identified either by purification or using molecular methods. Many of them, such as clusterin, GPX, lactoferrin, E-RABP, osidases (hexosaminidase, mannosidase or galactosidase), cholesterol transferase protein/HE1 and

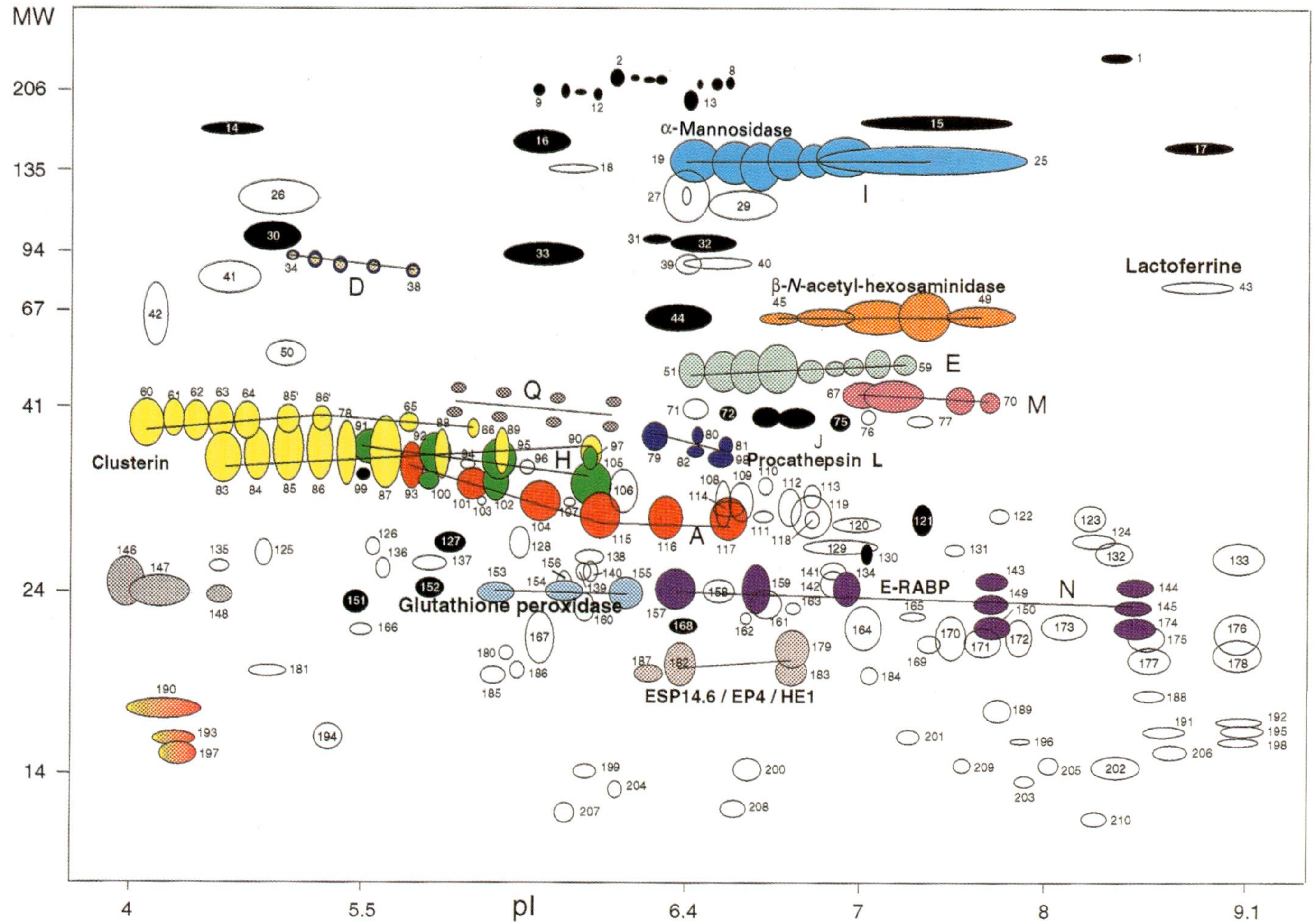

Fig. 2. Computer simulated diagram showing the location on a two-dimensional gel of proteins secreted by all regions of the epididymis of the boar. The diagram was determined by compiling information from two-dimensional gels of each of the epididymal regions on the abscissa of Fig. 3. The largest spots were reduced for better visualization of the other spots, and spots secreted outside the tubule are presented in black. Spots with the same colour belong to the same train (adapted from Syntin *et al.*, 1996).

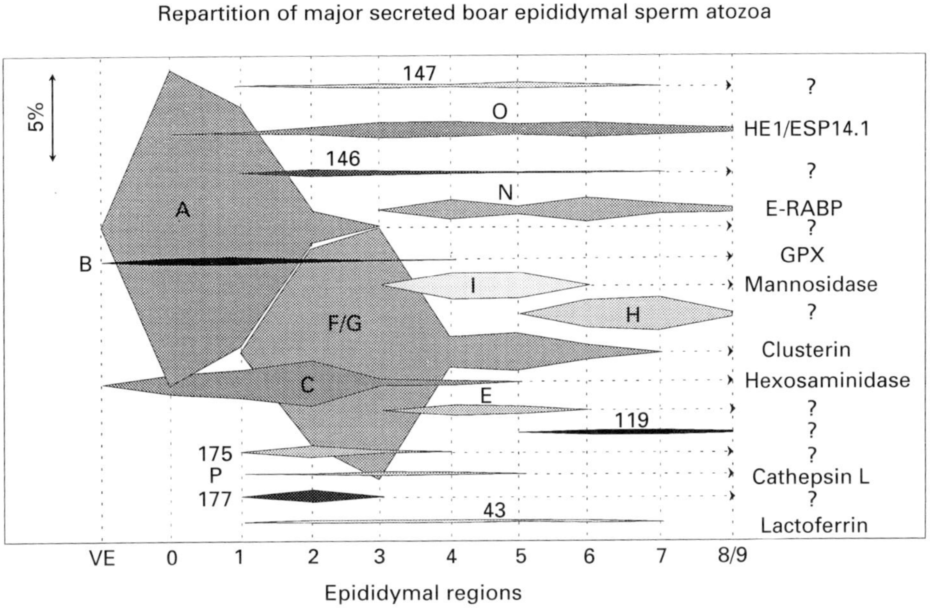

Fig. 3. Diagram showing the relative amount of some of the major proteins secreted by different regions of the epididymis of the boar. Protein secretion was determined by incubating sections of the epididymis *in vitro* and determining incorporation of [^{35}S]methionine. Amounts of protein secreted are expressed as a percentage of the total labelled protein which was secreted into the incubation medium. The values and identification numbers and letters are those used in Syntin *et al.*, 1996 and are the same as those used in Fig. 2.

prostaglandin D_2 synthase are present in almost all of the species studied (Syntin *et al.*, 1996; Druart *et al.*, 1994). There is also similarity among these proteins in terms of the change in their concentration in the lumen of the epididymal duct, the luminal concentration being a balance between secretion, reabsorption and degradation rates.

Several epididymal regions can therefore be defined by the species and the amount of protein secretion and concentration profile, each region being comparable between species. In domestic animals such as rams or horses, secretion in the proximal caput epididymis is characterized by glutathione peroxidase, clusterin and PGDS, and secretion in the distal caput epididymis and the corpus epididymis are characterized by clusterin, lactoferrin, osidase, retinol acid binding protein (RABP) and CTP/HE1-like secretions (Druart *et al.*, 1998; S. Fouchécourt, S. Metayer and J. L. Dacheux, unpublished).

From the data about epididymal proteins from different species, it appears that similar compounds are found in the same epididymal regions, suggesting that there may be a general pattern of secretion in mammals.

Epididymal Secretory Proteins and Sperm Maturation

The maturation of spermatozoa during epididymal transit is the result of a pattern of events probably controlled by epididymal activity. If there is such control, interactions between spermatozoa and epididymis should be mediated by sequential changes in the composition of the epididymal fluid. According to this hypothesis, correlating changes on the spermatozoa and changes in protein composition of the fluid should provide a way of determining the nature of the epididymal events that lead to sperm differentiation. Thus, for determining and understanding the origin of sperm differentiation, two approaches seem to be valuable and complementary: from the known sperm modifications it should be possible to interpret epididymal factors responsible for these modifications, and from the known protein changes in the fluid along the epididymis, it should be possible to deduce the sperm transformations induced by the proteins.

In the first approach, major sperm modifications in the epididymis are due mostly to the modifications of the surface of testicular spermatozoa. Most of the changes appear to be related to protease activation either on the sperm surface or in the epididymal fluid. Proteolytic enzymes such as procathepsin L, a lysosomal precursor of a highly active protease secreted in the distal caput epididymidis (Okamura *et al.*, 1995b), and ACE (Vanha-Pertulla *et al.*, 1985; Gatti *et al.*, 1998) have already been described in the epididymal fluid (Tomomasa *et al.*, 1994). However, strong inhibitors of these activities, such as α_2-macroglobulin, cystatin C and serine protease inhibitors, are also present in the fluid where proteolytic enzymes are detected (Cornwall *et al.*, 1992; Perry *et al.*, 1993b; Peloille *et al.*, 1997). A difference in concentration of an enzyme and its inhibitor may determine its proteolytic activity *in situ*. Serine protease activity has been involved in endoproteolysis of PH20, PH30 and CE9 (Jones *et al.*, 1996; Lum and Blobel, 1997), and in the secretase that liberates ACE from the sperm membrane (Gatti *et al.*, 1998). However, to date, no specific serine protease has been identified. The enzymes, which probably have high specificity toward their substrates, are present or are active only in very restricted regions of the epididymis. However, there have been few investigations on such region-specific epididymal proteins.

Sperm proteases are also involved in protein surface processing *in vivo*. They are either present on the cell surface, or reach the cell surface in the epididymis. In all cases, these enzymes are activated by unknown factors in specific epididymal regions. Major sperm protein surface modifications have not yet been associated with specific epididymal factors. These modifications may provide a useful assay for use in isolating and characterizing epididymal factors involved in the modifications (Lum and Blobel, 1997). If proteins secreted by the epididymis act on the sperm surface, modifications are probably induced on the gamete as soon as the protein is secreted in the fluid.

Several enzymes are secreted in the epididymis. In rams and rats, secretion of galactosidase in the corpus epididymidis coincides with the reduction in galactose residues on the sperm surface (X. Druart, J. L. Dacheux and F. Dacheux unpublished; Tulsiani *et al.*, 1995b). Most of these enzymes are found in very high concentrations and in active forms throughout the epididymis. Mannosidase and hexosaminidase in boars represent about 9% of the total protein secreted (Syntin *et al.*, 1996). Therefore, in spite of the rapid action of these enzymes on the sperm surface, it is probable that they have another function on the spermatozoa that has not yet been identified.

Several epididymal proteins bind to the sperm membrane, probably to induce direct or indirect changes on the sperm surface. Such effects are probably related to the degree of binding of the epididymal component on the sperm surface. For several proteins, the binding is transitory and occurs principally when the protein is most concentrated in the fluid, such as for GPX (Jimenez *et al.*, 1992; Okamura *et al.*, 1997), clusterin (Sylvester *et al.*, 1991) and lactoferrin (Jin *et al.*, 1997). The effects of these transitory interactions on the spermatozoa are unknown but could directly affect the membrane. Specific binding of one molecule (originating from fluid) on to its membrane receptor may activate an enzyme present on the sperm surface. Such a mechanism could be involved in activation of proteolysis of membrane proteins such as PH20 (Lum and Blobel, 1997).

Among the proteins that bind strongly to the sperm surface, some could be anchored by GPI linking (Moore *et al.*, 1989, Kirchhoff, 1996) or be integrated into the membrane by their hydrophobic properties. In various species, several epididymal proteins have been described as closely bound to the sperm membrane (Hall *et al.*, 1996). However, using an immunological approach, few sperm proteins seem to have a common antigen with epididymal proteins. In rams, an antiserum against the membrane of mature spermatozoa reveals only 17–30 kDa epididymal antigens in the last part of the epididymis. These epididymal proteins are minor in the fluid (low secretion rate) (J. L. Gatti, unpublished). The role of these sperm surface changes is probably more related to changes in motility pattern than to egg recognition. Similar interactions between the sperm surface and epididymal proteins have also been characterized in rats (Brown *et al.*, 1983) and boars (Dacheux *et al.*, 1989).

No direct changes on the spermatozoa can be correlated for most of the major proteins secreted into the epididymal lumen. For example, clusterin (Fritz *et al.*, 1983) and prostaglandin D_2 synthase

(Fouchécourt *et al.*, 1998) are secreted at successive epididymal sites and are also detected generally in the testicular fluid. The secretion rate of clusterin could reach about 30–50% of the total secretion of epididymal protein in rams and boars. The presence of these compounds is intriguing, as they appear not to affect spermatozoa, although several hypothetical functions such as lipophile compound exchange have been suggested for some of them. The absence of regionalization of these secreted proteins reduces their potentiality to trigger a sperm change in a specific region, so they may play a general role, such as protecting spermatozoa .

Among the other major proteins secreted, several probably have an indirect effect on spermatozoa by protecting them against superoxides, as for GGT (Hinton *et al.*, 1991), glutathione peroxidase (GPX) (Vernet *et al.*, 1997), superoxide dismutase (SOD) (Perry *et al*, 1993) and lactoferrin (Syntin *et al.*, 1996; Okamura *et al.*, 1997). The specific localization and successive secretion of these proteins in the epididymis are in agreement with the presence of a system of protection adapted to sperm metabolism throughout epididymal transit (Hinton *et al.*, 1995).

It is concluded that the search for the roles of the major epididymal proteins, starting from their respective secretory and concentration profiles throughout the organ, tends to indicate that the presence of these major components is more probably related to controlling the milieu of the spermatozoa to preserve their function than to induce sequential changes on the gametes. The epididymal proteins that are probably directly linked to sperm modification appear to be discrete secretions that are as yet unidentified.

Conclusion

The post-testicular differentiation of the sperm comprises a pattern of events that occur only in specific regions of the epididymis. The exact cellular events that are necessary to induce the principal functions of a mature spermatozoon such as motility and egg recognition are still unknown. Clearly the epididymis plays many roles in sperm maturation: (1) directly or indirectly by modifying pre-existing structures on the sperm surface, (2) providing new surface properties for the membrane and (3) preserving active sites on the sperm membrane. It is not easy to establish the relationship between an individual event on the spermatozoa and the importance of the event in sperm function because the function occurs only when other modifications have taken place. Nevertheless our knowledge about epididymal proteins has progressed rapidly in recent years. Among the 100–200 proteins that are estimated to be secreted by the epididymis, few have been identified. For the major ones already identified it appears that they are present in most of the species studied, and that their functions are related to protecting the sperm membrane and cellular vitality. Enzymes or related proteins that are directly involved in modifying the surface of testicular spermatozoa by endoproteolysis have to be identified.

Understanding sperm maturation and storage in the epididymis depends on the identification of sperm membrane and epididymal proteins and their roles. The combination of molecular biology and physiological approaches, such as gene modifications, should provide new ways of understanding what is necessary for a spermatozoa to be able to fertilize an oocyte *in vivo.*

The authors thank Dr RC Jones for his interest and help in the review of the manuscript. Results from the authors presented in this review were supported by ACC-SV Grant project 9504155.

References

Blobel CP, Myles DG, Primakoff P and White JM (1990) Proteolytic processing of a protein involved in sperm–egg fusion correlates with acquisition of fertilization competence *Journal of Cell Biology* **111** 69–78

Brooks DE (1981) Secretion of proteins and glycoproteins by the rat epididymis: regional differences, androgen-dependence, and effects of protease inhibitors, procaine, and tunicamicyin *Biology of Reproduction* **25** 1099–1117

Brown CR, von Glos KI and Jones R (1983) Changes in plasma membrane glycoproteins of rat spermatozoa during maturation in the epididymis *Journal of Cell Biology* **96** 256–264

Chatterjee T and Majumder GC (1989) Identification of membrane antigens of goat epididymal spermatozoa *Biochemical and Biophysical Research Communications* **162** 550–556

Chaturapanich G, Jones RC and Clulow J (1992) Protein synthesis and secretion by the epididymis of Tammar Wallaby, *Macropus eugenii* (Macropodidae: Marsupialia) *Reproduction, Fertility and Development* **4** 533–545

Cornwall GA, Vreeburg JT, Holland MK and Orgebin-Crist MC (1990) Interactions of labeled epididymal secretory proteins with spermatozoa after injection of ^{35}S-methionine in the mouse *Biology of Reproduction* **43** 1212–1219

Cornwall G, Orgebin-Crist MC and Hann SR (1992) The CRES gene: a unique testis-regulated gene related to the cystatin family is highly restricted in its expression to the proximal region of the mouse *Molecular Endocrinology* **6** 1653–1664

Dacheux JL and Voglmayr JK (1983) Sequence of sperm cell surface differentiation and its relationship to exogenous fluid proteins in ram epididymis *Biology of Reproduction* **29** 1033–1046

Dacheux JL, Dacheux F and Paquignon M (1989) Changes in sperm surface membrane and luminal protein fluid content during epididymal transit in the boar *Biology of Reproduction* **40** 635–651

Del-Rio AG (1979) Macromolecular secretion into various segments of the guinea pig epididymis *Archives of Andrology* **3** 231–237

Druart X, Gatti J, Dacheux F and Dacheux JL (1994) Analysis by two-dimensional gel electrophoresis of ram epididymal secreted proteins *Cellular and Molecular Biology* **40** 91–93

Druart X, Gatti J, Guérin Y, Dacheux F and Dacheux JL Characterization, identification and origin of major proteins present in ram epididymal fluid *Biology of Reproduction* (submitted)

Fouchécourt S, Dacheux F and, Dacheux JL Origin, secretion and regulation of glutathione independent prostaglandin D2 synthase in ram, stallion and boar epididymis *Biology of Reproduction* (submitted)

Fritz IB, Burdzy K, Setchell BP and Blaschuk O (1983) Ram rete testis fluid contains a protein (Clusterin) which influences cell–cell interactions *in vitro*. *Biology of Reproduction* **28** 1173–1188

Gatti JL, Druart X, Guerin Y, Dacheux F and Dacheux JL A 105–94 kDa protein in the epididymal fluid of ram, boar and stallion is angiotensin I-converting enzyme (ACE): evidence that sperm are the source of ACE. *Biology of Reproduction* (in press)

Hall JC, Tubbs CE, Li Y and Ashraf S (1996) Characterization of high-affinity protein D binding sites on the surface of rat epididymal spermatozoa *Biochemical Molecular Biological International* **40** 1003–1010

Hinton BT, Palladino MA, Mattmueller DR, Bard D and Good K (1991) Expression and activity of gamma-glutamyl-transpeptidase in the rat epididymis *Molecular Reproduction and Development* **28** 40–46

Hinton BT, Palladino MA, Rudolph D and Labus JC (1995) The epididymis as protector of maturing spermatozoa *Reproduction Fertility and Development* **7** 731–745

Jimenez C, Lefrançois AM, Ghyselinck NB and Dufaure JP (1992) Characterization and hormonal regulation of 24 kDa protein synthesis by the adult murine epididymis *Journal of Endocrinology* **133** 197–203

Jin YZ, Bannai S, Dacheux F, Dacheux JL and Okamura N (1997) Direct evidence for the secretion of lactoferrin and its binding to sperm in the porcine epididymis *Molecular Reproduction and Development* **47** 490–496

Jones R (1989) Membrane remodelling during sperm maturation in the epididymis *Oxford Reviews of Reproductive Biology* **11** 285–337

Jones R, Ma A, Hou ST, Shalgi R and Hall L (1996) Testicular biosynthesis and epididymal endoproteolytic processing of rat sperm surface antigen 2B1 *Journal of Cell Science* **109** 2561–2570

Jones RC and Clulow J (1994) Interactions of sperm and the reproductive ducts of the male tammar wallaby, *Macropus eugenii* (Macropodidae : Marsupiala) *Reproduction Fertility and Development* **6** 437–444

Kirchhoff C (1996) CD52 is the 'major maturation-associated' sperm membrane antigen *Molecular Human Reproduction* **2** 9–17

Lum L and Blobel CP (1997) Evidence for distinct serine protease activities with a potential role in processing the sperm protein fertilin *Developmental Biology* **191** 131–145

Moore A, White TW, Ensrud KM and Hamilton DW (1989) The major maturation glycoprotein found on rat cauda epididymal sperm surface is linked to the membrane via phosphatidylinositol *Biochemical and Biophysical Research Communication* **160** 460–468

Okamura N, Tamba M, Liao HJ, Onoe S, Sugita Y, Dacheux F and Dacheux JL (1995a) Cloning of complementary DNA encoding a 135-kilodalton protein secreted from porcine corpus epididymis and its identification as an epididymis-specific alpha-mannosidase *Molecular Reproduction and Development* **42** 141–148

Okamura N, Tamba M, Uchiyama Y, Sugita Y, Dacheux F, Syntin P and Dacheux JL (1995b) Direct evidence for the elevated synthesis and secretion of procathepsin L in the distal caput epididymis of boar *Biochimica et Biophysica Acta* **1245** 221–226

Okamura N, Iwaki Y, Hiramoto S, Tamba M, Bannai S, Sugita Y, Syntin P, Dacheux F and Dacheux JL (1997) Molecular cloning and characterization of the epididymis-specific glutathione peroxidase-like protein secreted in the porcine epididymal fluid *Biochimica et Biophysica Acta* **1336** 99–109

Olson GE and Hinton B (1985) Regional differences in luminal fluid polypeptides of the rat testis and epididymis revealed by two-dimensional gel electrophoresis *Journal of Andrology* **6** 20–34

Peloille S, Esnard A, Dacheux JL, Guillou F, Gauthier F and Esnard F (1997) Interactions between ovine cathepsin L, cystatin C and alpha 2-macroglobulin. Potential role in the genital tract *European Journal of Biochemistry* **244** 140–146

Perry AC, Jones R and Hall L (1993a) Isolation and characterization of a rat cDNA clone encoding a secreted superoxide dismutase reveals the epididymis to be a major site of its expression *Biochemistry Journal* **293** 21–25

Perry AC, Jones R and Hall L (1993b) Sequence analysis of monkey acrosin–trypsin inhibitor transcripts and their abundant expression in the epididymis *Biochimica et Biophysica Acta* **1172** 159–160

Petruszak JAM, Nehme CL and Bartles JR (1991) Endoproteolytic cleavage in the extracellular domain of the integral plasma membrane protein CE9 precedes its redistribution from the posterior to the anterior tail of the rat spermatozoon during epididymal maturation *Journal of Cell Biology* **115** 917–927

Phelps BM, Koppel CH, Primakoff P and Myles DG (1990) Evidence that proteolysis of the surface is an initial step in the mechanism of formation of sperm cell surface domains *Journal of Cell Biology* **11** 1839–1847

Primakoff P, Cowan AE, Hyatt H, Tredick-Kline J and Myles DG (1988) Purification of the guinea pig sperm preparations that cleaves PH-20 into two disulfide-linked fragments *Biology of Reproduction* **38** 921–934

Robitaille G, Sullivan R and Bleau G (1991) Identification of epididymal proteins associated with hamster sperm *Journal of Experimental Zoology* **258** 69–74

Shabonowitz RB and Killian GJ (1987) Two dimensional electrophoresis of proteins in principal cells, spermatozoa, and fluid associated with the rat epididymis *Biology of Reproduction* **36** 753–768

Sylvester SR, Morales C, Oko R and Griswold MD (1991) Localization of sulfated glycoprotein 2 (clusterin) on spermatozoa and in the reproductive tract of the male rat *Biology of Reproduction* **45** 195–207

Syntin P, Dacheux F, Druart X, Gatti JL, Okamura N and Dacheux JL (1996) Characterization and identification of proteins secreted in the various regions of the adult boar epididymis *Biology of Reproduction* **55** 956–974

Tomomasa H, Waguri S, Umeda T, Kois K, Kominami E and Uchiyama Y (1994) Lysosomal cysteine protease in rat epididymis *Journal of Histochemistry and Cytochemistry* **42** 417–425

Tulsiani DR, NagDas SK, Skudlarek MD and Orgebin-Crist MC (1995a) Rat sperm plasma membrane mannosidase: localization and evidence for proteolytic processing during epididymal maturation *Developmental Biology* **167** 584–595

Tulsiani DR, Skudlarek MD, Araki Y and Orgebin-Crist M-C (1995b) Purification and characterization of two forms of beta-D-galactosidase from rat epididymal luminal fluid: evidence for their role in the modification of sperm plasma membrane glycoprotein(s) *Biochemical Journal* **305** 41–50

Vanha-Perttula T, Mather JP, Bardin CW, Moss SB and Bellve AR (1985) Localization of angiotensin-converting enzyme activity in testis and epididymis *Biology of Reproduction* **33** 870–877

Vernet P, Faure J, Dufaure JP and Drevet JR (1997) Tissue and developmental distribution, dependence upon testicular factors and attachment to spermatozoa of GPX5, a murine epididymis-specific glutathione peroxidase *Molecular Reproduction and Development* **47** 87–98

Xu W, Ensrud KM and Hamilton DW (1997) The 26 kD protein recognised on rat cauda epididymal sperm by monoclonal antibody 4E9 has internal peptide sequence that is identical to the secreted form of epididymal protein E *Molecular Reproduction and Development* **46** 377–382

Journal of Reproduction and Fertility Supplement **53**, 109–118

Maturation of redox regulatory mechanisms in the epididymis

R. J. Aitken and P. Vernet

MRC Reproductive Biology Unit, 37 Chalmers Street, Edinburgh EH3 9EW, UK

As spermatozoa pass through the epididymis they complete a maturation process that enables these cells to participate in the process of fertilization. Epididymal maturation involves a complex cascade of changes involving the remodelling of the sperm surface, the induction of chromatin condensation, the acquisition of movement, and development of the potential for capacitation. In this review we shall consider how changes in the redox status of mammalian spermatozoa may contribute to the completion of these maturation events. Spermatozoa from all regions of the epididymis exhibit a spontaneous capacity for superoxide anion production which can be enhanced by exposure to NADPH, particularly in the caput region. It is hypothesized that this spontaneous free radical generating activity is mediated by a membrane-bound NADPH oxidase, the function of which is to generate the peroxides that are needed to serve as hydrogen acceptors for phospholipid hydroperoxide glutathione peroxidase in the induction of sperm chromatin condensation. As spermatozoa enter the cauda epididymidis they also express a capacity for hydrogen peroxide (H_2O_2) generation when released into simple, defined culture media. The onset of this activity is thought to be associated with the induction of sperm capacitation through stimulation of the tyrosine phosphorylation events involved in the attainment of a capacitated state. It is concluded that sperm maturation is a dynamic, redox regulated process, any imbalance in which could lead to the production of spermatozoa that are compromised in terms of their potential for fertilization and the integrity of their DNA.

Introduction

Spermatozoa that emerge from the testes are infertile and acquire the potential for fertilization only after they have completed a period of maturation in the epididymis. The acquisition of functional competence during epididymal transit appears to involve at least two major physiological changes. The first concerns the ability of the spermatozoa to exhibit movement. Spermatozoa from the caput epididymidis exhibit little or no motility but, as they pass through the corpus epididymidis, increases in percentage motility, curvilinear velocity and progressiveness are generally observed. The precise location within the corpus epididymidis where the potential for rapid progressive movement is acquired shows considerable inter-species variation. In primates, the change in motility expression is most marked as spermatozoa move from the distal caput to proximal corpus region of the epididymis; in the mouse the most marked changes are seen as spermatozoa pass through the mid-corpus region; in the hamster, it is the corpus to cauda transition where the potential for movement is fully realised (Soler *et al.*, 1994; Yeung *et al.*, 1994, 1996a).

The second major change associated with epididymal maturation concerns the ability of the spermatozoa to undergo capacitation. Capacitation is a physiological priming phenomenon whereby spermatozoa acquire the ability to acrosome react in response to the intracellular calcium signals generated when these cells make contact with the cumulus–oocyte complex. Thus, in uncapacitated human spermatozoa a physiological agonist such as progesterone can trigger a marked cytoplasmic calcium transient, but this signal does not precipitate an acrosome reaction. By contrast, when progesterone is administered to capacitated human spermatozoa, a similar calcium signal is generated, but this time it is followed by a rapid biological response (Aitken *et al.*, 1996). The inability of caput epididymal spermatozoa to capacitate is reflected by the lack of biological response observed when calcium signals are induced in such cells with agonists as powerful as A23187 (Yeung *et al.*, 1996b). Since capacitation is thought to be tightly coupled to the ability of the spermatozoa to exhibit a spontaneous increase in tyrosine phosphorylation (Visconti *et al.*, 1995), it is not surprising that the lack of responsiveness exhibited by spermatozoa from the caput epididymidis is correlated with their inability to exhibit high levels of tyrosine phosphorylation, at least in the mouse and bull (Visconti *et al.*, 1995; Vijayaraghavan *et al.*, 1997). In order to understand why immature spermatozoa from the caput epididymidis cannot undergo capacitation, it is necessary to review the biochemistry of this process and, in particular, the central role of redox regulated reactions in the attainment of a capacitated state (Aitken *et al.*, 1995; De Lamirande and Gagnon, 1993, 1995).

Redox Regulation of Sperm Capacitation

Studies with human spermatozoa have demonstrated that the tyrosine phosphorylation events associated with sperm capacitation are redox regulated (Aitken *et al.*, 1995, 1996; Leclerc *et al.*, 1997). An example of the evidence linking reactive oxygen species (ROS) generation, tyrosine phosphorylation and capacitation can be found in the behaviour of human spermatozoa incubated under bicarbonate-free conditions. In the absence of extracellular bicarbonate, human spermatozoa remain fully motile but appear incapable of ROS generation or the expression of tyrosine phosphorylation. As a consequence, the spermatozoa cannot capacitate and cannot exhibit functional responses to physiological agonists such as progesterone (Aitken *et al.*, 1998a). This effect is associated with a fall in intracellular pH. However, if cytoplasmic pH is buffered back into the normal range then, even though the medium may lack bicarbonate, ROS generation and tyrosine phosphorylation return to normal and, when progesterone is added, high rates of sperm–oocyte fusion are observed (Aitken *et al.*, 1998a). A direct involvement of ROS, particularly H_2O_2, in the induction of tyrosine phosphorylation can be deduced from the inhibitory effects of catalase, a specific scavenger of this oxidant, on both the expression of phosphotyrosine residues and capacitation (Aitken *et al.*, 1995, 1998b). Conversely, either exposure of human spermatozoa to low doses of H_2O_2, or the stimulation of endogenous H_2O_2 generation with NADPH, will accelerate the capacitation process (Aitken *et al.*, 1995). Similarly in the hamster, catalase is known to disrupt sperm capacitation, while exposure to low concentrations of H_2O_2 will enhance this process (Bize *et al.*, 1991).

The mechanisms by which H_2O_2 stimulates tyrosine phosphorylation in human spermatozoa probably include the inhibition of tyrosine phosphatase activity. Tyrosine phosphatases possess a conserved cysteine residue in their catalytic domain that must be in a reduced state for full activity to be expressed. Exposure of this class of enzyme to H_2O_2 leads to the suppression of phosphatase activity (Hecht and Zick, 1992) and a consequential enhancement of phosphotyrosine expression. In addition to the inhibition of tyrosine phosphatases, H_2O_2 is also capable of activating tyrosine kinase activity. For example, this oxidant can potentiate the tyrosine phosphorylation induced by insulin in Fao hepatoma cells (Heffetz and Zick, 1989) and has been implicated in the direct activation of tyrosine kinase activity in connection with such molecules as Lck, PLCγ or NF-κB (Kaul and Forman, 1996; Monteiro and Stern, 1996). In addition to the direct effects of ROS on the tyrosine phosphorylation system present in human spermatozoa, these molecules may also use supplementary mechanisms for controlling phosphotyrosine expression in these cells, through the increase of intracellular cAMP (Aitken *et al.*, 1998b). A similar enhancing effect of oxidative stress on adenylyl cyclase activity has recently been described in a vascular smooth muscle cell line by Tan *et al.* (1995). Thus the ability of human spermatozoa to control their tyrosine phosphorylation status through a redox regulated pathway is in keeping with an emerging body of data emphasizing the general importance of such mechanisms in the control of cellular function.

Although the induction of tyrosine phosphorylation is central to the capacitation process, the latter involves a variety of other biochemical changes to the spermatozoa including the loss of cholesterol from the sperm plasma membrane, increased intracellular calcium, zinc dispersal, decreased surface charge and rearrangements of surface antigens (de Lamirande *et al.*, 1997). As a consequence of these events the spermatozoa not only acquire the ability to acrosome react and fuse with the vitelline membrane of the oocyte but they also exhibit a particular form of vigorous, non-progressive movement, known as hyperactivation, which is characteristic of the capacitated state (Yanagimachi, 1994). A specific reactive oxygen metabolite, the superoxide anion, has been implicated in the induction of hyperactivated motility, although the mechanisms underlying this association remain obscure (de Lamirande *et al.*, 1997).

ROS may also contribute to the capacitation process by destabilizing the plasma membrane and thereby facilitating the induction of the acrosome reaction. Such destabilization could be achieved through the ability of lipid hydroperoxides to stimulate phospholipase A_2 (PLA_2) activity (Goldman *et al.*, 1992). The induction of this enzyme results in the formation of lysophospholipids in the sperm plasma membrane, which destabilise this structure and promote the membrane fusion events associated with the acrosome reaction (Parrish *et al.*, 1988).

Given the close association between the redox status of mammalian spermatozoa and capacitation, it is of interest to consider how acquisition of the potential to capacitate during epididymal maturation is associated with the ability of these cells to generate ROS.

The Epididymis and Redox Status

ROS generation in the epididymis

Mammalian spermatozoa recovered from the caput, corpus and caudal regions of the epididymis spontaneously generate lucigenin-dependent chemiluminescent signals, indicating the release of superoxide anion into the extracellular space (Fisher and Aitken, 1997). This activity is particularly intense with mouse and rat spermatozoa but does not vary significantly between different regions of the epididymis (Fig. 1). The presence of an NADPH oxidase-like activity in these cells was indicated by the ability of this coenzyme, but not $NADP^+$, to stimulate significant increases

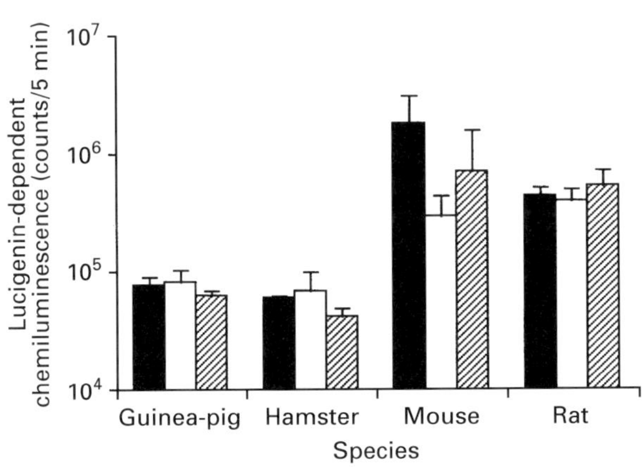

Fig. 1. Lucigenin-dependent chemiluminescence was exhibited by epididymal spermatozoa (■: caput; □: corpus; ▨: cauda) from all species tested; particularly intense signals were recorded for the rat and mouse. No significant relationship was apparent between the intensity of the chemiluminescent signal and the maturation status of the spermatozoa. (Reproduced with permission from Fisher and Aitken, 1997.)

in superoxide anion generation in epididymal spermatozoa from the hamster, mouse, rat and guinea-pig (Fig. 2). However, in the case of NADPH-induced ROS generation, a significant difference in activity was observed in different regions of the epididymis with caput epididymal spermatozoa exhibiting the greatest response in every species examined (Fig. 2).

Epididymal spermatozoa are also capable of generating H_2O_2 as detected by peroxidase-enhanced, luminol-dependent chemiluminescence (Fisher and Aitken, 1997). This activity also varies significantly with the stage of epididymal maturation, but in this case it is the mature cells recovered from the caudal epididymis that are the most active. Time-dependent analyses revealed

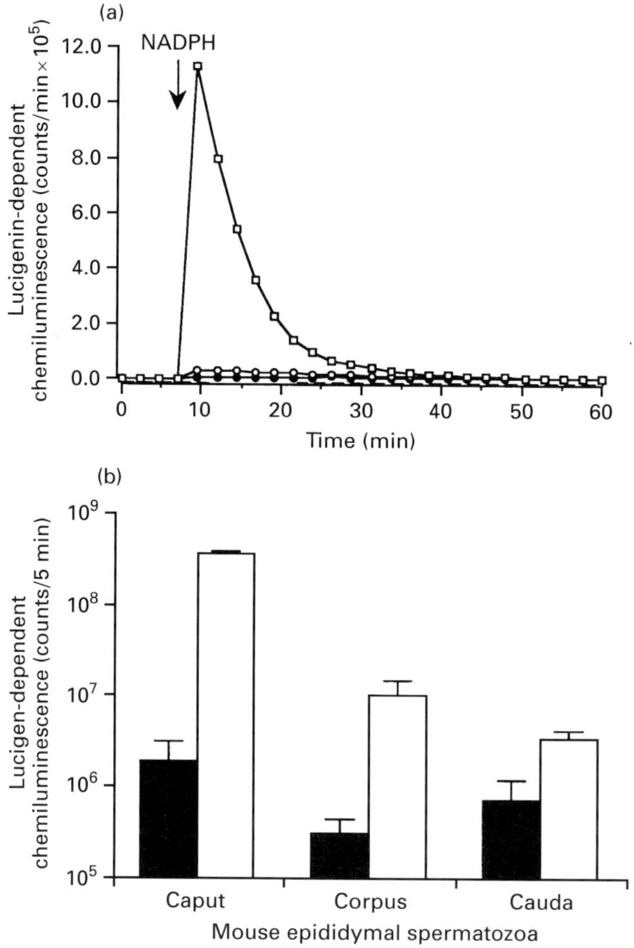

Fig. 2. The induction of superoxide generation in mouse epididymal spermatozoa after exposure to exogenous NADPH. (a) Longitudinal traces illustrating the pattern of lucigenin-dependent chemiluminescence elicited in mouse spermatozoa over 60 min; (□) caput spermatozoa; (○) corpus spermatozoa; (●) cauda spermatozoa; control incubations (---) contained the chemiluminescent probe and NADPH but no spermatozoa. (b) Mean (± SEM) responses for three independent experiments in which the chemiluminescent counts were integrated over 5 min after addition of NADPH (□); control (■). $P = 0.0001$ for between treatment effects. (Reproduced with permission from Fisher and Aitken, 1997.)

that H_2O_2 generation was initiated by caudal epididymal spermatozoa as soon as these cells were diluted into culture medium. However, after approximately 10 min, the rate of H_2O_2 generation stabilized and remained high for several hours, although the signal could be suppressed at any time by the addition of catalase (Fisher and Aitken, 1997).

The generation of H_2O_2 by spermatozoa from the cauda epididymidis could involve the activation of an enzyme complex capable of effecting the direct reduction of molecular oxygen. Alternatively, the generation of this oxidant may reflect the enhanced dismutation of superoxide anion to H_2O_2 by superoxide dismutase (SOD). The latter suggestion is supported by the observation that the cauda epididymidis secretes a unique form of SOD (Perry *et al.*, 1993), which may become associated with the sperm surface and facilitate the dismutation of superoxide anions reaching the extracellular space. A superficial location for the superoxide dismutase associated with spermatozoa from the cauda epididymidis is certainly suggested by the fact that a significant proportion of this activity can be removed by a simple washing procedure (Holland *et al.*, 1982).

Function of ROS generation in the epididymis

Capacitation. The sudden onset of H_2O_2 generation by spermatozoa released from the epididymis would be in keeping with a role for this particular oxidant in the induction of sperm capacitation. As indicated above, this conclusion is supported by the ability of catalase to inhibit the capacitation of both human and hamster spermatozoa and the complementary capacity of H_2O_2 to induce this process (Bize *et al.*, 1991; Aitken *et al.*, 1995, 1996, 1998b).

While the generation of H_2O_2 by spermatozoa from the cauda epididymidis may be associated with capacitation, this does not explain the functional significance of ROS generated spontaneously by spermatozoa recovered from the caput and corpus epididymides (Fisher and Aitken, 1997). Moreover the potential to exhibit NADPH oxidase activity seems to be gradually suppressed during epididymal maturation, not stimulated, caput spermatozoa generating significantly more ROS on exposure to NADPH than cells recovered from more distal regions of the epididymis (Fisher and Aitken, 1997). Given the susceptibility of spermatozoa to peroxidative damage such observations suggest that these cells must have a functional use for the ROS generated during the early stages of epididymal maturation. A possible hypothesis in this context would be that a low level of lipid peroxide formation during the early stages of epididymal maturation is necessary to achieve chromatin condensation (Godeas *et al.*, 1997).

Sperm chromatin condensation. Spermatozoa contain a form of glutathione peroxidase that is active against intact phospholipid hydroperoxides (as well as H_2O_2 and fatty acid hydroperoxides) known as phospholipid hydroperoxide glutathione peroxidase (PHGPx). This is a selenium containing enzyme that is tightly bound to both the mitochondria and the chromatin of mature spermatozoa (Roveri *et al.*, 1992; Godeas *et al.*, 1996, 1997). Moreover PH GPx from the spermatozoon exhibits thiol oxidase activity which is particularly effective in cross-linking protamines recovered from spermatozoa from the caput epididymidis (Godeas *et al.*, 1997). For this enzyme to function it requires an electron acceptor in the form of H_2O_2, fatty acid hydroperoxide or phospholipid hydroperoxide. We hypothesize that the NADPH oxidase activity detected in mammalian spermatozoa (Fisher and Aitken, 1997; Aitken *et al.*, 1997) during epididymal transit (Fisher and Aitken, 1997) generates these three peroxide species (Fig. 3) any one of which could support PL-GPx action in effecting the oxidation of protamine thiols and the induction of chromatin cross-linkage (Fig. 3). Although low amounts of H_2O_2 appear to be generated by spermatozoa from the caput and cauda epididymides, it should be recognized that the system used to detect this oxidant (peroxidase-enhanced, luminol-dependent chemiluminesence) is responsive only to H_2O_2 released into the extracellular space. The lack of a significant signal from spermatozoa from the caput epididymidis does not mean that H_2O_2 is not being produced by these cells. It may be produced intracellularly but prevented from reaching the extracellular space by glutathione peroxidase bound to the sperm surface in the proximal regions of the epididymis (Vernet *et al.*, 1997). ROS generated by the

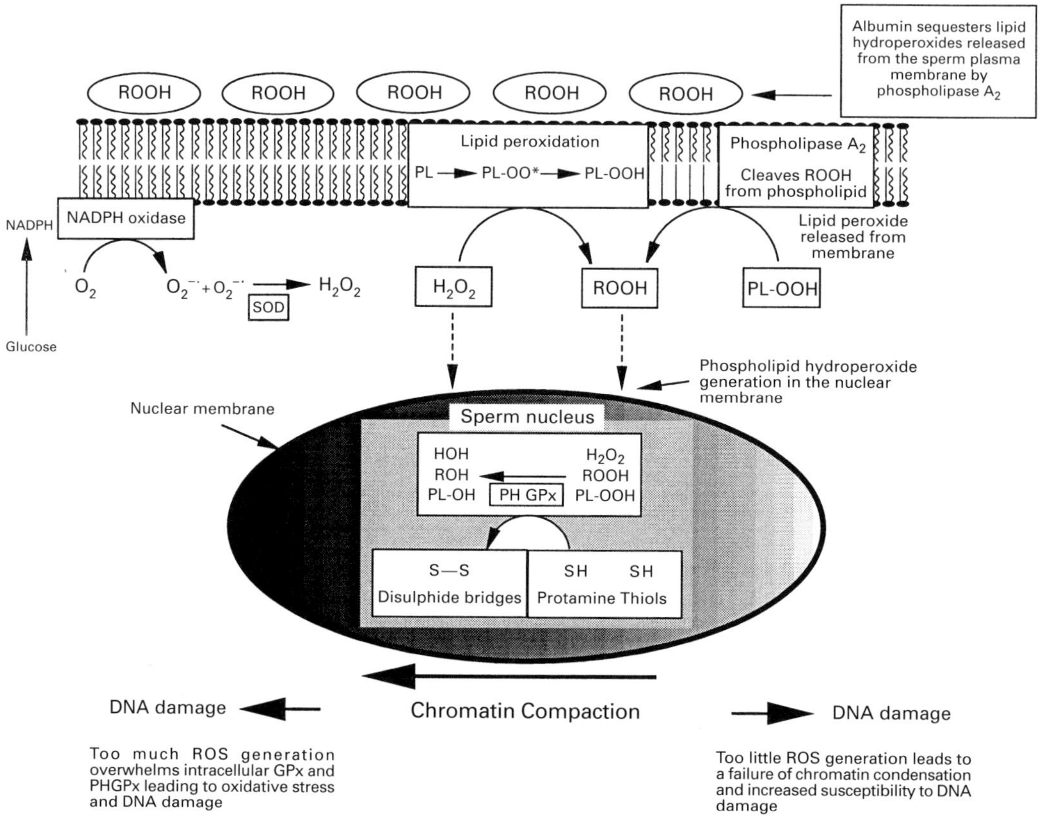

Fig. 3. Hypothesis for the functional significance of reactive oxygen species (ROS) in the facilitation of chromatin cross-linking during epididymal maturation. The central concept is built around the ability of epididymal spermatozoa to generate ROS (Fisher and Aitken, 1997) and the presence of a phospholipid hydroperoxide glutathione peroxidase (PH GPx) in the sperm nucleus capable of using hydrogen peroxide (H_2O_2), fatty acid peroxide (ROOH) and phospholipid hydroperoxide (PL-OOH) as hydrogen acceptors in the oxidation of thiol groups (SH) associated with sperm protamines (Godeas *et al.*, 1997). PH GPx thus plays a dual role in protecting the male genome by (a) metabolizing potentially damaging peroxides to the corresponding alcohols while (b) effecting the disulfide bond formation associated with chromatin compaction, which will also protect the male genome from oxidative stress.

proposed NADPH oxidase (Aitken *et al.*, 1997) system should also stimulate the formation of fatty acid peroxides in the plasma membrane that could be released from the parent phospholipids by PLA_2 and diffuse to the nucleus to support PH GPx in the induction of chromatin condensation (Fig. 3). PH GPx activity might also be promoted by phospholipid hydroperoxides generated in the nuclear membrane, as a result of lipid peroxidation cascades triggered by the fatty acid peroxides released from the plasma membrane or H_2O_2 itself (Fig. 3).

For the ROS-PH GPx system to be effective in the induction of chromatin cross-linking, it would have to be very carefully controlled. If ROS generation were inadequate, insufficient peroxide tone would be established to induce nuclear condensation and the resultant failure of sperm chromatin packaging would, in turn, render these cells susceptible to DNA damage (Bianchi *et al.*, 1993). On the other hand, if ROS generation was excessive, the limited antioxidant defences possessed by mammalian spermatozoa would be easily overwhelmed and DNA damage induced (Hughes *et al.*, 1996). Evidence that excessive oxidative stress can induce DNA damage in human spermatozoa has been obtained in experiments involving the direct exposure of these cells to H_2O_2, the stimulation of excessive endogenous ROS generation with NADPH and suppression of glutathione peroxidase activity with mercaptosuccinate (Hughes *et al.*, 1996; Twigg *et al.*, 1998). Thus in using lipid hydroperoxides as an electron recipient, PH GPx not only mediates sperm chromatin condensation but also protects the sperm DNA from peroxide mediated attack.

Antioxidant defences in the epididymis

Although spermatozoa appear to use redox mechanisms to control their physiology, this should not obscure the fact that epididymal spermatozoa are extremely vulnerable to oxidative stress. This vulnerability stems from the relative paucity of intracellular antioxidant enzymes in these cytoplasm-deficient cells, as well as the high concentrations of unsaturated fatty acids present in epididymal spermatozoa, particularly 22:5 and 22:6 (Awano *et al.*, 1993). The double bonds present in such molecules render them vulnerable to a lipid peroxidation cascade that is initiated by the extraction of a hydrogen atom to create a lipid radical which then combines with oxygen to generate a lipid peroxide. The peroxidative process damages the fluidity and integrity of the sperm plasma membrane and thereby precipitates a loss of sperm function (Aitken and Fisher, 1994). Given the susceptibility of mammalian spermatozoa to peroxidative damage, the ability of epididymal spermatozoa to generate ROS has clear implications for the viability of these cells and their potential for long term storage. In the light of these factors, it is not surprising that the epididymis is a rich source of antioxidant enzymes that scavenge any excess reactive oxygen metabolites released by the spermatozoa during epididymal transit. Thus northern blot analysis by Jow *et al.* (1993) revealed that the epididymis is a major site for the expression of a 0.77 kb transcript of the SOD gene. This enzyme catalyses the rapid removal of superoxide anion to form H_2O_2. Unfortunately the latter is extremely toxic to spermatozoa, inducing a rapid loss of fertilizing potential via mechanisms that involve the induction of lipid peroxidation and a loss of ATP (De Lamirande and Gagnon, 1992; Aitken *et al.*, 1992). Thus, if SOD is to serve as an effective antioxidant it must be coupled with the presence of enzyme systems, such as catalase and glutathione peroxidase, that rapidly remove the H_2O_2. Curiously the male reproductive tract, including the epididymis, possesses relatively low amounts of catalase RNA (Zini and Schlegel, 1996). However, the epididymis is a rich source of glutathione peroxidase, including both the conventional, selenium-containing plasma enzyme, GPX3 (Maser *et al.*, 1994; Schwaab *et al.*, 1995) and an epididymis-specific variant lacking a selenium binding component (GPX5; Vernet *et al.*, 1997). Despite the lack of selenium this epididymal enzyme does possess glutathione peroxidase activity, as judged by its capacity to protect transfected eukaryotic cells from oxidative stress (Vernet *et al.*, 1996). This enzyme is secreted by the caput epididymidis and becomes intimately associated with the sperm surface where it serves to remove any H_2O_2 generated by these cells as a consequence of SOD action.

An alternative strategy for dealing with the leakage of superoxide anion into the extracellular space would be to metabolise this molecule in such a way that H_2O_2 was not formed. An enzyme that is capable of achieving this objective, indoleamine dioxygenase, is present in the epididymis in extremely high concentrations and may play an important role protecting epididymal spermatozoa from oxidative stress (Yoshida *et al.*, 1980).

In addition to the secretion of antioxidant enzymes, the epididymis may also minimise the oxidative stress experienced by maturing spermatozoa by maintaining a relatively low pH in the lumen of the epididymal tubules. The epididymis possesses a proton pumping ATPase that generates an acidic intraluminal pH (Breton *et al.*, 1996) and thus helps maintain epididymal spermatozoa in a quiescent state. Since a low intracellular pH has also been shown to suppress NADPH oxidase activity in human spermatozoa incubated under bicarbonate-free conditions (Aitken *et al.*, 1998a), it seems likely that the acidic epididymal environment may also ensure that the generation of reactive oxygen metabolites is kept to a low, defensible level.

Antioxidant enzymes and low intraluminal pH are not the only strategies used by the epididymis to reduce oxidative stress. For example, the epididymis is a major site for the synthesis of lactoferrin (Jin *et al.*, 1997). This protein serves to bind free iron and prevent this transition metal from participating in the catalysis of lipid peroxidation chain reactions within the epididymal lumen. The epididymis also secretes albumin-like proteins (Carles *et al.*, 1992) that sequester toxic lipid peroxides with high efficiency and serve as sacrificial antioxidants. Other small molecular weight free radical scavengers such as vitamin C, glutathione and polyamines (Muscari *et al*, 1995; Khan *et al.*, 1992), are also present in epididymal plasma and contribute to the creation of a carefully engineered environment in which oxidative stress is kept to an absolute minimum (Hinton *et al.*, 1995), while permitting the intracellular redox chemistry that supports the maturation process.

Conclusions

Epididymal spermatozoa of all mammalian species examined generate reactive oxygen metabolites when incubated in simple defined culture media. In the caput and corpus epididymides the major species detected, but not necessarily the only species generated, is the superoxide anion. It is proposed that the ROS generated by spermatozoa in the proximal regions of the epididymis reflect the presence of NADPH oxidase activity in these cells and is of functional significance in the induction of chromatin condensation. The latter involves the oxidation of thiol groups in nuclear protamines mediated, it is proposed, by an intranuclear PH GPx using hydrogen-, fatty acid- and phospholipid peroxides as hydrogen acceptors. Spermatozoa from the cauda epididymidis that have completed the maturation process have simultaneously acquired the capacity to release H_2O_2. It is suggested that this activity is associated with the competence of spermatozoa from the cauda epididymidis to undergo capacitation, through the stimulation of a redox-regulated, tyrosine phosphorylation cascade. The epididymis is therefore an environment in which spermatozoa develop, and make functional use of, their ability to generate ROS. It is also an environment where oxidative stress is kept to a minimum through the secretion of a variety of antioxidant factors into the epididymal lumen. Characterizing the biochemical nature of the ROS generating systems in epididymal spermatozoa and understanding the way in which these pathways are controlled may be relevant to contraception as well as to our understanding of the aetiology of DNA damage and sperm dysfunction in the male germ line.

References

Aitken RJ and Fisher H (1994) Reactive oxygen species generation and human spermatozoa: the balance of benefit and risk *Bioessays* **16** 259–267

Aitken RJ, Buckingham D and Harkiss D (1992) Use of a xanthine oxidase oxidant generating system to investigate the cytotoxic effects of reactive oxygen species on human spermatozoa *Journal of Reproduction and Fertility* **97** 441–450

Aitken RJ, Paterson M, Fisher H, Buckingham DW and Van Duin M (1995) Redox regulation of tyrosine phosphorylation in human spermatozoa is involved in the control of human sperm function *Journal of Cell Science* **108** 2017–2025

Aitken RJ, Buckingham DW, Harkiss D, Fisher H, Paterson M and Irvine DS (1996) The extragenomic action of progesterone on human spermatozoa is influenced by redox regulated changes in tyrosine phosphorylation during capacitation *Molecular Cellular Endocrinology* **117** 83–93

Aitken RJ, Fisher H, Fulton N, Knox W and Lewis B (1997) Reactive oxygen species generation by human spermatozoa is induced by exogenous NADPH and inhibited by the flavoprotein inhibitors diphenylene iodonium and quinacrine *Molecular Reproduction and Development* **47** 468–482

Aitken RJ, Harkiss D, Knox W, Paterson M and Irvine DS (1998a) On the cellular mechanisms by which the bicarbonate ion mediates the extragenomic action of progesterone on human spermatozoa *Biology of Reproduction* **58** 186–196

Aitken RJ, Harkiss D, Knox W, Paterson M and Irvine DS (1998b) Cross talk between cAMP- and redox-regulated pathways controlling the tyrosine phosphorylation events associated with sperm capacitation *Journal of Cell Science* (in press)

Awano M, Kawaguchi A and Mohri H (1993) Lipid composition of hamster epididymal spermatozoa *Journal of Reproduction and Fertility* **99** 375–383

Bianchi P, Manicardi GC, Bizzaro D, Bianchi U and Sakkas D (1993) Effect of DNA protamination on fluorochrome staining and *in situ* nick-translation of murine and human mature spermatozoa *Biology of Reproduction* **49** 1038–1043

Bize I, Santander G, Cabello P, Driscoll D and Sharpe C (1991) Hydrogen peroxide is involved in hamster sperm capacitation *in vitro*. *Biology of Reproduction* **44** 389–403

Breton S, Smith PJ S, Lui B and Brown D (1996) Acidification of the male reproductive tract by a proton pumping ATPase *Nature Medicine* **2** 470–472

Carles C, Fournierdelpech S and Ribadeaudumas B (1992) Purification of an ovine, androgen dependent epididymal protein – evidence for a strong amino acid sequence homology with serum albumin *Reproduction, Nutrition and Development* **32** 277–284

De Lamirande E and Gagnon C (1992) Reactive oxygen species and human spermatozoa I. Effects on the motility of intact spermatozoa and on sperm axonemes *Journal of Andrology* **13** 368–378

De Lamirande E and Gagnon C (1993) A positive role for superoxide anion in triggering hyperactivation and capacitation of human spermatozoa *International Journal of Andrology* **16** 21–25

De Lamirande E and Gagnon C (1995) Capacitation-associated production of superoxide anion by human spermatozoa *Free Radical Biology and Medicine* **18** 487–495

De Lamirande E, Leclerc P and Gagnon C (1997) Capacitation as a regulatory event that primes spermatozoa for the acrosome reaction and fertilization *Molecular Human Reproduction* **3** 175–194

Fisher HM and Aitken RJ (1997) Comparative analysis of the ability of precursor germ cells and epididymal spermatozoa to generate reactive oxygen metabolites *Journal of Experimental Zoology* **277** 390–400

Godeas C, Tramer F, Micali F, Roveri A, Majorino M, Nisii C, Sandri G and Panfili E (1996) Phospholipid hydroperoxide glutathione peroxidase (PHGPx) in rat testis nuclei is bound to chromatin *Biochemical and Molecular Medicine* **59** 118–124

Godeas C, Tramer F, Micali F, Soranzo M, Sandri G and Panfili E (1997) Distribution and possible novel role of phospholipid hydroperoxide glutathione peroxidase in rat epididymal spermatozoa *Biology of Reproduction* **57** 1502–1508

Goldman R, Ferber E and Zort U (1992) Reactive oxygen species are involved in the activation of cellular phospholipase A_2 *FEBS Letters* **309** 190–192

Hecht D and Zick Y (1992) Selective inhibition of protein tyrosine phosphatase activities by H_2O_2 and vanadate *in vitro. Biochemical and Biophysical Research Communications* **188** 773–779

Heffetz D and Zick Y (1989) H_2O_2 potentiates phosphorylation of novel putative substrates for the insulin receptor kinase in intact Fao cells *Journal of Biological Chemistry* **264** 10126–10132

Hinton BT, Palladino MA, Rudolph D and Labus JC (1995) The epididymis as protector of maturing spermatozoa. In *Seventh International Symposium on Spermatology: Plenary Papers. Reproduction, Fertility and Development* **7** 73–88

Holland MK, Alvarez JG and Storey BT (1982) Production of superoxide and activity of superoxide dismutase in rabbit epididymal spermatozoa *Biology of Reproduction* **27** 1109–1118

Hughes CM, Lewis SEM, McKelvey-Martin VJ and Thompson W (1996) A comparison of baseline and induced DNA damage in human spermatozoa from fertile and infertile men using a modified comet assay *Molecular Reproduction and Development* **2** 613–620

Jin YZ, Bannai S, Dacheux F, Dacheux JL and Okamura N (1997) Direct evidence for the secretion of lactoferrin and its binding to sperm in the porcine epididymis *Molecular Reproduction and Development* **47** 490–496

Jow WW, Schlegel PN, Cichon Z, Phillips D, Goldstein M and Bardin CW (1993) Identification and localization of copper-zinc superoxide dismutase gene expression in rat testicular development *Journal of Andrology* **14** 439–447

Kaul N and Forman HJ (1996) Activation of NF-kappa-B by the respiratory burst of macrophages *Free Radical Biology and Medicine* **21,** 401–405

Khan AU, Mei YH and Wilson T (1992) A proposed function for spermine and spermidine: protection of replicating DNA against damage by singlet oxygen *Proceedings of the National Academy of Sciences USA* **89** 11426–11427

Leclerc P, de Lamirande E and Gagnon C (1997) Regulation of protein-tyrosine phosphorylation and human sperm capacitation by reactive oxygen derivatives *Free Radical Biology and Medicine* **22** 643–656

Maser RL, Magenheimer BS and Calvet JP (1994) Mouse plasma glutathione peroxidase cDNA sequence analysis and renal proximal tubular expression and secretion *Journal of Biological Chemistry* **269** 27066–27073

Monteiro HP and Stern A (1996) Redox regulation of tyrosine phosphorylation-dependent signal transduction pathways *Free Radical Biology and Medicine* **21** 323–333

Muscari C, Guarnieri C, Stefanelli C, Giaccari A and Caldarera CM (1995) Protective effect of spermine on DNA exposed to oxidative stress *Molecular and Cellular Biochemistry* **144** 125–129

Parrish JJ, Susko-Parrish JL, Winer MA and First NL (1988) Capacitation of bovine sperm by heparin *Biology of Reproduction* **38** 1171–1180

Perry AC, Jones R and Hall L (1993) Isolation and characterization of a rat cDNA clone encoding a secreted superoxide dismutase reveals the epididymis to be a major site of its expression *Biochemical Journal* **293** 21–25

Roveri A, Casasco A, Maiorino M, Dalan P, Calligaro A and Ursini F (1992) Phospholipid hydroperoxide glutathione-peroxidase of rat testes – gonadotrophin dependence and immunocytochemical identification *Journal of Biological Chemistry* **267** 6142–6146

Schwaab V, Baud E, Ghyselinck N, Mattei MG, Dufaure JP and Drevet JR (1995) Cloning of the mouse gene encoding plasma glutathione peroxidase – organization, sequence and chromosomal localization *Gene* **167** 25–31

Soler C, Yeung C-H and Cooper TG (1994) Development of sperm motility patterns in the murine epididymis *International Journal of Andrology* **17** 271–278

Tan CM, Xenoyannis S and Feldman RD (1995) Oxidant stress enhances adenylyl cyclase activation *Circulation Research* **77** 710–717

Twigg JP, Irvine DS and Aitken RJ (1998) Oxidative damage to DNA in human spermatozoa does not preclude pronucleus formation at ICSI *Human Reproduction* (in press)

Vernet P, Rigaudiere N, Ghyselinck N, Dufaure JP and Drevet JR (1996) *In vitro* expression of a mouse tissue specific glutathione peroxidase protein lacking selenocysteine can protect stably transfected mammalian cells against oxidative damage *Biochemistry and Cell Biology* **74** 125–131

Vernet P, Faure J, Dufaure JP and Drevet JR (1997) Tissue and developmental distribution, dependence upon testicular factors and attachment to spermatozoa of GPX5, a murine epididymis-specific glutathione peroxidase *Molecular Reproduction and Development* **47** 87–98

Vijayaraghavan S, Trautman KD, Goueli SA and Carr DW (1997) A tyrosine-phosphorylated 55-kilodalton motility-associated bovine sperm protein is regulated by cyclic adenosine 3′,5′-monophosphates and calcium *Biology of Reproduction* **56** 1450–1457

Visconti PE, Bailey JL, Moore GD, Pan D, Olds-Clarke P and Kopf GS (1995) Capacitation of mouse spermatozoa 1. Correlation between the capacitation state and protein tyrosine phosphorylation *Development* **121** 1129–1137

Yanagimachi, R (1994) Mammalian Fertilization. In *The Physiology of Reproduction* (2nd Edn) pp 189–317 Eds E Knobil and J D Neill. Raven Press, New York

Yeung C-H, Oberlander G and Cooper TG (1994) Maturation of hamster epididymal sperm motility and influence of the thiol status of hamster and rat spermatozoa on their motility patterns *Molecular Reproduction and Development* **38** 347–355

Yeung C-H, Morrell JM, Cooper TG, Weinbauer GF and Hodges JK (1996a) Maturation of sperm motility in the epididymis of the common marmoset (*Callithrix jacchus*) and the Cynomolgus monkey (*Macaca fascicularis*) *International Journal of Andrology* **19** 113–121

Yeung C-H, Cooper T G and Weinbauer G F (1996b) Maturation of monkey spermatozoa in the epididymis with respect to their ability to undergo the acrosome reaction *Journal of Andrology* **17** 427–432

Yoshida R, Nukiwa T, Watanabe Y, Fujiwara M, Hirata F and Hayaishi O (1980) Regulation of indoleamine 2,3-dioxygenase activity in small intestine and epididymis of mice *Archives of Biochemistry and Biophysics* **203** 343–351

Zini A and Schlegel PN (1996) Catalase messenger RNA expression in the male rat reproductive tract *Journal of Andrology* **17** 473–480

Journal of Reproduction and Fertility Supplement **53**, 119–136

Interactions between epididymal secretions and spermatozoa

T. G. Cooper

Institute of Reproductive Medicine of the University, Domagkstraße 11, D-48129 Münster, Germany

The interactions between spermatozoa and epididymal secretions are reviewed with respect to the nature of the interactions, the maturity of the spermatozoa and the environment in which spermatozoa mature. The estimated ionic strength of epididymal fluid is low enough for all peripheral proteins to be in close contact with the membrane. Two sorts of interactions are evident, those dependent on the state of the maturity of the spermatozoa (for example peripheral proteins and some integral proteins) and those independent of it (many integral proteins). For the former, a change in the sperm membrane charge must occur to permit recognition of peripheral proteins and the insertion of secreted charged integral membrane proteins may precede the interaction with more distally secreted products. For integral proteins, partition into the membrane may depend on the composition of the plasma membrane. Changes in the sterol content of particular domains have been documented and an array of lipid-binding proteins secreted by the epididymis may mediate these changes. The dependence of the transfer of lipid-anchored proteins to spermatozoa on membranous vesicles invites reassessment of the situation of spermatozoa within the epididymis and their contact with membranous vesicles and merocrine secretions that may be crucial to promoting physiological changes in spermatozoa.

Introduction

The widespread and rapid introduction of molecular biology techniques has driven epididymal research forwards at a rapid pace. Together with increased understanding of the behaviour of membrane lipids, it has secured a better appreciation of the complexities of changes occurring to spermatozoa in the epididymis. Nevertheless, the intricacies of forever changing domains on spermatozoa make an exact description of the maturation process unfeasible at present and understanding the regulation of the sequential processes remains to be elucidated. This article reviews some of the myriad processes that occur to spermatozoa during epididymal transit that involve interaction with mainly proteinaceous epididymal secretions against a background of long-established observations on epididymal anatomy and physiology.

By way of introduction, Fig. 1 is a simplified account of the sites of some gene and protein expression in the rat epididymis, taken as the most investigated species. It serves to highlight that some proteins are expressed in epithelial cells proximally only, some distally only, and some throughout the duct system. As would be expected, cellular sites of gene expression determined by *in situ* hybridization are those where proteins are localized by immunohistochemical procedures; secretion is indicated by reaction product over the epithelial cell microvilli and luminal spermatozoa. It is clear that as they move through the duct system spermatozoa come into sequential contact with different proteins, some of the functions of which are required for fertilization. Other proteins may alter the spermatozoa to permit the association or insertion of proteins from more distal parts of the tract and thus indirectly facilitate the development of fertilizing capacity (see Fig. 1).

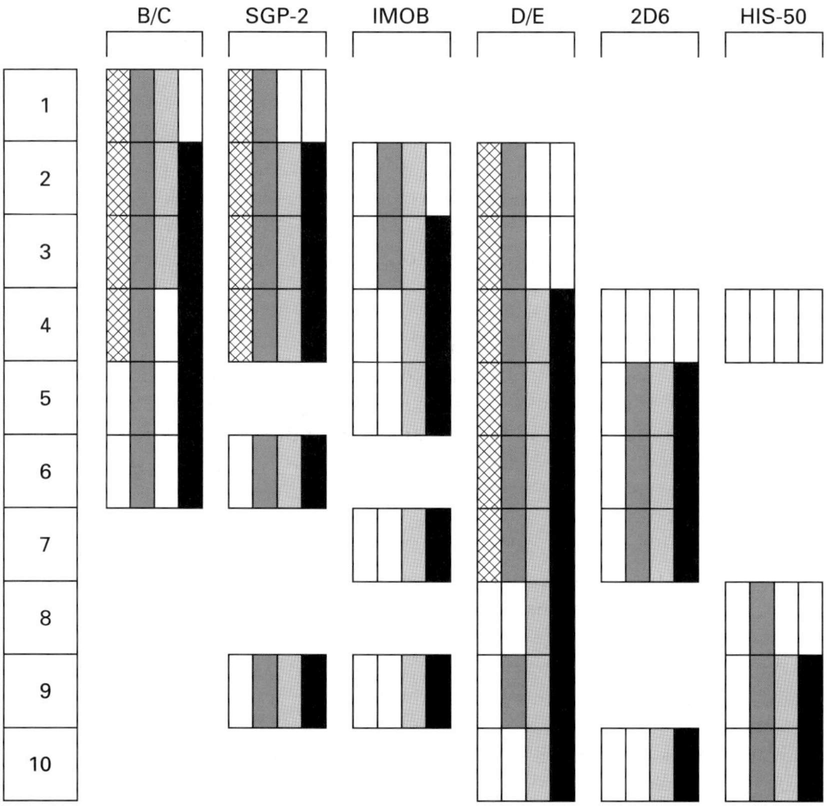

Fig. 1. Schematic representation of the localization (from left to right for each protein) of the genes (hatched boxes) and proteins located histochemically in principal cells (mid-grey boxes), on their microvilli (light grey boxes) and on spermatozoa in the lumen (black boxes) of different regions of the rat epididymis (after Moore *et al.*, 1990, 1 = initial segment and proximal (2,5,8), middle (3,6,9) and distal (4,7,10) regions of the caput, corpus and cauda epididymidis, respectively). (According to Reid and Cleland (1957): 1 = zone 1; 2 = zone 2; 3 = zone 3; 4 = proximal zone 4; 5 = mid-zone 4; 6 = distal zone 4 and proximal zone 5; 7 = middle zone 5; 8 = distal zone 5; 9 = terminal zone 5; 10 = zone 7.) Clear boxes indicate epididymal regions and compartments that were examined but found to be negative for the components studied. Sequential interaction of maturing spermatozoa with B/C (retinoic acid modification, membrane modelling?) → SGP-2 (glycoprotein modification, membrane modelling?) → IMOB (preventing motility) → D/E (zona binding? vitellus fusion?) → 2D6 (vitellus fusion?) → HIS-50 (decapacitation?) is shown.

Similar diagrams could be drawn for other species, although different locations of similar proteins may be found. For example β-hexosaminidase can be demonstrated histochemically in principal cells along the length of the rat epididymis (Hermo *et al.*, 1997) but one boar antagglutinin (subsequently identified as β-hexosaminidase: Syntin *et al.*, 1996) is not found beyond the mid-corpus in this species (Dacheux and Dacheux, 1988). Such inter-species comparisons are complicated by the difficulty in identifying analogous regions of the epididymis across species.

Nature of Proteins Secreted in Epididymal Fluid

An exhaustive list of epididymal-specific proteins found in many species is beyond the scope of this review and Table 1 is limited to listing major secreted proteins, most of which interact with spermatozoa, that can be recognized by function or amino acid or nucleotide sequence. It is evident that many similar proteins are found in epididymal secretions of several species whereas others are specific to one species. Some of the former have been demonstrated to function as carrier molecules for lipid-soluble ligands (for example phospholipids (PLBP), glycolipids (SGP-2), sterols (HE-1), iron (lactoferrin), retinoic acid (ESP-1)) and their presence across species attests to an active involvement of epididymal secretions with membrane remodelling. For the latter, for example ASF, detected solely in the rabbit, may perform similar functions to completely different proteins in other species or may be necessitated by peculiarities of the rabbit epididymis (for example higher scrotal temperature and high luminal magnesium concentration).

The multiplicity of enzymes secreted into epididymal fluid has been shown by direct measurement of activity with artificial substrates, although for most, the natural substrate (whether spermatozoa or proteins of epididymal or testicular origin) is unknown. Furthermore, some proteins that share either nucleotide or amino acid sequence homology with known proteins in databases may not perform the anticipated functions. For example, the epididymal secretory glutathione peroxidase in three species lacks the selenocysteine codon; the molecule itself contains no selenium and the enzyme activity is less than 0.1% of that of the cytosolic enzyme. In addition, the concentration of its substrate, glutathione, in epididymal fluid is far less than optimal (Okamura *et al.*, 1997). These authors have postulated another, protective, role for the protein that is found on the plasma membrane over the acrosome in two species.

Location of Secreted Proteins on Spermatozoa

In histochemical sections fixation will have precipitated luminal proteins upon luminal spermatozoa as well as microvilli, so that while providing evidence that after secretion there is a distal migration of protein, sometimes at the same regions as the protein is observed in the principal cells (*e.g.* HIS-50), or a little more distally (for example protein E), it provides no information on whether such proteins are truly sperm coating proteins *in situ*. Figure 2 shows a mature rat spermatozoon and the various locations on it where various secreted epididymal proteins have been reported. The localization of secreted proteins on sperm cells removed from the tract is difficult to ascertain, owing to the necessity of washing the cells to remove loosely adherent material (that may yet play a role *in situ*, see below), the fragility of their membranes to handling, the influence of fixatives, all of which may lead to exposure of intracellular organelles, as well as the nature and quality of antibodies used. Nevertheless, regional locations on spermatozoa are apparent, with some proteins (for example HIS-50) binding only to the sperm head and others (for example 2D6) only to the tail (Phillips *et al.*, 1991). Neither Brooks and Tiver (1983) nor Rankin *et al.* (1992) detected firm binding of protein B/C to spermatozoa from rats and mice under conditions *in vitro*, respectively. A report of binding of proteins D/E to the acrosomal region in uncapacitated rat spermatozoa (Rochwerger and Cuasnicú, 1992) conflicts with the post-acrosomal location of D/E (Brooks and Tiver, 1983) and purified protein E (Xu *et al.*, 1997). This highly selective targeting of proteins to sperm membranes reflects the nature of the protein, the membrane domain involved and the nature of the interaction between the two, and there is increasing evidence that the epididymis is involved in these changes.

Interactions of Epididymal Proteins with Spermatozoa and Uptake of Epididymal Proteins

Sperm coating proteins are usually considered as either peripheral or integral membrane proteins, depending on the ease with which they are extracted from the sperm cell *in vitro* (see Table 1 and Roy Jones, this supplement) and for some proteins this is unknown or unclear.

Table 1. Proteins secreted by the epididymis that are associated with spermatozoa in several species

Name/synonym*	kDa [subunits]	pI	CHO†	Interaction‡	Species	References§
ASF	360[290]			P	rabbit (not monkey, man, bull, horse, dog,	1–4
	(2 × 180[129])			P	hamster, guinea-pig, ram, mouse, rat)	
B/C, Lipocalin, Epididymal secretory protein I (ESP1), luminal retinoic acid binding protein (RBP), E-RABP, MEP-10						
	18–21	4.9–6.0		none?	rat, mouse, guinea-pig, pig	5–9
CD52, Major maturation antigen, SmemG, RB7, HE5, CE5, EP-1						
	18, 24 (32–37)		y	GPI	rat, mouse, man, monkey, chimpanzee, dog	10–19
		5.4–4.9 (3.8)				
		5.5–5.6 Caput				
		5.0–5.5 Cauda	I			
D/E, CRISP1, AEG, MEP-7, major acidic secretory glycoprotein, AEGL1						
	27–37	4.1–5.1		P? I?	rat, mouse, man	5,8,20–22
D	30			I?	rat	23,24
E, 4E9	26,38–26,32	3.8–4.0		I, not GPI	rat	23,25,26
E-GPX	24 (4 × 23)			?	mouse, rat, pig	9,27–31,70
E-SOD				?	rat	31,70
EP	61.4		y	P	hamster	32
EP3	23.8		y	P	hamster	32
EP4	20.4		y	P	hamster	32
EP21	21			?	rabbit	33
EP35	35			?	rabbit	33
ESA152	18			I, not GPI	ram	34,35
FMP	37			I?	bull, hamster	36–38
HIS-50/100	50/100		y	P	rat	39
GP17	17	2.0	y	P,I	rat	40
GP49	49			?	mouse	41
GP83	83			?	mouse	41
HE1, CE1, ESP14.6, EP-1						
	27			?	pig, man, monkey, bull, ram, dog, chimpanzee	9,17,18,42–44
HE2	10			?	man	45
HE3	14.9			?	man	46

Table 1. (*Cont*).

Name/synonym*	kDa [subunits]	pI	CHO†	Interaction‡	Species	References§
HE4, CE4	10	4.3		?	man, dog	17,18,47,48
immobilin	5 × 106		y	?	rat, hamster, guinea-pig	49
lactoferrin	70			?	pig, mouse	9,50
mannosidase	135 (sperm 27)			?	pig (not monkey, rabbit, dog, guinea-pig, hamster, rat)	51
PLBP,MEP-9	25	6.0		none?	mouse, rat + PLBP	8,52,53
p26h, p34H	26,34			GPI	hamster, man	71,72
procathepsin L	40			?	pig	54
R1		3.45		?	rabbit	55,56
R2		4.15		?	rabbit	55,56
R3		4.65		?	rabbit	55,56
SEP (40% DE)			y	P	rat	57,58
sialoprotein	30–34		y	?	rat	59
SGP2, Clusterin	66–70 (27–32, 35–41)	4.2–6.7 (4.8–7.2, 3.7–6.5)	?		pig, rat, ram	5,9,60
SMA4, T21, GP-49, GP-83)	54(49), 85(83)		y	S?	mouse	41,61–63
uteroglobin					rabbit	33
α		4.65		?	rabbit	64
β		4.25		?	rabbit	64
γ		4.15		?	rabbit	64
2D6	23.3	4.0–6.0		I?	rat	65
?	26			?	mouse	66
? (CD52?)	24			GPI	ram	35,67
?	23			?	rat, hamster (not rabbit, bull, mouse, guinea-pig)	68
?	26	4.0		I?	rat	69

* ASF, acrosome stabilizing factor; CD, cluster of differentiation; E-GOX, (epididymal) glutathione peroxidase; E-SOD, (epididymal) superoxide dismutase; EP, epididymal protein; ESA, epididymal specific antigen; FMP, forward motility protein; HIS, high ionic strength; GP, glycoprotein; HE, human epididymal; PLBP, phospholipid binding protein; R, rabbit; SEP, specific epididymal protein; SGP2, sulphated glycoprotein-2; SMA, sperm maturation antigen ; † carbohydrate: y, yes;
‡ nature of interaction with spermatozoa: P, peripheral; I, integral; S, disulphide, GPI, glycosylphosphatidylinositol anchor.
§ Key to References is in Appendix 1.

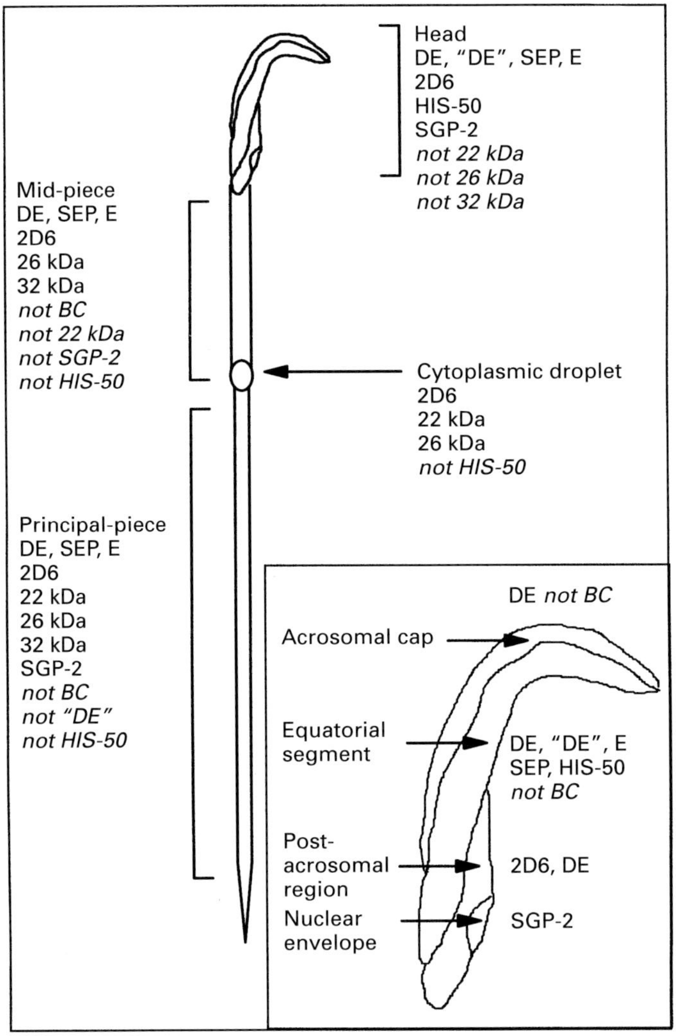

Fig. 2. Schematic immunocytochemical location on the rat spermatozoon of secreted epididymal proteins. For each cell compartment (head, mid-piece, tail) selective localization of proteins is found. For example, HIS-50 is found only on the head, 22 kDa (PLBP) is found only on the cytoplasmic droplet and principal piece but not the mid-piece or head; protein B/C is not associated with spermatozoa. There is debate over whether protein D/E is localized on the acrosomal or post-acrosomal membranes. Labelling of the sperm head with 2D6 antibody represents binding to an intracellular, not surface, site.

Peripheral proteins eluted with high ionic strength

The extent to which peripheral proteins are bound to spermatozoa may be reflected *in vitro* by use of different ionic strength solutions ($\mu = \frac{1}{2}\Sigma c.i^2$, where c = molar concentration and i = the charge on the species). For example, ASF is lost from mature rabbit spermatozoa as the ionic strength is raised from 0.335 to 0.410 (Oliphant and Singhas, 1979) but hamster proteins EP, EP3, EP4 are eluted from mature spermatozoa with ionic strengths greater than 0.5 (González-Echeverría *et al.*, 1982) and

HIS-50 is not eluted from rat cauda spermatozoa at ionic strengths below 0.8 (Rifkin and Olson, 1985). The finding that higher ionic strength media are required to elute SEP (a mixture of proteins C,D,E) from caput and corpus than from cauda spermatozoa (Kohane *et al.* 1980) indicates that changes occur to either the plasma membrane or the protein, or both, during maturation to decrease binding affinity for both proteins.

The nature of the substrates to which the proteins are held is not clear. Holt (1980) demonstrated increasing electronegative charge and thickness of a neuraminidase-sensitive glycocalyx in maturing spermatozoa from the bull and ram, but a residual negative charge remained on caudal membranes after neuraminidase treatment, similar to that of untreated caput spermatozoa, that was probably due to glycolipids, sulphates and phosphates. Suzuki and Nagano (1980) similarly demonstrated the presence of a glycocalyx on both the caput and cauda epididymidal spermatozoa, to which transient attachment of a variable glycocalyx material was observed as spermatozoa moved through the epididymis. Iusem *et al.* (1989) suggested that an acidic glycophosphoprotein with high mannose-type oligosaccharide (pI < 2) secreted by the caput epididymidis could be responsible for the increasing electronegativity of whole cells upon maturation. Species differences in membrane charge may explain the various affinities between homologous proteins and spermatozoa demonstrated by the weak association of CRISP-1 and mouse spermatozoa (Rankin *et al.*, 1992) and AEGL1 and human spermatozoa (Krätzschmar *et al.*, 1996).

Ionic strength of epididymal luminal fluid

Estimates of the ionic strength surrounding luminal spermatozoa can be made from data obtained by micropuncture in the rat because the molar concentration of ionic and organic osmolytes almost totally account for the osmotic pressure measured (Hinton 1990). They are 0.130, 0.100 and 0.085 in the caput, corpus and cauda epididymidis, respectively. These are extremely low compared with most solutions used to study spermatozoa *in vitro* (for example buffered saline μ = 0.310) and suggest that proteins considered loosely attached to spermatozoa *in vitro* may well be closely adherent *in situ*. However, there is no selective accumulation of proteins B/C, considered loosely adherent from *in vitro* studies, within the epididymal canal of tissue fixed *in situ* (Vierula *et al.*, 1995).

Uptake of peripheral proteins by spermatozoa

Spermatozoa from the corpus, but not caput, take up HIS-50 protein *in vitro* (Rifkin and Olson, 1985). This protein is held electrostatically to cauda spermatozoa, implying that caput spermatozoa have not yet acquired the binding sites that permit the uptake of HIS-50. Certain hamster cauda epididymidal proteins can be eluted from mature spermatozoa with high ionic strength and be transferred to the corpus epididymidis in lower ionic strength medium. The binding is sufficiently firm for them to remain on the spermatozoa during subsequent manipulation to improve their zona binding capacity *in vitro* (Cuasnicú *et al.*, 1984) and fertilizing capacity *in vitro* and *in vivo* (González-Echeverría *et al.*, 1984).

Causes of maturational changes in the uptake of peripheral membrane proteins

Modification of surface proteins could be responsible for the increased adherence of peripheral proteins upon maturation (for example HIS-50). This could be achieved by extrinsic, secreted enzymes, or by the activity of the spermatozoon itself. The activity of several glycosyltransferases associated with intact epididymal spermatozoa from the rat and mouse change as spermatozoa mature: galactosyltransferases (GT: Hamilton and Gould, 1982; Scully *et al.*, 1987), fucosyltransferase (FT: Cossu and Boitani, 1984) and sialyltransferase (ST: Bernal *et al.* 1980). Activities expressed per whole sperm cell are about the same for caput and cauda cells for GT, but FT and ST activities are higher in caput spermatozoa with the loss of FT activity on maturation due to a decrease in enzyme activity on the tail. Extensive work in rats by Tulsiani *et al.* (1993) has indicated a decreasing activity of ST, a peak in FT activity in the caput and more or less constant activity per cell of GT and GlcNAc transferase. In addition to expressing enzyme activity, rat spermatozoa are also acceptors for the sialyl and fucosyl residues transferred by sperm enzymes, cauda cells more than caput cells (Bernal *et al.*, 1980; Tulsiani *et al.*, 1993). Glycosidase activity is also associated with rat epididymal spermatozoa and caput spermatozoa again show more activity towards substrates of β-hexosaminidase and fucosidase (Hancock *et al.*, 1993).

External anchoring of proteins by disulphide bonds

Brooks (1985) was the first to suggest that binding of an epididymal protein (22 kDa PLBP) to spermatozoa may be via disulphide bridges, from evidence of the relative amounts of SH and SS on proteins in the fluid and on the spermatozoa. If such associations occur, the activity of epididymal sulphydryl oxidase may be important. A similar conclusion was drawn by Feuchter *et al.* (1988) for the binding of mouse epididymal SMA4 but this was not confirmed by Vernon *et al.* (1987).

Integral proteins of the membrane

Proteins that are not eluted from the sperm surface with high ionic strength media may be removed with chaotropic agents or detergents. The necessity for such treatment implies a tight relationship with the membrane, with hydrophobic regions inserting or otherwise being linked to the bilayer leaflets of the sperm membrane. Purified rat protein E reveals a tight association reminiscent of integral membrane proteins (Moore *et al.*, 1994; Xu *et al.*, 1997).

A debate surrounds the galactose oxidase-sensitive glycoprotein of rat cauda spermatozoa that appears first on corpus spermatozoa as a major maturation antigen. Whereas Hamilton *et al.* (1986) consider that the nonglycosylated peptide is found on spermatozoa entering the epididymis and becomes glycosylated during epididymal transit, the presence of a similar protein (32 kDa, pI 4.2) in epididymal fluid of the distal corpus and cauda (Jones *et al.*, 1981) and the crossreaction of an antibody against the fluid protein with the membrane (Brown *et al.*, 1983) suggested to these authors the acquisition of the protein on spermatozoa from a secreted epididymal product. This work was further confused by the uncertainty about whether the galactose oxidase-sensitive glycoproteins in rat epididymal fluid (32 kDa, pI 3.8) and spermatozoa (32 kDa, pI 4.9-5.4) differed (Brown *et al.*, 1983) or arose as an artefact from the sperm membrane (Goldin *et al.*, 1989).

Evidence supporting the view that there is modification by glycosylation *in situ* of pre-existing proteins on the sperm surface (Hamilton *et al.*, 1986) is the demonstration of galactose transfer to caput spermatozoa *in vitro* in the presence of rete testis fluid (a source of galactosyltransferase: Hamilton, 1980), or by spermatozoa galactosyltransferase itself (Hamilton and Gould, 1982). Could this reflect a physiological event in the epididymis? For detectable conversion in short *in vitro* incubations a source of UDP-galactose and Mn^{2+} is required and neither has been documented within the epididymal canal. Conversion could of course occur more slowly *in situ* (over the days it takes to progress through the caput epididymidis) in the absence of these factors. On the other hand, such factors may be present in the lumen if apocrine secretion by the epididymis is extensive (see below). The recent demonstration of zinc in the epididymis (Stoltenberg *et al.* 1996) may herald identification of other divalent metal ions in the epididymis.

More recent work on this galactose oxidase-sensitive major maturation antigen of spermatozoa has shown it to be linked to the sperm surface by a glycosylphosphatidyl anchor (Moore *et al.*, 1989). Analysis of peptide fragments of SMemG (Eccleston *et al.*, 1994) produced the amino acid sequence predicted from the cDNA of a rat epididymal specific gene product (Kirchhoff, 1994) that is homologous to the human gene product HE5, previously identified as the peptide backbone of the small (26 kDa) highly glycosylated lymphocyte antigen CD52 (Hale *et al.*, 1993; Kirchhoff *et al.*, 1993; Kirchhoff , 1996). This is considered by Kirchhoff and Hale (1996) to be secreted and inserted into the membrane with its lipid anchor intact, for which there is now evidence (see below).

Uptake of integral membrane proteins by spermatozoa

Ovine testicular spermatozoa can absorb a highly glycosylated 24 kDa protein during incubation for 2–6 h with cauda epididymidal fluid. Since this is a GPI-linked, galactose oxidase-sensitive protein that contains sialic acid (Voglmayr *et al.*, 1980, 1982, 1983, 1985; Weaver *et al.*, 1993), it resembles the GPI-linked major galactose oxidase-sensitive integral membrane protein CD52. Human seminal CD52 is an acidic (pI 2.5–3.0) glycoprotein (Diekmann *et al.*, 1977) of epididymal origin that can be transferred from diluted human epididymal fluid and seminal fluid to testicular, efferent duct and corpus epididymidal spermatozoa (Yeung *et al.*, 1997).

By contrast, no interaction was discernible between the rat galactose oxidase sensitive protein and testicular (Brown *et al.* 1983) or caput epididymidal spermatozoa (Zeheb and Orr, 1984), although the former are capable of binding another acidic rat caput epididymidal phosphoprotein (GP17, 17 kDa, pI 2.0) from cauda epididymidal fluid during *in vitro* incubation for up to 4 h (Iusem *et al.*, 1989). The uptake of this protein is low, but is more specific (44% can be inhibited by excess antigen) than that shown by caput (12%), corpus (2%) or cauda (9%) spermatozoa, suggesting a saturation of binding sites even in caput spermatozoa.

Forward motility protein (FMP), a bovine epididymal protein of caudal origin purported to promote forward motion of stimulated immature spermatozoa, can be extracted from caudal spermatozoa by detergents and caput, but not cauda, epididymidal spermatozoa can remove FMP from bovine seminal plasma in bulls (Acott and Hoskins, 1981) and hamsters (Raynaud and Kann, 1986). Rat caput spermatozoa can bind a 26 kDa protein (pI 4.0) extracted by detergents from rat cauda sperm membranes during incubation for 1 h in PBS (Olson *et al.*, 1987).

A 27 kDa chimpanzee epididymal sperm protein (EP-1) is taken up by caput spermatozoa during 1 h incubation at 34°C in (low ionic strength) cauda epididymidal fluid (Young *et al.*, 1987) by an unknown mechanism. Several 27 kDa proteins occur (Young *et al.* 1994), one of them being a sterol-binding protein (Fröhlich and Young, 1996) that may be responsible for modifying membrane sterol content.

Causes of maturational changes in the uptake of integral membrane proteins

As the nature of the lipid bilayer of membranes influences the partition of hydrophobic or GPI-linked anchors into them, maturational changes in membrane composition could be responsible for the differences in uptake of integral membrane proteins on maturation, for example, the failure of caput, as opposed to corpus, epididymidal spermatozoa from the monkey to take up CD52 (Yeung *et al.*, 1997). Domain-specific changes in membrane lipids can be visualized by examination of spermatozoa incubated with filipin. This antibiotic forms a complex with sterols visible in freeze fracture images of definite membranes of the spermatozoa. Figure 3 reveals that the number of sterol molecules per unit area of plasma membrane overlying the acrosome of four species during maturation in the epididymis is not consistent. The biphasic pattern in the hamster may reflect first the loss of cholesterol and then uptake of sterol sulphates upon maturation (Legault *et al.*, 1978; Bleau and vandenHeuvel, 1974), since these are not distinguished by the antibiotic.

Peripheral and integral membrane binding

In the mouse, proteins D/E and PLBP are also extracted by low salt and detergents indicating two forms of attachment (Rankin *et al.*, 1992). Similarly, rat protein GP17 can be removed from cauda spermatozoa by both high salt ($\mu = 1.0$, 40%) and detergent (60%) (Iusem *et al.*, 1989).

Significance of Membrane Vesicles in the Epididymis

It is imperative to chart the origin of vesicles of epithelial origin within the epididymal lumen, as they are a prerequisite for membrane-mediated transfer to the spermatozoa of epididymal proteins secreted with their lipid anchor intact. Merocrine secretion (the reverse of endocytosis) has long been

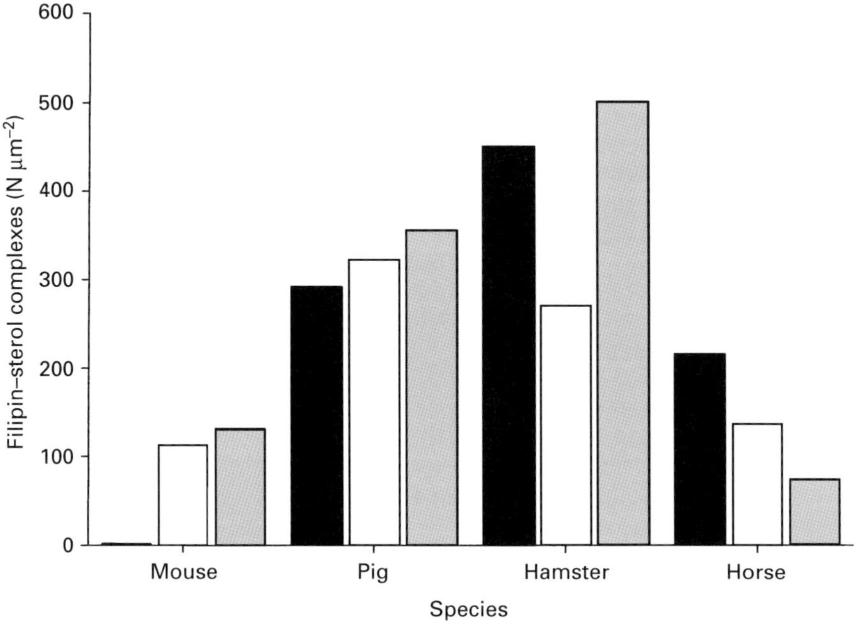

Fig. 3. Number of filipin–sterol complexes per μm^2 of plasma membrane over the acrosome of maturing spermatozoa from the mouse, pig , hamster and horse (black, caput; white, corpus; grey, cauda). Data from Toshimori *et al.*, 1985; Seki *et al.*, 1992; Suzuki, 1988; and Lopez and de Souza, 1991.

considered the major mode of secretion in the epididymis for proteins conventionally synthesized in RER and transported through the Golgi apparatus (Nicander and Malmqvist, 1977), but there is increasing evidence for apocrine secretion playing a role in the male reproductive tract. This alternative route, in which cell 'blebbing' and loss of cytoplasmic components into the lumen, could give rise to vesicles pinched off the microvilli. Whereas the original observations of organelle-poor cytoplasm extending into the lumen and blebbing (for example, Agrawal and Vanha-Perttulla, 1988) were considered by some anatomists to be indicative of inadequate, often immerse, fixation of large organs with resultant poor tissue preservation, the persistence of these structures in rapidly and well-fixed epididymal tissue of monkeys, cats and rats (see Fornés and De Rosas, 1991) supports the view that apocrine secretion is a normal phenomenon in the epididymis. There is strong evidence in the murine vas deferens that this route is taken by proteins lacking a signal sequence to gain entry to the lumen (Marin *et al.*, 1995). Antigenic similarity between prostasomes in human, semen and components in the epididymis has lead to the suggestion that these vesicles be called 'seminosomes' or 'aposomes' to indicate their multifarious origin (Renneberg *et al.*, 1997), but neither prostasomes nor evidence for diacytosis (an unusual route of passage of membrane bound 'prostasomes' through prostate and coagulating gland epithelial cells) have been observed in the epididymis. If apocrine secretion of vesicles with cytoplasmic contents in the epididymis is extensive, a whole new aspect of epididymal function comes to light: for example, the disruption of aposomes in the lumen would release cytoplasmic components (for example nucleoside sugars essential for glycosylation of proteins) and thus may provide the necessary cofactors for sperm surface glycosylation.

Ultrastructural Evidence for Interaction of Spermatozoa with Luminal Contents

During epididymal transit soluble and vesicular secretions of the epididymal epithelium will be thoroughly mixed with vital and degenerating spermatozoa which at some time may come into contact with the epithelial microvilli. Epididymal secretions may be involved in these interactions.

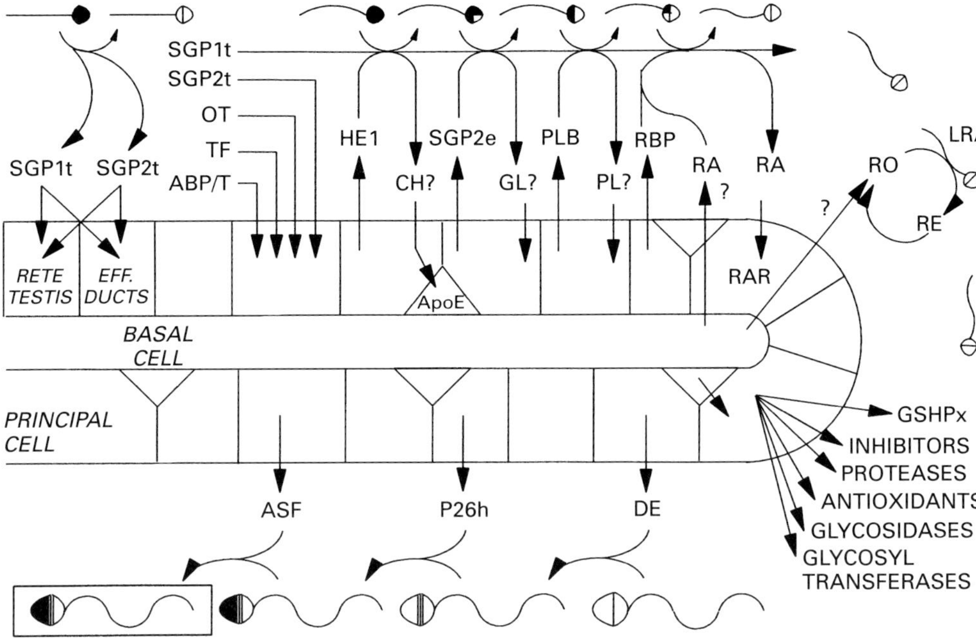

Fig. 4. Speculative scheme of the epididymal involvement in sperm maturation and storage. Spermatozoa are first modified by proteins in testicular and epididymal fluid and later acquire coating proteins in specific locations to facilitate sperm–egg and sperm–zona binding and to necessitate capacitation. ABP/T, androgen-binding protein–testosterone complex; ApoE, apolipoprotein E (involved in sterol transport); ASF, acrosome stabilizing factor; CH, cholesterol; DE (CRISP-1, see Table 1); GL, glycolipid; Eff. Ducts, efferent ducts; GSHPx, glutathione peroxidase; HE1, sterol-binding protein; LRAT, lecithin-retinol acyltransferase; OT, oxytocin; P26h (see Table 1); PL, phospholipid; PLB, phospholipid-binding protein; RA, retinoic acid; RAR, retinoic acid receptor α; RBP, retinoic acid binding protein (see Table 1); RE, retinyl esters; RO, retinol; SGP1t, sulphated glycoprotein-1 (testicular form); SGP2t/e, testicular and epididymal forms of sulphated glycoprotein-2; TF, transferrin. From Cooper, 1998.

Contact between spermatozoa and epididymal proteins in situ

Temporary association *in situ* between spermatozoa and a variable glycocalyx material (VGM) has been demonstrated in ultrastructural studies by Suzuki and Nagano (1980). Attachment occurs in the mid-caput but separation begins in the distal caput epididymidis and is complete in the cauda epididymidis. Neither the nature of the protein nor the interaction is known (CRISP1 was considered) and a relationship to the transient changes in distinct membrane topography suggests that coincident, and possibly causal, changes occur at the time.

Contact between spermatozoa and membrane vesicles and epithelial microvilli

The Chinese hamster displays an obvious maturation-dependent association with intraluminal membranous vesicles (Yanagimachi *et al.*, 1985). These first appear in close apposition to the plasma membrane over the acrosome of spermatozoa, but no other sperm domains, in the distal caput. The number of vesicles decreases in the distal cauda and they are absent from vasal spermatozoa despite their presence in the lumen. No evidence of fusion with the membrane was observed and they were easily removed from spermatozoa by washing in Tyrode's solution ($\mu = 0.349$). Contact between vesicles and spermatozoa within the epididymal lumen, but less specific (heads and tails), has been documented in rats (Fornés and De Rosas, 1991). Electron micrographs of well fixed epididymal material do occasionally indicate the contact of luminal spermatozoa with the microvilli, but it is generally considered that this is a fortuitous event unrelated to their acquisition of secretions. By contrast, in the South American guinea-pig *Galea musteloides,* there is extensive contact of sperm acrosomes in the cauda epididymidis with microvilli (Guttierez *et al.*, 1995). Even in this species, the chances are small that all luminal spermatozoa would experience such contact and the role, if any, for the privileged few spermatozoa is obscure.

Contact between components of the epithelial cells (microvilli and vesicles related to or stemming from them) could mediate transfer of lipid components, or lipid-anchored proteins, to and from the sperm membrane. Transfer of other GPI-anchored proteins between membrane vesicles and mature (human ejaculated) spermatozoa has been demonstrated by Rooney *et al.* (1996) for which contact and fusion of the vesicles and spermatozoa is not required.

Interaction between spermatozoa

A feature of many New World species is agglutination of spermatozoa within the epididymal canal in rouleaux that persist outside it. A role for the epididymis in induction of these rouleaux in guinea-pigs is suggested by the dispersion of these sperm agglutinates by WH-30 antibody (Flaherty *et al.*, 1993) which clearly recognizes antigens on the membranes involved in the cell association. As it also detects determinants on testicular spermatozoa in this species (Myles and Primakoff, 1983), but spermatozoa from the caput do not agglutinate (Hoffer and Greenberg, 1978), there must be either changes to the WH-30 antigen during epididymal maturation or secretion of (unknown) 'agglutinins' that bridge WH-30 of adjacent spermatozoa. For species in which association of spermatozoa within the epididymal duct has been observed, the biological significance is thought to lie beyond the male tract in protecting the large acrosome (guinea-pigs) or promoting flagellation in viscous media. In contrast, spermatozoa released from the epididymis may initially form small 'rosettes' of head–head agglutination upon release from the epididymis that rapidly disperse (Fornés and Burgos, 1990). Epididymal secretion D/E has been demonstrated in this adhesion between spermatozoa in the epididymal lumen (Fornés and Burgos, 1994).

Evidence from other species has indicated that epididymal fluid contains proteins that prevent the agglutination of immature spermatozoa that occurs once they are removed from the tract and diluted. These 'antagglutinins' have been associated with 17 and 18.5 kDa FMP in the hamster (Raynaud and Kann, 1986) and with 65 kDa (Dacheux and Dacheux, 1988) and 25 kDa (Harayama *et al.*, 1996) proteins in the boar. They presumably associate with surface moieties that have affinity for each other on spermatozoa but the physiological importance of this is obscure since immature spermatozoa are not normally removed from the tract – they may merely highlight changes in the surface properties of the spermatozoa during maturation that are not obvious within the epididymal duct in the microscope. Similar reasoning may explain the visible agglutination of immature spermatozoa in the caput of the loris epididymis which is not evident in the cauda (Phillips and Bedford, 1987).

In contrast to the association of live spermatozoa, aggregates ('clusters') of non-viable spermatozoa detected within the epididymal lumen are first detected in the proximal cauda of rats and other species (see Fornés and Burgos, 1990) and increase in size and number distally. Epididymal protein D/E can be immunolocalized in these clusters (Fornés and Burgos, 1994) but it may not be the sole epididymal protein sequestered there. The presence of epididymal glycoproteins may merely reflect the charged, adhesive nature of intracellular sperm components exposed within these masses. They may nevertheless play a role in the accretion of effete spermatozoa into masses separate from viable cells.

Conclusion

The interaction of spermatozoa with epididymal secretions during their sojourn in the epididymis occurs in a low ionic strength environment in which proteins free in solution and lipid-anchored proteins bound to membrane vesicles come into contact with spermatozoa whose surface glycoproteins and membrane lipids are undergoing constant change. Epididymal secretions are responsible for activating and inhibiting luminal and sperm-bound enzymes that further modify membrane components, thus indirectly influencing the state of the membrane. As a consequence of these membrane changes occurring proximally, other more distal epididymal secretions are able to interact with the membrane to provide specific components required for fertilization or to provide stability to a potentially unstable membrane.

Appendix 1. Key to References in Table 1

1 Reynolds AB and Oliphant G (1984) Production and characterization of monoclonal antibodies to the sperm acrosome stabilizing factor (ASF): utilization for purification and molecular analysis of ASF *Biology of Reproduction* **30** 775–786; **2 Reynolds AB and Oliphant G** (1986) Quantitation of the rabbit sperm acrosome stabilizing factor utilizing a sensitive immunoradiometric assay *Biology of Reproduction* **35** 705–715; **3 Oliphant G and Singhas CA** (1979) Iodination of rabbit sperm plasma membranes: relationship of specific surface proteins to epididymal function and sperm capacitation *Biology of Reproduction* **21** 937–944; **4 Reynolds AB, Thomas TS, Wilson WL and Oliphant G** (1989) Concentration of acrosome stabilising factor (ASF) in rabbit epididymal fluid and species specificity of anti-ASF antibodies *Biology of Reproduction* **40** 673–680; **5 Cooper TG** (1992) Epididymal proteins and sperm maturation *Spermatogenesis, Fertilization, Contraception. Molecular, Cellular and Endocrine Events in Male Reproduction* pp 285–318 Ed. E Nieschlag and U-F Habenicht. Springer Verlag, Berlin; **6 Flickinger CJ, Herr JC and Eril KE** (1986) Identification and isolation of epididymal luminal proteins of the mouse *Journal of Andrology* **7** 163–168; **7 Rankin TL, Ong DE and Orgebin-Crist M-C** (1992) The 18 kDa mouse epididymal protein (MEP 10) binds retinoic acid *Biology of Reproduction* **46** 767–771; **8 Rankin TL, Tsuruta KJ, Holland MK, Griswold MD and Orgebin-Crist M-C** (1992) Isolation, immunolocalization and sperm-association of three proteins of 18, 25 and 29 kilodaltons secreted by the mouse epididymis *Biology of Reproduction* **46** 747–766; **9 Syntin P, Dacheux F, Druart X, Gatti J-L, Okamura N and Dacheux J-L** (1996) Characterization and identification of proteins secreted in the various regions of the adult boar epididymis *Biology of Reproduction* **55** 956–974; **10 Eccleston ED, White TW, Howard JB and Hamilton DW** (1994) Characterization of a cell surface glycoprotein associated with maturation of rat spermatozoa *Molecular Reproduction and Development* **37** 110–119; **11 Kirchhoff C** (1994) A major messenger ribonucleic acid of the rodent epididymis encodes a small glycosylphosphatidylinositol-anchored lymphocyte surface antigen *Biology of Reproduction* **50** 896–902; **12 Perry ACF, Jones R and Hall L** (1992) Identification of an abundant monkey epididymal transcript encoding a homologue of human CAMPATH-1 antigen precursor *Biochemica et Biophysica Acta* **1171** 122–124; **13 Kirchhoff C, Krull N, Pera I and Ivell R** (1993) A major mRNA of the human epididymis principal cells, HE5, encodes the leucocyte differentiation CDw52 antigen peptide backbone *Molecular Reproduction and Development* **34** 8–15; **14 Kirchhoff C** (1996) CD52 is the 'major maturation-associated' sperm membrane antigen *Molecular Human Reproduction* **2** 9–17; **15 Hamilton DW, Wenstrom JC and Baker JB** (1986) Membrane glycoproteins from spermatozoa: partial characterization of an integral *Mr* – c 24,000 molecule from rat spermatozoa that is glycosylated during epididymal maturation *Biology of Reproduction* **34** 925–936; **16 Zeheb R and Orr GA** (1984) Characterization of a maturation-associated glycoprotein on the plasma membrane of rat caudal epididymal sperm *Journal of Biological Chemistry* **259** 839–848; **17 Ellerbrock K, Pera I, Hartung S and Ivell R** (1994) Gene expression in the dog epididymis: a model for human epididymal function *International Journal of Andrology* **17** 314–323; **18 Pera I, Ivell R and Kirchhoff C** (1994) Regional variation of specific gene expression in the dog epididymis as revealed by in-situ transcript hybridization *International Journal of Andrology* **17** 324–330; **19 Diekman AB, Westvrook-Cae VA, Naaby-Hansen S, Klotz KL, Flickinger CJ and Herr JC** (1997) Biochemical characterisation of sperm agglutination antigen-1, a human sperm surface antigen implicated in gamete interactions *Biology of Reproduction* **57** 1136–1144; **20 Goldin BF, Voulalas PJ and Orr GA** (1989) Characterization of the maturation-associated galactose oxidase-sensitive glycoproteins of rat caudal sperm plasma membrane and epididymal fluid *Archives of Biochemistry and Biophysics* **270** 208–218; **21 Hayashi M, Fujimoto S, Takano H, Ushika T, Abe K, Ishikura H, Yochida MC, Kirchhoff C, Ishibashi T and Kasahara M** (1996) Characterization of a human glycoprotein with a potential role in sperm–egg fusion: cDNA cloning, immunohistochemical localization and chromosomal assignment of the gene AEGL1 *Genomics* **32** 367–374; **22 Flickinger CJ** (1988)

Immunocytochemical localization of the major glycoprotein of epididymal fluid from the cauda in the epithelium of the mouse epididymis *Cell and Tissue Research* **251** 603–610; **23 Xu W and Hamilton DW** (1996) Identification of the rat epididymis-secreted 4E9 antigen as protein E: further biochemical characterization of the highly homologous epididymal secretory proteins D and E *Molecular Reproduction and Development* **43** 347–357; **24 Moore A, White TW, Ensrud KM and Hamilton DW** (1989) The major maturation glycoprotein found on rat cauda epididymal sperm surface is linked to the membrane via phosphatidylinositol *Biochemical and Biophysical Research Communications* **160** 460–468; **25 Xu W, Ensrud KM and Hamilton DW** (1997) The 26kDA protein recognised in rat cauda epididymal sperm by monoclonal antibody 4E9 has internal peptide sequence that is identical to the secreted form of epididymal protein E *Molecular Reproduction and Development* **46** 377–382; **26 Moore A, Ensrud K, White TW, Frethem CD and Hamilton DW** (1994) Rat epididymis-specific sperm maturation antigens. I. Evidence that the 26 kDa 4E9 antigen found on rat caudal epididymal sperm tail is derived from a protein secreted by the epididymis *Molecular Reproduction and Development* **37** 181–194; **27 Perry ACF, Jones R, Ninang LSP, Jackson RM and Hall L** (1992) Genetic evidence for an androgen-regulated epididymal secretory glutathione peroxidase whose transcript does not contain a selenocysteine codon *Biochemical Journal* **284** 863–870; **28 Ghyselinck NB, Jimenez C and Dufaure JP** (1991) Sequence homology of androgen-regulated epididymal proteins with glutathione peroxidase in mice *Journal of Reproduction and Fertility* **93** 461–466; **29 Jimenez C, Ghyselinck NB, Depeiges A and Dufaure J-P** (1990) Immunocytochemical localization and association with spermatozoa of androgen-regulated proteins of Mr 24 000 secreted by the mouse epididymis *Biologie Cellulaire* **68** 171–174; **30 Okamura N, Iwaki Y, Hiramoto S, Tamba M, Bannai S, Sugita Y, Syntin P, Dacheux F and Dacheux J-L** (1997) Molecular cloning and characterization of the epididymis-specific glutathione peroxidase-like protein secreted in the porcine epididymal fluid *Biochemica et Biophysica Acta* **1336** 99–109; **31 Perry AC, Jones R and Hall L** (1993) Isolation and characterization of a rat cDNA clone encoding a secreted superoxide dismutase reveals the epididymis to be a major site of its expression *Biochemical Journal* **293** 21–25; **32 González Echeverriá FM, Cuasnicú PS and Blaquier JA** (1982) Identification of androgen-dependent glycoproteins in the hamster epididymis and their association with spermatozoa *Journal of Reproduction and Fertility* **64** 1–7; **33 Garcia C, Regaldo F, Lopez de Haro MS and Nieto A** (1988) Ultrastructural localization of epididymal secretory proteins associated with the surface of spermatozoa from rabbit cauda epididymis *Histochemical Journal* **20** 708–714; **34 McKinnon CA, Weaver FE, Yoder JA, Fairbanks G and Wolf DE** (1991) Cross-linking a maturation-dependent ram sperm plasma membrane antigen induces the acrosome reaction *Molecular Reproduction and Development* **29** 200–207; **35 Weaver FE, Gaffney KJ, Dono JE, Germain BJ and Fairbanks G** (1990) Hydrophobic anchoring of maturation-dependent surface proteins of ram spermatozoa *Fertilization in Mammals* pp 423 Ed. BD Bavister, J Cummins and ERS Roldan. Serono Norwell, Massachusetts; **36 Acott TS and Hoskins DD** (1981) Bovine sperm forward motility protein: binding to epididymal spermatozoa *Biology of Reproduction* **24** 234–240; **37 Acott TS, Johnson DT, Brandt H and Hoskins DD** (1979) Sperm forward motility protein: tissue distribution and species cross reactivity *Biology of Reproduction* **20** 247–252; **38 Serres C and Kann ML** (1984) Motility induction in hamster spermatozoa from caput epididymidis: effects of forward motility protein (FMP) and calmodulin inhibitor *Reproduction, Nutrition and Development* **24** 81–89; **39 Rifkin JM and Olson GE** (1985) Characterization of maturation-dependent extrinsic proteins of the rat sperm surface *Journal of Cell Biology* **100** 1582–1591; **40 Iusem ND, Pineiro L, Blaquier JA and Belocopitow E** (1989) Identification of a major secretory protein from rat epididymis: interaction with spermatozoa *Biology of Reproduction* **40** 307–336; **41 Liu H-W, Shang S-T, Chao C-F and Muller C** (1991) The secretion of two sperm maturation-related glycoproteins in BALB/c mouse epididymis *Cell and Tissue Research* **265** 409–414; **42 Kirchhoff C, Osterhoff C and Young L** (1996) Molecular cloning and characterization of HE1, a major secretory protein of the human epididymis *Biology of Reproduction* **54** 847–856; **43 Perry ACF, Jones R and Hall L** (1995) The monkey ESP14.6 mRNA, a novel transcript expressed at high levels in the epididymis *Gene* **153** 291–292; **44 Nolan JP and Hammerstedt RH** (1997) Regulation of membrane stability and the acrosome reaction in mammalian sperm *FASEB Journal* **11** 670–682; **45 Osterhoff C, Kirchhoff C, Krull N and Ivell R** (1994) Molecular cloning and characterization of a novel human sperm antigen (HE2) specifically expressed in the proximal epididymis *Biology of Reproduction* **50** 516–525; **46 Kirchhoff C, Pera L, Rust W and Ivell R** (1994) Major human epididymis-specific gene product, HE3, is the first representative of a novel gene family *Molecular Reproduction and Development* **37** 130–137; **47 Kirchhoff C, Habben I, Ivell R and Krull N** (1991) A major human epididymis-specific cDNA encodes a protein with sequence homology to extracellular proteinase inhibitors *Biology of Reproduction* **45** 350–357; **48 Perry ACF, Jones R and Hall L** (1993) Sequence analysis of monkey acrosin-trypsin inhibitor transcripts and their abundant expression in the epididymis *Biochemica et*

Biophysica Acta **1172** 159–160; **49 Ruiz-Bravo N** (1988) Tissue and cell specificity of immobilin biosynthesis *Biology of Reproduction* **39** 901–911;**50 Yu L-C and Chen Y-H** (1993) The development profile of lactoferrin in mouse epididymis *Biochemical Journal* **296** 107–111; **51 Okamura N, Tamba M, Liao HJ, Onoe S, Sugita Y, Dacheux F and Dacheux J-L** (1995) Cloning of complementary DNA encoding a 135-kilodalton protein secreted from porcine corpus epididymis and its identification as an epididymal-specific alpha-mannosidase *Molecular Reproduction and Development* **42** 141–149; **52 Perry ACF, Hall L, Bell AE and Jones R** (1994) Sequence analysis of a mammalian phospholipid-binding protein from testis and epididymis and its distribution between spermatozoa and extracellular secretions *Biochemical Journal* **301** 235–242; **53 Araki Y, Vierula ME, Rankin TL, Tulsiani DRP and Orgebin-Crist M-C** (1992) Isolation and characterization of a 25-kilodalton protein from mouse testis: sequence homology with a phospholipid-binding protein *Biology of Reproduction* **47** 832–843; **54 Okamura N, Tamba M, Uchiyama Y, Sugita Y, Dacheux F, Syntin P and Dacheux J-L** (1995) Direct evidence for the elevated synthesis and secretion of procathepsin L in the distal caput epididymis of boar *Biochemica et Biophysica Acta* **1245** 221–226; **55 Moore HDM** (1980) Localization of specific glycoproteins secreted by the rabbit and hamster epididymis *Biology of Reproduction* **22** 705–718; **56 Moore HDM** (1981) Glycoprotein secretions of the epididymis in the rabbit and hamster: localization on epididymal spermatozoa and the effect of specific antibodies on fertilization in vivo *Journal of Experimental Zoology* **215** 77–85; **57 Garberi JC, Fontana JD and Blaquier JA** (1982) Carbohydrate composition of specific rat epididymal protein *International Journal of Andrology* **5** 619–626; **58 Kohane AC, Cameo MS, Pineiro L, Garberi JC and Blaquier JA** (1980) Distribution and site of production of specific proteins in the rat epididymis *Biology of Reproduction* **23** 181–187; **59 Yamamoto Y, Serizawa O and Uto N** (1991) *Limas flaxis* lectin specifies the maturation-related sialoglycoprotein in epididymal spermatozoa of rat *Zoological Science* **8** 329–337; **60 Mattmueller DH and Hinton BT** (1991) *In vivo* secretion and association of clusterin (SGP-2) in luminal fluid with spermatozoa in the rat testis and epididymis *Molecular Reproduction and Development* **30** 62–69; **61 Feuchter FA, Tabet AJ and Green MF** (1988) Maturation antigen of the mouse sperm flagellum. I. Analysis of its secretion, association with sperm and function *American Journal of Anatomy* **181** 67–76; **62 Vernon RB, Miller CH and Eddy EM** (1987) Further characterization of a secreted epididymal glycoprotein in mice that binds to sperm tails *Journal of Andrology* **8** 123–128; **63 Toshimori K, Araki S, Tanii I and Oura C** (1992) Masking the cryptodeterminant on the 54-kilodalton mouse sperm surface antigen *Biology of Reproduction* **47** 1161–1167; **64 Jones R, von Glos KI and Brown CR** (1981) Characterization of hormonally regulated secretory proteins from the caput epididymidis of the rabbit *Biochemical Journal* **196** 105–114; **65 Jones R and Brown CR** (1987) Identification and characterization of the 2D6 and Mr 23000 antigens on the plasma membrane of rat spermatozoa *Biochemical Journal* **241** 353–360; **66 Murphy GJP and Carroll J** (1987) Detection and localization of antigens on the surface of mouse spermatozoa. Antigen synthesis in the epididymis *Biochemical Journal* **241** 379–387; **67 Voglmayr JK, Fairbanks G, Jackowitz MA and Colella JR** (1980) Post-testicular developmental changes in the ram sperm cell surface and their relationship to luminal fluid proteins of the reproductive tract *Biology of Reproduction* **22** 655–667; **68 Hoos PC and Olson GE** (1988) Characterization of a 23kDa sperm-binding protein polypeptide of the golden hamster epididymis *Biology of Reproduction* **39** 131–140; **69 Olson GE, Lifsics MR, Winfrey VP and Rifkin JM** (1987) Modification of rat sperm flagellar plasma membrane during maturation in the epididymis *Journal of Andrology* **8** 129–147; **70 Zini A and Schlegel PN** (1997) Identification and characterization of antioxidant enzyme mRNAs in the rat epididymis *International Journal of Andrology* **20** 86–91; **71 Bégin S, Bérubé B, Boué F and Sullivan R** (1995) Comparative immunoreactivity of mouse and hamster sperm proteins recognized by an anti-P26h hamster sperm protein *Molecular Reproduction and Development* **41** 249–256; **72 Boué F, Blais J and Sullivan R** (1996) Surface localization of P34H, an epididymal protein, during maturation, capacitation, and acrosome reaction of human spermatozoa *Biology of Reproduction* **54** 1009–1017

References

Acott TS and Hoskins DD (1981) Bovine sperm forward motility protein: binding to epididymal spermatozoa *Biology of Reproduction* **24** 234–240

Agrawal Y and Vanha-Perttula T (1988) Electron microscopic study of the secretion process in bovine reproductive organs *Journal of Andrology* **9** 307–316

Bernal A, Torres J, Reyes A and Rosado A (1980) Presence and regional distribution of sialyl transferase in the epididymis of rat *Biology of Reproduction* **23** 290–293

Bleau G and vandenHeuvel WJA (1974) Desmosterol sulphate and desmosterol in hamster epididymal spermatozoa *Steroids* **24** 549–556

Brooks DE (1985) Characterization of a 22kDa protein with widespread tissue distribution but which is uniquely present in secretions of the testis and epididymis and on the surface of spermatozoa *Biochemica et Biophysica Acta* **841** 59–70

Brooks DE and Tiver K (1983) Localization of epididymal secretory proteins on rat spermatozoa *Journal of Reproduction and Fertility* **69** 651–657

Brown C, vonGlos KI and Jones R (1983) Changes in plasma membrane glycoproteins of rat spermatozoa during maturation in the epididymis *Journal of Cell Biology* **96** 256–264

Cooper TG (1998) Epididymis. In *Encyclopaedia of Reproduction* Vol. 2 pp. 1–17 Eds E Knobil and JD Neill. Academic Press, San Diego

Cossu G and Boitani C (1984) Lactosaminoglycans synthesised by mouse male germ cells are fucosylated by an epididymal fucosyltransferase *Developmental Biology* **102** 402–408

Cuasnicú PS, González Echeverría F, Piazza AD, Piñeiro L and Blaquier JA (1984) Epididymal proteins that mimic the androgenic effect on zona pellucida recognition by immature hamster spermatozoa *Journal of Reproduction and Fertility* **71** 427–431

Dacheux F and Dacheux JL (1988) Immunocytochemical localization of antagglutinin in the boar epididymis *Cell Tissue Research* **252** 329–337

Diekman AB, Westvrook-Cae VA, Naaby- Hansen S, Klotz KL, Flickinger CJ and Herr JC (1997) Biochemical characterisation of sperm agglutination antigen-1, a human sperm surface antigen implicated in gamete interactions *Biology of Reproduction* **57** 1136–1144

Eccleston ED, White TW, Howard JB and Hamilton DW (1994) Characterization of a cell surface glycoprotein associated with maturation of rat spermatozoa *Molecular Reproduction and Development* **37** 110–119

Feuchter FA, Tabet AJ and Green MF (1988) Maturation antigen of the mouse sperm flagellum I. Analysis of its secretion, association with sperm, and function *American Journal of Anatomy* **181** 67–76

Flaherty SP, Swann NJ, Primakoff P and Myles DG (1993) A role for the WH-30 protein in sperm–sperm adhesion during rouleaux formation in the guinea pig *Developmental Biology* **156** 243–252

Fornés MW and Burgos MH (1990) Sperm association in the rat epididymis *Microscopica Electronica Biologica Cellular* **14** 115–130

Fornés MW and Burgos MH (1994) Epididymal glycoprotein involved in rat sperm association *Molecular Reproduction and Development* **38** 43–47

Fornés MW and De Rosas JC (1991) Interaction between rat epididymal epithelium and spermatozoa *Anatomical Record* **231** 193–200

Fröhlich O and Young LG (1996) Molecular cloning and characterization of EP-1, the major protein in chimpanzee (*Pan troglodytes*) cauda epididymal fluid *Biology of Reproduction* **54** 857–864

Goldin BF, Voulalas PJ and Orr GA (1989) Characterization of the maturation-associated galactose oxidase-sensitive glycoproteins of rat caudal sperm plasma membrane and epididymal fluid *Archives of Biochemistry and Biophysics* **270** 208–218

González-Echéverría FM, Cuasnicú PS and Blaquier JA (1982) Identification of androgen-dependent glycoproteins in the hamster epididymis and their association with spermatozoa *Journal of Reproduction and Fertility* **64** 1–7

Gutierrez LS, Burgos MH and Brengio SD (1995) Cauda epididymis of *Galea musteloides* in periods of reproduction and gonadal regression 1. Ultrastructural and cytochemical studies *Biocell* **19** 141–151

Hale G, Rye PD, Warford A, Lauder I and Brito-Babapulle A (1993) The glycosylphosphatidylinositol-anchored lymphocyte antigen CDw52 is associated with the epididymal maturation of human spermatozoa *Journal of Reproductive Immunology* **23** 189–205

Hamilton DW (1980) UDP-galactose:*N*-acetylglucosamine galactosyltransferase in fluids from rat rete testis and epididymis *Biology of Reproduction* **23** 377–385

Hamilton DW and Gould RP (1982) Preliminary observations on enzymatic galactosylation of glycoproteins in the surface of rat caput epididymal spermatozoa *International Journal of Andrology* Supplement **5** 73–80

Hamilton DW, Wenstrom JC and Baker JB (1986) Membrane glycoproteins from spermatozoa: partial characterization of an integral Mr ≈ c 24,000 molecule from rat spermatozoa that is glycosylated during epididymal maturation *Biology of Reproduction* **34** 925–936

Hancock LW, Raab LS and Aronson NN (1993) Synthesis and processing of rat sperm-associated α-L-fucosidase *Biology of Reproduction* **48** 1228–1238

Harayama H, Kato S and Hammerstedt RH (1996) Electrophoretic characterization of boar antiagglutinin *Biology of Reproduction* **55** 325–332

Hermo L, Adamali HA, Mahuran D, Gravel RA and Trasler JM (1997) β-Hexosaminidase immunolocalization and α- and β- subunit gene expression in the rat testis and epididymis *Molecular Reproduction and Development* **46** 227–242

Hinton BT (1990) The testicular and epididymal luminal amino acid microenvironment in the rat *Journal of Andrology* **11** 498–505

Hoffer AP and Greenberg J (1978) The structure of the epididymis, efferent ductules and ductus deferens of the guinea pig: a light microscope study *Anatomical Record* **190** 659–678

Holt WV (1980) Surface-bound sialic acid on ram and bull spermatozoa: deposition during epididymal transit and stability during washing *Biology of Reproduction* **23** 847–857

Iusem ND, Piñeiro L, Blaquier JA and Belocopitow E (1989) Identification of a major secretory protein from rat epididymis: interaction with spermatozoa *Biology of Reproduction* **40** 307–336

Jones R, Pholpramool C, Setchell BP and Brown CR (1981) Labelling of membrane glycoproteins in rat spermatozoa collected from different regions of the epididymis *Biochemical Journal* **200** 457–460

Kirchhoff C (1994) A major messenger ribonucleic acid of the rodent epididymis encodes a small glycosyl-phosphatidylinositol-anchored lymphocyte surface antigen *Biology of Reproduction* **50** 896–902

Kirchhoff C (1996) CD52 is the 'major maturation-associated' sperm membrane antigen *Molecular Human Reproduction* **2** 9–17

Kirchhoff C and Hale G (1996) Cell-to-cell transfer of glycosylphosphatidylinositol-anchored membrane proteins during sperm maturation *Molecular Human Reproduction* **2** 177–184

Kirchhoff C, Krull N, Pera I and Ivell R (1993) A major mRNA of the human epididymis principal cells, HE5, encodes the leucocyte differentiation CDw52 antigen peptide backbone *Molecular Reproduction and Development* **34** 8–15

Kohane AC, González-Echéverría FMC, Piñeiro L and Blaquier JA (1980) Interaction of proteins of epididymal origin with spermatozoa *Biology of Reproduction* **23** 737–742

Krätzschmar J, Haendler B, Eberspaecher U, Roosterman D, Donner P and Schleuning WD (1996) The human cysteine-rich secretory protein (CRISP) family. Primary structure and tissue distribution of CRISP-1, CRISP-2 and CRISP-3 *European Journal of Biochemistry* **236** 827–836

Legault Y, vandenHeuvel WJA, Arison B, Bleau G, Chapdelaine A and Roberts KD (1978) 5α-Cholesta-7,24-dien-3β-ol as a major sterol of the male hamster reproductive tract *Steroids* **32** 649–658

Lopez A ML and de Souza W (1991) Distribution of filipin–sterol complexes in the plasma membrane of stallion spermatozoa during the epididymal maturation process *Molecular Reproduction and Development* **28** 158–168

Marin M, Lecher P, Martinez A, Tournadre S and Jean C (1995) Exportation of mouse vas deferens protein, a protein without a signal peptide, from mouse vas deferens epithelium: a model of apocrine secretion *Biology of Reproduction* **52** 50–62

Moore A, White TW, Ensrud KM and Hamilton DW (1989) The major maturation glycoprotein found on rat cauda epididymal sperm surface is linked to the membrane via phosphatidylinositol *Biochemical Biophysical Research Communications* **160** 460–468

Moore A, Ensrud KM, White TW, Frethem C and Hamilton DW (1994) Rat epididymis-specific sperm maturation antigens. I. Evidence that the 26kD 4E9 antigen found on rat caudal epididymal sperm tail is derived from a protein secreted by the epididymis *Molecular Reproduction and Development* **37** 181–194

Myles DG and Primakoff P (1983) Establishment of sperm surface topography during development analyzed with monoclonal antibodies. In *The Sperm Cell* pp 127–139 Ed. J Andre. Martinus Nijhoff, The Hague

Nicander L and Malmqvist M (1977) Ultrastructural observations suggesting merocrine secretion in the initial segment of the mammalian epididymis *Cell and Tissue Research* **184** 487–490

Okamura N, Iwaki Y, Hiramoto S *et al* . (1997) Molecular cloning and characterization of the epididymis-specific glutathione peroxidase-like protein secreted in the porcine epididymal fluid *Biochemica et Biophysica Acta* **1336** 99–109

Oliphant G and Singhas CA (1979) Iodination of rabbit sperm plasma membranes: relationship of specific surface proteins to epididymal function and sperm capacitation *Biology of Reproduction* **21** 937–944

Olson GE, Lifsics MR, Winfrey VP and Rifkin JM (1987) Modification of the rat sperm flagellar plasma membrane during maturation in the epididymis *Journal of Andrology* **8** 129–147

Phillips DM and Bedford JM (1987) Sperm–sperm associations in the loris epididymis *Gamete Research* **18** 17–25

Phillips DM, Jones R and Shalgi R (1991) Alterations in distribution of surface and intracellular antigens during epididymal maturation of rat spermatozoa *Molecular Reproduction and Development* **29** 347–356

Rankin TL, Tsuruta KJ, Holland MK, Griswold MD and Orgebin-Crist MC (1992) Isolation, immunolocalization, and sperm-association of three proteins of 18, 25, and 29 kilodaltons secreted by the mouse epididymis *Biology of Reproduction* **46** 747–766

Raynaud P and Kann M-L (1986) Forward motility protein (FMP): localization in hamster epididymal spermatozoa *International Journal of Andrology* **9** 371–380

Reid BL and Cleland KW (1957) The structure and function of the epididymis I. The histology of the rat epididymis *Australian Journal of Zoology* **5** 223–246

Renneberg H, Konrad L, Dammhäuser I, Seitz J and Aumüller G (1997) Immunohistochemistry of prostasomes from human semen *Prostate* **30** 98–106

Rifkin JM and Olson GE (1985) Characterization of maturation-dependent extrinsic proteins of the rat sperm surface *Journal of Cell Biology* **100** 1582–1591

Rochwerger L and Cuasnicú PS (1992) Redistribution of a rat sperm epididymal glycoprotein after *in vitro* and *in vivo* capacitation *Molecular Reproductions and Development* **31** 34–41

Rooney IA, Heuser JE and Atkinson JP (1996) GPI-anchored complement regulatory proteins in seminal plasma. An analysis of their physical condition and the mechanisms of their binding to exogenous cells *Journal of Clinical Investigation* **97** 1675–1686

Scully NF, Shaper JH and Shur BD (1987) Spatial and temporal expression of cell surface galactosyltransferase during mouse spermatogenesis and epididymal maturation *Developmental Biology* **124** 111–124

Seki N, Toyoma Y and Nagano T (1992) Changes in the distribution of filipin–sterol complexes in the boar sperm head plasma membrane during epididymal maturation and in the uterus *Anatomical Record* **232** 221–230

Stoltenberg M, Ernst E, Andreasen A, and Danscher G (1996) Histochemical localization of zinc ions in the epididymis *Histochemical Journal* **28** 175–185

Suzuki F (1988) Changes in the distribution of intramembranous particles and filipin–sterol complexes during epididymal maturation of golden hamster spermatozoa *Journal of Ultrastructure and Molecular Structure Research* **100** 39–54

Suzuki F and Nagano T (1980) Epididymal maturation of rat spermatozoa studies by thin sectioning and freeze fracture *Biology of Reproduction* **22** 1219–1231

Syntin P, Dacheux F, Druart X, Gatti J-L, Okamura N and Dacheux J-L (1996) Characterization and identification of protein secreted in the various regions of the adult boar epididymis *Biology of Reproduction* **55** 956–974

Toshimori K, Higashi R and Oura C (1985) Distribution of intramembranous particles and filipin–sterol complexes in mouse sperm membranes: polyene antibiotic filipin treatment *American Journal of Anatomy* **174** 455–470

Tulsiani DRP, Skudlarek MD, Holland MK and Orgebin-Crist M-C (1993) Glycosylation of rat sperm plasma membrane during epididymal maturation *Biology of Reproduction* **48** 417–428

Vernon RB, Miller CH and Eddy EM (1987) Further characterization of a secreted epididymal glycoprotein in mice that binds to sperm tails *Journal of Andrology* **8** 123–128

Vierula ME, Rankin TL and Orgebin-Crist M-C (1995) Electron microscopic immunolocalization of the 18 and 29 kilodalton secretory proteins in the mouse epididymis: evidence for their differential uptake by clear cells *Microscopy Research and Technique* **30** 24–36

Voglmayr JK, Fairbanks G, Jackowitz MA and Colella JR (1980) Post-testicular developmental changes in the ram sperm cell surface and their relationship to luminal fluid proteins of the reproductive tract *Biology of Reproduction* **22** 655–667

Voglmayr JK, Fairbanks G, Vespa DB and Colella JR (1982)

Studies on the mechanisms of surface modifications in ram spermatozoa during the final stages of differentiation *Biology of Reproduction* **26** 483–500

Voglmayr JK, Fairbanks G and Lewis RG (1983) Surface glycoprotein changes in ram spermatozoa during epididymal maturation *Biology of Reproduction* **29** 767–775

Voglmayr JK, Sawyer RF and Dacheux JL (1985) Glycoproteins: a variable factor in surface transformation of ram spermatozoa during epididymal transit *Biology of Reproduction* **33** 165–176

Weaver FE, Dione JE, Germain BJ, Wolf DE and Fairbanks G (1993) Biochemical characterization and epididymal localization of the maturation-dependent ram sperm surface antigen ESA152 *Molecular Reproduction and Development* **35** 293–301

Xu W, Ensrud KM and Hamilton DW (1997) The 26 kDA protein recognised in rat cauda epididymal sperm by monoclonal antibody 4E9 has internal peptide sequence that is identical to the secreted form of epididymal protein E *Molecular Reproduction and Development* **46** 377–382

Yanagimachi H, Kamiguchi Y, Mikamo K, Suzuki F and Yanagimachi R (1985) Maturation of spermatozoa in the epididymis of the Chinese hamster *American Journal of Anatomy* **172** 317–330

Yeung CH, Schröter S, Wagenfeld A *et al.* (1997) Interaction of the human epididymal protein CD52 (HE5) with epididymal spermatozoa from men and cynomolgus monkeys *Molecular Reproduction and Development* **48** 267–275

Young LG, Gould KG and Hinton BT (1987) Changes in binding of a 27-kilodalton chimpanzee cauda epididymal protein glycoprotein component to chimpanzee sperm *Gamete Research* **18,** 163–178

Young LG, Hinton BT, Smithwick EB and Gould KG (1994) Sodium, potassium, and protein concentrations and 2D-SDS-PAGE of epididymal luminal and ejaculated seminal fluids of the adult chimpanzee (*Pan troglodytes*) *American Journal of Primatology* **34** 249–259

Zeheb R and Orr GA (1984) Characterization of a maturation-associated glycoprotein on the plasma membrane of rat caudal epididymal sperm *Journal of Biological Chemistry* **259** 839–848

Journal of Reproduction and Fertility Supplement **53**, 137–147

Receptor tyrosine kinase c-*ros* knockout mice as a model for the study of epididymal regulation of sperm function

C. H. Yeung[1], E. Sonnenberg-Riethmacher[2] and T. G. Cooper[1]

[1]*Institute of Reproductive Medicine of the University, D-48129 Münster; and* [2]*Max-Delbrück-Centre for Molecular Medicine, D-13122 Berlin, Germany*

Despite recent advances in understanding sperm function and characterization of epididymal secretion products, little is known about the mechanisms regulating the fertilizing capacity of spermatozoa during maturation. The recently produced receptor tyrosine kinase c-*ros* knockout mouse has provided the first transgenic model for such study. The only abnormalities in these transgenic mice are shown in homozygous mutant males whose epididymis fails to develop the initial segment. Normal matings by these mice do not result in oocyte fertilization, but *in vitro* fertilization is successful. Detailed analysis of the development of sperm motility *per se* did not reveal any gross abnormalities that could explain infertility *in vivo*. Studies on c-*ros*, which is expressed temporarily in a few embryonic organs but solely and at high levels in the epididymis in adults, are few and nothing is known about its putative ligand or substrates. Review of the literature on other family members of receptor tyrosine kinases throws hardly any light on its role in epididymal function affecting sperm maturation. The preliminary observations that the majority of motile spermatozoa exhibit angulation in the tail and further findings suggest a defect in the volume regulation mechanism which would normally develop during sperm maturation. This finding has provided a starting point for further research to establish the link between abnormal epididymides and sterility.

Introduction

With the rapid development of techniques in molecular biology for the design and production of transgenic mice, it has become the method of choice for studying the role of particular sperm factors that contribute critically to successful fertilization. Such animals have been produced using targeted gene mutations, such as the deletion of acrosin required for egg-investment penetration (Adham *et al.*, 1997) and β-galactosyltransferase for binding to the zona pellucida (Lu and Shur, 1997). On the other hand, sterile males produced by any knockout animals may yield information on the regulation of the fertilizing capacity of spermatozoa, providing spermatogenesis still occurs. The first and only transgenic mice produced so far in which male infertility is caused by abnormal post-testicular development, namely in the epididymis, was reported by Sonnenberg-Riethmacher *et al.* (1996). These receptor tyrosine kinase c-*ros* knockout mice have presented us with a unique model for studying the role of the epididymis in the regulation of sperm function.

The c-*ros* Gene and Its Expression

The c-*ros* receptor gene belongs to the family of proto-oncogenes containing the intracellular tyrosine kinase catalytic domain and is very conserved, and it is homologous to the *Drosophila sevenless* tyrosine kinase receptor responsible for the morphogenesis of compound eyes. In mammalian cells, it was first discovered in a human mammary tumour cell line identified in a transfection tumorigenicity assay (Birchmeier *et al.*, 1986). The deduced amino acid sequence of the *c-ros* protein is very similar among humans, mice, rats and chickens (see Riethmacher *et al.*, 1994). In view of the similarity to other tyrosine kinase receptor proto-oncogenes that are expressed in specific epithelia predominantly or exclusively during embryonic development, such as *ret, met, neu* (erbB2) and the keratinocyte growth factor receptor (KGFR), a similar role in growth induction, differentiation or morphogenesis during early development was putatively assigned to c-*ros* (see Birchmeier and Birchmeier, 1993).

In the developing mouse, the c-*ros* gene is mainly expressed in the kidney, lung and intestine in specific temporal patterns (Sonnenberg *et al.*, 1991; Tessarollo *et al.*, 1992). Expression of c-*ros* in the embryo starts with the ureter bud and continues throughout morphogenesis of the metanephric kidney. It persists postnatally for one or two weeks, and then mRNA declines markedly to become undetectable before adulthood. Expression in the intestine reaches a peak at the late embryonic and neonatal stages but is absent around puberty. There is also moderate expression of c-*ros* in the lung, most obviously in newborn mice, but it is not detectable or expression is minimal in adults. In the genital system, c-*ros* is only temporally expressed in the Wolffian duct when the ureter bud grows out to meet the metanephric mesenchyme (Sonnenberg *et al.*, 1991). In prepubertal mice, upregulated *in situ* hybridization signals in the epididymal epithelium are detected between day 16 and 21, and are confined to the proximal region of the caput epididymidis which starts differentiating into the characteristic initial segment (Sonnenberg-Riethmacher *et al.*, 1996). High and moderate expression in the initial segment and the remaining caput region, respectively, persist in the adult (Fig. 1), and there is a lack of expression in the corpus and cauda epididymides, the efferent ducts, vas deferens and seminal vesicles which also derive from the Wolffian duct. The testis shows no expression detectable by northern blot analysis until adult life, but the c-*ros* transcript produced is truncated such that it lacks the extracellular domain and is not translated (Sonnenberg *et al.*, 1991, 1996). Although *in situ* hybridization has shown that spermatids and spermatozoa are responsible for this testicular expression (Tessarollo *et al.*, 1992), similar techniques did not detect a signal in the spermatozoa within the epididymal lumen (Sonnenberg-Riethmacher *et al.*, 1996).

There have been few studies on the human c-*ros* and these have been confined to the glioblastoma tumour cell lines (Birchmeier *et al.*, 1990). The expression is thought to be ectopic since it has not been found in normal murine neural tissues.

Specific Epididymal Abnormality and Infertility of c-*ros* Knockout Male Mice

The homozygous, as well as the heterozygous, mutant mice develop normally into healthy adults, and the females are fertile. However, homozygous males, which lack the regionalized high expression of c-*ros* in the epididymis and do not contain the c-*ros* protein, fail to develop the initial segment which in normal mice is morphologically distinguishable from the rest of the caput by enriched vascularization, and histologically by tall epithelial cells with long stereocilia extending into the tubule lumen (Fig. 1). These males contain normal numbers of potentially motile spermatozoa in the epididymis and can copulate normally, but fail to impregnate wild type females; eggs were not fertilized after mating (Sonnenberg-Riethmacher *et al.*, 1996). By contrast, heterozygous male mice show neither abnormal phenotype nor subfertility. Retrieval of spermatozoa from the female tract after mating revealed differences between heterozygous and homozygous knockout male mice. Whereas the number of spermatozoa in the uterus after mating was not different between the different genotypes, there were no spermatozoa in the oviduct in 40% of females mated with the homozygous knockout mice. Numbers of spermatozoa in the remaining 60% of females were within the lower range found in females mated to the heterozygous males. The overall difference between the fertile and infertile mutants was significant (Fig. 2a). When oocytes were incubated directly with spermatozoa recovered from the cauda epididymidis of the homozygous mutants by conventional *in vitro* fertilization, fertilization was achieved at success rates similar to those obtained in the heterozygous or wild type animals (Fig. 2b) and embryo transfer resulted in healthy offspring (Sonnenberg-Riethmacher *et al.*, 1996).

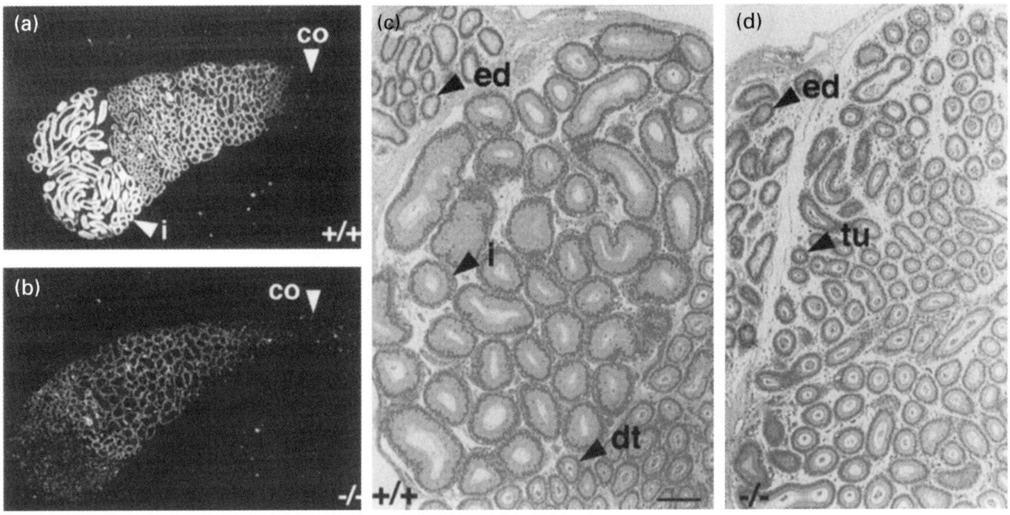

Fig. 1. Photomicrographs of the caput epididymidis of the wild type (+/+; a and c) and homozygous c-*ros* knockout (–/–; b and d) mice. *In situ* hybridization (a and b) shows high expression of c-*ros* in the initial segment (i) and lower expression in the remaining caput region of the wild type, whereas expression in the knockout mostly disappears; no expression is shown in the corpus (co) of either genotype. Histology of the epididymal head (c and d; scale bar represents 50 µm) shows initial segment (i) in the wild type characterized by the tall epithelium and larger tubule size than the more distal tubule (dt), whereas similar distal tubule and efferent ducts (ed) are found in the knockout but the region for initial segment is filled by the small tubules (tu) resembling dt. Reproduced from Sonnenberg-Riethmacher *et al.* (1996) with permission.

These findings suggest that spermatozoa passing through an epididymis that lacks an initial segment fail to accomplish certain facets of normal development and as a result are unable to negotiate the female tract to reach the oocytes; other functional and genetic aspects contributing to fertilization and embryo development should be intact in these mutant spermatozoa. The important question is whether the epididymis of the homozygous transgenic mice is solely responsible for the infertility, or whether the epididymal abnormality and sterility *in vivo* are parallel consequences of c-*ros* knockout.

Is the Epididymis Solely Responsible for the Infertility?

Evidence from previous studies is outlined in this section, indicating that in the knockout mice the sperm defect is derived solely from epididymal factors and is not of testicular origin or autonomous to the spermatozoa.

Except for the missing vascularized zone indicating the initial segment of the epididymis, the testis and the reproductive tract of knockout and wild type mice appear identical. The cauda epididymidis of the knockout mice is full of spermatozoa that are motile *in vitro* and fertile by IVF and these mice copulate normally (they are successfully used to replace vasectomized animals to stimulate females for embryo transfer). This result indicates normal basic testicular function. Nevertheless, there is expression of c-*ros* by the adult testis in mice (Sonnenberg *et al.*, 1991; Tessarollo *et al.*, 1992), rats (Matsushime and Shibuya 1990) and chickens (Chen *et al.*, 1994). However, except in the chicken, the testicular transcripts are truncated forms of the 8 kb full length to 5.2 or 4.5 kb in mice and 2.4 or 1.9 kb in rats, lacking the N-terminal (extracellular) domain. As expected, the knockouts targeting only the extracellular locus, which results in epididymal abnormality and infertility, do not affect the expression of the testicular c-*ros* in the mutant mice

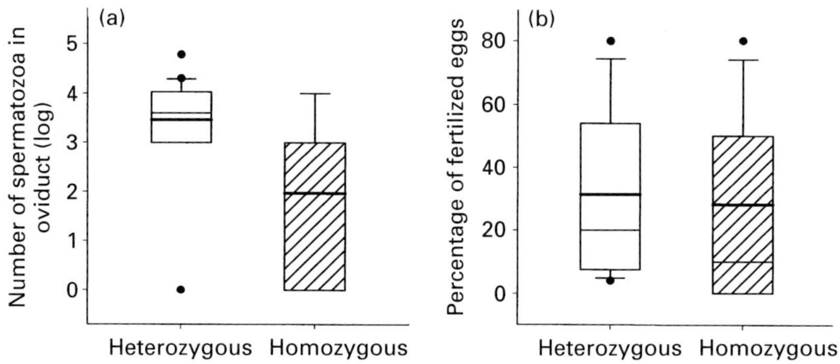

Fig. 2. Box and whisker plots showing greater numbers of spermatozoa recovered from the oviduct of females after mating with fertile heterozygous (open box, $n = 17$) compared with infertile homozygous (hatched box, $n = 22$) c-*ros* knockout male mice (a), but no difference in percentage of eggs fertilised *in vitro* (b, $n = 9$ for both groups). Each box encloses data within the upper and lower quartiles and the bars at the end of the two whiskers show the 95% confidence interval, with outliers indicated by individual data points; the thick line in the box indicates the mean and the thin line the median value.

(Sonnenberg-Riethmacher *et al.*, 1996). Furthermore, using antibodies against the C-terminal peptides, no c-*ros* protein can be detected in testicular tissues, confirming that such truncated transcripts are not functional .

Wild type spermatozoa do not have the c-*ros* protein as detected by western blots of testicular or cauda epididymidal tissues which contain plenty of sperm cells. Is c-*ros* required intrinsically by spermatozoa or germ cells at all, in a cell-autonomous manner, for spermatogenesis and sperm function? This has been clarified using chimaeric mice (generated by fusion of c-*ros* −/− and +/+ morulae) which produce both +/+ and −/− germ cells in each individual (Sonnenberg-Riethmacher *et al.*, 1996). These chimaeric males, when mated with +/+ females, sire offspring of +/+ and −/+ genotypes in equal proportions, indicating no inferiority in fertilization of spermatozoa produced by −/− germ cells and matured in a normal epididymal phenotype.

In Search of the Role of c-*ros* in Epididymal Development

Little is known about the function of c-*ros*. Knowledge about the large family of receptor tyrosine kinases has highlighted the following general characteristics (see van der Geer *et al.*, 1994). The N-terminal extracellular domains, which consist of different combinations of characteristic domains, encode the signal peptide and the ligand binding site. Ligand binding leads to dimerization and autophosphorylation of the receptor, resulting in binding and phosphorylation of cytoplasmic substrates which elicit signal transduction. Yet for c-*ros*, neither its ligand nor substrates are identified. As a receptor tyrosine kinase, c-*ros* may form a subfamily of its own, but it has been classified under the subfamily of insulin receptors by some authors (Van der Geer *et al.*, 1994) based on the molecular phylogeny of the cytoplasmic tyrosine kinase domains, which may suggest similar substrates among members. In this respect the IGF-I receptor, a close homologue of c-*ros*, belongs to this subfamily and IGF-I has been detected in the rat epididymis (Leheup and Grignon, 1993). Since most of these receptor tyrosine kinases are growth factor receptors, the putative ligand for c-*ros* is probably a peptide. Nevertheless, steroids are also candidates, since oestradiol binds to and activates autophosphorylation of the receptor encoded by the proto-oncogene *neu* (Matsuda *et al.*, 1993). On the other hand, no ligand is required for the function of the lymphocyte tyrosine kinase (Ltk), another member of the insulin receptor subfamily. Ltk is not located on the plasma membrane but on the endoplasmic reticulum and is activated under oxidative stress by disulphide cross-linking of the extramembrane domain which may serve as a sensor for the redox status of the cytoplasm (Bauskin *et al.*, 1991).

Since the ligand for c-*ros* is unknown, information on the functional role of this receptor has so far been obtained indirectly from two methods of study, by applying antisense-oligonucleotide inhibition of transcription by organs in culture, or designing chimaeric receptors to be expressed in cell lines that normally do not express the proteins. When metanephric explants from fetal mice were used, blocking of the phosphotyrosine kinase domain resulted in merely 10% inhibition of expression of c-*ros* protein, concomitant with decreases in synthesis of extracellular matrix glycoproteins including heparin sulphate proteoglycan and laminin (Kanwar *et al.*, 1995; Liu *et al.*, 1996), suggesting a role of c-*ros* in the interaction between epithelial and mesenchymal cells. In the second approach, chimaeric receptors have been generated by replacing the extracellular domain of the c-*ros* gene with that of another tyrosine kinase receptor gene (trkA or EGFR) so that transfected cells expressing such chimaeric receptors (NIH3T3 fibroblasts: Riethmacher *et al.*, 1994 and Xiong *et al.*, 1996; or MDCK epithelial cells: Sachs *et al.*, 1996) can be stimulated with known ligands (nerve growth factor for trkA-ros chimaera and epidermal growth factor for EGFR-ros chimaera). Responses are manifested as activated mitosis and morphological transformation, induction of epithelial cell scattering and migration, phosphorylation or activation of early signalling proteins including mitogen activating protein kinase, insulin receptor substrate 1, phospholipase Cγ and inositol triphosphate kinase. Therefore c-*ros* protein could have diverse functions in mediating certain effects of growth factors on cell growth and differentiation. Other tyrosine kinase receptors involved in growth and morphogenesis that also show restricted expressions in embryonic epithelia of kidney, liver, lung and neural tissues, and are often studied or mentioned in parallel with c-*ros* in the literature, include *ret, met, neu* and KGFR. However, in contrast to the knocking out of these proto-oncogenes that results in death of embryos or severely damaged organogenesis (see Sachs *et al.*, 1996), functional deletion of c-*ros* allows general growth and development of the epididymal epithelium but inhibits prepubertal zonal differentiation. Another difference is the persistent expression of c-*ros* in the adult. Therefore the downstream signal transduction and substrates for the activated receptor tyrosine kinase may be quite different.

It is possible that the trigger of the prepubertal upregulation of c-*ros* expression in the proximal epididymis as well as the putative receptor ligand, if there is one, is of testicular origin such as the rete testis fluid which first enters the epididymis at about the time of the differentiation of the initial segment. The initial segment would be primed to provide factors necessary for sperm maturation when spermatozoa first arrive in the tubule lumen. For facilitating the search of the potentially diverse functions of c-*ros* in reproduction, the molecular basis of the sperm defects should first be characterized and defined.

Characterization of Sperm Defects in c-*ros* Knockout Mice

Motility

The observations of complete infertility *in vivo* combined with successful *in vitro* fertilization prompted speculation that a motility defect resulted in failure of spermatozoa to reach the oocytes *in vivo*, but was compensated for *in vitro* by direct contact with the oocytes in medium supplemented with exogenous glycolytic and oxidative substrates. Therefore the motility and swimming pattern of the epididymal spermatozoa and the profile of change as they mature was investigated in these mice using the computer-assisted sperm analysis system as in Soler *et al.* (1994).

When a medium that contained glucose, lactate and pyruvate at an osmolality of 310 mosm kg^{-1} water was used, spermatozoa released from various regions along the length of the epididymis of the homozygous knockout mice showed percentages of motile spermatozoa similar to those from the heterozygous or wild type animals, and exhibited no apparent difference in the profile of development for forward motility. Incubation of both the knockout and control spermatozoa over

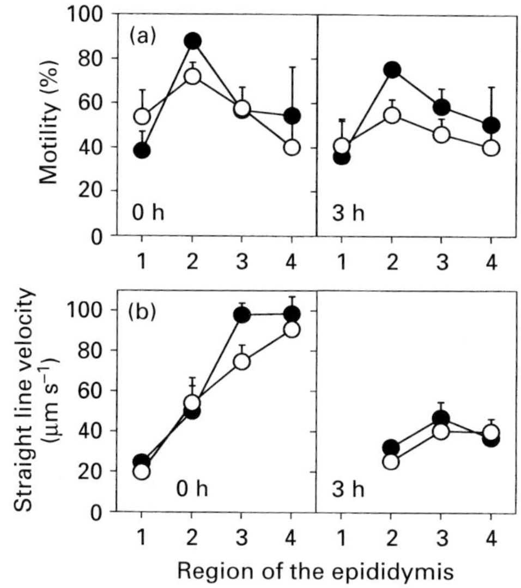

Fig. 3. Motility (a) and straight line velocity (b) of spermatozoa from various regions of the epididymis (1, distal caput; 2, proximal corpus; 3, proximal cauda; 4, distal cauda) of heterozygous (filled circles, $n = 3$) and homozygous (open circles, $n = 5$) mice analysed immediately (0 h) and after 3 h incubation.

3 h resulted in the same extent of decline in the straight line velocities with similar maintenance of percentage motility (Fig. 3). Since glucose metabolism is crucial for the fertilization process, and mature epididymal spermatozoa showing normal motility characteristics in fully supplemented medium fail to fertilize oocytes *in vivo* after the male animals are fed ornidazole which impairs sperm glycolysis (Yeung *et al.*, 1995; Oberländer *et al.*, 1996), the above experiments were repeated in medium containing glucose but no oxidative substrates, to check for any similar metabolic defect. No appreciable differences were detected in any motility parameters measured in the two media for both the control and knockout mice. There were no differences between control and knockout spermatozoa in either medium.

The shape of motile spermatozoa

During the motility experiments, it was observed that a large proportion of spermatozoa from the homozygous knockout mice, particularly mature spermatozoa from the cauda epididymidis, swam with an angulation of the tail at the site of the cytoplasmic droplet, which in the corpus and cauda spermatozoa is located at the junction of the midpiece and principal piece. The extent of the tail bending was various, the extreme being a sperm cell in a hair-pin form with the head and midpiece folded back, resulting in 'backwards' swimming. Hairpin forms were more common in motile than in immotile spermatozoa. When first released in the control medium (310 mosm kg^{-1} water), tail angulation was observed in cauda, corpus and caput epididymidal spermatozoa, with gradually lower extents towards the more proximal epididymal regions (zero time points in Fig. 4a), such that only a minority of mature spermatozoa swam without kinked tails (zero time points in Fig. 4b). In heterozygous transgenic mice, most of the spermatozoa swam with straight tails upon release, although further incubation resulted in a transient or slight occurrence of tail kinking in the

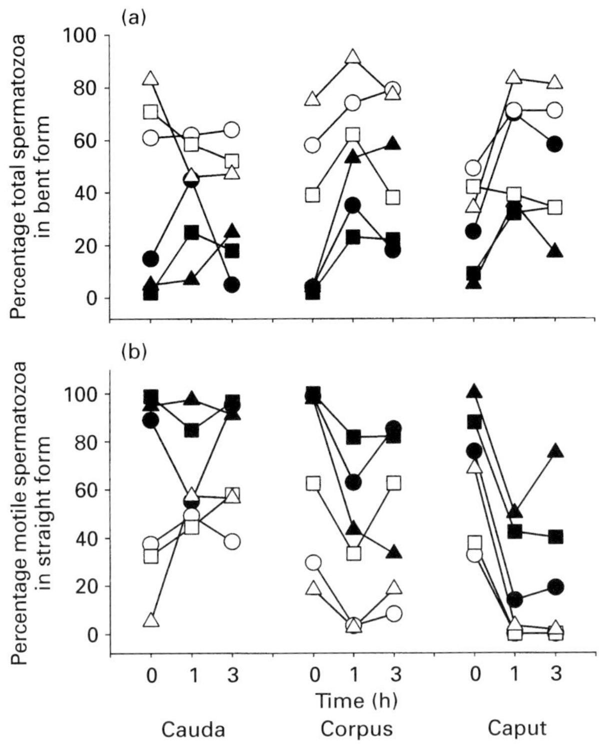

Fig. 4. Proportions of bent or unbent (straight) forms of spermatozoa (as a percentage of total or motile cells) from three regions of the epididymis (cauda, corpus and caput) upon release and incubation over 3 h. Different symbols represent individual mice; filled symbols represent heterozygous and open symbols represent homozygous knockout mice.

mature spermatozoa. In the corpus and caput spermatozoa, kinking appeared to greater extents and more persistently with time, such that they differ less from the c-*ros* knockout spermatozoa than at the start of the incubation (1 and 3 h in Fig. 4).

Susceptibility of sperm tail to angulation as a characteristic of immature spermatozoa

Whereas mature spermatozoa swimming with kinked tails upon release from the epididymis into physiological medium is an abnormal phenomenon, angulation in motile caput spermatozoa with induced forward motility has been observed in hamsters by Serres and Kann (1984) and Cornwall *et al.* (1986). The former authors suggested that such angulation is caused by osmotic swelling at the cytoplasmic droplet, as demonstrated in rodent spermatozoa using glycerol as the permeant osmotically active molecule (Cooper, 1985). This explanation is supported by the absence of such kinking when forward motility is induced in the naked flagellum of caput hamster spermatozoa in which cell volume is abolished by demembranation (Yeung 1984). On the other hand, Cornwall *et al.* (1988) suggested that this is due to the presence of fewer disulphide bonds and therefore a less stiff flagellum in the immature than in the mature spermatozoa, as angulation could be induced in the cauda spermatozoa by treatment with dithiothreitol to render the flagellum more

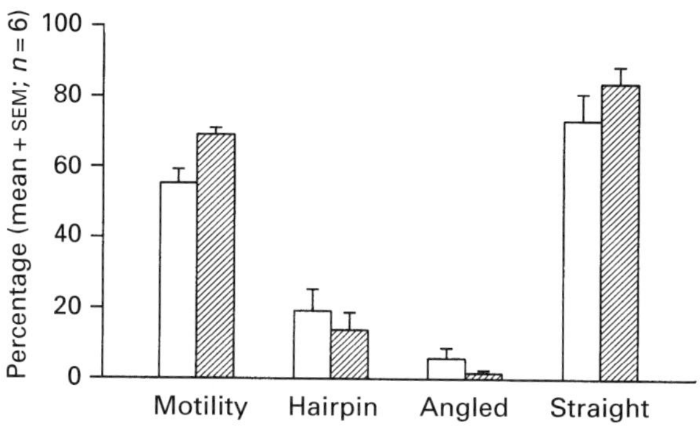

Fig. 5. Incubation of cauda spermatozoa from wild type mice for 45 min with sulphydryl oxidizing agent (5 μmol diamide l^{-1}, open bars) or thiol-reducing agent (0.5 mmol dithiothrietol l^{-1}, hatched bars) shows no difference in percentage motility or in the different forms of the motile spermatozoa (hair-pin, angled or straight); $n = 6$.

flexible, albeit only achieved in a high potassium and low sodium solution. When cauda spermatozoa from wild type mice were incubated to examine the effect of agents that oxidise (diamide) or reduce (dithiothrietol) sulphydryl or disulphide bonds, there was no difference in the extent of flagellar angulation (Fig. 5).

Defective response of cauda spermatozoa from c-ros *knockout mice to osmolarity*

Swelling of mature spermatozoa in hypotonic media resulting in coiling or folding back of the sperm tail has been well characterized in bulls (Drevius and Eriksson, 1966; Drevius, 1972). Although no data are available in mice, studies from other laboratory animals have indicated high osmolarity of epididymal luminal fluids ranging from 330 to 420 mosm kg^{-1} water, and is highest in the corpus (see Cooper, 1986). Kinking of the mutant infertile spermatozoa when diluted with the experimental medium might be an *in vitro* response to changes from some abnormal luminal environment not experienced by normal fertile spermatozoa. However, increasing the osmolality of the medium to which cauda spermatozoa were released up to 510 mosm kg^{-1} water did not abolish angulation, whereas control spermatozoa in hypotonic media showed swelling-induced kinking, as expected, which was markedly decreased at 310 mosm kg^{-1} water and further at hyperosmolarity (Fig. 6). Normal mouse spermatozoa are readily permeable to water and behave as ideal osmometers since their cell volumes vary linearly with the reciprocal of external osmolality over a very wide range from 75 to 1200 mosm kg^{-1} water (Du *et al.*, 1994; Willoughby *et al.*, 1996). Although tail angulation in hypo-osmotic solution has been observed in these studies, the relationship between cell volume and cell shape has not been examined.

Tail angulation as an in situ *defect in homozygous mutant spermatozoa*

The persistence of tail angulation in hypertonic media suggests that it was unlikely to be an *in vitro* response. Cauda spermatozoa fixed within seconds of release already revealed the kinked form in most cells. The possibility that kinking could have occurred instantaneously at the moment of dilution with physiological medium before fixation was eliminated by directly releasing luminal content into the fixative and sperm clumps were mechanically dispersed for observation. Identical percentages of kinked spermatozoa were found (74 ± 7% in homozygous versus 4 ± 2% in heterozygous control mice, mean ± SD of six samples from two animals in each group, with data pooled from the different sperm preparation methods).

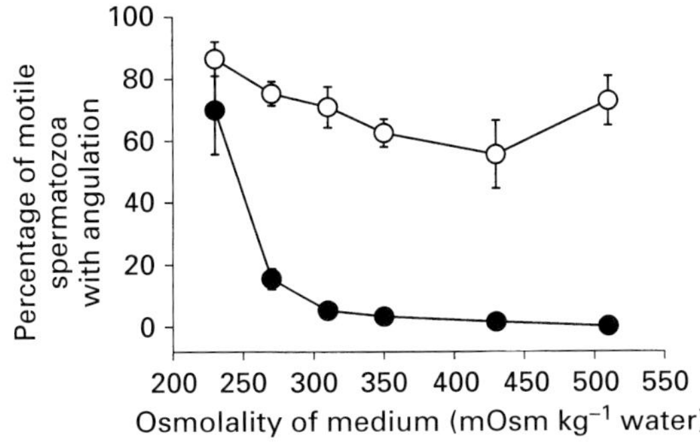

Fig. 6. The lack of response of cauda spermatozoa from homozygous knockout mice (open circles) to increasing osmolalities of the dilution medium in contrast to wild type mice (filled circles), as shown by the persistently high percentages of motile spermatozoa with angulation of the tail (including hair-pin form).

Is a Defect In Cell Volume Regulation A Possible Cause Of Infertility?

The association of infertility in domestic animals with swollen sperm tails has long been known. The presence of coiled spermatozoa in semen was first identified as a condition associated with sterility in some bulls bred as stud animals (Koefoed-Johnsen and Pederson 1971; Wenkoff 1978), the so-called 'Dag' defect after the name of the first animal studied. It arises as an abnormality in the epididymis and has subsequently been identified in boars (Holt 1982), dogs (Kawakami *et al.*, 1988) and stallions (Hellander *et al.*, 1991). Analyses of epididymal fluid (in the boar and bull) have not indicated the cause of the defect (see Cooper, 1992).

The swelling of epididymal spermatozoa could be a consequence of an imbalanced epididymal milieu, or a defect in volume regulation of the sperm cell. The control of water fluxes to achieve cell volume homeostasis is a ubiquitous cell function. In somatic cells, swelling induces rapid effluxes of osmolytes, leading to a regulatory volume decrease (RVD) to re-establish optimal cell volume. Different cell types in different species use different effectors of volume regulation. The best studied RVD pathways include K^+/Cl^- cotransport and the Cl^--independent K^+ channels, for example in erythrocytes (see Cossins and Gibson, 1997), Ca^+-sensitive K^+ channels (see McCarty and O'Neil, 1992; Woll *et al.*, 1996; O'Neil and Leng, 1997), separate Cl^- and K^+ channels, voltage-gated Cl^- channels, and VSOAC (volume-sensitive organic osmolyte anion channels) (see Strange *et al.*, 1996; Okada 1997). The mechanisms of activation of these channels are current topics of research in many laboratories, while their molecular identities are largely unknown besides three cloned proteins as candidates for the anion channels (see Okada 1997). It is interesting to note that efflux of amino acids, myo-inositol, betaine and glycerophosphocholine through the VSOAC has been demonstrated in renal epithelial cells which are sensitive to anion blockers (see Strange and Jackson, 1995). Large amounts of all these organic osmolytes (betaine being the precursor of carnitine) are secreted by the epididymis (see Hinton and Palladino, 1995). Understanding the characteristics of cell volume regulation by spermatozoa from the wild type and c-*ros* knockout mice and the influence of the epididymis could help to elucidate the link between epididymal abnormality and sperm infertility.

Conclusion

In the homozygous c-*ros* receptor tyrosine kinase knockout sterile mice, the most proximal region of the epididymis fails to differentiate into the initial segment, where both c-*ros* mRNA and protein are highly expressed in the wild type. Evidence so far suggests normal testicular function in these knockout animals and intact fertilizing capacity of spermatozoa carrying mutant alleles in chimaeric mice that have normal epididymides. This distinct and restricted epididymal abnormality as the only altered phenotype, accompanied by complete infertility *in vivo*, provides us with a unique model for the study of the role of the epididymis in the regulation of sperm development. For this research, it is necessary to characterize the relevant defects in sperm function and to define the crucial epididymal deficiencies at molecular levels to establish the cause–effect relationship. The abnormal angulation of sperm tail observed in the preliminary studies, which may explain the impairment of sperm transport in the female tract, postulates a defect in sperm volume regulation. This aspect of sperm maturation in the normal epididymis is still to be characterized. One speculation is that the lack of epididymal c-*ros* with the subsequent lack of a differentiated initial segment could result in missing epididymal elements which would normally respond to testicular factors to provide the necessary conditions for normal sperm maturation. Much effort is needed to investigate the developmental expression of c-*ros* in the epididymis, the nature and source of the ligand and substrates of the receptor protein, and the presumably many intermediate steps involved in its regulation of sperm function.

C. H. Yeung is supported by a research grant (Ni130/15-4) from the Deutsche Forschungsgemeinshaft.

References

Adham IM, Nayernia K and Engel W (1997) Spermatozoa lacking acrosin protein show delayed fertilization *Molecular Reproduction and Development* **46** 370–376

Bauskin AR, Alkalay I and Ben-Neriah Y (1991) Redox regulation of a protein tyrosine kinase in the endoplasmic reticulum *Cell* **66** 685–696

Birchmeier CD and Birchmeier W (1993) Molecular aspects of mesenchymal–epithelial interactions *Annual Reviews of Cell Biology* **9** 511–540

Birchmeier C, Birnbaum D, Waitches G, Fasano O and Wigler M (1986) Characterization of an activated human ros gene *Molecular and Cell Biology* **6** 3109–3116

Birchmeier C, O'Neill K, Riggs M and Wigler M (1990) Characterization of ROS1 cDNA from a human glioblastoma cell line *Proceedings of the National Academy of Sciences USA* **87** 4799–4803

Chen J, Zong CS and Wang LH (1994) Tissue and epithelial cell-specific expression of chicken proto-oncogene c-ros in several organs suggests that it may play roles in their development and mature functions *Oncogene* **9** 773–780

Cooper TG (1985) Prevention of hypo-osmotic swelling by detergents provides clues to the membrane structure of rat sperm *International Journal of Andrology* **8** 159–167

Cooper TG (1986) *The Epididymis, Sperm Maturation and Fertilisation* p240 Springer-Verlag, Berlin

Cooper TG (1992) The epididymis as a site of contraceptive attack *Spermatogenesis, Fertilization, Contraception. Molecular, Cellular and Endocrine Events in Male Reproduction* pp 419–460 Schering Foundation Workshop 4 Springer-Verlag, Berlin

Cornwall GA, Smyth TB, Vindivich D, Harter C, Robinson J and Chang TSK (1986) Induction and enhancement of progressive motility in hamster caput epididymal spermatozoa *Biology of Reproduction* **35** 1065–1074

Cornwall GA, Vindivich D, Tillman S and Chang TSK (1988) The effect of sulfhydryl oxidation on the morphology of immature hamster epididymal spermatozoa induced to acquire motility *in vitro. Biology of Reproduction* **39** 141–155

Cossins AR and Gibson JS (1997) Volume-sensitive transport systems and volume homeostasis in vertebrate red blood cells *Journal of Experimental Biology* **200** 343–352

Drevius LO (1972) Osmotic behaviour, membrane permeability and mobility mechanisms in bull spermatozoa *Acta Universitatis Upsaliensis, Abstracts of Uppsala Dissertations From the Faculty of Science* **195** 1–20

Drevius LO and Eriksson H (1966) Osmotic swelling of mammalian spermatozoa *Experimental Cell Research* **42** 136–156

Du J, Tao J, Kleinhaus FW, Mazur P and Critser JK (1994) Water volume and osmotic behaviour of mouse spermatozoa determined by electron paramagnetic resonance *Journal of Reproduction and Fertility* **101** 37–42

Hellander JC, Samper JC and Crabo BG (1991) Fertility of a stallion with low sperm motility and a high incidence of an unusual sperm tail defect *Veterinary Record* **128** 449–451

Hinton BT and Palladino MA (1995) Epididymal epithelium: its contribution to the formation of a luminal fluid microenvironment *Microscopy Research Technique* **30** 67–81

Holt WV (1982) Epididymal origin of a coiled-tail sperm defect in a boar *Journal of Reproduction and Fertility* **64** 485–489

Kanwar YS, Liu ZZ, Kumar A, Wada J and Carone FA (1995) Cloning of mouse c-ros renal cDNA: its role in development and relationship to extracellular matrix glycoprotiens *Kidney International* **48** 1646–1659

Kawakami E, Tsutsui T and Ogasa A (1988) Two cases of acrosome and folded tail abnormality in dog spermatozoa *Japanese Journal of Veterinary Science* **50** 1274–1276

Koefoed-Johnsen HH and Pederson H (1971) Further observations on the Dag-defect of the tail of the bull spermatozoon *Journal of Reproduction and Fertility* **26** 77–83

Leheup BP and Grignon G (1993) Immunohistochemical localization of insulin-like growth factor I (IGF-I) in the rat epididymis *Journal of Andrology* **14** 159–163

Liu ZZ, Wada J, Kumar A, Carone FA, Takahashi M and Kanwar YS (1996) Comparative role of phosphotyrosine kinase domains of c-ros and c-ret protooncogenes in metanephric development with respect to growth factors and matrix morphogens *Developmental Biology* **178** 133–148

Lu QX and Shur BD (1997) Sperm from beta 1,4-galactosyltransferase-null mice are refractory to ZP3-induced acrosome reactions and penetrate the zona pellucida poorly *Development* **124** 4121–4131

McCarty NA and O'Neil RG (1992) Calcium signaling in cell volume regulation *Physiological Reviews* **72** 1037–1061

Matsuda S, Kadowaki, Ichino M, Akiyama TTK and Yamamoto T (1993) 17β-Estradiol mimics ligand activity of the c-erbB2 protooncogene product *Proceedings of the National Academy of Sciences USA* **90** 10803–10807

Matsushime H and Shibuya M (1990) Tissue-specific expression of rat c-ros-1 gene and partial structural similarity of its predicted products with sev protein of *Drosophila melanogaster. Journal of Virology* **64** 2117–2125

Oberländer G, Yeung CH and Cooper TG (1996) Influence of oral administration of ornidazole on capacitation and the activity of some glycolytic enzymes of rat spermatozoa. *Journal of Reproduction and Fertility* **106** 231–239

Okada Y (1997) Volume expansion-sensing outward-rectifier Cl-channel: fresh start to the molecular identity and volume sensor *American Journal of Physiology – Cell Physiology* **42** C755–C789

O'Neil RG and Leng LJ (1997) Osmo-mechanically sensitive phosphatidylinositol signaling regulates a Ca^{2+} influx channel in renal epithelial cells *American Journal of Physiology:Renal Physiology* **42** F120–F128

Riethmacher D, Langholz O, Gödecke S, Sachs M and Birchmeier C (1994) Biochemical and functional characterization of the murine ros protooncogene *Oncogene* **9** 3617–3626

Sachs M, Weidner KM, Brinkmann V, Walter I, Obermeier A, Ulrich A, and Birchmeier W (1996) Mitogenic and morphogenic activity of epithelial receptor tyrosine kinases *Journal of Cell Biology* **133** 1095–1107

Serres C and Kann M-L (1984) Motility induction in hamster spermatozoa from caput epididymidis: effects of forward motility protein (FMP) and calmodulin inhibitor *Reproduction Nutrition and Development* **24** 81–94

Soler C, Yeung CH and Cooper TG (1994) Development of sperm motility patterns in the murine epididymis *International Journal of Andrology* **17** 271–278

Sonnenberg E, Gödecke A, Walter B, Bladt F and Birchmeier C (1991) Transient and locally restricted expression of the ros1 protooncogene during mouse development *EMBO Journal* **10** 3693–3702

Sonnenberg-Riethmacher E, Walter B, Riethmacher D, Gödecke S and Birchmeier C (1996) The c-ros tyrosine kinase receptor controls regionalization and differentiation of epithelial cells in the epididymis *Gene Development* **10** 1184–1193

Strange K and Jackson PS (1995) Swelling-activated organic osmolyte efflux: a new role for anion channels *Kidney International* **48** 994–1003

Strange K, Emma F and Jackson PS (1996) Cellular and molecular physiology of volume-sensitive anion channels *American Journal of Physiology* **270** C711–C730

Tessarollo L, Nagarajan L and Parada LF (1992) c-ros: the vertebrate homolog of the sevenless tyrosine kinase receptor is tightly regulated during organogenesis in mouse embryonic development *Development* **115** 11–20

van der Geer P, Hunter T and Lindberg RA (1994) Receptor protein-tyrosine kinases and their signal transduction pathways *Annual Review of Cell Biology* **10** 251–337

Wenkoff MS (1978) A sperm mid-piece defect of epididymal origin in two Hereford bulls *Theriogenology* **10** 275–281

Willoughby CE, Mazur P, Peter AT and Critser JK (1996) Osmotic tolerance limits and properties of murine spermatozoa *Biology of Reproduction* **55** 715–727

Woll E, Ritter M, Haller T, Volkl H and Lang F (1996) Calcium entry stimulated by swelling of Madin-Darby canine kidney cells *Nephron* **74** 150–157

Xiong Q, Chan JL, Zong CS and Wang LH (1996) Two chimeric receptors of epidermal growth factor receptor and c-ros that differ in their transmembrane domains have opposite effects on cell growth *Molecular Cell Biology* **16** 1509–1518

Yeung CH (1984) Effects of cyclic AMP on the motility of mature and immature hamster epididymal spermatozoa studied by reactivation of the demembranated cells *Gamete Research* **9** 99–114

Yeung CH, Oberlander G and Cooper TG (1995) Effects of the male antifertility agent ornidazole on sperm function *in vitro* and in the female genital tract *Journal of Reproduction and Fertility* **103** 257–264

Journal of Reproduction and Fertility Supplement **53**, 149–155

The MDC family of proteins and their processing during epididymal transit

J. Frayne, J. A. Jury, H. L. Barker and L. Hall*

Bristol Molecular Reproductive Biology Group, Department of Biochemistry, University of Bristol, School of Medical Sciences, Bristol BS8 1TD, UK

All members of the MDC family of integral membrane proteins contain a metalloproteinase-like domain, a disintegrin-like domain and a cysteine-rich domain. They have been identified in a wide range of mammalian tissues and many are abundantly expressed in the male reproductive tract. We have previously cloned and sequenced several MDC transcripts expressed in the testes of the macaque (*Macaca fascicularis*). Using polyclonal antisera we have localized a number of these MDC proteins (fertilin α, fertilin β, tMDC I, tMDC II and tMDC III) to spermatogenic cells and demonstrated that they are processed as spermatozoa pass through the epididymis, yielding proteins that retain their disintegrin domain on mature, fertilization-competent cauda spermatozoa. In rodents, two of these MDC proteins (fertilin β and tMDC I) have been implicated in egg recognition, mediated by a disintegrin–integrin interaction. It is possible that the additional MDC proteins expressed on macaque spermatozoa may also be involved in this process.

Introduction

Spermatozoa are highly differentiated cells which acquire well defined surface domains during spermiogenesis; each domain is characterized by a unique distribution of surface antigens. After spermiation, spermatozoa undergo considerable remodelling of their plasma membrane components during epididymal transit, including the modification and relocation of a number of sperm surface antigens. Intriguingly, many proteins that undergo modification are considered important in gamete interactions during fertilization (Jones *et al.*, 1996); fertilin α and β represent two particularly well characterized examples (reviewed by Myles and Primakoff, 1997). Both of these proteins are synthesized as large precursor proteins in the testis; fertilin α is then cleaved to produce its mature form in the testis, whereas fertilin β is processed during epididymal transit. Fertilin α and β are members of a novel family of multidomain, integral membrane proteins, all of which possess a metalloproteinase-like domain, a disintegrin-like domain and a cysteine-rich domain (the MDC family; alternatively referred to as ADAMs, proteins with a disintegrin and metalloprotease domain). In the guinea-pig, fertilin α and β exist as a heterodimeric complex (Blobel *et al.*, 1990); fertilin β is implicated in sperm–egg binding by virtue of its disintegrin domain, and fertilin α is postulated to mediate membrane fusion via a putative fusogenic region within the cysteine-rich domain. To date over 20 members of the MDC protein family have been identified in a variety of species, and many are expressed abundantly in the testis (Frayne *et al.*, 1997; 1998), suggesting a role in reproductive function. Of particular interest in this context is the expression of a number of MDC proteins on spermatozoa and their potential involvement in gamete interactions at fertilization. These include the fertilin α and β subunits, tMDC I (also known as cyritestin), tMDC II and tMDC III.

Here we review the molecular structure, distribution and proposed roles of the mammalian MDC proteins. Moreover, with a view to studying their function in a more closely related human

*Correspondence

model, we include information on the macaque *(Macaca fascicularis)* MDC orthologues and present data demonstrating their expression by spermatogenic cells and their subsequent proteolytic processing during epididymal transit.

Molecular Structure

A remarkable feature of the MDC proteins is their striking sequence similarity to a number of snake venom haemorrhagic components that possess zinc metalloproteinase activity (capable of hydrolysing basement membranes) and disintegrin activity (which prevents fibrinogen binding and platelet aggregation by binding to the $\alpha_{IIb}\beta_3$ receptor on platelets) (see Hall, 1997). Within some snake venoms, for example that of habu *(Trimeresurus flavoviridis)*, the disintegrin activity and the metalloproteinase activity may reside within discrete polypeptides. In other snake venoms, such as jararhagin (from the pit viper, *Bothrops jararaca*), the disintegrin and metalloproteinase activities are present as domains within a single mosaic haemorrhagic protein composed of a prodomain, a metalloproteinase domain, a disintegrin domain and a cysteine-rich domain (Fig. 1). All of the MDC proteins sequenced to date also contain this distinct domain organization, but, unlike the soluble snake venom proteins, almost all are integral membrane proteins possessing a single transmembrane domain immediately C-terminal to the cysteine-rich domain, followed by a further hydrophilic (intracellular) domain (see Fig. 1) of variable length depending on the particular MDC protein. Furthermore, when the amino acid sequences of these MDC proteins are aligned, many conserved cysteine residues are seen throughout a large proportion of the coding region, suggesting a similar structural organization.

Metalloproteinase-like Domain

Snake venom metalloproteinases (or reprolysins as they are now generally termed) all possess a 'catalytic centre' consensus sequence, HEXXHXXGXXH, a feature they share with many other classes of zinc metalloproteinase, including the astacins, serralysins and matrixins (see Hall, 1997). Some of the mammalian MDC proteins also possess this consensus sequence within their metalloproteinase domain (Fig. 2): these include fertilin α, metargidin (Krätzschmar *et al.*, 1996), MDC 9 (Weskamp *et al.*, 1996), meltrin α (Yagami-Hiromasa *et al.*, 1995), MADM (Howard *et al.*, 1996), TACE (Black *et al.*, 1997) and KUZ (Pan and Rubin, 1997). However, although these MDC proteins may have the potential to act as metalloproteinases, proteolytic activity has been demonstrated only for the last three and a physiological function established for the last two: TACE, which cleaves tumour necrosis factor α (TNF-α) as part of the inflammatory response and KUZ, which cleaves NOTCH in *Drosophila* and *Xenopus*, as part of a pathway that mediates lateral inhibition of neuronal cell fate during neurogenesis. In contrast, many of the other MDC proteins, including most of those abundantly expressed in the male reproductive tract, lack the catalytic centre consensus residues characteristic of the snake venom reprolysins. However, the possibility that these catalytically inactive MDC proteins might function as specific, endogenous proteinase inhibitors, as has been shown for a mutant KUZ protein lacking protease activity (Pan and Rubin, 1997), should be borne in mind.

Disintegrin-like Domain

The disintegrin-like domain is a particularly highly conserved region within the MDC family of proteins, with almost complete conservation of the fourteen cysteine residues, indicative of a common tertiary structure, similar to that of the snake-venom disintegrins, and implying functional importance. However, although many snake venom disintegrins contain an RGD tripeptide motif, involved in integrin-binding, most of the MDC proteins sequenced to date contain the tripeptide

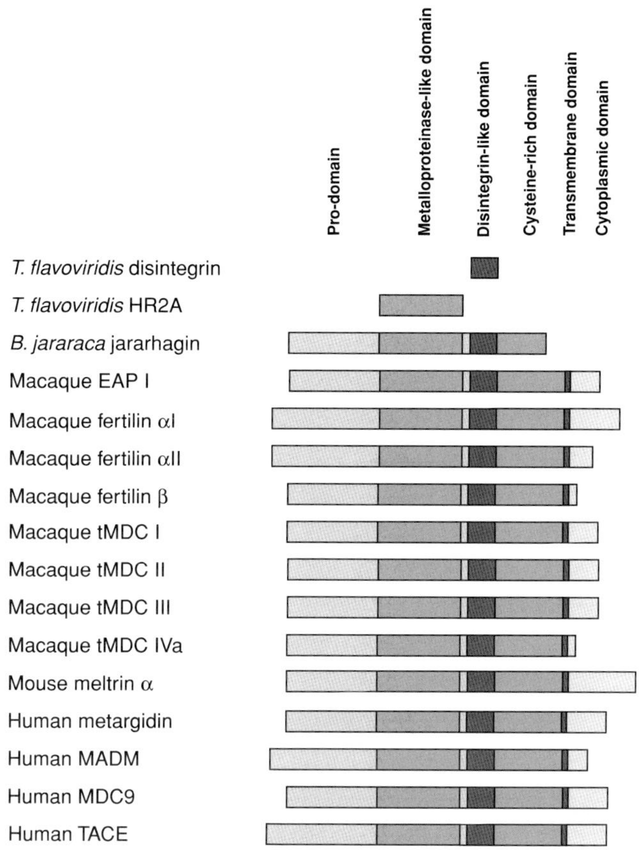

Fig. 1. Diagrammatic representation of the MDC family of proteins showing their homology to snake venom haemorrhagic proteins.

XCD (often ECD), in a similar position (Fig. 3). ECD is also the most common alternative tripeptide in snake venom disintegrins that do not contain RGD. Interestingly, the only MDC proteins that lack this XCD motif are TACE, MADM and KUZ, the three MDC proteins of proven metalloproteinase activity.

By analogy with the integrin binding activity of the snake venom disintegrins, it has been postulated that the disintegrin-like domains of the MDC proteins may also interact with integrins, but possibly with different specificities. Integrin receptors are found on nearly all cells and have important roles in both cell–cell adhesion events and the attachment of cells to the extracellular matrix. Among the integrins expressed on the oocyte plasma membrane, $\alpha_6\beta_1$ has been shown to function as a sperm receptor in mice (Almeida *et al.*, 1995), and more recent data support a role for the β_1 subunit in this context (Evans *et al.*, 1997). Similarly, the β_1 integrin subunit has been implicated in sperm–egg binding in humans. Indirect evidence for an interaction between the disintegrin domain of fertilin β and an egg integrin initially came from the demonstration that synthetic peptides corresponding to part of the disintegrin domain inhibit sperm–egg membrane interactions *in vitro* (Almeida *et al.*, 1995), while more recent studies, using a recombinant fertilin β protein representing the extracellular domain, directly implicate fertilin β in sperm–egg membrane binding, via an interaction with the β_1 integrin on the egg plasma membrane (Evans *et al.*, 1997). Similarly, synthetic peptides corresponding to part of the disintegrin domain of mouse cyritestin have recently been shown to inhibit strongly sperm–egg binding *in vitro* (Yuan *et al.*, 1997); indeed

[a] *Trimeresurus flavoviridis* HR2A	H	E	I	G	H	N	L	G	M	E	H
[a] *Bothrops jararaca* jararhagin	H	E	M	G	H	N	L	G	I	H	H
[a] Human TACE	H	E	L	G	H	N	F	G	A	E	H
[a] *Drosophila* KUZ	H	E	I	G	H	N	F	G	S	P	H
[a] Human MADM	H	E	V	G	H	N	F	G	S	P	H
[b] Macaque fertilin α	H	E	L	G	H	N	L	G	I	Q	H
[b] Human metargidin	H	E	L	G	H	S	L	G	L	D	H
[b] Human MDC9	H	E	L	G	H	N	L	G	M	N	H
[b] Mouse meltrin α	H	E	L	G	H	N	F	G	M	N	H
Macaque EAP I	H	Q	L	G	H	N	L	G	M	Q	H
Macaque tMDC I	Q	L	L	G	I	N	L	G	L	T	Y
Macaque tMDC II	Q	L	L	G	L	N	L	G	L	T	Y
Macaque tMDC III	Q	L	L	G	L	N	V	G	L	T	Y
Macaque fertilin β	Q	L	L	S	L	S	M	G	I	P	Y
Macaque tMDC IVa	Q	T	L	M	R	S	M	G	V	E	Y

Fig. 2. Comparison of the 'catalytic centre' of the metalloproteinase-like domain of a number of MDC proteins (all obtained from protein sequence databases) with those of snake venom reprolysins. Conserved residues important for activity are shaded. Proteins with proven metalloproteinase activity (a), or potential activity (b), are grouped.

cyritestin-based synthetic peptides appear to be more potent than those derived from fertilin β. A role for the other mammalian MDC proteins that are abundantly expressed in reproductive tissues has yet to be established.

Tissue Distribution

Although some of the MDC proteins are expressed in a wide range of tissues, other proteins demonstrate a much more restricted and specific pattern of expression. A number of rodent MDC proteins, namely fertilin α, fertilin β, tMDC I (also known as cyritestin), tMDC II (ADAM 5), tMDC III, tMDC IV (ADAM 6) and tMDC V (ADAM 4) are all expressed by spermatogenic cells (Frayne *et al.*, 1997) and in some cases (for example, fertilin β and tMDC I/cyritestin) expression appears to be exclusive to this cell type. Similarly, in macaques, fertilin α and β, tMDC I, tMDC II and tMDC III are all expressed by spermatogenic cells (Frayne *et al.*, 1998). However, although fertilin β expression is exclusively restricted to germ cells in macaques, tMDC I has been found, by sensitive PCR analysis, to be expressed by other tissues (Frayne *et al.*, 1998), albeit at much reduced levels. Furthermore, the fertilin α gene is non-functional in humans (Jury *et al.*, 1997) and gorillas (Jury *et al.*, 1998). These findings clearly emphasize the dangers of generalizing between species and highlight the problems that can arise when using rodent models for elucidating the functions of MDC proteins in humans.

Processing of MDC Proteins

All of the MDC proteins characterized to date are initially synthesized as large precursor proteins with an N-terminal pro-domain preceding the metalloproteinase-like domain, similar to the organization within the mosaic snake venom reprolysins (see Fig. 1). Cleavage of the pro-domain from the snake venom reprolysins serves to activate the metalloproteinase domain via a 'cysteine switch' mechanism; prior to this cleavage a single cysteine residue in the pro-domain interacts with

'RGD' motif																*R*	*G*	*D*					
Trimeresurus flavoviridis disintegrin	C	R	F	K	K	K	T	G	I	C	R	I	A	-	-	R	G	D	F	P	D	D	R
Bothrops jararaca jararhagin	C	K	F	S	K	S	G	T	E	C	R	A	S	M	S	-	E	C	D	P	A	E	H
Macaque fertilin α	C	T	F	R	R	K	G	F	L	C	R	P	T	Q	D	-	E	C	D	L	P	E	Y
Macaque fertilin β	C	L	F	M	S	Q	E	R	V	C	R	P	S	F	D	-	E	C	D	L	P	E	Y
Macaque tMDC I	C	T	I	Y	A	R	G	H	V	C	R	K	S	I	D	-	M	C	D	F	P	E	Y
Macaque tMDC II	C	K	F	K	P	A	N	T	I	C	R	K	S	V	D	V	E	C	D	F	T	E	F
Macaque tMDC III	C	E	L	S	I	V	G	T	P	C	R	K	S	V	D	P	E	C	D	F	T	E	Y
Macaque tMDC IVa	C	S	F	S	A	Q	G	T	L	C	R	P	I	Q	N	-	I	C	D	L	P	E	Y
Macaque EAP I	C	Q	I	K	K	A	G	S	I	C	R	P	A	E	D	-	E	C	D	F	P	E	M
Mouse meltrin α	C	Q	L	K	P	P	G	T	A	C	R	G	S	S	N	-	S	C	D	L	P	E	F
Human MDC9	C	R	F	L	P	G	G	T	L	C	R	G	K	T	S	-	E	C	D	V	P	E	Y
Human metargidin	C	Q	L	R	P	S	G	W	Q	C	R	P	T	R	G	-	D	C	D	L	P	E	F
Human MADM	C	A	F	K	S	K	S	E	K	C	R	D	D	S	-	-	D	C	A	R	E	G	I
Human TACE	C	Q	F	E	T	A	Q	K	K	C	Q	E	A	I	N	A	T	C	K	G	V	S	Y
Drosophila KUZ	C	T	F	V	P	T	S	Y	H	Q	K	C	K	E	E	T	E	C	S	W	S	S	T
'XCD' motif																	*X*	*C*	*D*				

Fig. 3. Comparison of the integrin binding loop and adjacent residues of a series of MDC proteins (all obtained from protein sequence databases) with those of snake venom disintegrins. The 'RGD' and 'XCD' motifs (see text) are boxed. Shaded residues are highly conserved throughout the MDC family.

the zinc ion at the catalytic site thereby maintaining the proenzyme in a latent state. A similar mechanism has been proposed for a number of MDC proteins including metargidin (Kratzchmar *et al.*, 1996), MDC9 (Weskamp *et al.*, 1996), TACE (Black *et al.*, 1997) and MADM (Howard *et al.*, 1996), although metalloproteinase activity has as yet been demonstrated only for TACE and MADM. The pro-sequences of these proteins end with a furin-like protease cleavage motif suggesting that cleavage of the pro-domain is likely to occur intracellularly within the Golgi complex. In addition, many of the MDC proteins (for example, fertilin α, fertilin β, tMDC I/cyritestin and meltrin α) are further cleaved between the metalloproteinase- and disintegrin-like domains, to yield mature proteins retaining the disintegrin domain at their N-terminus. Such cleavage of the metalloproteinase-like domain may regulate the activity of the disintegrin domain within the mature protein, for example, cleavage of the metalloproteinase-like domain of fertilin β correlates with the acquisition of fertilizing competence, exposes an epitope that is recognized by a function-blocking monoclonal antibody and may be required for relocalization of fertilin from the whole head of testicular spermatozoa to the posterior head on mature spermatozoa (Myles and Primakoff, 1997). Similarly, in the case of meltrin α, which plays a role in myoblast fusion, over-expression of a truncated form of the protein lacking the metalloproteinase-like domain leads to an increase in myoblast fusion, whereas over-expression of the full-length protein leads to a decrease in the observed fusion (Yagami-Hiromasa *et al.*, 1995).

To determine whether the MDC proteins expressed on macaque spermatozoa undergo similar proteolytic processing, we raised polyclonal antisera to bacterially expressed, recombinant MDC proteins representing the region from the end of the disintegrin domain through to the natural C-terminus (a region of maximum disparity between individual MDC proteins). These antisera were then used to probe Western blots of proteins derived from membrane preparations of macaque testicular cells and caput and cauda epididymidal spermatozoa. From examination of the data presented in Fig. 4 it can be seen that (i) all of the MDC proteins are processed from large precursor proteins in the testis; (ii) fertilin β, tMDC II and III are processed in two stages, the sizes consistent with an initial loss of the pro-domain and subsequent loss of the metalloproteinase-like domain; and (iii) processing of these MDC proteins is not co-incident, suggesting differential regulation; fertilin α losing both its pro- and metalloproteinase-like domain in the testis, tMDC I and III losing both

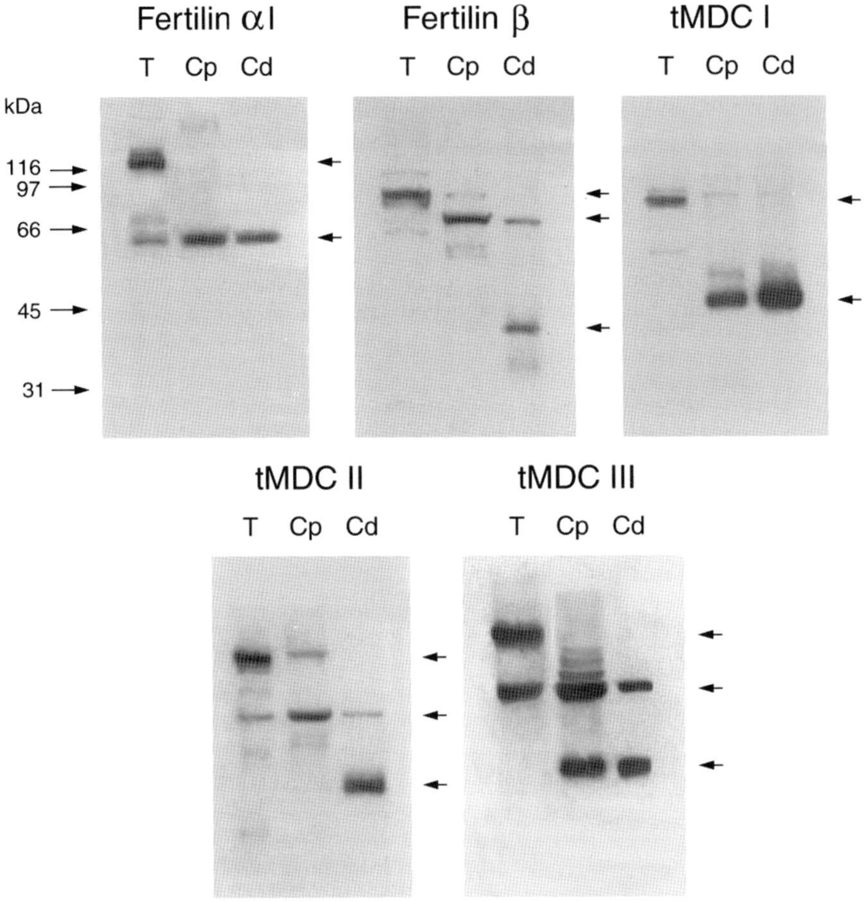

Fig. 4. Processing of the MDC proteins during epididymal transit. Western blots of detergent-extracted membrane proteins from macaque testicular cells (T) and from spermatozoa from the caput (Cp) and caudal (Cd) epididymides were probed with specific antisera raised against bacterially expressed recombinant (fertilin α1, fertilin β, tMDC I, tMDC II and tMDC III) fusion proteins. (Reproduced with permission from Frayne *et al.*, 1998.)

domains by the time spermatozoa reach the caput epididymidis and fertilin β and tMDC II by the time spermatozoa reach the cauda region.

The endoproteases responsible for processing the MDC proteins have yet to be identified; however, Lum and Blobel (1997) have provided new information on the potential enzymes involved in the cleavage of guinea-pig fertilin α and β. First, it was shown that fertilin α is probably cleaved intracellularly within the Golgi apparatus by virtue of the presence of a basic furin-like protease cleavage site at the boundary of the metalloproteinase- and disintegrin-like domains. Second, studies *in vitro* on the processing of fertilin β suggest that at least some of the enzymes involved are serine proteinases which are present in spermatozoa. As an interesting parallel, rat 2B1, a sperm surface glycoprotein implicated in sperm–zona binding, is also endoproteolytically processed during epididymal transit, this processing also occurs *in vitro* on washed testicular spermatozoa (implying the proteinase is of testicular, rather than epididymal origin) and is prevented by serine proteinase inhibitors (Jones *et al.*, 1996).

After leaving the testis, spermatozoa are transcriptionally inactive and can no longer synthesize new surface proteins. Hence, endoproteolytic processing of sperm surface antigens within the epididymis must represent the cleavage of pre-existing, membrane-inserted precursors, rather than intracellular processing during synthesis prior to targeting to the sperm surface.

Conclusion

In conclusion, the mammalian MDC proteins form a fascinating family with diverse functions ranging from myoblast fusion to processing of TNF-α and sperm–egg binding. Although a role for many of the MDC proteins has yet to be established, it is possible that those expressed on the surface of spermatozoa may be involved in gamete interaction by virtue of their disintegrin-like domains, possibly following 'unmasking' as a result of endoproteolytic processing in the epididymis. It is possible that sperm–egg binding may be a multistep process and that the disintegrin-like domains of a number of different MDC proteins may participate in one or more of these binding steps.

References

Almeida EAC, Huovilla APJ, Sutherland AE, Stephens LE, Calarco PG, Shaw LM, Mercurio AM, Sonnenberg A, Primakoff P, Myles DG and White JM (1995) Mouse egg integrin $\alpha_6\beta_1$ functions as a sperm receptor *Cell* **81** 1095–1104

Black RA, Rauch CT, Kozlosky CJ *et al.* (1997) A metalloproteinase disintegrin that releases tumour-necrosis factor-α from cells *Nature* **385** 729–733

Blobel CP, Myles DC, Primakoff P and White JM (1990) Proteolytic processing of a protein involved in sperm–egg fusion correlates with acquisition of fertilizing competence *Journal of Cell Biology* **111** 69–78

Evans JP, Kopf GS and Schultz RM (1997) Characterisation of the binding of recombinant mouse sperm fertilin β subunit to mouse eggs: evidence for adhesive activity via an egg β1 integrin-mediated interaction *Developmental Biology* **187** 79–93

Frayne J, Jury JA, Barker HL and Hall L (1997) Rat MDC family of proteins: sequence analysis, tissue distribution and expression in prepubertal and adult rat testis *Molecular Reproduction and Development* **48** 159–167

Frayne J, Jury JA, Barker HL, Perry ACF, Jones R and Hall L (1998) Macaque MDC family of proteins: sequence analysis, tissue distribution and proteolytic processing in the male reproductive tract *Molecular Human Reproduction* **4** 429–437

Hall L (1997) Fertilin and the MDC family of related proteins. In *Cell-Surface Peptidases in Health and Disease* pp 263–273 Ed. J Kenny and CM Boustead, BIOS Scientific Publications Ltd, Oxford

Howard L, Lu X, Mitchell S, Griffiths S and Glynn P (1996) Molecular cloning of MADM: a catalytically active mammalian disintegrin-metalloprotease expressed in various cell types *Biochemical Journal* **317** 45–50

Jones R, Ma A, Hou ST, Shalgi R and Hall L (1996) Testicular biosynthesis and epididymal endoproteolytic processing of rat sperm surface antigen 2B1 *Journal of Cell Science* **109** 2561–2570

Jury JA, Frayne J and Hall L (1997) The human fertilin α gene is non-functional: implications for its proposed role in fertilization *Biochemical Journal* **321** 577–581

Jury JA, Frayne J and Hall L (1998) Sequence analysis of a variety of primate fertilin α genes: evidence for non-functional genes in the gorilla and man *Molecular Reproduction and Development* **51** 92–97

Krätzschmar J, Lum L and Blobel CP (1996) Metargidin, a membrane-anchored metalloprotease–disintegrin protein with an RGD integrin binding sequence *Journal of Biological Chemistry* **271** 4593–4596

Lum L and Blobel CP (1997) Evidence for distinct serine protease activities with a potential role in processing the sperm protein fertilin *Developmental Biology* **191** 131–145

Myles DG and Primakoff P (1997) Why did the sperm cross the cumulus? To get to the oocyte. Functions of the sperm surface proteins PH-20 and fertilin in arriving at, and fusing with, the egg *Biology of Reproduction* **56** 320–327

Pan D and Rubin GM (1997) Kuzbanian controls proteolytic processing of Notch and mediates lateral inhibition during *Drosophila* and vertebrate neurogenesis *Cell* **90** 271–280

Weskamp G, Kråtzschmar J, Reid MS and Blobel CP (1996) MDC9, a widely expressed cellular disintegrin containing cytoplasmic SH3 ligand domain *Journal of Cell Biology* **132** 717–726

Yagami-Hiromasa T, Sato T, Kurisaki T, Kamijo K, Nabeshima Y-I and Fujisawa-Sehara A (1995) A metalloprotease–disintegrin participating in myoblast fusion *Nature* **377** 652–656

Yuan R, Primakoff P and Myles DG (1997) A role for the disintegrin domain of cyritestin, a sperm surface protein belonging to the ADAM family, in mouse sperm–egg plasma membrane adhesion and fusion *Journal of Cell Biology* **137** 105–112

Journal of Reproduction and Fertility Supplement **53**, 157–162

Characterization, regulation of the expression and putative roles of two glutathione peroxidase proteins found in the mouse epididymis

V. Schwaab, J-J. Lareyre[†], P. Vernet[††], E. Pons, J. Faure, J-P. Dufaure and J. R. Drevet*

CNRS UMR 6547 - GEEM, Reproduction & Développement, Université Blaise Pascal, 24, avenue des Landais, 63177 Aubière Cedex, France

Two glutathione peroxidase genes (*gpx5* and *gpx3*) were found to be expressed in the mouse epididymis. *Gpx5* was shown to be epididymis specific and restricted to the caput epididymidis, while *gpx3* was found to be expressed in a wide array of tissues including the caput, corpus and cauda epididymides. Both single copy genes are regulated by androgens as well as being developmentally regulated during postnatal ontogenesis of the epididymis. In this report data collected to date concerning the mechanisms by which these genes are regulated in the mouse epididymis are summarized. The putative roles of these antioxidant enzymes in the sperm maturation process are discussed.

Introduction

In the search for markers of the secretory activity of the mammalian epididymis, we have cloned two cDNAs encoding secreted glutathione peroxidase proteins (GPX) from the mouse epididymis. GPX together with catalase and superoxide dismutase are part of the enzymatic defence system that is used by cells to resist free radical-mediated attacks resulting from normal oxygen metabolism. Antibodies were generated against each protein and used to analyse their synthesis and subcellular localization. The corresponding genes (*gpx5* and *gpx3*) were cloned (Ghyselinck *et al.*, 1993; Schwaab *et al.*, 1995), mapped on the mouse chromosomes (Dufaure *et al.*, 1996) and the characteristics of their expression were investigated (Lareyre *et al.*, 1997; Drevet *et al.*, 1998). Experiments to identify their putative roles in the sperm maturation process have been undertaken (Vernet *et al.*, 1996, 1997).

Materials and Methods

Tissues were obtained from male mice of the swiss strain CD1 (Charles River, Cléon, France) raised in the laboratory under constant conditions of temperature, daylight and feeding. Northern blot analyses were carried out as described by Sambrook *et al.* (1989). For the identification of DNA-binding proteins found within the promoter of the GPX5 gene, DNase-1 footprinting experiments, gel shift assays and transient transfection experiments were carried out as described by Lareyre *et al.* (1997) and Drevet *et al.* (1998). Immunohistochemical analyses of the localization of GPX5 and GPX3 within the cauda epididymidis and on spermatozoa were performed using a polyclonal antiserum directed against GPX3 or GPX5 as described by Faure *et al.* (1991) with the modifications reported in

* Correspondence:
[†]Present address: Center for Reproductive Biology Research, Vanderbilt University, School of Medicine, Nashville, Tennessee 37232–2633, USA.
[††] Present address: MRC Reproductive Biology Unit, 37 Chalmers Street, Edinburgh EH3 9EW, UK.

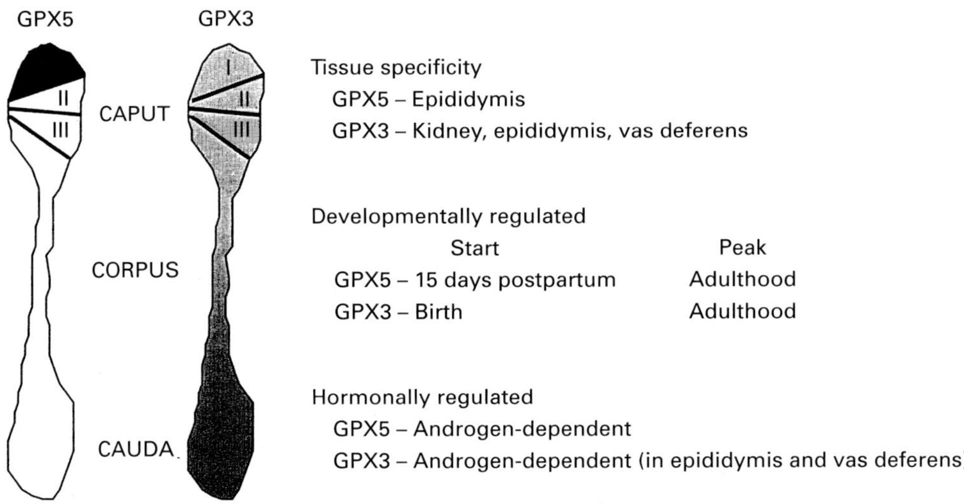

Fig. 1. Schematic representation of the epididymal distribution of mRNAs encoding GPX5 and GPX3 and characteristics of the expression of the corresponding genes. Segments I, II and III within the caput epididymidis are as originally defined by Abe *et al.* (1983).

Vernet *et al.* (1997). For optimum results, a goat anti-rabbit IgG labelled with 1 nm gold particles (BioCell) was used as the secondary antibody (dilution: 1/100) and the sections were subsequently silver contrasted.

Results

The GPX5 gene was strongly expressed exclusively in the caput epididymidis (segment I or initial segment as described in Abe *et al.*, 1983) while the expression of the GPX3 gene was low throughout the epididymis (Fig. 1). Both single-copy genes were cloned and mapped to mouse chromosomes 13 and 11, for the *gpx5* and *gpx3* genes, respectively. Both genes were found to be androgen dependent in the epididymis, while the GPX3 gene was found to be androgen independent in the kidney, its major site of expression (Fig. 2). A functional ARE (Androgen Response Element) was identified within the distal promoter of the GPX5 gene (see Fig. 3) and may partly explain the impact of androgen deprivation after castration on the transcription of *gpx5* (Faure *et al.*, 1991). A DNA-binding protein, polyoma enhancer activator 3 (PEA3), belonging to the *Ets* family of oncogene proteins that was shown to be restricted to the caput epididymidis (Xin *et al.*, 1992; Lan *et al.*, 1997; Drevet *et al.*, 1998) was shown *in vitro* to bind to and modulate the activity of the GPX5 gene promoter (Fig. 3. and Drevet *et al.*, 1998). As indicated in Fig. 3, the accumulation of mRNA encoding PEA3 was also found to be controlled by androgens and testicular factors (Lan *et al.*, 1997; Drevet *et al.*, 1998). As shown in Fig. 3., other putative DNA-binding proteins were found to interact with the GPX5 promoter such as NF1-like protein in the vicinity of the androgen receptor target sequence and a GATA-like DNA-binding protein within the proximal promoter. Both DNA-binding activities are presently under investigation.

To date, the GPX5 protein has been found in the epididymal lumen and it binds strongly to transiting spermatozoa (Fig. 4a,c). In parallel, studies *in vitro* have shown that, although the GPX5 protein does not contain the selenocysteine residue known to be critical for GPX function, it can protect stably transfected mammalian tissue-culture cells against H_2O_2-mediated peroxidative damage. In contrast, the GPX3 protein was found to have a cellular localization in the cauda epididymidis (Fig. 4b) and was not detected on spermatozoa or in the epididymal fluid (Fig. 4d and Schwaab *et al.*, in press).

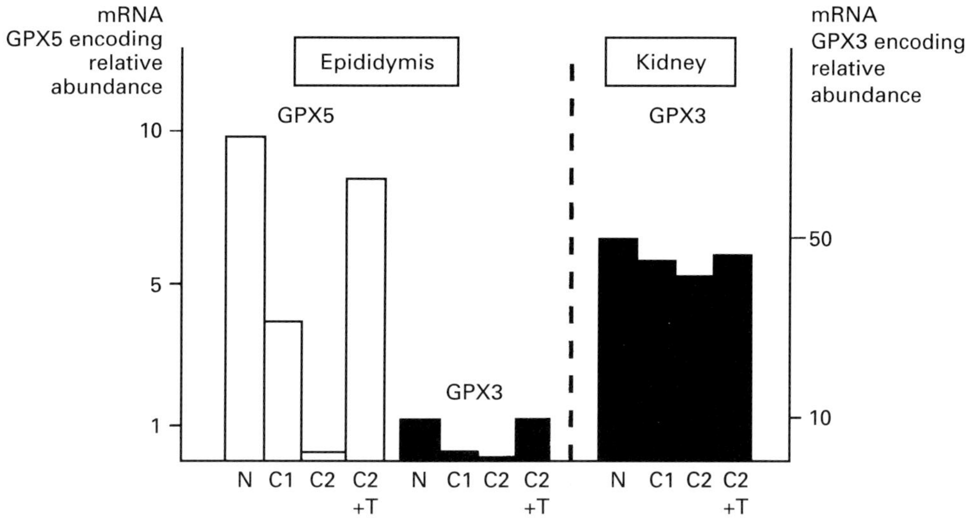

Fig. 2. Densitometric analyses of northern blot hybridizations of GPX5 (□) and GPX3 (■) carried out with either a GPX5 or a GPX3 cDNA probe on total epididymis or kidney RNA from normal (N), 10 days castrated (C1), 20 days castrated (C2) and 20 days castrated + testosterone reinjected (C2 + T) 60-day-old male mice. Numbers on *y*-axes correspond to arbitrarily chosen values reflecting the relative abundance of mRNAs encoding GPX5 and GPX3 within the epididymis (left *y*-axis) or of the GPX3 mRNA within the kidney (right *y*-axis).

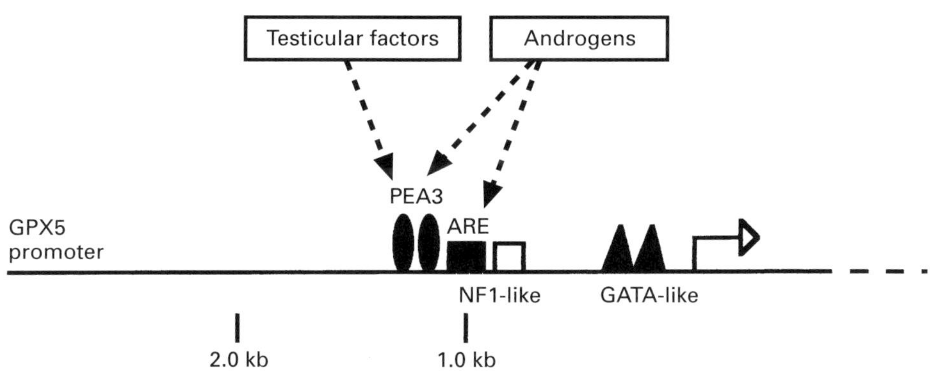

Fig. 3. Schematic representation of the key *cis*-acting elements and *trans*-acting factors identified to date on the *gpx5* promoter. Functional evidence of the involvement of the ARE (Androgen Response Element) and the PEA3 (polyoma enhancer activator 3) motifs in the fine tuning of the GPX5 gene expression were obtained *in vitro* using gel shift assays, footprinting experiments, run-on assays and transient expression experiments with heterologous cell lines (Lareyre *et al.*, 1997; Drevet *et al.*, 1998). NF1: nuclear factor 1.

Discussion

The characterization and cloning from the mouse epididymis of two differentially expressed genes encoding secreted GPXs provided us with a powerful model for analysing the mechanisms governing organ-, region- as well as development- and hormone-specific gene expression in mammals. Thus far, at the molecular level, data collected quite exclusively on the GPX5 gene suggest that androgen control of *gpx5* is partly exerted at the transcriptional level via an androgen response element located within the distal promoter of the gene. Regarding the organ- and region-specific pattern of expression of *gpx5*, the prevailing view is that the restriction of expression of *gpx5* to the

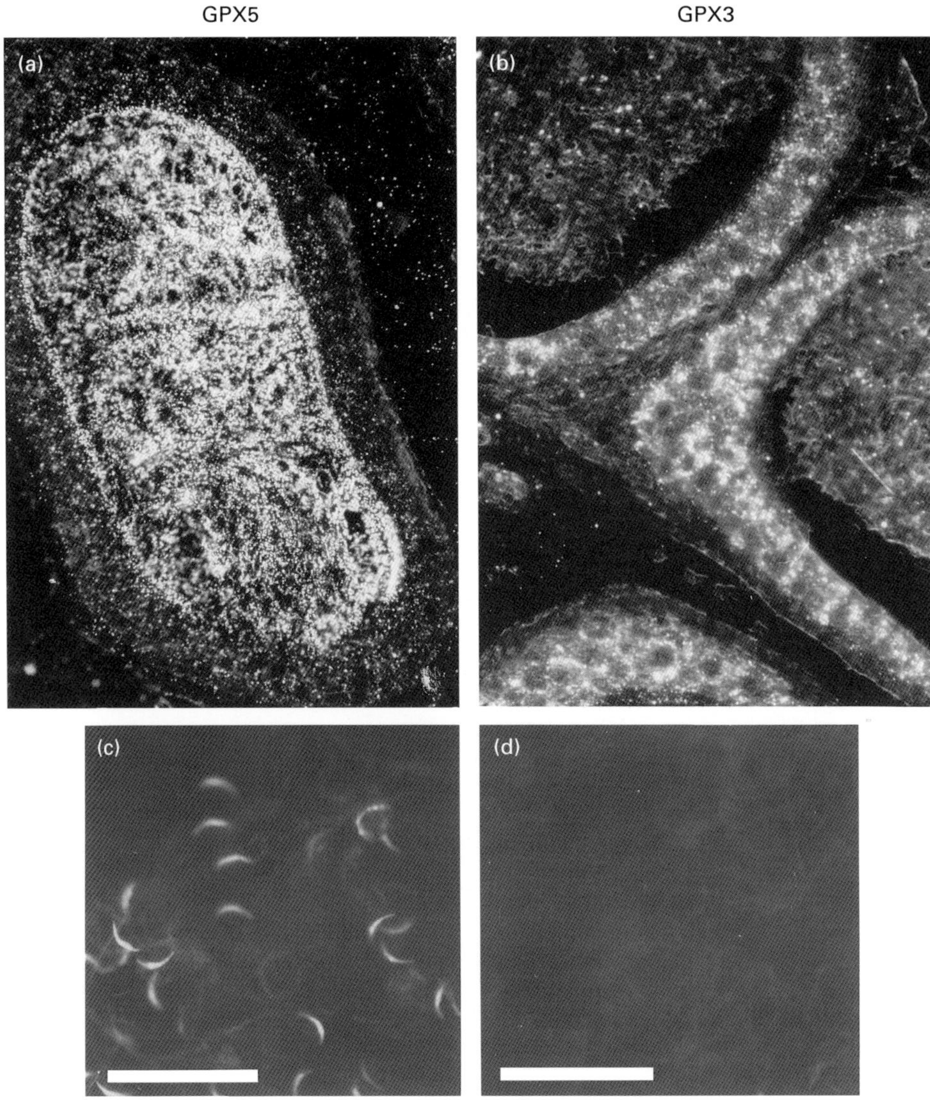

Fig. 4. Localization of GPX5 and GPX3 within the mouse cauda epididymidis and on spermatozoa recovered from cauda epididymidis of 60-day-old male mice. Immunodetection of GPX5 (a and c) and GPX3 (b and d) in cauda epididymidis (a and b) and on epididymal spermatozoa (c and d) using the GPX5 or GPX3 immune serum and either silver-enhanced immunogold-labelled anti-IgG visualized by darkfield micrographs (a and b) or fluorescein isothiocyanate conjugated with anti-IgG as a secondary antibody (c and d). Scale bars represent 50 μm.

epididymis, and within the organ itself to the caput epididymidis, is most likely controlled by tissue- or segment-specific *trans*-acting factor(s). Among these tissue-specific *trans*-acting factors PEA3 appeared to be a good candidate to explain the regionalization of *gpx5,* as well as other caput expressed genes, to the initial segment of the caput epididymidis (Lan *et al.*, 1997; Drevet *et al.*, 1998). Regarding the putative role(s) played by these secreted GPXs in the mammalian epididymis, we are conducting experiments to verify the hypothesis that GPX5 and GPX3 protect spermatozoa from peroxidative damage and from H_2O_2-mediated premature capacitation. On the one hand, it is well documented that spermatozoa in transit through the epididymis, and also during storage within the

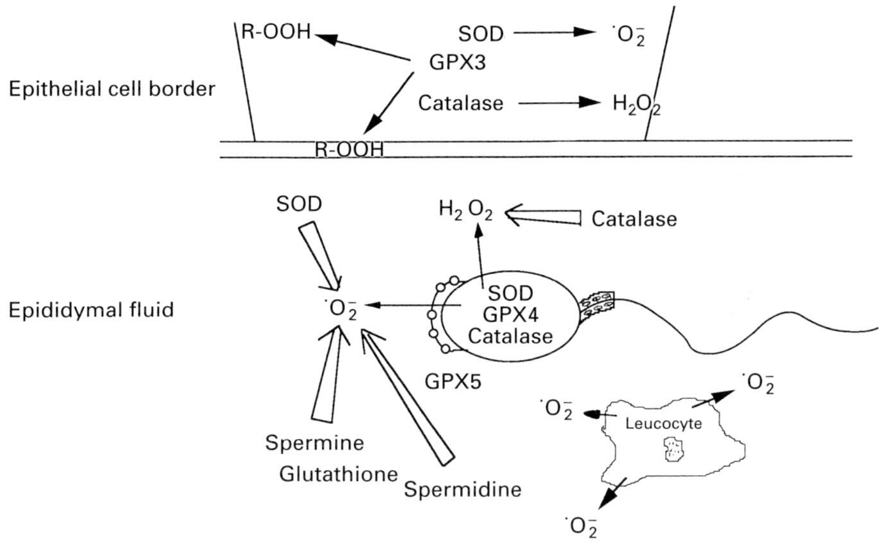

Fig. 5. Reactive oxygen species and their principal enzymatic scavengers within the epididymal epithelium and luminal environment. Primary antioxidants such as spermine, spermidine and glutathione found in the epididymal fluid are shown together with secondary antioxidants such as superoxide dismutase (SOD), catalase and glutathione peroxidase (GPX) taking into account their respective localization: epididymal fluid, sperm-membrane bound and cauda epididymidis epithelial cell. Sources of reactive oxygen species such as $\cdot O_2^-$, H_2O_2 and R–OOH are also indicated by arrows.

cauda epididymidis, are constantly challenged by high concentrations of reactive oxygen species (ROS). Reactive oxygen species, if not controlled, may lead to cell death mainly because of the high content of polyunsaturated fatty acids in spermatozoa (Gagnon and de Lamirande, 1994). Ubiquitous and tissue-specific GPXs along with superoxide dismutase (SOD) and catalases present in the luminal environment could limit free radical mediated attacks on spermatozoa (see Fig. 5). Thus, we hypothesize that the presence of a secreted GPX protein, such as GPX5, is required to increase sperm survival. On the other hand, at the onset of capacitation, a sudden increase in H_2O_2 was observed suggesting that ROS might to some extent be necessary for sperm capacitation and the acrosome reaction (Fisher and Aitken, 1997). Hence, numerous activities involved in recycling H_2O_2 are necessary to limit precocious maturation of spermatozoa. Moreover, it is suspected that spermatozoa can produce ROS and since spermatozoa are stored within the cauda epididymidis, it may be necessary to protect the cauda epithelial cells from the damaging effect of the ROS produced by spermatozoa. Thus, it is likely that the cellular GPX3 found in the cauda epididymidis might act in this respect. The contention that glutathione peroxidase has a role in sperm maturation is also strengthened by the recent observation that the testis-expressed phospholipid hydroperoxide glutathione peroxidase (GPX4 or PHGPx) is present in rat epididymal spermatozoa (see Fig. 5 and Godeas *et al.*, 1997). We are curently attempting to generate knock-out mice for GPX5 and GPX3 to test the hypothesis that both GPXs are involved in the maturation of spermatozoa.

References

Abe K, Takano H and Ito T (1983) Ultrastructure of the mouse epididymal duct with special reference to the regional differences of the principal cells *Archives Histology of Japan* **46** 51–68

Drevet JR, Lareyre J-J, Schwaab V, Vernet P and Dufaure J-P (1998) The PEA3 protein of the *Ets* oncogene family is a putative transcriptional modulator of the mouse epididymis-specific glutathione peroxidase gene gp*x*5. *Molecular Reproduction and Development* **49** 131–140

Dufaure J-P, Lareyre J-J, Schwaab V, Mattei M-G and Drevet JR

(1996) Structural organization, chromosomal localization, expression and phylogenetic evaluation of mouse glutathione peroxidase encoding genes *Comptes Rendus de l'Académie des Sciences série III* **319** 559–568

Faure J, Ghyselinck N, Jimenez C and Dufaure J-P (1991) Specific distribution of messenger ribonucleic acids for 24-kilodalton proteins in the mouse epididymis as revealed by *in situ* hybridization: developmental expression and regulation in the adult *Biology of Reproduction* **44** 13–22

Fisher HM and Aitken RJ (1997) Comparative analysis of the ability of precursor germ cells and epididymal spermatozoa to generate reactive oxygen metabolites *Journal of Experimental Zoology* **227** 390–400

Gagnon C and De Lamirande E (1994) Detrimental and beneficial effects of reactive oxygen species on sperm function *Perspective in Assisted Reproduction* **4** 121–127

Ghyselinck N, Dufaure I, Lareyre J-J, Rigaudière N, Mattei M-G and Dufaure J-P (1993) Structural organization and regulation of the gene for androgen-dependent glutathione peroxidase-like protein specific to the mouse epididymis *Molecular Endocrinology* **7** 258–272

Godeas C, Tramer F, Micali F, Soranzo M, Sandri G and Panfili E (1997) Distribution and possible novel role of phospholipid hydroperoxide glutathione peroxidase in rat epididymal spermatozoa *Biology of Reproduction* **57** 1502–1508

Lan ZJ, Palladino MA, Rudolph DB, Labus JC and Hinton BT (1997) Identification, expression, and regulation of the transcriptional factor polyomavirus enhancer activator 3, and its putative role in regulating the expression of gamma-glutamyl transpeptidase mRNA-IV in the rat epididymis *Biology of Reproduction* **57** 186–193

Lareyre J-J, Claessens F, Rombauts W, Dufaure J-P and Drevet JR (1997) Characterization of an androgen response element within the promoter of the epididymis-specific murine glutathione peroxidase 5 gene, gpx5. *Molecular and Cellular Endocrinology* **129** 33–46

Schwaab V, Baud E, Ghyselinck N, Dufaure J-P and Drevet JR (1995) Cloning of the mouse gene encoding plasma glutathione peroxidase: organization, sequence and chromosomal localization *Gene* **167** 25–31

Sambrook J, Fritsch EF and Maniatis T (1989) *Molecular Cloning: a Laboratory Manual* (2nd Edn) Cold Spring Harbor Laboratory, Cold Spring Harbor, New York

Vernet P, Rigaudière N, Ghyselinck N, Dufaure J-P and Drevet JR (1996) *In vitro* expression of a mouse tissue-specific glutathione peroxidase-like protein lacking the selenocysteine can protect stably transfected mammalian cells against oxidative damage *Biochemistry and Cell Biology* **74** 125–131

Vernet P, Faure J, Dufaure J-P and Drevet JR (1997) Tissue and developmental distribution, dependence upon testicular factors and attachment to spermatozoa of GPX5, a murine epididymis-specific glutathione peroxidase *Molecular Reproduction and Development* **47** 87–98

Xin JH, Cowie A, Lachance P and Hassel JA (1992) Molecular cloning and characterization of PEA3, a new member of the Ets oncogene family that is differentially expressed in mouse embryonic cells *Genes and Development* **6** 481–496

Journal of Reproduction and Fertility Supplement **53**, 163–181

Evolution of the vertebrate epididymis

R. C. Jones

Department of Biological Sciences, University of Newcastle, NSW 2308, Australia

This review examines the structure and function of the extratesticular sperm ducts of vertebrates in terms of their evolutionary development and adaptive significance. The primitive extratesticular duct system of Chondrichthyes is described as an example of the vertebrate archetype. Adaptations of the duct system in higher vertebrates have involved a loss of some structures and specialization of others. The duct system probably evolved as a homeostatic mechanism to facilitate fertilization and some embryological development under conditions protected from the external environment. However, it is argued that the ducts also play an important role in the competition between males to achieve paternity. In vertebrates that practise internal fertilization the ducts are involved in post-testicular maturation and storage of spermatozoa. The biological significance of post-testicular sperm maturation has not been resolved. By contrast, sperm storage is essential in most male vertebrates because of the slow rate of spermatogenesis, particularly in ectotherms. Sperm storage is also important in the competition between males for paternity as it enables a male to mate a 'partner' a number of times during an oestrus in order to reduce the prospect of being cuckolded by another male. The extent of sperm maturation and storage in the epididymis of particular vertebrates depends on the relative roles of the testis and its extragonadal ducts in the competition between males for paternity. These roles depend on a number of factors, including allometric limitations to testis size, metabolic rate and the development of endothermy, and the reproductive strategy of females of the species.

Introduction

It is generally recognized that in mammals the extratesticular duct system plays two important roles in reproduction as well as transporting spermatozoa from the testis. It is essential for the survival of a species as spermatozoa are not capable of fertilizing an ovum when they leave the testis, and only acquire the capacity when they pass through the extratesticular ducts. The ducts also play an important role in an individual's strategy to achieve paternity, by accumulating and storing spermatozoa available for use. This maximises the number of spermatozoa that can be delivered at each mating, and the number of effective matings that are possible during a day (Jones and Lin, 1993a). These roles of the mammalian sperm ducts are accomplished by a highly differentiated system that is involved in fluid and solute transport and protein secretion and reabsorption, and the process of post-testicular sperm maturation is dependent on the androgen-dependent secretion of protein (Orgebin-Crist and Jahad, 1979). Although there is a growing knowledge of the sperm ducts in mammals, our knowledge of the ducts in other vertebrates is poor. There is no consistent terminology for the ducts among vertebrates, and there is little knowledge of their role in vertebrate evolution.

It is generally recognized that the primitive condition of both the male and female reproductive systems of vertebrates is the occurrence of paired gonads situated between the kidneys, but no extragonadal ducts to transport gametes. For example, the extant Agnatha (lampreys and hagfish) produce and store gametes in their gonad (the left and right are fused in adults), and spawning gametes are released into the peritoneal cavity and pass outside through a peritoneal funnel in the body wall. Extragonadal ducts probably evolved in male and female vertebrates as a homeostatic mechanism to allow fertilization and some development to occur under conditions protected from the external environment. Development of these capacities has allowed animals to exploit a wide range of reproductive strategies. In association with internal fertilization, a long and highly differentiated extratesticular sperm duct system has evolved in male Chondrichthyes and amniotes, in which some post-testicular maturation seems to be essential for spermatozoa to achieve the capacity to fertilize ova (Bedford, 1979). On the other hand, in osteichthyians and amphibians which practise external fertilization the ducts only act as conduits and are short and lined by a simple epithelium (Marshall, 1986; Chase, 1923). As the evolution of the extratesticular sperm ducts has involved the testes taking over excretory ducts for reproductive functions (Romer, 1970) it is informative to assess the relative roles of the testes and the sperm ducts in the reproductive strategies of male vertebrates.

Male Reproductive Strategies

It is suggested that internal fertilization increases the potential for paternity to be determined by natural selection. This is because it reduces the requirement for precise synchrony in both sexes shedding their gametes and it consequently provides opportunities for inter-male competition to deliver spermatozoa closest to ovulation, and for competition between spermatozoa within the female tract to achieve fertilization. Increased opportunity for natural selection of males is significant as in birds, for example, mutation rates of the two types of sex chromosome account for a four to seven times faster mutation rate in males than females, suggesting 'that evolution is driven by males' (Ellegren and Fridolfsson, 1997). Associated with this potential for natural selection is the occurrence of considerable competition between males to achieve paternity (sperm competition). Sperm competition has been demonstrated in a number of vertebrates and it is important even in monogamous species (Parker, 1984). In general, it is considered that it is the last male that mates before ovulation which achieves paternity. Consequently, there are selective advantages in having: (1) a high rate of sperm production, (2) the capacity to store spermatozoa so that a reserve is available for mating, and (3) the production of spermatozoa which, in the female reproductive tract, can successfully compete with spermatozoa from other males in achieving fertilization. However, selection for these parameters would be constrained by allometric limitations to testis size, metabolic rate, temperature and the development of endothermy.

Ectothermic animals produce spermatozoa at a much slower rate than homoeothermic endotherms (Table 1). Consequently, ectotherms are very dependent on establishing a store of spermatozoa in the epididymis for use during the mating season (which may be shorter than the duration of spermatogenesis). On the other hand, endotherms can produce spermatozoa at a daily rate equivalent to the number in one or two ejaculates for a mammal (man, for example, is an exception taking 2.5 days to produce enough spermatozoa for one ejaculate: Bedford, 1990), and up to 25 ejaculates for a bird (Jones and Lin, 1993a), so that they are continually replenishing their epididymal store of spermatozoa during the mating season. Comparison of a nonpasserine bird and a scrotal mammal illustrates how metabolic rate, and the reproductive pattern of females, may determine the strategy of sperm production in males (Fig. 1). Whereas mammals ovulate all eggs contributing to a litter over a few hours, birds ovulate about once a day during a week or more to produce a clutch of eggs. Consequently, although spermatozoa deposited at one mating may be stored by a hen for many days to ensure she produces young (her insurance for achieving maternity), a male may have to mate a partner many times around the time of ovulation in order to compete with other males to achieve paternity, and this competition must continue over weeks for a bird compared with a day or so for mammals. Nonpasserine birds achieve the capacity to mate frequently for many weeks by rapid spermatogenesis (four times the rate of mammals) producing spermatozoa that are almost mature (Howarth, 1983), and rapid transit of spermatozoa through the extratesticular ducts. On the other hand, mammalian testes produce immature spermatozoa that are modified (matured) during a slow passage through the epididymis, and mature spermatozoa

Table 1. Comparison of the duration of spermatogenesis, and transit and survival times for spermatozoa in the extratesticular ducts of some vertebrate ectotherms and endotherms. The duration of spermatogenesis in the ectotherms may include a period of diapause, and may also vary with environmental temperature

	Chondrichthyian[a]	Reptile[b]	Eutherian mammal[c]	Non-passerine bird[c]
Spermatogenesis (days)	260	90–270	38	10
Spermatozoa in the extratesticular ducts:				
Transit time (days)	42	–	8.4	1
Survival time (days)	–	–	42	≤7

[a]Olsen (1954); [b]Reynolds (1943), Badir (1958); [c]Jones and Lin (1993a).

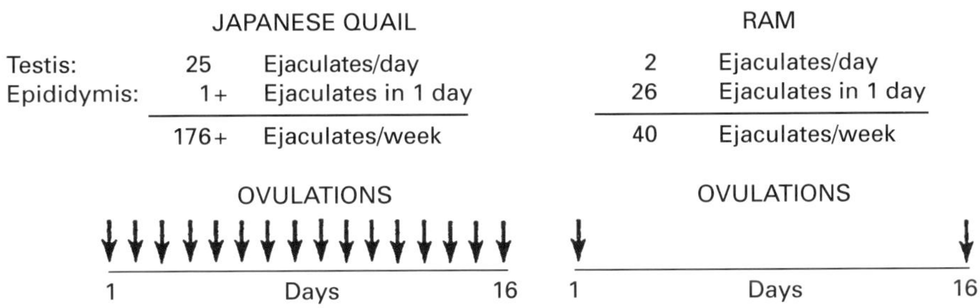

Fig. 1. The process of sperm production of a bird (Japanese quail) and mammal (ram) is related to the ovulatory pattern of the females. Quail hens ovulate daily, and cock birds produce enough spermatozoa for many matings each day by rapid production of spermatozoa in the testis and transit through the epididymal ducts. Ewes ovulate once every 16 days, and rams have a much lower output of spermatozoa from the testis, but accumulate and store enough spermatozoa in the epididymis for many matings during a day. Note that hens also store spermatozoa to ensure that their eggs are fertilized, but that is an adaptation of the female to ensure maternity whereas this figure considers adaptations of males to ensure paternity in a competitive mating system.

accumulate in a region where they store and are available for many matings. Passerine birds are more specialised for flight than non-passerines. Consequently, they have smaller testes, but they have developed a sperm store in the epididymis (see below).

Primitive Arrangement and Adaptations of the Extratesticular Sperm Ducts

The primitive condition of the extratesticular duct system is displayed in some of the Chondrichthyes, and this general plan has been modified during evolution (Fig. 2 and Table 2) for the other major vertebrates that practise internal fertilization. There is general agreement about the

Table 2. Comparison of the terminology commonly used for structurally distinct regions of the testicular sperm ducts of various vertebrates, and proposed homologies[a]. The regions of the duct system have been grouped according to their embryological origin and because they have a distinct structure which changes abruptly between adjacent regions

Embryological origin	Elasmobranchs (Stanley, 1963; Jones and Jones, 1982)	Reptiles (Volsøe, 1944; St Girons, 1957)	Birds (Budras and Sauer, 1975; Tingari, 1971)	Mammals (Roosen-Runge, 1961; Reid and Cleland, 1957)
Gonadal blastema	Connecting ducts	–	–	–
	Central canal of testis	–	Intratesticular rete	Intratesticular rete testis
	–	–	Intracapsular rete testis	–
Rete blastema	Marginal canal of kidney[b]	Tubuli efferentes	Extratesticular rete testis	Extratesticular rete testis
Mesonephric tubules	Ductuli efferentes	Ductuli epididymides – proximal	Ductuli efferentes proximales	Ductuli efferentes - initial zone
	–	Ductuli epididymides – distal	Ductuli efferentes distales	Ductuli efferentes - coni vasculosi
Connecting tubule of mesonephric duct[a]	Ductuli epididymides	–	Ductuli conjugentes[c]	Ductus epididymidis - initial segments
Mesonephric duct	Ductus epididymidis	Ductus epididymidis	Ductus epididymidis	Ductus epididymidis
	Ductus deferens	Ductus deferens	Ductus deferens[d]	Ductus epididymidis
	–	–	Receptaculum ductus deferentis	–
	–	–	–	Ductus deferens

[a] Segmental kidney tubule (Stanley, 1963).
[b] Also called the longitudinal canal of epididymis, and Bidder's duct.
[c] Immunologically similar to the ductus epididymidis and not ductuli efferentes (Croisille, 1981).
[d] Seminal sac is formed in passerine birds (Riddle, 1927; Bailey, 1953).

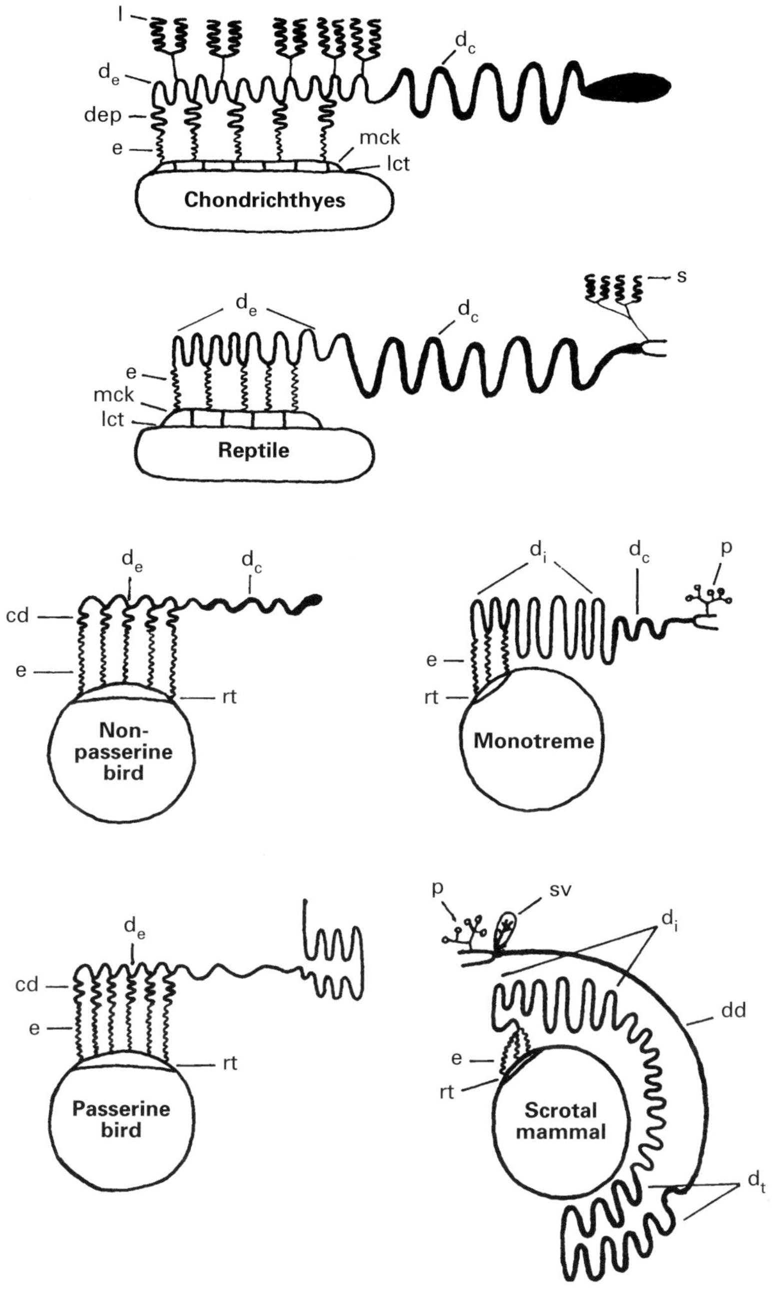

Fig. 2. The proposed primitive arrangement of the extratesticular sperm ducts in Chondrichthyes, reptiles, birds (non-passerine) and mammals (monotreme), and the arrangement in a passerine bird and scrotal (eutherian) mammal that display the development of a storage region for spermatozoa in the ductus epididymidis. The primitive arrangement of the ductuli efferentes and epididymal ducts is displayed in Chondrichthyes: numerous ductuli efferentes leave the rete testis and each ductulus efferens courses for a distance, then continues as a ductulus epididymidis which independently joins the main ductus epididymidis. e, ductuli efferentes; cd, connecting ducts; d_e, d_c, d_i, and d_t, epididymal, caudal, initial segment and terminal segment respectively of the ductus epididymidis; dd, ductus deferens; dep, ductuli epididymides; l, Leydig gland; lct, longitudinal canal of the testis; mck, marginal canal of the kidney; p, prostate gland; sv, seminal vesicles; rt, rete testis; s, sexual gland of the kidney.

homologies of the regions, except for the contribution of the mesonephric tubules (including Bowman's capsule) to regions at either end of the ductuli efferentes. It is suggested that the ductuli epididymides of Chondrichthyes correspond to the connecting tubules of the domestic rooster which develop into the ductuli conjugentes (Budras and Sauer, 1975) and to the initial segment of the epididymis of mammals (Benoit, 1926) which has many characteristics similar to the ductuli epididymides.

The following description of the primitive duct system in Chondrichthyes (Fig. 2) is mainly based on structural and functional studies of the Port Jackson shark, *Heterodontus portusjacksoni* (Jones and Jones, 1982; Jones *et al.*, 1984a; Jones and Lin, 1993b). Spermatogenesis in this class occurs in spermatogenic cysts which evacuate remnants of Sertoli cells (Sertoli cell bodies and Sertoli cell cytoclasts) as well as spermatozoa into the rete testis. The Sertoli cell bodies disappear from the lumen of the proximal ductus epididymidis, whereas the Sertoli cell cytoclasts persist throughout the sperm ducts. The cytoclasts have the capacity to convert cholesterol to 11-deoxycorticosterone (Simpson *et al.*, 1964) and so could be involved in local regulation of the duct epithelium by a mechanism analogous to the way that luminal fluid from the testis regulates the initial segment of the epididymis of mammals (see below).

Noteworthy features of the extratesticular ducts of Chondrichthyes are: transport of bodies through the ducts is dependent on cilia as they are lined by a ciliated epithelium, and only the terminal ampullary region of the ductus epididymidis has a muscular tunic; and protein synthesized in the epithelium is stored in granules in contrast to the merocrine secretion characteristic of the mammalian epididymis. The rete testis consists of narrow ducts lined by ciliated cuboidal cells with little cytoplasm, and numerous intraepithelial leucocytes. The ductuli efferentes are narrow and lined by a low columnar epithelium composed of ciliated cells that possess a moderate number of organelles indicating the occurrence of some heterophagic digestion. The epithelium contains numerous intraepithelial leucocytes. The ductuli epididymides are wider than the ductuli efferentes, and spermatozoa are more concentrated in the lumen than in the ductuli efferentes. Their epithelium is very tall consisting mainly of nonciliated cells specialised for the synthesis and secretion of protein. It also contains some ciliated cells and few intraepithelial leucocytes. The ductus epididymidis is wider than the ductuli epididymides. The duct mucosa is a low, columnar, ciliated epithelium which contains intraepithelial leucocytes, and two regions can be recognized. The proximal region is characterized by ciliated epithelial cells, specialised for heterophagic digestion and by the presence of numerous intraepithelial leucocytes. The Sertoli cell bodies disappear from the duct lumen in this region. Caudally, the duct widens, there are very few intraepithelial leucocytes, the ciliated cells are moderately specialised for protein synthesis and secretion, and the epithelium is thrown into folds. The duct terminates in an ampulla. In the lumen, spermatozoa form into bundles and numerous Leydig cell bodies are present. The bodies are nonmembranous protein secretions of the Leydig glands. The glands develop from the mesonephric tubules and form the anterior opisthonephros (which has only a reproductive function).

Among the Chondrichthyes the number of ductuli efferentes varies from 1 to 7 and the number of ductuli epididymides is the same or fewer than the number of ductuli efferentes (Jones and Jones, 1982). The considerable variation in the arrangement of the epididymal ducts among reptiles is illustrated in Fig. 14 of Volsøe (1944). Snakes display the primitive condition with ductuli leaving the rete testis along the entire length of the testis, with up to 33 connections (Volsøe, 1944). Lizards are most specialized with 5–9 ductuli reported in some species and a single ductulus in others (Alverdes, 1928). Reports on reptiles have referred to the rete testis as tubule efferentes, and the ductuli efferentes as ductuli epididymides (Table 2). The latter are differentiated into proximal ductuli with unciliated, secretory epithelium and distal ductuli with ciliated epithelium in *Vipera aspis* (St Girons, 1957). It is doubtful whether reptiles have a homologue of the ductuli epididymides in Chondrichthyes.

Birds seem to have retained the primitive condition with numerous ductuli efferentes leaving along the whole dorsal surface of the testis (Table 3) and continuing as connecting ducts. The proximal region of the ductuli is cavernous and develops from Bowman's capsule; the distal region

Table 3. Fluid reabsorption by the ductuli efferentes of the Japanese quail and Wistar rat showing how the ducts cope with different rates of sperm output. Reabsorption is expressed as % total testicular output, rate for the whole duct system and rate per unit area of wall of ductuli

Parameter	Quail[a]	Rat[b]
Mass of animal (g)	150	560
Daily sperm production ($\times 10^{-6}$ spermatozoa)	93	19
Number of ductuli efferentes	43	6–7
Fluid reabsorption:		
Percentage total testicular plasma output	99	96
$\mu l\ h^{-1}$ (all ductuli)	219	45
$\mu l\ cm^{-1}\ h^{-1}$	130	16

[a] Clulow and Jones (1988); [b] Clulow *et al.* (1994).

is tubular and develops from the rest of the mesonephric tubule (Budras and Sauer, 1975; Budras and Meier, 1981). Mammalian ductuli efferentes develop from the ductular part of the mesonephric tubules and are fewer than in comparably sized birds (Table 3). The ductuli are fairly straight in the initial zone, but follow a highly sinuous path and anastomose with one another in the distal zone (coni vasculosi). The anastomoses often result in a reduction in the number of ductuli (Benoit, 1926). In some small marsupials only one ductulus efferens leaves the testis (Hughes, 1965; Noqueira *et al.*, 1977). As the main function of the ductuli in mammals is fluid reabsorption (see below) the reduced number, and presumably a reduced total length of ductulus, may be associated with a reduced output of spermatozoa and fluid from the testis.

Early anatomists distinguished between the derivative of the mesonephric duct which lies on the testis (epididymal region) and the more caudal regions by referring to these regions as the ductus epididymidis and ductus deferens, respectively. However, Glover and Nicander (1971) argued that the 'ductus deferens' of Chondrichthyes, reptiles, birds and testicond mammals has an equivalent function to the cauda epididymidis of scrotal mammals, sperm storage. The term 'ductus deferens' is only appropriate for the muscular conduit which transports spermatozoa from the epididymis during ejaculation of scrotal and large testicond mammals, and passerine birds. The epididymis of these animals has a specialised region for sperm storage, which is displaced from the copulatory organ (Glover, 1973; Bedford, 1977). Work on the rat indicates that the ductus deferens normally contains few spermatozoa, and any remaining after ejaculation are retrogradely moved back to the ductus epididymidis by the action of the muscular tunic (Prins and Zandeveldt, 1980). The common shrew appears to be an exception in this regard since its 'ductus deferens' has a terminal dilation packed with spermatozoa (Suzuki and Racey, 1984).

Function of the Ductuli Efferentes in Mammals and Birds

Some micropuncturists have confounded the functions of the ductuli efferentes and initial segments of the epididymis and consequently have suggested incorrectly that the initial segments are responsible for reabsorbing most of the fluid leaving the testis (Jones *et al.*, 1987). Work using the tammar wallaby, *Macropus eugenii*, for micropuncture studies, and the rat for stereological (Jones and Jurd, 1987) and microcannulation (Clulow *et al.*, 1994) studies, indicates that the ductuli efferentes are a distinct functional unit of the excurrent duct system. They play a major role in the excurrent duct system by reabsorbing most of the fluid leaving the testes (96% in the rat), so that spermatozoa are delivered in a small volume of fluid to the ductus epididymidis where its composition is modified. It is interpreted that fluid reabsorption by the ductuli efferentes is iso-osmotic as between the rete testis and ductus epididymidis there is no change in luminal concentration of the major inorganic cations (Na^+ and K^+) or osmotic pressure. However, there is an increase in osmotic pressure in the initial zone of the ductuli (see Clulow *et al.*, 1998). The ductuli efferentes also reabsorb 50% (tammar) to 80% (rat) of the protein leaving the testis, and the uptake is receptor mediated (Hermo and Morales, 1984).

The mucosa lining the ductuli efferentes of birds is also specialised for fluid reabsorption. The rate of reabsorption is much higher than for mammals (Table 3), reflecting the higher rates of metabolism and sperm production of birds.

Derivatives of the Mesonephric Duct in Reptiles

In reptiles, the ductus epididymidis is lined by a pseudostratified, columnar epithelium consisting of principal cells and basal cells. It is tall in the epididymal region, but reduces to cuboidal in the caudal region (Haider and Rai, 1987; Saint Girons, 1957; Mesure *et al.*, 1991). The caudal region has a thicker muscular tunic than the epididymal region. There is considerable variation between species in the amount of eosinophilic material which is formed and secreted into the duct, ranging from no obvious eosinophilia (but, hypertrophied epithelium) to voluminous secretions and numerous granules within the epithelium (Dufaure and St Girons, 1984). It is suggested that this variation may be a reflection of the mechanism of protein secretion, as granules, or as a merocrine secretion as in the mammalian epididymis, and this in turn may be related to differences in preferred body temperature (and hence metabolic rate) of the different species. Reports on some species indicate that the duct epithelium is differentiated along its length into four regions (Haider and Rai, 1987). However, there is no definitive evidence that the epididymis of reptiles has an initial segment as in mammals. The main androgen-dependent protein secreted into the lumen of *Lacerta* has a molecular mass of of 17.2 kDa and has significant similarities with retinoic acid binding protein (Morel *et al.*, 1993).

Derivatives of the Mesonephric Duct in Birds

In birds, the ductuli conjugentes join the ductuli efferentes to the ductus epididymidis. The ductuli conjugentes and ductus epididymidis are lined by a low, pseudostratified, columnar epithelium consisting of nonciliated cells and basal cells, and there is no variation in epithelial structure along these ducts (Tingari, 1971; Aire *et al*, 1979). The ductus epididymidis has a muscular tunic, and is short in nonpasserine birds compared with mammals (72 cm in the Japanese quail and 339 cm in the Wistar rat: Clulow and Jones, 1988; Jones and Jurd, 1987). There is a terminal dilation (receptaculum ductus deferentis) which enters the cloaca through an ejaculatory duct (papilla ductus deferentis) (Tingari, 1971; Hess *et al.*, 1976; Aire *et al.*, 1979). In passerines, the duct extends caudally and forms an enlarged region (the seminal sac or seminal vesicle) structurally similar to the cauda epididymidis of scrotal mammals; this duct protrudes into the body wall below the rectum where its temperature is less than deep body temperature (Riddle, 1927; Bailey, 1953; Wolfson, 1954). Only one androgen-dependent protein (17 kDa) has been identified in secretions of the ductus epididymidis of the Japanese quail (Kidd, 1982).

Derivatives of the Mesonephric Duct in Mammals

The ductus epididymidis of mammals is more complex than its homologue in other vertebrates. The mucosa is unciliated and composed of principal cells, apical cells, narrow (mitochondria rich) cells, light cells, basal cells and halo cells (intraepithelial leucocytes) (Reid and Cleland, 1957; Sun and Flickinger, 1980; Hoffer *et al.*, 1973a), and it is adapted for protein secretion and reabsorption, and fluid and solute transport. In all the mammals that have been studied the ductus is structurally

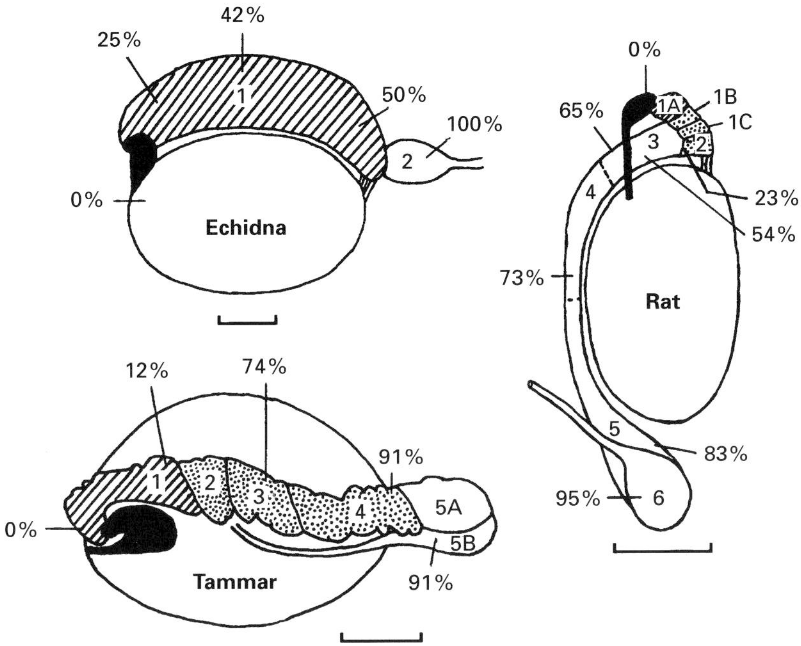

Fig. 3. Structural differentiation of the extratesticular sperm ducts of a monotreme (echidna), marsupial (tammar wallaby) and eutherian (rat) mammal showing the relationship between the histologically distinct zones and sperm maturation as indicated by the development of the capacity for motility (the rate of forward motility is expressed as a percentage). The ductuli efferentes are black, the initial segment proper is striped and the distal initial segments are speckled. The numerics show all the structurally distinct zones of the epididymal duct that have been described (echidna – Djakiew and Jones, 1981; tammar – Jones *et al.*, 1984b; rat – Reid and Cleland, 1957). Note that the location of zone 2 in the rat is correct in this figure and in Nicander *et al.* (1983), but inaccurate in Reid and Cleland (1957): it is interpreted that Hermo *et al.* (1991) refer to zone 1A as the 'proximal zone', zones 1B and 1C as 'distal zones' and zone 2 as the 'intermediate zone' of the initial segment. The number (and location) of zones that have been described in other mammals are: 4 in the European mole (Suzuki and Racey, 1976) and African elephant (Jones and Brosnan, 1981); 4 to 6 in macaques (Ramos and Dym, 1977; Alsum and Hunter, 1978); 5 in the mouse (Abe *et al.*, 1983); 6 in the ram, stallion and bull (Nicander, 1958), and hamster (Nicander and Glover, 1973); 7 in the South American opossum (Orsi *et al.*, 1980); and 8 in the rabbit (Nicander, 1957; Jones *et al.*, 1979) and human (Holstein, 1969).

differentiated along its length in terms of the duct mucosa, the muscular tunic and the microvasculature. However, in marsupials and eutherian mammals the changes in structure of the mucosa along the duct are gradual, and there are no reports of abrupt changes like those reported for the junctions between the structures in each row of Table 2. Nevertheless, *in situ* hybridization studies have shown that each gene exhibits its own distinctive expression along the epididymis (Douglass *et al.*, 1991; Winer *et al.*, 1993; Cornwall and Hann, 1995), several genes exhibiting abrupt changes in mRNA whilst others exhibit a more gradual increase or decrease in expression between regions.

The mucosa is structurally differentiated into two zones in monotremes and four to eight in marsupials and eutherian mammals (Fig. 3). Glover and Nicander (1971) provided a common nomenclature for this zonation to facilitate comparisons among species. Their classification is based on the hamster epididymis (Nicander and Glover, 1973) and knowledge of some eutherian mammals, but it requires qualification to be applied to some species, such as rats (L. Nicander, personal communication). They proposed that the zonation reflects a division of labour along the duct into a proximal region involved in sperm maturation, and a distal region specialised for the storage of 'mature' spermatozoa. However, the proximal region probably plays an important role protecting spermatozoa against oxidative and possibly other damage (see Hinton and Pallidino, 1995), and preparing them for storage (Bedford, 1991). The two regions are best distinguished by the structure and innervation of the muscular tunic (Baumgarten *et al.*, 1971). Slender muscle cells coat the entire duct, and additional layers of thick muscle cells coat the storage region (most of the cauda epididymidis). Repeated ejaculation does not affect the rate of sperm passage through the proximal region, whereas it increases the rate through the storage region, and could empty it (Kirton *et al.*, 1967). There is considerable variation in the location of the storage region in testicond mammals (Glover, 1973; Bedford, 1977).

Benoit (1926) drew attention to the occurrence of an initial segment in the epididymis of the six species of mammal that he studied, and described it as a region of the ductus with a wide diameter, a tall, actively secretory epithelium and containing few spermatozoa in the lumen. It is also characterized by the occurrence of narrow cells (Sun and Flickinger, 1980), and the ultrastructure of the principal cells (Nicander and Glover, 1973; Fawcett and Hoffer, 1979). The characteristics are present in the initial segment of all mammals that have been studied: including monotremes (Djakiew and Jones, 1982) and marsupials (Jones *et al.*, 1984b). The only qualifications to Benoit's criteria are that in the human (Holstein, 1969), common shrew (Suzuki and Racey, 1984) and tammar wallaby (Jones *et al.*, 1984b) the epithelium is not very tall as in the rat and hamster. The initial segment has been identified in a monotreme (Jones *et al.*, 1992) and marsupial (Jones *et al.*, 1988) by the presence of other unique characteristics of the region: its dependence on luminal fluids from the testis, and high activity of 5α-reductase compared with the rest of the epididymis (see below). Additional unique features of the initial segment include the relatively high blood flow and density and permeability of blood capillaries (Kormano, 1968; Abe *et al.*, 1984), and the susceptibility to drugs, such as cadmium and α-chlorhydrin (Hoffer *et al.*, 1973b).

The initial segment is dependent on a luminal connection with the testis. If this connection is interrupted by orchidectomy or ligation of the ductuli efferentes, the initial segment epithelium regresses severely impairing its secretory capacity even when systemic testosterone concentrations are maintained (Gustafsson, 1966; Fawcett and Hoffer, 1979). There has been little work on the nature of the regulator which supports the initial segment epithelium. Early suggestions that it may be androgen-binding protein, or the high concentration of testosterone in the luminal fluid from the testis, are unfounded as: (1) fluid leaving the testis of the boar contains no androgen-binding protein (Setchell, 1978); (2) increasing the concentration of systemic testosterone to that present in fluid leaving the testis of the rat does not prevent regression of the initial segment epithelium following efferent duct ligation (Fawcett and Hoffer, 1979); and (3) structural signs of regression occur within 6 h of efferent duct ligation (Nicander *et al.*, 1983) which is much earlier than expected if a steroid were involved. There is some evidence that the regulator is a growth factor (Brown *et al.*, 1983; Sujarit *et al.*, 1990; Hinton *et al.*, this supplement).

Another unique feature of the initial segment is the 5α-reductase activity which is three to five times higher than in the rest of the epididymis (Aafjes and Vreeburg, 1972; Robaire *et al.*, 1977). The enzyme converts testosterone to dihydrotestosterone (DHT) while throughout the epididymis a second enzyme is present (3α-hydroxysteroid dehydrogenase) which converts DHT to 5α-androstane-3α,17β-diol (3α-diol). The androgens are retained within the ductus at higher concentrations than in blood. In rats, for example, the concentration of testosterone in systemic blood, and luminal fluid from the caput and cauda epididymidis were 1.20, 5.38 and 7.72 ng ml^{-1}, respectively, and concentrations of DHT were 0.12, 58.73 and 4.40 ng ml^{-1}, respectively (Turner *et al.*, 1984). The occurrence of the androgen converting enzymes is not confined to the ductus

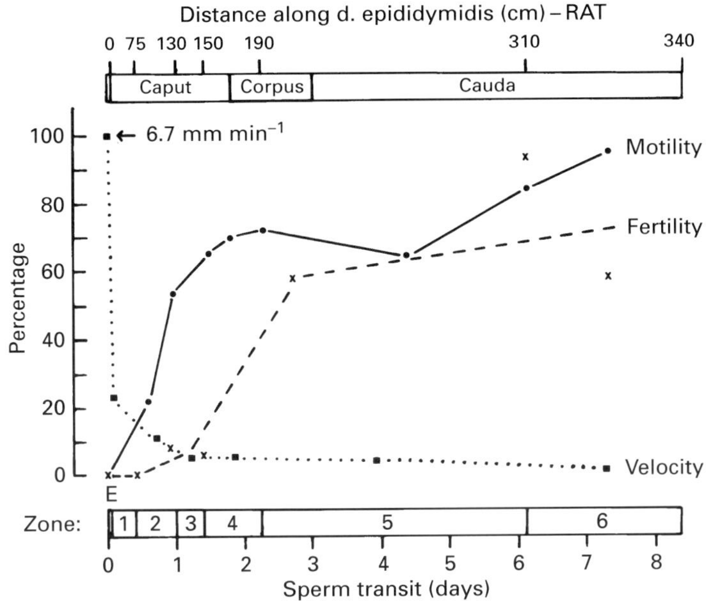

Fig. 4. Sperm maturation and transit in relation to epididymal structure in the rat. The zones shown in the abscissa are numbered according to Reid and Cleland (1957). E indicates the ductuli efferentes. Reproduced with permission from Jones and Clulow (1987).

epididymidis of mammals. They have been demonstrated in a lizard (Dufaure and Gigon, 1975), and 5α-reductase activity has been demonstrated in a bird (Japanese quail: G.M. Stone and R.C. Jones, unpublished). The luminal androgens must contribute to regulating the duct mucosa, and may explain why the epididymis can be maintained when systemic androgen concentrations are low (Jones, 1989). They may also explain why spermatozoa retained in the cauda epididymidis by a caudal ligature survived three times as long as spermatozoa retained in the same region but prevented from receiving luminal fluid by a ligature proximal to the site of retention (Paufler and Foote, 1968).

In rats the initial segment described by Benoit (1926) corresponds to zone 1A described by Reid and Cleland (1957). However, Fawcett and Hoffer (1979) showed that the part of the duct dependent on luminal factors also includes zones 1B, 1C and 2, and proposed that zone 1A be referred to as the 'initial segment proper'. For the purpose of comparison between species, it is suggested (Jones *et al.*, 1987) that zones 1B, 1C and 2 be referred to as the 'distal initial segments' and zones 1 and 2 inclusive as 'initial segments'. The structure of the epithelium lining the distal initial segments is similar to that of the initial segment proper except that the cells are less active and the epithelium is lower (Fawcett and Hoffer, 1979), but taller than more caudally (Reid and Cleland, 1957; Jones *et al.*, 1984b). The occurrence of distal initial segments has been demonstrated in hamsters (Moniem, Glover and Lubicz-Nowrocki, 1978), rabbits (Jones *et al.*, 1981), rams (Jones *et al.*, 1982) and a marsupial, the tammar (Jones *et al.*, 1988), as well as rats. They have not been recognized in mice (Abe and Takano, 1989) or monotremes (Jones *et al.*, 1992).

Jones *et al.* (1987) proposed that the initial segments of the epididymis play an important role in sperm maturation in mammals. Spermatozoa develop much of their capacity for motility during passage through the initial segments of a monotreme, marsupial and eutherian which have been studied as models of their subclass of Mammalia (Fig. 3). In the monotreme model, structural signs of maturation develop in the first few centimeters of ductus beyond the initial segment proper. In the marsupial, spermatozoa leaving the initial segments have developed their full capacity for motility. In the eutherian model (Figs 3 and 4) there is substantial sperm maturation in the initial segments, and when the "initial segment" is absent, as in the mouse with a targetted mutation of the c-ros tyrosine kinase receptor, animals are sterile even though spermatogenesis is unaffected (Sonnenberg-Riethmacher *et al.*, 1996).

The significance of zones 3, 4 and the proximal end of 5 in rats (and equivalent regions in other eutherians) has not been resolved. They may relate to the need for sperm capacitation (Bedford, 1991) and so be an adaptation of eutherian mammals towards increasing the competitive ability of spermatozoa in the female tract. Although spermatozoa transit slowly through these zones (Fig. 4), it is interpreted that they are not specialized for storage as spermatozoa in these zones are not recruited for ejaculation. Nothing is known of the capacity of the cauda epididymidis of monotremes to store spermatozoa. Studies on the tammar (Chaturapanich *et al.*, 1992a) indicate that spermatozoa can retain the capacity for motility in this marsupial for up to 9 weeks which is at least as long as in eutherians such as rats (6 weeks: White, 1932) and rabbits (4–6 weeks, Paufler and Foote, 1968).

It is generally recognized that the initial segments reabsorb fluid. In tammars (Jones, 1987; Chaturapanich and Jones, 1991), for example, they reabsorb more than 80% of the fluid that enters the ductus epididymidis, but at a rate (0.33 $\mu m\ cm^{-1}\ h^{-1}$ for the initial segment proper and 0.02 $\mu m\ cm^{-1}\ h^{-1}$ for the distal initial segments) which is much lower than that in the ductuli efferentes (8.86 $\mu m\ cm^{-1}\ h^{-1}$). There are substantial changes in the intraluminal concentrations of solute in the initial segment proper (Fig. 5) and in zone 5 of the tammar.

The initial segments are also engaged in receptor mediated pinocytotic uptake of protein (Pelliniemi *et al.*, 1981; Djakiew *et al.*, 1986). On the other hand, protein reabsorption is probably a function of all the epididymal epithelium, and may be involved in regulating the structural differentiation of the duct mucosa (Abe *et al.*, 1984).

The initial segment proper is the major site of net protein secretion in the epididymis of the tammar, and the distal initial segments and zone 5 (Fig. 3) carry out net reabsorption of protein (Fig. 5). These findings are in general agreement with reports on rats (Jones *et al.*, 1980; Brooks, 1981). Studies of the incorporation of [^{35}S]methionine indicate that there is little difference between zones of the epididymis in the rate of protein synthesis in most species. However, there are differences between zones in the electrophoretic pattern of secreted proteins, which are least for tammars (Chaturapanich *et al.*, 1992b) and rams (Jones *et al.*, 1982) and greatest in rats (Jones *et al.*, 1980; Brooks, 1981), rabbits (Jones *et al.*, 1981) and mice (Holland and Orgebin-Crist, 1988).

The proteins secreted by the epididymis are essential for post-testicular sperm maturation (Orgebin-Crist and Jahad, 1979). These proteins may have a number of important functions: (1) regulation of the function of the duct downstream; (2) protection of spermatozoa against oxidative or other chemical changes; (3) protection of spermatozoa against the immune system; (4) modification of other luminal proteins; (5) contributing to sperm maturation by modifying sperm membrane proteins or becoming incorporated into the membrane. Reports on the identification of epididymal proteins in eutherian mammals have been reviewed (Hinton and Palladino, 1995). Of particular interest to the present discussion is the report that the six major proteins secreted by the epididymis of the echidna (Djakiew and Jones, 1983), and the tammar are only secreted by the initial segments (Chaturapanich *et al.*, 1992b).

Conclusions

It is proposed that the extratesticular sperm ducts develop in vertebrates coincident with the development of internal fertilization, and that the evolutionary history of the duct system follows a pattern similar to that of other vertebrate structures. The basic plan can be recognized in extant

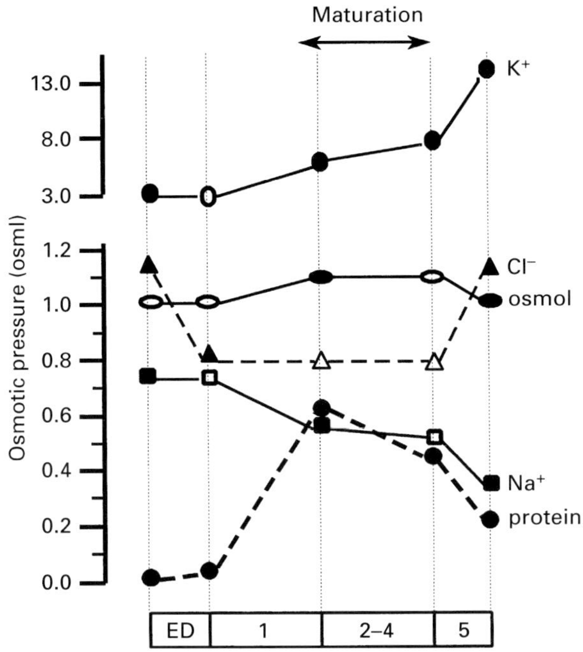

Fig. 5. Diagrammatic representation of the changes in composition of the luminal plasma along the extratesticular sperm ducts of the tammar wallaby. The ordinate shows the concentration of Na^+, K^+, Cl^- and protein, and osmotic pressure (osml) as a proportion of values for peripheral blood plasma. The abscissa indicates the length of each region of the duct(s) relative to the total length of the ductuli efferentes and ductus epididymidis. The length shown for the ductuli efferentes (ED) is the combined length of all the ductuli. The structurally distinct zones of the epididymis are (Fig. 3) zone 1, initial segment proper, zones 2–4, the distal initial segments and zone 5, the cauda epididymidis. Open symbols indicate no statistically significant change in concentration from the adjacent proximal sampling site and closed symbols indicate a statistically significant change. Values at the left of the graph are for samples from the rete testis. The horizontal line at the top of the graph (with arrows at each end) indicates the region of the epididymis where spermatozoa develop the capacity for motility or show changes in structure. Reproduced from Jones and Clulow (1994).

Chondrichthyes, and there has been a reduction and specialization of certain regions of the system during subsequent evolution. The ductuli efferentes are specialized for fluid and solute transport, and in endotherms they cope with considerable fluid output from the testes (Table 3). The ductus epididymidis is specialized for sperm storage in vertebrates in which internal fertilization occurs, and this is an important adaptation in the competition between males to achieve paternity (Parker,

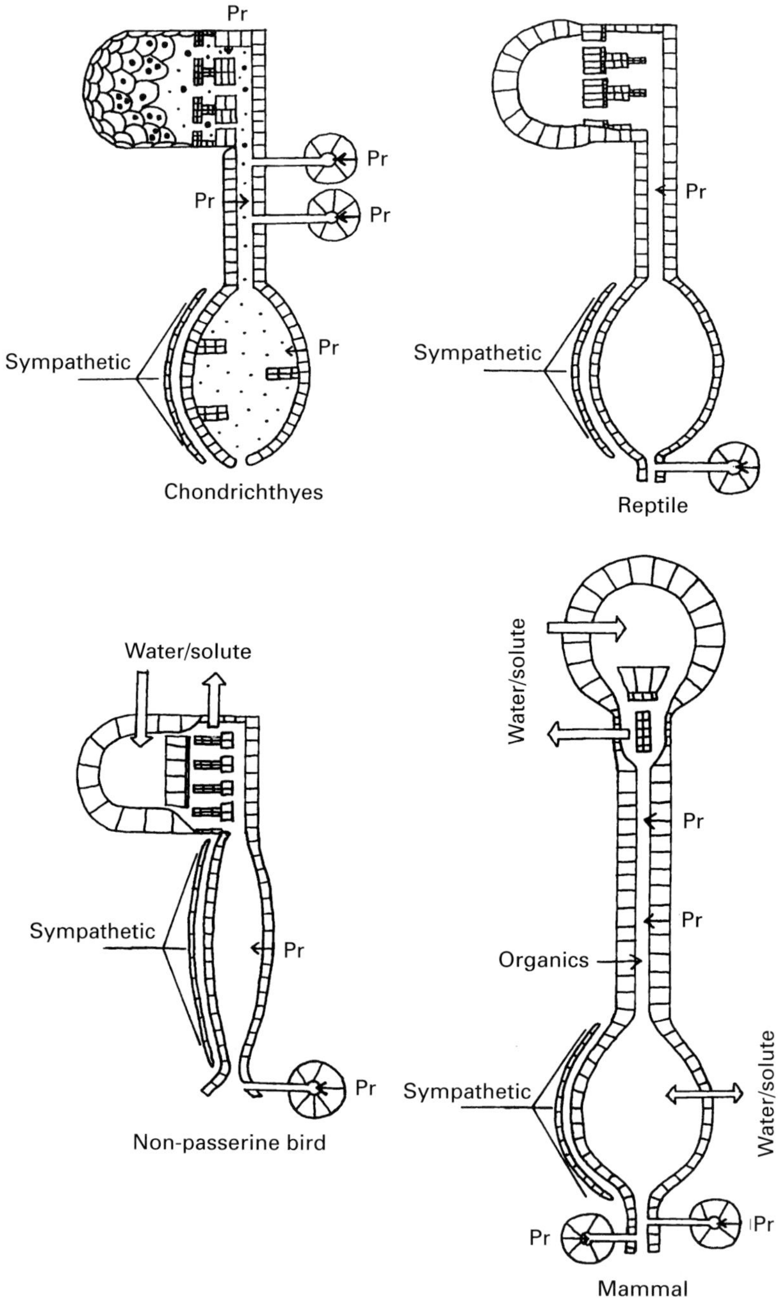

Fig. 6. Models of the male reproductive system of the major vertebrate classes that practise internal fertilization summarizing the structure and function of the main units of the systems: the testis (represented by a sphere or hemisphere) containing seminiferous cysts (Chondrichthyes) or represented by a seminiferous tubule (other vertebrates), leading into the rete testis (lined by a low epithelium), the ductuli efferentes (low epithelium except in reptiles in which it is moderately high proximally and low distally), the ductuli epididymides in Chondrichthyes (very tall epithelium), and the ductus epididymidis. The structural differentiation of the ductus epididymidis (for example see Fig. 3) is not shown except for an expanded distal (storage) region where spermatozoa are mature and may be recruited by the neuromuscular effectors involved in ejaculation. Accessory glands are represented by double circles (for example Leydig's gland in Chondrichthyes, sexual gland of the kidney in reptiles, cloacal glands in birds, and the seminal vesicles and prostate in mammals). Pr, epithelium is secreting protein.

1984). The processes involved in sperm storage have been modified in mammals with the development of endothermy, but in non-passerine birds the sperm storage role has been largely surpassed by an increase in the rate of sperm production in order to cope with the different ovulatory pattern in birds compared with mammals. The ductus epididymidis is also adapted to complete sperm maturation in vertebrates in which internal fertilization occurs. However, the value of post-testicular sperm maturation has not been resolved. It may be an adaptation which makes spermatozoa more competitive in the female reproductive tract. Bedford (1979) considers that it is a more extensive process in marsupials and eutherian mammals than in other vertebrates, and related its development in eutherian mammals to the development of a resistant zona pellucida coating the ovum. However, this does not explain why the epididymis of marsupials seems to be as well developed as in eutherians. In addition, it does not explain why monotreme mammals, which have reptilian-like spermatozoa, have an epididymis with an initial segment involved in sperm maturation and which is nearly as long, as the ductus epididymidis of marsupials and eutherians. Identification of the proteins secreted by the epididymides of these mammalian groups may be important in assessing differences in their functions.

It is proposed that the role and degree of specialization of the different parts of the extratesticular duct system, and its relation to testicular function, depends on the reproductive strategy of a species. Factors that determine the relation and function of the ducts are: allometric considerations, metabolic rate and the nature of the reproductive pattern of the females of the species. A model showing the main structural units of the male reproductive system of the major vertebrate classes in which internal fertilization occurs is given (Fig. 6) to provide a basis for comparing the structure and function of the extratesticular duct system among vertebrates. The models are partly interpreted from our knowledge of the mammalian system, and emphasise the close relation between the testis and excurrent duct system. The mammalian model illustrates the considerable production of fluid and solute by the seminiferous tubules, and the unitary role of the ductuli efferentes in reabsorbing most of the secretion (including specific proteins) so that spermatozoa are delivered to the ductus epididymidis in a small volume of fluid. The proximal region of the ductus epididymidis is involved in the maturation and preparation of spermatozoa for storage, and secretion of considerable protein. The transport of non-proteinaceous organics (carnitine, inositol and glycerylphosphoryl choline) into the duct in the proximal region has been demonstrated in all eutherians that have been studied, although their concentration in the lumen varies widely. Their role in the epididymis has not been resolved, and they have not been identified in the epididymis of marsupials or monotremes. The sperm storage region is where sperm transit is slowed by widening of the ductus epididymidis and occlusion of the end by the collapsed ductus deferens. The region has a neuromuscular effector system to recruit spermatozoa during ejaculation. Much of the activity of the mucosa in the region must be involved in maintaining a suitable milieu for the spermatozoa which are very concentrated in the lumen.

The model for non-passerine birds is dominated by a larger number of ductuli efferentes which cope with the greater production of spermatozoa and fluid by the testes. The ductus epididymidis is relatively short, it may secrete only one androgen-dependent protein, and has no region where spermatozoa may be stored for many days. The model for Chondrichthyes indicates the considerable capacity of cystic spermatogenesis to evacuate a large number of spermatozoa from a row of mature cysts. The ductuli epididymides (as well as the ductuli efferentes) are arranged in parallel with one another to cope with this output, and the Leydig glands are arranged to secrete considerable protein into a length of ductus epididymidis which is relatively short compared with mammals. Products of Sertoli cells are released into the rete testis as well as spermatozoa and may be involved in regulating the function of the epididymal epithelium.

The reptilian model shows the development from spermatogenesis in cysts in the Chondrichthyes to tubules in the higher vertebrates with a concomitant loss of 'kidney' (Leydig) glands secreting into the ductus epididymidis and development of accessory glands (sexual gland of the kidney) which evacuate during ejaculation. A secretory portion of the ductuli efferentes has been described, but to date attention has been focussed on the secretion of only one epididymal protein.

I am indebted to colleagues who have collaborated with me and are coauthors of reports on the epididymis of a variety of vertebrates. I am also indebted to Lennart Nicander, Michael Bedford and Brian Setchell for discussions on comparative aspects of the epididymis, and to Brian Setchell for commenting on this manuscript.

References

Aafjes JH and Vreeburg JTM (1972) Distribution of 5α-dihydrotestosterone in the epididymis of bull and boar, and its concentration in rat epididymis after ligation of efferent testicular duct, castration and unilateral gonadectomy *Journal of Endocrinology* **53** 85–93

Abe K and Takano H (1989) Cytological response of the principal cells in the initial segment of the epididymal duct to efferent duct cutting in mice *Archivum Histologicum Cytologicum* **52** 321–326

Abe K, Takano H and Ito T (1983) Ultrastructure of the mouse epididymal duct with special reference to the regional differences of the principal cells *Archivum Histologicum Japonicum* **46** 51–68

Abe K, Takano H and Ito T (1984) Interruption of the luminal flow in the epididymal duct of the corpus epididymis in the mouse, with special reference to differentiation of the epididymal epithelium *Archivum Histologicum Japonicum* **47** 137–147

Aire TA Ayeni JS and Olowo-Okorun MO (1979) Structure of the excurrent ducts of the guinea-fowl (*Numidia meleagris*). *Journal of Anatomy* **129** 633–643

Alsum DJ and Hunter AG (1978) Regional histology and histochemistry of the ductus epididymis in the Rhesus monkey (*Macaca mulatta*). *Biology of Reproduction* **19** 1063–1069

Alverdes K (1928) Die epididymis der sauropsiden im vergleich zu saugetier und mensch *Zeitschrift fur Mikroskopisch- Anatomisch Forschung Leipzig* **15** 405–471

Badir N (1958) Seasonal variation of the male urogenital organs of *Scincus scincus* L. and *Chalcides ocellatus* Forsk *Zeitschrift fuer Wissenschaftliche Zoologie* **160** 290–351

Bailey RE (1953) Accessory reproductive organs of male fringillid birds: seasonal variations and response to various sex hormones *Anatomical Record* **115** 1–19

Baumgarten HG, Holstein AF and Rosengren E (1971) Arrangement, ultrastructure, and adrenergic innervation of smooth musculature of the ductuli efferentes, ductus epididymidis and ductus deferens of man *Cell and Tissue Research* **120** 37–79

Bedford JM (1977) Evolution of the scrotum: the epididymis as the prime mover? In *Reproduction and Evolution* pp 171–182 Eds JH Calaby and CH Tyndale-Biscoe. Australian Academy of Science, Canberra

Bedford JM (1979) Evolution of the sperm maturation and sperm storage functions of the epididymis. In *The Spermatozoan: Maturation, Motility, Surface Properties and Comparative Aspects* pp 7–21 Eds DW Fawcett and JM Bedford. Urban and Schwarzenberg Inc., Baltimore-Munich

Bedford JM (1990) Sperm dynamics in the epididymis. In *Gamete Physiology* pp 53–67 Eds RH Ash, JP Balmaceda and I Johnson. Norwell, Massachusetts

Bedford JM (1991) The coevolution of mammalian gametes. In *A Comparative Overview of Mammalian Fertilization* pp 3–35 Eds B Dunbar and M O'Rand. Plenum Press, New York

Benoit J (1926) Recherches anatomiquès, cytologiques et histologiques sur les voies excrètes du testicule, chez les mammifères *Archives d'Anatomie, d'Hstologie et d'Embryologie* **5** 173–412

Brooks DE (1981) Secretion of proteins and glycoproteins by the rat epididymis: regional differences, androgen-dependence, and efforts of protease inhibitors, procaine and tunicamycin *Biology of Reproduction* **25** 1099–1110

Brown DV, Amann RP and Wagley LM (1983) Influence of rete testis fluid on the metabolism of testosterone by cultured principal cells isolated from the proximal or distal caput of the rat epididymis *Biology of Reproduction* **28** 1257–1268

Budras K-D and Meier V (1981) The epididymis and its development in ratite birds (ostrich, emu, rhea) *Anatomy and Embryology* **162** 281–299

Budras K-D and Sauer T (1975) Morphology of the epididymis of the cock (*Gallus domesticus*) and its effect upon the steroid sex hormone synthesis. I. Ontogenesis, morphology and distribution of the epididymis *Anatomy and Embryology* **148** 175–196

Chase SW (1923) The mesonephros and urogenital ducts of *Necturus maculosus*, rafinesque *Journal of Morphology* **37** 457–531

Chaturapanich G and Jones RC (1991) Morphometry of the epididymis of the tammar, *Macropus eugenii*, and estimation of some physiological parameters *Reproduction Fertility and Development* **3** 651–658

Chaturapanich, G Jones RC and Clulow J (1992a) Role of androgens in the survival of spermatozoa in the epididymis of the tammar wallaby, *Macropus eugenii*. *Journal of Reproductiion and Fertility* **95** 421–429

Chaturapanich G, Jones RC and Clulow J (1992b) Protein synthesis and secretion by the epididymis of the tammar wallaby, *Macropus eugenii* (Macropodidae: Marsupialia) *Reproduction Fertility and Develepent* **4** 533–545

Clulow J and Jones RC (1988) Studies of fluid and sperm transport in the extratesticular ducts of the Japanese quail *Journal of Anatomy* **157** 1–11

Clulow J, Jones RC and Hansen LA (1994) Micropuncture and cannulation studies of fluid composition and transport in the ductuli efferentes testis of the rat: comparisons with the homologous metanephric proximal tubule *Experimental Physiology* **79** 915–928

Clulow J, Jones RC, Hansen LA and Man SY (1998) Fluid and electrolyte reabsorption in the ductuli efferentes testis *Journal of Reproduction and Fertility Supplement* **53** 1–14

Cornwall GA and Hann SR (1995) Specialized gene expression in the epididymis *Journal of Andrology* **16** 379–383

Croisille Y (1981) Differentiation of the epididymis in birds, with particular reference to the rooster. In *Progress in Reproductive Biology Epididymis and Fertility: Biology and Pathology* **8** pp 1–11 Eds C Bollack and A Clavert. Karger, Basel

Djakiew D and Jones RC (1981) Structural differentiation of the male genital ducts of the echidna, *Tachyglossus aculeatus*. *Journal of Anatomy* **132** 187–202

Djakiew D and Jones RC (1982) Ultrastructure of the ductus epididymidis of the echidna, *Tachyglossus aculeatus*. *Journal of Anatomy* **135** 625–634

Djakiew D and Jones RC (1983) Sperm maturation, fluid transport and secretion and absorption of protein in the epididymis of the echidna, *Tachyglossus aculeatus*. *Journal of Reproduction and Fertility* **68** 445–456

Djakiew D, Griswold MD, Lewis DM and Dym M (1986) Micropuncture studies of receptor-mediated endocytosis of transferrin in the rat epididymis *Biology of Reproduction* **34** 691–699

Douglass J, Garrett S and Garrett J (1991) Differential gene expression in the adult rat epididymis *Annals of the New York Academy of Sciences* **637** 384–398

Dufaure JP and Gigon A (1975) Action des hormones androgens sur l'epididyme d'un reptile lacertilian, *Lacerta vivipara* Jacquin. Effects de la testosterone et de ses principaux metabolites en culture organotypique *General and Comparative Endocrinology* **25** 112–120

Dufaure JP and Saint Girons H (1984) Histologie comparee de l'epididyme et de ses secretions chez les reptiles (lezards et serpents) *Archive d'Anatomie microscopique* **73** 15–26

Ellegren H and Fridolfsson A-K (1997) Male driven evolution of DNA sequences in birds *Nature Genetics* **17** 182–184

Fawcett DW and A Hoffer (1979) Failure of exogenous androgen to prevent regression of the initial segments of the rat epididymis after efferent duct ligation or orchidectomy *Biology of Reproduction* **20** 162–181

Glover TD (1973) Aspects of sperm production in some East African mammals *Journal of Reproduction and Fertility* **35** 45–53

Glover TD and Nicander L (1971) Some aspects of structure and function in the mammalian epididymis *Journal of Reproduction and Fertility Supplement* **13** 13–51

Gustafsson B (1966) Luminal contents of the bovine epididymis under conditions of reduced spermatogenesis, luminal blockage and certain sperm abnormalities *Acta Veterinaria Scandinavica Supplementum* **17** 1–80

Haider S and Rai U (1987) Epididymis of the Indian wall lizard (*Hemidactylu flaviviridеs*) during the sexual cycle and in response to mammalian pituitary gonadotrophins and testosterone *Journal of Morphology* **191** 151–160

Hermo L and Morales C (1984) Endocytosis in nonciliated epithelial cells of the ductuli efferentes in the rat *American Journal of Anatomy* **171** 59–74

Hermo L, Wright J, Oko R and Morales C R (1991) Role of epithelial cells in the male excurrent duct system of the rat in the endocytosis or secretion of sulfated glycoprotein-2 (clusterin) *Biology of Reproduction* **44** 1113–1131

Hess RA, Thurston RJ and Biellier HV (1976) Morphology of the epididymal region and ductus deferens of the turkey (*Meleagris gallopavo*). *Journal of Anatomy* **122** 241–252

Hinton BT and Palladino MA (1995) Epididymal epithelium: its contribution to the formation of a luminal fluid microenvironment *Microscopy Research Technique* **30** 67–81

Hoffer AP, Hamilton DW and Fawcett DW (1973a) The ultrastructure of the principal cells and intraepithelial leucocytes in the initial segment of the rat epididymis *Anatomical Record* **175** 169–202

Hoffer AP, Hamilton DW and Fawcett DW (1973b) The ultrastructural pathology of the rat epididymis after administration of α-chlorhydrin (U-5897). I. Effects of a single high dose *Anatomical Record* **175** 203–230

Holland MK and Orgebin-Crist M-C (1988) Characterization and hormonal regulation of protein synthesis by the murine epididymis *Biology of Reproduction* **38** 487–496

Holstein A-F (1969) Morphologische Studien am Nebenhoden des Menschen. In *Zwanglose Abhandlungen aus dem Gebiet der normalen und pathologischen Anatomie* pp 77–91 Eds W Bargmann and W Doerr. G Thieme, Stuttgart

Howarth B (1983) Fertilizing ability of cock spermatozoa from the testis, epididymis and vas deferens following intramagnal insemination *Biology of Reproduction* **28** 586–590

Hughes RL (1965) Comparative morphology of spermatozoa from five marsupial families *Australian Journal of Zoology* **13** 533–543

Jones N and Jones RC (1982) The structure of the male genital system of the Port Jackson shark, *Heterodontus portusjacksoni*, with particular reference to the genital ducts *Australian Journal of Zoology* **30** 523–543

Jones R, Hamilton DW and Fawcett DW (1979) Morphology of the epithelium of the extratesticular rete testis, ductuli efferentes and ductus epididymidis of the adult male rabbit *American Journal of Anatomy* **156** 373–400

Jones R, Brown CR, von Glós KI and Parker MG (1980) Hormonal regulation of protein synthesis in the rat epididymis *Biochemical Journal* **188** 667–676

Jones R, von Glos KI and Brown CR (1981) Characterization of hormonally regulated secretory proteins from the caput epididymidis of the rabbit *Biochemical Journal* **196** 105–114

Jones R, Fournier-Delpech S and Willadsen SA (1982) Identification of androgen-dependent proteins synthesised *in vitro* by the ram epididymis *Reproduction, Nutrition, Développment* (Paris) **22** 495–504

Jones RC (1987) Changes in protein composition of the luminal fluids along the epididymis of the tammar, *Macropus eugenii*. *Journal of Reproduction and Fertility* **80** 193–199

Jones RC (1989) Reproduction in male Macropodidae. In *Kangaroos, Wallabies and Rat Kangaroos* pp 287–305 Eds G Grigg, P Jarman and ID Hume. Surrey Beatty and Sons, Chipping North, NSW

Jones RC and Brosnan M (1981) Studies of the deferent ducts from the testis of the African elephant, *Loxodonta africana*. I. Structural differentiation *Journal of Anatomy* **132** 371–386

Jones RC and Clulow J (1987) Fluid absorption and sperm maturation and storage in the mammalian epididymis. In *Proceedings of the 1st Asian and Oceanian Physiological Society, Bangkok* pp 229–240 Eds C Pholpramool and R Sudsuang. The Physiological Society (Thailand)

Jones RC and Clulow J (1994) Interactions of sperm and the reproductive tract of the male tammar wallaby, *Macropus eugenii* (Macropodidae: Marsupialia) *Reproduction Fertility and Development* **6** 437–444

Jones RC and Jurd KM (1987) Structural differentiation and fluid reabsorption in the ductuli efferentes testis of the rat *Australian Journal of Biological Sciences* **40** 79–90

Jones RC and Lin M (1993a) Spermatogenic cycle in birds and mammals *Oxford Reviews of Reproductive Biology* **15** 233–264

Jones RC and Lin M (1993b) Structure and functions of the genital ducts of the male Port Jackson shark, *Heterodontus portusjacksoni*. *Environmental Biology of Fishes* **38** 127–138

Jones RC, Jones N and Djakiew D (1984a) Luminal composition and maturation of spermatozoa in the male genital ducts of the Port Jackson shark, *Heterodontus portusjacksoni*. *Journal of Experimental Zoology* **230** 417–426

Jones RC, Hinds LA and Tyndale-Biscoe CH (1984b) Ultrastructure of the epididymis of the tammar, *Macropus eugenii*, and its relationship to sperm maturation *Cell and Tissue Research* **237** 525–535

Jones RC, Clulow J, Stone GM and Setchell BP (1987) The role of the initial segments of the epididymis in sperm maturation in mammals. In *New Horizons in Sperm Cell Research* pp 63–74 Ed. H Mohri. Japan Sci. Press, Gordon and Breach Sci. Pubs

Jones RC, Stone GM, Hinds LA and Setchell BP (1988) Distribution of 5α-reductase in the epididymis of the tammar wallaby, *Macropus eugenii*, and the dependence of the epididymis on systemic testosterone and luminal fluids from the testis *Journal of Reproduction and Fertility* **83** 779–783

Jones RC, Stone GM and Zupp J (1992) Reproduction in the male echidna. In *Platypus and Echidnas* pp 115–126 Ed. ML Augee. Royal Society of New South Wales, Sydney

Kidd G (1982) Protein secretion by the epididymis of the Japanese quail (*Coturnix coturnix japonica*). Honours thesis submitted to the Department of Biological Sciences, University of Newcastle, Australia

Kirton KT, Desjardins C and Hafs HD (1967) Distribution of sperm in male rabbits after various ejaculation frequencies *Anatomical Record* **158** 287–292

Kormano M (1968) Penetration of intravenous trypan blue into the rat testis and epididymis *Acta Histochemica* **30** 133–136

Marshall WS (1986) Sperm duct epithelium of brook trout: Na^+ transport and seminal plasma composition *Canadian Journal of Zoology* **64** 1827–1830

Mesure M, Chevalier M, Depeiges A, Faure J and Dufaure JP (1991) Structure and ultrastructure of the epididymis of the viviparous lizard during the annual hormonal cycle: changes of the epithelium related to secretory activity *Journal of Morphology* **210** 133–145

Morel L, Dufaure JP and Depeiges A (1993) LESP, an androgen-regulated lizard epididymal secretory protein family identified as a new member of the lipocalin superfamily *Journal of Biological Chemistry* **268** 10274–10281

Moniem KA, Glover TD and Lubicz-Nawrocki CW (1978) Effects of duct ligation and orchidectomy on histochemical reactions in the hamster epididymis *Journal of Reproduction and Fertility* **54** 173–176

Nicander L (1957) On the regional histology and cytochemistry of the ductus epididymis in rabbits *Acta Morphologica Neerlando-Scandinavica* **1** 99–118

Nicander L (1958) Studies on the regional histology and cytochemistry of the ductus epididymidis in stallions, rams and bulls *Acta Morphologica Neerlando-Scandinavica* **1** 337–362

Nicander L and Glover TD (1973) Regional histology and fine structure of the epididymal duct in the golden hamster *Journal of Anatomy* **114** 347–364

Nicander L, Osman DI, Ploen L, Bugge HP and Kvisgaard KA (1983) Early effects of efferent ductule ligation on the proximal segment of the rat epididymis *International Journal of Andrology* **6** 91–102

Noqueira JC, Godinho HP and Cardoso FM (1977) Microscopic anatomy of the scrotum, testis with its excurrent duct system and spermatic cord of *Didelphis azarae*. *Acta Anatomica* **99** 209–219

Olsen AM (1954) The biology, migration and growth rate of the school shark, *Galeorhinus australis* (Macleay) (Carchorhanidae), in south-eastern Australian waters *Australian Journal of Marine and Freshwater Research* **5** 353–410

Orgebin-Crist M-C and Jahad N (1979) Maturation of rabbit epididymal sperm in organ culture: stimulation by epididymal cytoplasmic factors *Biology of Reproduction* **21** 511–515

Orsi AM, De Mello VR, Ferreira AL and Campos VJM (1980) Morphology of the epithelial cells of the epididymal duct of the South American opossum (*Didelphis azarae*). *Anatomischer Anzeiger* (Jena) **148** 7–13

Parker GA (1984) Sperm competition and the evolution of animal mating strategies. In *Sperm Competition and the Evolution of Animal Mating Systems* pp 1–60 Ed RL Smith Academic Press, Orlando, San Diego, New York, London, Toronto

Paufler SK and Foote RH (1968) Morphology, motility and fertility of spermatozoa recovered from different areas of ligated rabbit epididymides *Journal of Reproduction and Fertility* **17** 125–137

Pelliniemi LJ, Dym M, Gunsalus GL, Musto NA, Bardin CW, Hamilton DW and Fawcett DW (1981) Immunocytochemical localization of androgen-binding protein in the male reproductive tract *Endocrinology* **108** 925–931

Prins GS and Zaneveld LJD (1980) Contractions of the rabbit vas deferens following sexual activity: a mechanism for proximal transport of spermatozoa *Biology of Reproduction* **23** 904–909

Ramos AS and Dym M (1977) Fine structure of the monkey epididymis *American Journal of Anatomy* **149** 501–531

Reid BL and Cleland KW (1957) The structure and function of the epididymis. I. The histology of the rat epididymis *Australian Journal of Zoology* **5** 223–426

Reynolds AE (1943) The normal seasonal reproductive cycle in the male *Eumeces fasciatus* together with some observations on the effects of castration and hormone administration *Journal of Morphology* **72** 331–377

Riddle O (1927) The cyclical growth of the vesicula seminalis in birds is hormone controlled *Anatomical Record* **30** 1–11

Robaire B, Ewing LL, Zirkin BR and Irby DC (1977) Steroid $delta^4$-5α-reductase and 3α-hydroxysteroid dehydrogenase in the rat epididymis *Endocrinology* **101** 1379–1390

Romer AS (1970) *The Vertebrate Body* (4th Edn) W.B. Saunders Co., Philadelphia, London, Toronto

Roosen-Runge EC (1961) The rete testis in the albino rat. Its structure, development and morphological significance *Acta Anatomica* (Basel) **45** 1–30

Saint Girons H (1957) Le cycle sexuel chez *Vipera aspis* (L.) dans l'ouest de la France *Bulletin Biologiques de la France et de la Belgique* **91** 1–67

Setchell BP (1978) *The Mammalian Testis* Paul Elek, London

Simpson TH, Wright RS and Renfrew J (1964) Steroid biosynthesis in the semen of dogfish (*Sqalus acanthias*). *Journal of Endocrinology* **31** 11–20

Sonnenberg-Riethmacher E, Walter B, Riethmacher D, Godecke S, and Birchmeier C (1996) The c-ros tyrosine kinase receptor controls regionalization and differentiation of epithelial cells in the epididymis *Genes and Development* **10** 1184–1193

Stanley HP (1963) Urogenital morphology in the chimaeroid fish *Hydrolagus collici*. *Journal of Morphology* **112** 99–128

Sujarit S, Jones RC, Setchell BP, Chaturapanich G, Lin M and Clulow J (1990) Stimulation of protein secretion in the initial segment of the rat epididymis by fluid from the rete testis *Journal of Reproduction and Fertility* **88** 315–321

Sun EL and Flickinger CJ (1980) Morphological characteristics of cells with apical nuclei in the initial segment of the adult rat epididymis *Anatomical Record* **196** 285–293

Suzuki F and Racey PA (1976) Fine structural changes in the epididymal epithelium of moles (*Talpa europaea*) throughout the year *Journal of Reproduction and Fertility* **47** 47–54

Suzuki F and Racey PA (1984) Light and electron microscopical observations on the male excurrent duct system of the common shrew (*Sorex araneus*). *Journal of Reproduction and Fertility* **70** 419–428

Tingari MD (1971) On the structure of the epididymal region and ductus deferens of the domestic fowl (*Gallus domesticus*). *Journal of Anatomy* **109** 423–435

Turner TT, Jones CE, Howards SS, Ewing LL, Zegeye B and Gunsalus GL (1984) On the androgen microenvironment of maturing spermatozoa *Endocrinology* **115** 1925–1932

Volsøe H (1944) Structure and seasonal variation of the male reproductive organs of *Vipera berus* (L.) *Spolia Zoologica Musei Hauniensis, Copenhagen Universitet-Skrifter* **5** 1–157

White WE (1932) The effect of hypophysectomy on the survival of spermatozoa in the male rat *Anatomical Record* **54** 253–273

Winer M, Wadewitz A and Wolgemuth D (1993) Members of the raf gene family exhibit segment-specific patterns of expression in mouse epididymis *Molecular Reproduction and Development* **35** 16–23

Wolfson A (1954) Sperm storage at lower-than-body temperature outside the body cavity on some birds *Science* **120** 68–71

Journal of Reproduction and Fertility Supplement **53**, 183–195

Development and use of surgical procedures to bypass selected regions of the mammalian epididymis: effects on sperm maturation

P. D. Temple-Smith[1,2], S. S. Zheng[3], T. Kadioglu[4] and G. J. Southwick

Department of Anatomy, Monash University, Clayton, Victoria 3168, Australia

Microsurgical procedures have been used to examine the function of selected regions of the epididymis. Vasoepididymostomy in the rabbit and rat confirmed that spermatozoa require some exposure to the epididymal environment for normal development of motility and fertilizing ability. In both of these species surgical redirection of spermatozoa from a region just distal to the initial segment into the vas deferens resulted in a significant reduction in sperm viability, motility and fertility compared with untreated animals. Surgical bypass of the distal cauda epididymidis in the rabbit did not significantly reduce the number of spermatozoa in ejaculates or the total sperm output accumulated during exhaustive ejaculations. The capacity of these bypass animals to store spermatozoa may be explained by the post-surgical formation of convolutions in the normally straight segment of the rabbit vas deferens. Vas autografts in the rabbit and rat were used to bypass selected epididymal segments. In rabbits, vascularized grafts were used as bridges to bypass the distal caput and proximal corpus epididymidis. Despite high rates of graft survival and patency in this species, the motility and viability of ejaculated spermatozoa were similar to those observed following high level vasoepididymostomy. In rats, non-vascularized vas grafts also showed a high survival and patency rate. There was a transitory reduction in sperm viability and motility 2 weeks after surgery which was associated with structural changes, especially in the epithelium, in vas bridge autografts during revascularization. Longer term observations (3 and 6 months) showed recovery of epithelial morphology and by three months after surgery, no difference was observed in sperm motility, sperm viability or fertility between experimental groups and controls. Similar results were obtained when epididymoepididymostomy was used as the surgical procedure to bypass the same regions of the epididymis. The evidence considered in this review clearly shows that the proximity of vasoepididymal bypass to the testis is inversely related to the state of maturity of ejaculated spermatozoa. More surprisingly, perhaps, it reveals that exposure of spermatozoa to the distal caput and proximal corpus regions of the epididymis in the rat is not obligatory for spermatozoa to develop a level of maturation in the remaining regions of the epididymis sufficient to ascend the female tract and fertilize ova. This finding suggests that the epididymis is more flexible in its functions than had been considered previously and that sperm maturation may not be as dependent on specific regional functions of the epididymis as had been previously proposed.

Current addresses: [1]Conservation and Research Unit, Zoological Parks and Gardens Board, Parkville, Victoria 3052, Australia; [2]Department of Zoology, University of Melbourne, Parkville, Victoria 3052, Australia; [3]Institute of Reproduction and Development, Monash Medical Centre, Clayton 3168, Australia; and [4]Department of Urology, Istanbul Medical Faculty, Istanbul University, Capa, Istanbul, Turkey

Introduction

Martin and co-workers (see Thomas, 1987) and Young (1929, 1931) provided the first evidence that the mammalian epididymis had a more important function than simply transporting spermatozoa from the testis to the vas deferens for ejaculation. However, it was the pioneering work of Bedford (1963, 1966) and Orgebin-Crist (1967) using various laboratory species that provided data to corroborate this notion. These and subsequent studies have shown that, under normal circumstances, passage through the mammalian epididymis is required for sperm maturation and that the caudal region of the epididymis in mammals also functions as a pre-ejaculatory storage region for matured spermatozoa.

The process of sperm maturation involves the transformation, by exposure to sequential epididymal environments, of essentially immotile, non-fertile testicular spermatozoa into mature motile and fertile epididymal spermatozoa (see Robaire and Hermo, 1988). In a detailed study of mice, Lacham and Trounson (1991) confirmed that spermatozoa from the testis and the proximal caput epididymidis were immotile or showed only vibratory movements of the tail and that in more distal regions of the epididymis, spermatozoa developed the capacity for direct forward progressive motility. As expected from previous studies in the mouse and other species (Horan and Bedford, 1972; Pavlok, 1974; Hoppe, 1975; Holtz and Smidt, 1976; Moore, 1981), spermatozoa from the testis, initial segment and caput epididymidis were essentially incapable of fertilization (Lacham and Trounson, 1991). However, increasing fertilization rates were observed in spermatozoa from the proximal and distal corpus regions and these were either maintained or improved in sperm samples from the cauda epididymidis. These data coincide with results from motility, viability and fertilization studies in various other species, including the rabbit and rat (Temple-Smith *et al.*, 1989; Sapountzis, 1996). However, although parts of this process of maturation have been identified, the exact nature and sequence of the events that produce changes in maturing spermatozoa to confer the ability for progressive motility and fertilizing ability, and even the changes themselves, are still poorly defined or disputed.

As indicated previously (Southwick and Temple-Smith, 1994) it had been assumed that the principles of sperm maturation reported in mammals, including primates (Moore 1981), would also apply to human epididymal spermatozoa. However, data on the motility and fertilizing ability of testicular and caput epididymal spermatozoa have created controversy about the importance of the human epididymis in fertility (Silber 1988, 1989b; Silber *et al.*, 1988; Cooper, 1991). For example, pregnancies have been recorded from high-level vasoepididymal bypass patients (Schoysman and Bedford, 1986; Silber, 1988, 1989a,b) and from epididymal sperm aspiration patients (Temple-Smith *et al.*, 1985; Southwick and Temple-Smith, 1988; Silber *et al.*, 1988). Although the motility of testicular spermatozoa and those aspirated from the head of the epididymis is poor (Silber *et al.*, 1988), it is often better than may have been predicted from animal studies. Similarly, the incidence of oocytes fertilized by spermatozoa taken from similar sites is often reported to be greater in obstructive azoospermic patients than might have been anticipated from animal studies. However, without stimulation of motility and sperm selection procedures, which can improve the IVF rate to more than 30%, fertilization rates are often less than 10% (see Southwick and Temple-Smith, 1994). For spermatozoa aspirated from the caput regions of the epididymis, fertilization rates of 30–40% are usually only achieved *in vitro* if sperm density is increased at least tenfold over that required of normal men in IVF programmes (P. Temple-Smith, C. Yates, B. Downing, D. de Kretser and G. Southwick, unpublished).

Cooper (1991) and others have logically suggested that the structure and function of the epididymis above the site of absence or obstruction in these obstructive azoospermic patients may differ from the normal, unobstructed human epididymis. The observations by Moore *et al.* (1983) on motility and oocyte-penetrating capacity of spermatozoa from various levels in the human epididymis appear to support this conclusion. Pregnancies have been reported following attachment of the vasa deferentia to the vasa efferentia or directly to the testis (Silber, 1988). In these cases it is possible that the human vas deferens may, in some as yet unknown way, compensate for the absent distal epididymal regions by a process of 'epididymalization'. This would enable it to mimic at least some of the maturation functions of the normal epididymis. However, despite the observation of structural change in the rabbit vas deferens following vasoepididymostomy (Temple-Smith *et al.*, 1989), there is little evidence from experimental surgery of the epididymis in laboratory mammals that the maturation quality of spermatozoa improves with time after surgery. This also appears to be the case in man (Southwick and Temple-Smith, 1994), despite the encouraging findings to the contrary reported by Silber (1989b) of improved sperm motility after surgery.

Those interested in determining the importance of exposure of spermatozoa to the changing regional environments of the epididymis have found it difficult to establish experimental protocols *in vivo* or *in vitro* that reflect the dynamic nature of the epididymal environment and the sequential process of sperm maturation. The development and successful application of microsurgical techniques in the treatment of epididymal obstruction in man have provided techniques for experimental manipulation of the epididymis to examine the role of specific regions on the maturation of transiting spermatozoa. This review outlines the development of surgical procedures, including microsurgical vasoepididymostomy, vas bridge autografts and epididymoepididymostomy, which provide the means for 'surgical knockout' of selected epididymal regions. The effects of experimental bypass of selected epididymal regions on the motility of the spermatozoa excluded from the bypassed regions are then explored with a critical evaluation of each technique and its outcome.

Development of Surgical Techniques for Epididymal Manipulation

It is unusual for surgical techniques to be developed first in man and then applied experimentally in animals. However, for male reproductive tract surgery this sequence of development occurred. Before the development of IVF, epididymal sperm microaspiration procedures and sperm microinjection techniques, the only treatment option for infertile men diagnosed with obstructive azoospermia was to provide a surgical bypass of the obstructed region (Lespinosse, 1918; Bayle, 1952, 1966; Silber, 1978; Schoysman, 1981; Thomas, 1987; Southwick and Temple-Smith, 1988, 1994).

Initially macrosurgical attachment of the vas deferens to the epididymis above the site of obstruction – the Bayle technique – was the only technique available for treating epididymal obstruction. These techniques usually relied on fistula formation between the vas and the epididymal tissue which would provide passage for spermatozoa into the vas. Although less accurate than later techniques, sperm-containing ejaculates were reported in patients who had never previously produced ejaculated spermatozoa and pregnancies were achieved (Thomas, 1987).

Microsurgical vasoepididymal anastomosis

Advances in microsurgical techniques during the past 20 years improved the accuracy and success of vasoepididymal anastomosis (Silber, 1978; Thomas, 1987; Southwick and Temple-Smith, 1988). Microsurgical techniques provided the means for pursuing experimental surgical interventions that were difficult, if not impossible, to achieve previously – for example the termino-terminal anastomosis of two epididymal tubules (epididymoepididymostomy) (Krylov and Borovikov, 1984; Temple-Smith *et al.*, 1989; MeClatchey *et al.*, 1991; Zheng, 1995). A significant advantage of this experimental procedure is that its *in vivo* nature avoids criticisms that have been directed at past attempts to elucidate epididymal function using static or less dynamic *in vitro* approaches.

Vasoepididymostomy: Specific Level Bypasses of the Epididymis and Effects on Sperm Quality and Fertility

Rabbits

Short- and long-term studies examined the effects of vasoepididymal bypass from the proximal caput, distal caput and mid-corpus epididymidis (that is regions 2/3, 4 and 5/6, respectively of Jones *et al.*, 1979) on ejaculate characteristics, sperm quality and fertility in rabbits (Temple-Smith and

Southwick, 1985, Temple-Smith *et al.*, 1989). These studies have confirmed the observations of others that regional-specific changes occur in the motility and fertilizing ability of spermatozoa during passage through the epididymis. Spermatozoa in ejaculates collected into an artificial vagina from rabbits with vasoepididymal bypasses from the proximal (region 2/3) and distal (region 4) caput epididymidis were poorly motile. Both the percentage motility and the motility index (WHO Handbook, 1980) of ejaculated spermatozoa from animals bypassed from the proximal caput epididymidis were not significantly different from spermatozoa that were collected from the proximal caput epididymidis of normal animals and examined *in vitro*. For animals with bypasses from both the proximal (Fig. 1a) and distal caput epididymidis (regions 2/3 and 4), the motility of spermatozoa in ejaculates was significantly reduced after vasoepididymostomy and no long-term improvement was observed. However, vasoepididymostomy from the mid-corpus epididymidis did not result in a significant long-term reduction in sperm motility compared with pre-operative controls (Fig. 1b). These observations in the rabbit contrasted with reports on men (Silber, 1989b) which indicated that the maturation state of ejaculated spermatozoa improves with time after surgery. In the rabbit, double-mating was used to test the fertility of males (each male was mated twice over a period of about 2 h to each female), with bypasses from the proximal and distal caput epididymidis. These studies showed an increase in fertilization rate (6 and 18%, respectively) with increased distance of the anastomosis from the testis (Table 1). However, this fertilization rate was still considerably lower than for a group of normal males (71%). Interestingly, IVF tests with ejaculated spermatozoa from the four males with the vasoepididymal bypasses at proximal caput epididymidis showed that their fertilization rates were no higher *in vitro* (Table 2) than *in vivo* (Table 1). This finding implies that the requirement for ejaculated spermatozoa to ascend the female reproductive tract following natural matings did not result in a negative impact on fertility compared with washed ejaculated spermatozoa from the same males placed in close proximity to oocytes *in vitro*.

Although the caudal storage region of the rabbit epididymis was bypassed in the groups receiving vasoepididymostomy from the proximal caput, distal caput and mid-corpus epididymidis, the numbers of spermatozoa in ejaculates from these animals were much the same before and after surgery (Temple-Smith *et al.*, 1989). Even exhaustive ejaculation studies on these animals were not able to distinguish any significant change in cumulative sperm output either after the collection of ejaculates daily over 5 days or collection of four ejaculates during a 6–8 h period each for 5 days (Fig. 2). This rather unexpected result may be explained in three ways: (i) a propensity for the straight portion of rabbit vas deferens to become convoluted after surgery, (ii) larger than usual accumulations of spermatozoa in the vas deferens, or (iii) a combination of these two factors.

Rats

Recent studies on the effects of vasoepididymal bypass on sperm motility and fertility in rats (Sapountzis, 1996) have produced similar data to that collected from the rabbit model. In this study, groups of rats were set up with vasoepididymal bypasses immediately below the initial segment and at the distal caput, proximal corpus and distal corpus epididymidis (zones 1, proximal 3, and proximal and distal 4, respectively of Reid and Cleland, 1957). The effects of level of bypass on sperm motility (percentage and index, WHO 1980) and vitality (using a dye-exclusion test) was examined using samples taken from above and below the bypass. Fertility was tested by pairing each male with two females and comparing the mean sizes of litters in each group.

The greatest effects of bypass surgery on spermatozoa were seen in animals bypassed from below the initial segment of the epididymis. Spermatozoa from the vas deferens of these animals below the anastomosis site showed significant reductions in percentage motility and motility index and there was a significant increase in the number of dead spermatozoa. This phenomenon was similar to that seen in the rabbit and suggests that immature spermatozoa in both the rabbit and rat are not able to survive well in the luminal environment of the vas deferens. As with the rabbit, distance of the vasoepididymal bypass from the testis was related to an increase in the motility and survival of spermatozoa in the vas deferens below the anastomosis. Unlike in the rabbit, there was no evidence of post-surgical convolutions of the straight portion of the vas deferens used in the

Table 1. *In vivo* fertilization rates and motility characteristics of spermatozoa in semen collected into an artificial vagina from rabbits in which the vas deferens was surgically anastomosed with the proximal or distal caput epididymidis of the rabbit

Bypass (from)	*n*	Number of females/ mating trial[a]	Motility (mean ± SD) %	Motility (mean ± SD) Index	Ova fertilized/ collected	% fertilized
Proximal caput	4	19	21 ± 4	28 ± 7	13/208	6
Distal caput	4	19	28 ± 11	44 ± 27*	35/206	18
Untreated animals	5	20	71 ± 8**	172 ± 27*	78/109	71

[a] Each female was mated twice in succession by the same male, given 100 IU bCG i.v., killed 18 h later and oocytes flushed from the oviduct for assessment of fertilization using standard criteria. *n* = number of bucks $*P < 0.05$; $**P < 0.01$. (E. Herrera Castaneda, P. D. Temple-Smith and G. J. Southwick, unpublished).

Table 2. *In vitro* fertilization success and motility characteristics of ejaculated spermatozoa in rabbits after vasoepididymostomy from the proximal caput epididymidis

Buck	Number does/ mating trial	Number of ova fertilized	% fertilized	% motility	Motility index
1	5	3/47	6.3	18 ± 3	21 ± 2
2	5	2/56	4.5	21 ± 2	29 ± 3
3	5	4/68	5.8	25 ± 5	34 ± 10
4	4	4/45	8.8	22 ± 1	28 ± 1

Modified from Temple-Smith *et al.* (1989).

anastomosis. The basis of this species difference in the response of the vas deferens to vasoepididymostomy remains unexplained.

In rats, in contrast to rabbits, the two high-level bypass groups (from below the initial segment and from the distal caput epididymidis) did not sire any litters from natural matings (Fig. 3). However, the groups in which the bypass started below the proximal and distal corpus were able to sire normal sized litters after natural matings.

This need for spermatozoa to pass through all the caput epididymidis of the rat before achieving the capacity to fertilize an ovum contrasts with the acquisition of some fertilizing capacity more proximally in the rabbit, and the gradual increase in fertility with distance of the vasoepididymal bypass from the testis. This difference may be explained by different maturation dynamics operating on epididymal sperm populations in these two species. However, the effects of differences in histological differentiation of the duct mucosa (Reid and Cleland, 1957; Jones *et al.*, 1979) remain to be explored and the possibility of a stochastic effect from the small group sizes also cannot be ignored.

Advances Using Vas Grafts for Selective Regional Bypasses

Although experimental vasoepididymal surgery, as described in these two animal models, has provided some important insights into the dynamic function of the epididymis, it has limitations as an experimental procedure. Vasoepididymostomy can only be used to reduce in a sequential way the distance that spermatozoa traverse the proximal epididymidis. New surgical innovations were required to provide methods for bypassing selected regions of the epididymis so that the importance of those regions in sperm maturation could be determined.

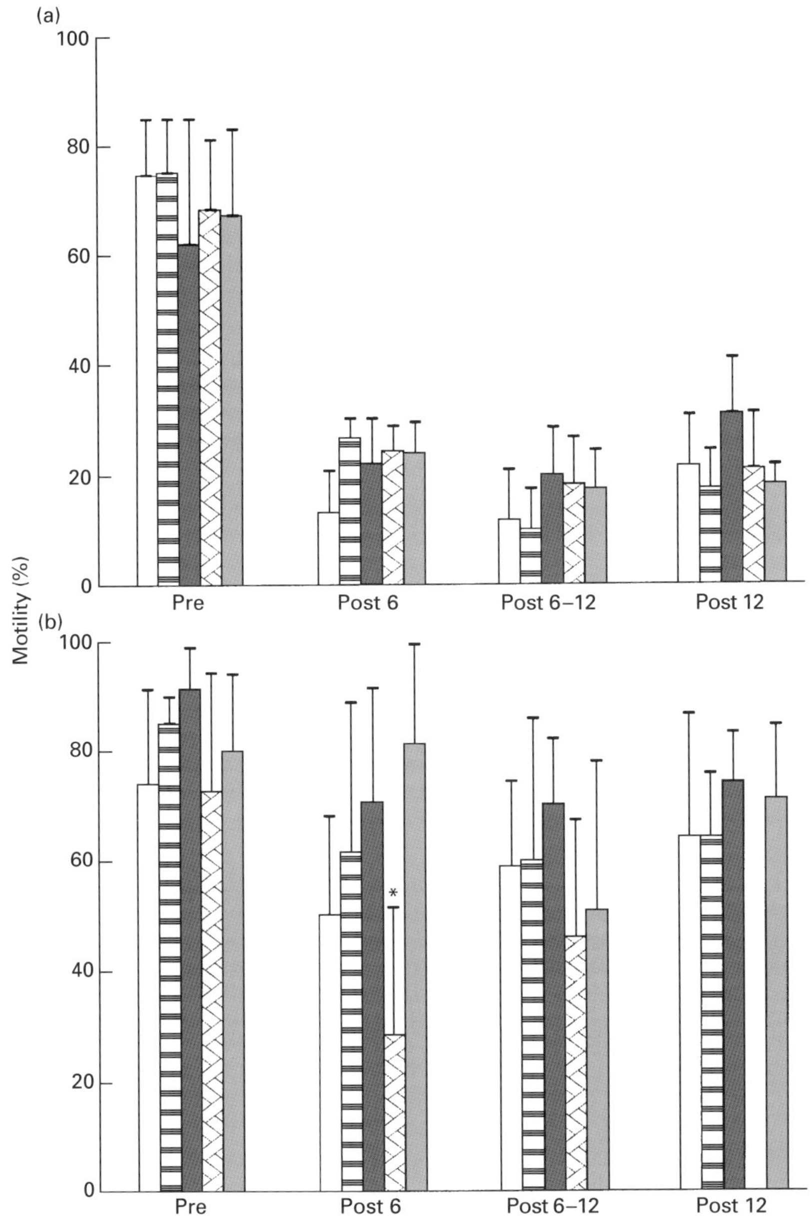

Fig. 1. Long-term effects of vasoepididymostomy from (a) the proximal caput and (b) mid-corpus epididymidis of the rabbit on sperm motility (mean ± SD). The data for each panel (a and b) are from five rabbits (results from individual rabbits are identified by a particular pattern) and compare, for each male, the percentage of motile spermatozoa in ejaculates (n = 6) taken during periods of 6 months (Post 6), 6–12 months (Post 6–12) and >12 months (Post 12) after vasoepididymal surgery with pre-operative sperm motility (Pre). Sperm motility assessments from all post-operative periods in the group bypassed from the proximal caput epididymidis were significantly different (P < 0.01) from pre-operative values. A transient reduction in sperm motility (P < 0.05) was observed during the 6 months after surgery in one male (*) receiving a vasoepididymostomy from the mid-corpus epididymidis. No Post 12 data were available from this male which died during the Post 12 period.

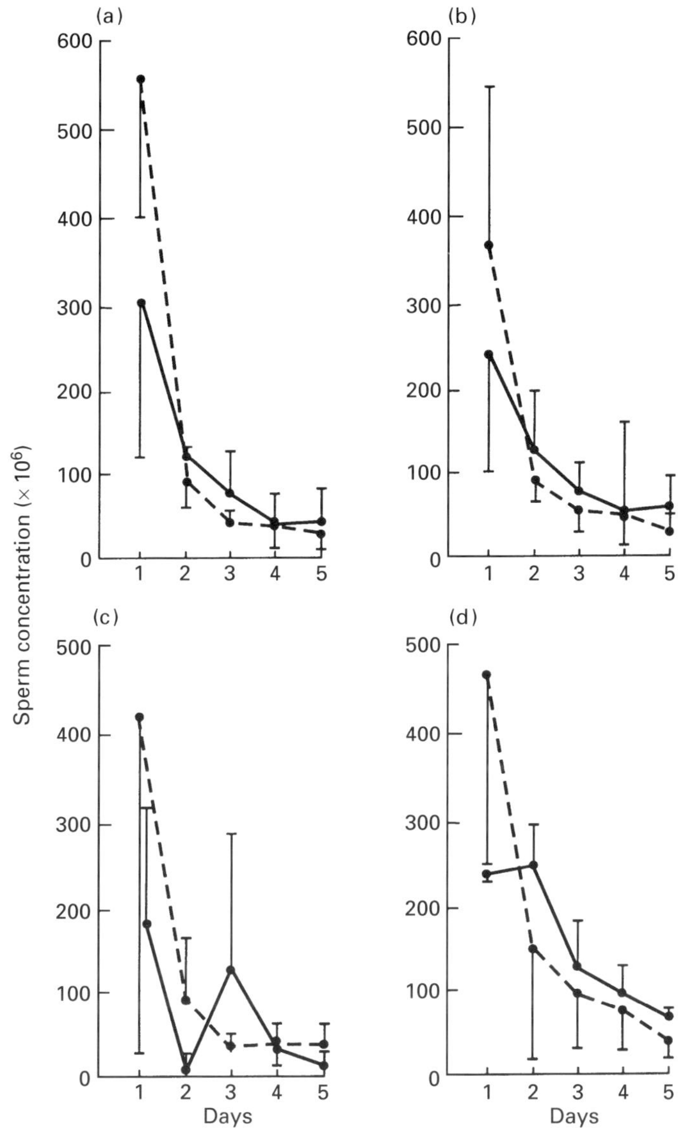

Fig. 2. Comparison of the effect of collecting one (---) or four (—) semen samples per day from the rabbit using a teaser female and artificial vagina, on daily sperm output (mean ± SD) in three groups receiving (a) proximal caput, (b) distal caput and (c) mid-corpus (regions 2/3, 4 and 5/6; Jones *et al.*, 1979) vasoepididymal bypasses (n = 4 per group) compared with (d) a normal unoperated (control) group (n = 4).

Two methods of vas grafting have been developed to bypass regions of the epididymis. Initially, a vascularized graft was successfully used in the rabbit to examine the effects on sperm maturation (Temple-Smith *et al.*, 1989). Later, because of the difficulty of raising vascular pedicies with vas grafts for these experiments in rats, a non-vascularized vas autograft procedure was developed (T. Kadioglu, G. Southwick and P. Temple-Smith, unpublished; Zheng, 1995).

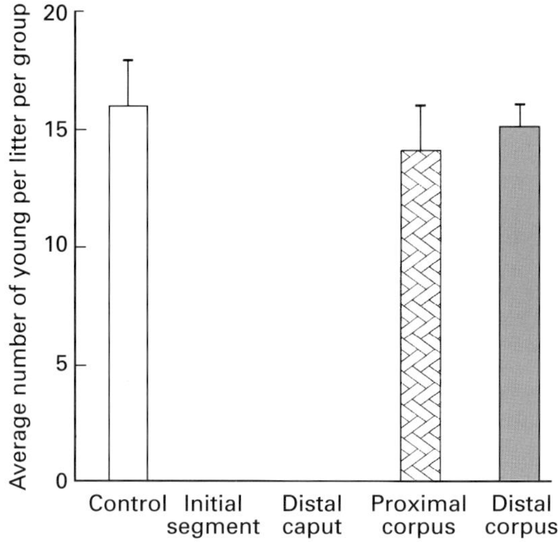

Fig. 3. Comparison of the siring success (litter size (mean ± SD) after natural mating) of a control (unoperated) group of rats (n = 5) and four groups receiving vasoepididymal bypasses (n = 5) from below the level of the initial segment, and in the distal caput, proximal corpus and distal corpus epididymides.

Vascularized vas grafts

Vascularized vas grafts were developed and tested in rabbits (Temple-Smith *et al.*, 1989). In this study segments of the vas, 1 cm long, were isolated with an intact vascular pedicle and used as a bridge to bypass the region between the proximal caput and the mid-corpus epididymidis. This procedure prevented exposure of spermatozoa to the luminal environment of the distal caput and proximal corpus epididymidis (regions 4 and 5/6, Jones *et al.*, 1979) which are important regions for sperm maturation. Despite the need to have three functional anastomoses – two vasoepididymostomies and a vasovasostomy to repair the gap from which the vas bridge was mobilized – for spermatozoa to transit the epididymis successfully, the vas grafts in all three rabbits on this pilot experiment survived and were patent.

However, spermatozoa collected by ejaculation from these animals – even more than one year after surgery – were always dead and degenerating with large numbers of decapitated spermatozoa present in all ejaculates. Examination of sperm samples aspirated from above, inside and below the vas bridge in these animals indicated that spermatozoa died inside the vas graft (Temple-Smith *et al.*, 1989). This provided further evidence that immature spermatozoa have a poor capacity to survive in the luminal environment of the vas deferens. However, care needs to be taken in this interpretation because no physiological comparison between the normal and vas graft environments has yet been made. These grafts show similar convolutions to those observed in the rabbit following vasoepididymal surgery. Histological observations indicated that the vas epithelium hypertrophied, and perhaps proliferated, following grafting suggesting that the graft environment may be different from that of the normal vas deferens.

Non-vascularized vas grafts

Although vascularized vas grafts in rabbits had a high rate of survival and patency, this advantage in studies of epididymal function was greatly diminished by the degenerative changes to spermatozoa during passage through the graft. For economic and other reasons, the rat was chosen as the animal model in which to explore further the use of vas grafts to bypass specific regions of the epididymis. However, because of a more intimate relationship between the deferential artery and the vas deferens in the rat it was necessary to develop a non-vascularized vas graft for this study in a similar way to the use of vascular autografts in vascular surgery (Wylie, 1965; Leather *et al.*, 1981). Although vascular autografts are now in routine clinical use, no previous attempts had been made to use free autografts of the vas deferens in experimental or clinical situations.

In the initial studies, the survival and function of free vas grafts in the rat (T. Kadioglu, G. Southwick and P. Temple-Smith, unpublished) were examined. Isolated vas segments (2.5 cm) were used as bilateral autografts in 15 rats. Each graft was anastomosed between the two transected ends of the contralateral vas deferens (cross-grafting) and the effects were examined one month later. All grafts survived (30/30; 100%) and remained patent. Sperm granulomata were observed adjacent to the proximal suture line in 10% of grafts (3/30); however, these had no effect on postoperative function of the vas grafts. Vas graft survival was associated with mild to severe changes in graft structure including reshaping of the lumen, reduction in epithelial height and stereocilial length, loss of periductal smooth muscle, increased periluminal fibrosis and hypervascularization. However, no significant difference was observed in sperm motility between grafted and control animals.

The high rate of survival and patency of these interpositional free vas autografts one month after the operation and the observation that sperm motility was not affected adversely by the procedure provided the impetus to proceed with further studies of this technique. Polarity reversal of the vas segment, which was used in the unsuccessful rabbit vas graft experiment, was proposed as an explanation for the small number of viable spermatozoa retrieved from the distal end of the grafts. Consequently, graft polarity was studied again in this rat model. Histological evaluation of the vas grafts three months after surgery and fertility assessment of the study population were performed post-operatively as measures of the success of the model.

This study showed that 70% (14/20) of the vas autografts were patent and viable 90 days after the operation. Polarity of the autograft appeared to be inconsequential for all the parameters studied. Minimal fluid leakage was observed at five (25%) of the proximal anastomotic sites in those rats that were mated and achieved pregnancies, but there was no adverse effect of this leakage on graft patency or survival. Prominent neovascularity was seen in all surviving autografts at 90 days.

This new vascular supply was continuous with the adventitial blood supply of the proximal and distal native vas segments. Examination of tissue sections from the mid-portions of the viable autografts under the light microscope showed that they had all undergone some degeneration of the smooth muscle layers and the normal stellate configuration of the vas lumen was lost. Eight (57%) of the grafts showed moderate structural changes and six (43%) showed severe changes.

Six of the ten (60%) rats with patent vas grafts established pregnancies by natural mating. This finding indicated that the structural changes seen in the vas grafts did not significantly affect the viability, motility and fertility of transiting spermatozoa. The mean size of the litters sired by the cross-grafted males was 9.5 (range 7–15) pups with a mean time from cohabitation to producing litters of 38 (range 29–55) days. No significant difference was observed between these fertility rates and those from unoperated rats.

Results of the rabbit vascularized vas graft study suggested that sperm death was caused by the exposure of immature spermatozoa to an environment in the vas graft that would not support their survival. Therefore, an experiment was designed to determine whether mature spermatozoa entering the cauda epididymidis (mid-zone 5 to mid-zone 6, Reid and Cieland, 1957) in the rat would be more resistant to any deleterious effects of the vas graft environment than spermatozoa that had not passed through the distal caput epididymidis (zone 3 of Reid and Cieland, 1957; Zheng, 1995). This experiment established a vas bridge bypass procedure in the cauda epididymidis of the rat. The study investigated the survival, structure and function of non-vascular vas bridge autografts and examined the effects of the vas bridge environment on viability of mature caudal spermatozoa. The study also included a group of rats with vas grafts that bypassed the distal caput region of the epididymis to compare the outcome of this level of bypass on rat spermatozoa with previous data from the rabbit.

The survival and structure of vas autografts, 1cm long, in the rat epididymis were examined at 2 weeks and at 3 and 6 months after surgery. The survival rate of free vas autografts was high in both the caput (41/42) and cauda epididymidis (31/42) groups and the success rate of the bypass surgery was 58% in the caput and 50% in the cauda (Zheng, 1995). Re-vascularization of the grafts occurred from blood vessels on the surface of the epididymis; however, the surviving grafts showed significant structural change similar to those reported in the vas cross-graft experiments. Peripheral fibrosis and degeneration of smooth muscle cells were found to be irreversible but epithelial cells, which were reduced in height 2 weeks after surgery, had recovered their normal structure by 6 months after surgery. After bypass of the cauda epididymidis, the only effect observed was a significant reduction in sperm motility index, suggesting that the bypassed segment of the cauda epididymidis plays a role in maintaining directed motility.

Two weeks after bypass of the distal caput epididymidis, an increase was observed in the incidence of dead and degenerating spermatozoa in the distal cauda epididymidis and vas deferens, and this correlated with transient changes in vas bridge histology. However, data on sperm structure and function from the 3 and 6 month experimental groups were similar to those of controls, suggesting normalization of vas bridge function in the long term. Surviving vas grafts in both the distal caput and cauda epididymidis functioned satisfactorily in transporting spermatozoa without affecting sperm viability and maturation. In addition, the fertility of rats 6 months after bypass of the distal caput or cauda epididymidis, as measured by comparison of litter sizes, did not significantly differ from the controls. This indicated that spermatozoa were still able to acquire normal fertilizing ability without exposure to the bypassed regions in the distal caput or cauda epididymidis once the graft had re-established and the blood supply stabilized. The result of the caudal bypass was, perhaps, not surprising. However, the observation that bypassing the distal caput epididymidis had no effect on any of the sperm maturation parameters examined, in particular viability, was in contrast to previous observations in the rabbit.

Epididymoepididymostomy

The technique of epididymoepididymostomy, like vasoepididymostomy, was first attempted in infertile men, in this case with focal obstruction in the caudal region of the epididymis (Krylov and Borovikov, 1984). Although its use in clinical situations has not been reported subsequently, perhaps because of the poor outcome, it is a technique that was quickly recognized as having relevance to basic studies of epididymal function in mammals (see Temple-Smith *et al.*, 1989).

Rabbits

The first use of this technique in animals was by Temple-Smith *et al.* (1989) who reported the results of unilateral epididymoepididymostomices in a pilot study of seven rabbits. In each male rabbit a small part (2–3 mm) of epididymis was excised and an end-to-side anastomosis performed between the two severed ends of the epididymis to reconnect the duct. The contralateral epididymis was obstructed to prevent this from contributing spermatozoa to the ejaculate. Four (57%) of these epididymal anastomoses were successful and those rabbits produced ejaculates containing large numbers of live spermatozoa with normal motility parameters. Three of these rabbits were successful in fertilizing oocytes (62%, 62% and 100%) after single matings with one female each at least 3 month after surgery. The fourth male rabbit died before fertility testing was performed.

Rats

The use of epididymostomy in the rat was first reported by MeClatchey *et al.* (1991). A similar procedure was used to that described for the rabbit and similar success rates for patency of the anastomosis were described. Litter sizes sired by the male rats used in this study were also normal. Zheng (1995) made a more detailed study of the effects of epididymoepididymostomy in rats. This

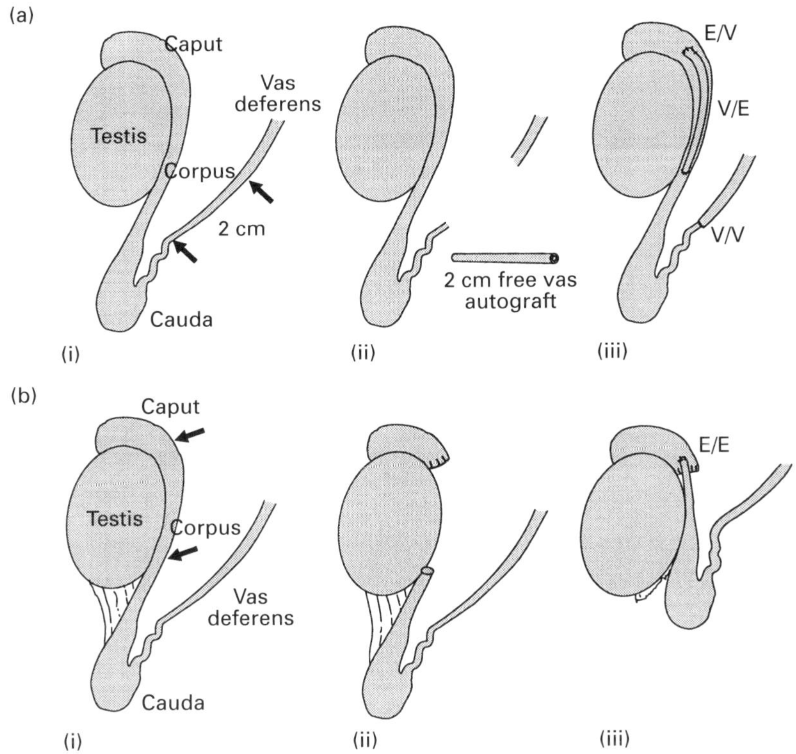

Fig. 4. Surgical bypass procedures in the rat epididymis. (a) Bypass of the distal caput and proximal corpus epididymidis (zone 3 and proximal half of zone 4; Reid and Cleland, 1957) using a 2 cm non-vascularized vas autograft: (i) before surgery showing the epididymis, testis and vas deferens and the 2 cm segment of the vas selected for grafting, (ii) excision of the vas autograft, (iii) position of the vas autograft after surgery and repair of the vas deferens. (b) Bypass of the distal caput and proximal corpus epididymidis zone 3 and proximal half of zone 4 (Reid and Cleland, 1957) using epididymoepididymostomy (i) prior to surgery showing the region selected for excision (ii) excision of the distal caput and proximal corpus epididymidis (iii) direct microsurgical attachment of the mid-corpus epididymidis to the distal caput epididymidis. E/E: epididymoepididymostomy; V/E: vaso-epididymostomy; V/V: vasovasostomy.

study was a continuation of work using non-vascularized vas grafts to examine the function of the epididymis. The experiment used bilateral epididymoepididymostomy to exclude a 2 cm region from the proximal caput epididymidis to the mid-corpus epididymidis (zone 3 and proximal half of zone 4, Reid and Cleland, 1957; see Fig. 4b) and determined the effect of this exclusion on the maturation status of the spermatozoa passing through the epididymis. The data from this study were also compared with a bilateral bypass procedure using 2 cm vas grafts which excluded transiting spermatozoa from a similar region of the epididymis (Fig. 4a). As with previous vas graft studies, sperm motility and viability in both experimental groups were significantly reduced in segments below the bypass at 2 weeks after surgery when compared with controls. However, further assessment of sperm quality at 3 and 6 months showed that motility and viability had returned to control values. This transition in sperm quality during the experimental period was closely related to structural changes in the vas grafts, in particular the epithelium, at 2 weeks and the normalization of epithelial structure at 3 and 6 months. Mating studies at 6 months after surgery showed no significant differences in litter sizes between any of the three experimental groups and controls.

This is convincing evidence that exposure of rat spermatozoa to the distal caput and proximal corpus regions of the epididymis are not obligatory for the normal development of sperm motility and the acquisition of the capacity for fertilization. The study also supports the conclusion that sperm maturation may not be as regionally dependent as had been previously proposed.

Conclusion

These studies demonstrate the value of using surgical perturbation of the epididymis to develop a more comprehensive understanding of the complex interactions between the epididymis and sperm maturation. The studies *in vivo* reviewed here have provided new and interesting information about epididymal function using relatively gross measures of sperm function to monitor the effects of surgical manipulation of the epididymis. Future experiments that combine these surgical techniques with a detailed examination of physiological and molecular changes in the luminal environment and the molecular changes in the maturing sperm plasma membrane will provide an even more robust method for deciphering the influence of the epididymis on the maturation of spermatozoa.

The authors thank Sue Simpson for preparing the diagrams, Rita Ellis for assistance with preparing the manuscript, and Russell Jones and Michael Holland for helpful comments and editorial suggestions on the manuscript.

References

Bayle H (1952) Les Azoospermies d'origine excrétoire *Bulletin de la Fédération Société de Gynécologie et d'Obstétrique* **4** 481

Bayle H (1966) Anastomose épididymo-déférentielle *Encyclopédie Médico-Chirurgicale (Paris)* **41** 435

Bedford JM (1963) Morphological changes in rabbit spermatozoa during passage through the epididymis *Journal of Reproduction and Fertility* **5** 169–177

Bedford JM (1966) Development of the fertilising ability of spermatozoa in the epididymis of the rabbit *Journal of Experimental Zoology* **163** 319–329

Bedford JM (1990) Sperm dynamics in the epididymis. In *Gamete Physiology* pp 53–68 Eds RH Asch, JP Balmaceda, and I Johnston Serono Symposia, Norwell, Massachusetts

Cooper TG (1991) In defense of a function for the human epididymis *Fertility and Sterility* **54** 965–975

Fogdestam I, Fall M and Nilsson S (1986) Microsurgical epididymovasostomy in the treatment of occlusive azoospermia *Fertility and Sterility* **46** 925–929

Hagner FR (1936) The operative treatment of sterility in the male *Journal of the American Medical Association* **107** 1851–1853

Holstein A-F (1969) Morphologische Studien am Nebenhoden des Menschen. In *Zwanglose Abhandlungen aus dem Gebiet der normalen und pathologischen Anatomie* Eds W Bargmann and W Doerr. Thieme, Stuttgart

Holstein A-F (1976) Structure of the human epididymis. In *Human Semen and Fertility Regulation in Men* pp 23–30 Ed. ESE Hafez Mosby, Saint Louis

Holtz W and Smidt D (1976) The fertilising capacity of epididymal spermatozoa in the pig *Journal of Reproduction and Fertility* **46** 227–229

Hoppe PC (1975) Fertilising ability of mouse spermatozoa from different epididymal regions and after washing and centrifugation *Journal of Experimental Zoology* **192** 219–222

Horan AH and Bedford JM (1972) Development of the fertilising ability of spermatozoa in the epididymis of the Syrian hamster *Journal of Reproduction and Fertility* **30** 417–423

Jones R, Hamilton DW and Fawcett DW (1979) *American Journal of Anatomy* **156** 373–400

Krylov VS and Borovikov AM (1984) Microsurgical method of reuniting ductus epididymidis *Fertility and Sterility* **41** 418–423

Lacham O and Trounson AO (1991) Fertilising capacity of epididymal and testicular spermatozoa microinjected under the zona pellucida of the mouse oocyte *Molecular Reproduction and Development* **29** 85–93

Leather RP , Shah DM , Buchbinder D , Annest SJ and Karmody AM (1981) Further experience with the saphenous vein used in situ for arterial bypass *American Journal of Surgery* **142** 506–511

Lespinasse VD (1918) Obstructive sterility in the male: Treatment by direct vaso-epididymostomy *Journal of the American Medical Association* **70** 448

McClatchey M, Temple-Smith PD and Southwick GJ (1991) Animal models for epididymo-epididymostomy: developing an alternative microsurgical procedure for vasoepididymostomy *British Journal of Urology* **68** 524–530

Moore HDM (1981) An assessment of the fertilising ability of spermatozoa in the epididymis of the marmoset monkey (*Callithrix jacchus*) *International Journal of Andrology* **4** 321–330

Moore HDM, Hartman TD and Pryor JP (1983) Development of the oocyte-penetrating capacity of spermatozoa in the human epididymis *International Journal of Andrology* **6** 310–316

Orgebin-Crist M-C (1967) Sperm maturation in the rabbit epididymis *Nature* **216** 816–818

Pavlok A (1974) Development of the penetration activity of mouse epididymal spermatozoa *in vivo* and *in vitro*. *Journal of Reproduction and Fertility* **36** 203–205

Reid BL and Cleland KW (1957) The structure and function of the epididymis *Australian Journal of Zoology* **5** 223–246

Robaire B and Hermo L (1988) Efferent ducts, epididymis, and vas deferens: structure, functions, and their regulation. In

The Physiology of Reproduction pp 999–1080 Eds E Knobil and J Neill Raven Press, New York

Sapountzis J (1995) *The Effects of Vasoepididymal Bypass on the Rat Epididymis in View of Sperm Maturation and Fertilisation* BSc Honours thesis, Department of Anatomy, Monash University, Clayton,

Schoysman R (1981) Epididymal causes of male infertility: pathogenesis and management. In *Pathology and Pathophysiology of the Epididymis Progress in Reproductive Biology* Vol. 8 pp 102–119 Eds CG Bollack and A Clavert. Karger, Basel

Schoysman R and Bedford JM (1986) The role of the human epididymis in sperm maturation and sperm storage as reflected in the consequences of epididymovasostomy *Fertility and Sterility* **46** 293–299

Silber SJ (1978) Microscopic vasoepididymostomy: specific microanastomosis to the epididymal tubule *Fertility and Sterility* **30** 565–571

Silber SJ (1988) Pregnancy caused by sperm from the vasa efferentia *Fertility and Sterility* **49** 373–375

Silber SJ (1989a) Apparent fertility of human spermatozoa from the caput epididymidis *Journal of Andrology* **10** 263–269

Silber SJ (1989b) Results of microsurgical vasoepididymostomy: role of epididymis in sperm maturation *Human Reproduction* **4** 298–303

Silber SJ, Balmaceda J, Borrero C, Ord T and Asch R (1988) Pregnancy with sperm aspiration from the proximal head of the epididymis: a new treatment for congenital absence of the vas deferens *Fertility and Sterility* **50** 525–528

Southwick GJ and Temple-Smith PD (1988) Epididymal microsurgery: current techniques and new horizons *Microsurgery* **9** 266–277

Southwick GJ and Temple-Smith PD (1994) Seminal tract microsurgery: vasoepididymostomy, epididymoepididymostomy and sperm microaspiration with *in vitro* fertilization (SMART IVF) In *Progress in Reproductive Biology and Medicine* Vol. 16 pp 49–79, Eds G Colpi and D Pozza. Karger, Basel

Temple-Smith PD and Southwick GJ (1985) Vasoepididymostomy in the rabbit: effects of level of anastomosis on semen quality and fertility *Journal of Andrology* **6** 30

Temple-Smith PD, Southwick GJ, Yates CA, Trounson AO and de Kretser DM (1985) Human pregnancy by *in vitro* fertilisation (IVF) using sperm aspirated from the epididymis *Journal of In Vitro Fertilisation and Embryo Transfer* **2** 199–122

Temple-Smith PD, Southwick GJ, Herrera Castaneda E, Hamer J and McClatchey M (1989) Surgical manipulation of the epididymis: an experimental approach to sperm maturation. In *Perspectives in Andrology* Vol. 63 pp 281–290 Ed. M Serio Serono Symposia Publications, Raven Press, New York

Thomas AJ (1987) Vasoepididymostomy. Male infertility *Urologic Clinics of North America* **14** 527–538

WHO (1980) In *Laboratory Manual for the Examination of Human Semen and Semen–Cervical Mucus Interaction* Eds MA Belsey, KS Moghissi, R Eliasson, CA Paulsen, AJ Gallegos and MRN Prasad. World Health Organisation Special Programme of Research, Development and Research Training in Human Reproduction. Press Concern, Singapore

Wylie EJ (1965) Vascular replacement with arterial autografts *Surgery* **57** 14–19

Young WC (1929) A study of the function of the epididymis. I. Is the attainment of full spermatozoon maturity attributable to some specific action of the epididymal secretion? *Journal of Morphology and Physiology* **47** 479–495

Young WC (1931) A study of the function of the epididymis. III. Functional changes undergone by spermatozoa during their passage through the epididymis and vas deferens in the guinea pig *Journal of Experimental Biology* **8** 151–162

Zheng SS (1995) *Survival, Structure and Function of Vas Bridge Autografts and the Effects of Bypassing the Epididymis in the Rat* Master of Reproductive Sciences Thesis, Institute of Reproduction and Development, Monash University, Clayton

Journal of Reproduction and Fertility Supplement **53**, 197–210

The specificity of epididymal secretory proteins

M. K. Holland[1] and B. Nixon[2]

Vertebrate Bio-Control Co-operative Research Center,
[1]CSIRO Division of Wildlife and Ecology, PO Box 284 Canberra, ACT 2601, Australia and
[2]Department of Biological Sciences, University of Newcastle, NSW 2308, Australia

Early studies in which the electrophoretic profiles of fluid from different regions of the epididymis were compared with other body fluids, such as blood serum, suggested that many proteins present in epididymal fluid were not found in other secretions and thus might be tissue specific. Comparative studies of epididymal fluid from different species further emphasized differences so that some epididymal proteins are considered both tissue and species specific. Such proteins are the putative molecular agents responsible for the array of changes undergone by spermatozoa during maturation. Thus a complete characterization of all the specific proteins secreted by the epididymis would yield important information for understanding the molecular events of maturation. Comparison of these proteins across species would determine whether the proteins and mechanisms at the centre of changes such as acquisition of fertilizing ability are conserved during evolution. This review critically examines the evidence for both tissue and species specificity of epididymal secreted proteins, describes how advances in molecular biology can be used to clarify this issue and concludes with a description of some preliminary work with different lagomorph species involving the REP 52 protein, an epididymal secretory protein that binds specifically to spermatozoa in New Zealand white rabbits.

Introduction

The role of the epididymis is to provide an environment in which structurally and functionally immature spermatozoa leaving the testis can be converted into fully functional cells. Spermatozoa are then stored here before ejaculation (for review see Cooper, 1986). Proteins synthesized and secreted into the lumen from the epididymal epithelium, some under the influence of systemic androgens, fill important roles in both this functional maturation and in maintaining spermatozoa before ejaculation (for reviews see Hedge, 1997 and Orgebin-Crist, this supplement). Epididymal specific proteins are probably also important for storage, although as yet there is little direct evidence for this. Comparative studies indicate that many of these proteins cannot be detected in other tissues (Table 1) or are present in the epididymis as specific isoforms.

New technologies such as proteome studies, creation of expressed sequence tag libraries and tissue-specific subtractive hybridization will result in identification of most , if not all, of the proteins synthesized and secreted by the epididymis. For proteins with specific activities, identification alone could be sufficient for elucidating their role. Comparison of these proteins across species will indicate whether this function is conserved. For other proteins, searches of the expanding molecular databases will determine putative tissue and species specificity. As a significant amount of sequence data from epididymal proteins from a number of species become available both conserved and putatively species-specific proteins will be identified. In addition, new molecular approaches provide, through analysis of these sequences for particular motifs (for example DNA binding domains), important information that can assist in determining the role of the protein. More focused direct attempts to elucidate their function(s) can then be made. Thus a clear and critical understanding of both the applications and limitations of these molecular technologies is essential for understanding of the role that epididymal specific proteins play in maturation.

Table 1. Epididymal proteins conserved among species

Protein	Species				
	Rat	Mouse	Rabbit	Human	Other
DE / AEG	32[1,2]	29 (CRISP-1)[3,4]	–	30 (ARP)[5,6]	guinea-pig[3]
BC / E-RABP	18.5[1]	18 (MEP10)[3,7]	21 (EP21)[8]	–	17.2 lizard (LESP IV)[9]
Immobilin	> 100[10]	–	–	–	–
GGT*	70 (nr)[11]	–	–	–	–
GST*	X[12,13]	–	–	–	–
SGP-2	41, 32[14]	–	–	X[15]	pig[16],horse[17], sheep[18]
E-GPX*	4 x 23[19]	24 (GPX5)[3,20,21,]	–	–	pig[22], monkey[19]
E-SOD*	64[23]	–	–	–	–
β-D-galactosidase*	84[24]	–	–	–	–
N-acetyl-β-hexosaminidase*	63, 55, 31[25]	–	–	–	pig[26], cow[27]
E-β-lactalbumin*	18[28]	–	–	–	–
Oxytocin*	X[29]	–	–	–	sheep[30]
Proenkephalin*	X[31]	–	–	–	hamster[31]
GP17	17[32]	–	–	–	–
B109	22, 24[33]	–	–	–	–
ADAM7	–	X[34]	–	–	–
M53*	X[35]	24[35]	X[35]	X[35]	pig[35], sheep[35]
SMA 4	–	85[36,37]	–	–	–
SF/HGF*	–	82[38]	–	–	–
CRES	–	19, 14[39]	–	–	–
Guanidino-benzoatase*	–	71[40]	–	–	–
EP20	–	–	20[41]	–	–
EP140	–	–	140 (nr)[42]	–	–
Uteroglobin*	–	–	15[43]	–	–
ASF	–	–	260 (nr)[44]	–	–
REP38	20[45]	–	38, 77[45]	–	–
R1	–	–	58[46]	–	–
R2	–	–	20[46]	–	–
R3	–	–	20[46]	–	–
P26h	–	–	–	26	guinea- pig[47]
P34H	–	–	–	34[48]	–
FMP	–	–	–	–	hamster[49],34.5 bull[50]
HE1	–	–	–	25, 27[51]	primates (EPI-1[52], ESP14.6[53]), dog (CE1)[54]
HE2	–	–	–	10[55]	–
HE3				14.9[56]	pig[16]
HE4	–	–	20 (BE-20)[57]	10[58]	pig[59],bull[59],horse[59], dog (CE4)[54]
HE5 / CDw52*	–	–	–	26[60]	dog (CE5)[54]
HE6	–	–	–	X[61]	human, dog, pig, bull[61]
GZS–1	–	–	–	21–25, 31, 51–54, 62[62]	–
1G12	–	–	–	15–25[63]	–
NW21	–	–	–	18[64]	–
α-mannosidase*	135[65]	X[66]	–	–	pig (135)[16, 67]
Antagglutinin	–	–	–	–	pig (65)[68]
Lactoferrin*	–	–	–	–	pig (70)[16]
Procathepsin*	–	–	–	–	pig (40)[16]

X, protein present but molecular weight unknown; *proteins present in other tissue besides the epididymis; –, indicates that a corresponding protein has not been identified in the epididymis of a particular species; nr, molecular weight of the protein resolved under non-reducing conditions
Key to References is in Appendix 1.

Table 2. Advantages and disadvantages to current procedures for studying epididymal protein synthesis and secretion

Technique	Advantage	Disadvantage	References
Fluid	Rapid, easy, inexpensive and yields much information	Highly dependent on purity of sample. Optimal with micropuncture but this requires expertise. Varies with resolution of separation and sensitivity of detection	Koskimies and Kormano, 1975; Huang and Johnson, 1975; Brooks and Higgins, 1980; Olson and Hinton, 1985; Jones, 1987.
In vitro labelling	Relatively easy, conditions and components of incubation can be varied so key factors can be identified, different tracers can be used	Relevance of *in vitro* to *in vivo*. Release of protein from damaged cells/tissue compared with true secretion.	Brooks, 1981; Jones *et al.*, 1980; Holland and Orgebin-Crist, 1988; Brooks, 1986; Klinefelter and Hamilton, 1984.
In vivo labelling	Permits direct study of secretion *in vivo*. Combined with micropuncture produces high quality data. Permits direct study of protein interaction with spermatozoa	Isotope expensive, difficulties with handling and disposal of radioactive animals, injection into epididymal artery is difficult.	Vreeburg *et al.*, 1990, 1992.
Gene cloning	Detailed information about protein encoded by a specific gene	Can only readily deal with single genes/proteins	Kirchoff *et al.*, 1990.

Key to references is in Appendix 2.

New Approaches to the Characterization of Epididymal Proteins

Most of the proteins present within the fluid compartment of the epididymal lumen originate from either the testis or are synthesized or secreted by the epididymal epithelium. A very small percentage are not synthesized by the epididymis and originate from serum, lymph or extracellular fluid (for reviews see Hegde, 1997; Cooper, 1986). A number of these epididymal luminal proteins (Table 1) have been characterized with various degrees of completeness across a range of species using a number of approaches each with its own advantages and limitations (Table 2). Some proteins are epididymal isoforms of proteins present in other tissues (Table 1) but a smaller number are putatively characteristic of the epididymis. The expanding armoury of molecular technologies will provide direct answers to the question of tissue (and even species) specificity of epididymal proteins. This will enable dissection of the process of maturation and its comparison across species. Therefore, it is important to understand both the potential and limitations of these new techniques and what information they can provide on the question of specificity.

Differential screening

In this approach, pioneered by Kirchhoff, Ivell and colleagues (Kirchhoff *et al.*, 1990) an epididymal cDNA expression library was screened with cDNA to epididymis using testis as negative control. Only those clones specifically hybridizing to epididymal cDNA were subjected to a second round of screening. In this second round, testis cDNA was replaced by cDNA from liver and brain. Positive clones were those encoding genes expressed in epididymis but not testis, liver or brain. This was confirmed by northern blots of RNA from a range of tissues resulting in four clones that appeared specific for the epididymis.

When used as described above, the aim is to identify genes that are expressed only in the epididymidis and not in other tissues (that is, tissue-specific genes). Alternatively, it could be refined to provide additional information about regional specificity of gene expression. If a library were made from the caput epididymidis and cDNA from corpus and cauda epididymides used to eliminate common genes, the result would be genes specifically expressed in the caput epididymidis. Judicious application of this approach would enable identification of genes expressed only in regions where specific physiological changes of interest are occurring in spermatozoa. This approach could be adapted to search for species-specific epididymal genes. For example, cDNA from mouse epididymis could be subtracted from a rat epididymal cDNA library to yield genes specifically expressed in the rat.

Besides the experiments of Kirchoff and colleagues (Ivell, this supplement) alluded to earlier, no experiments have been performed using this technology. The limitation to these approaches is the degree of homology between the gene in the cDNA library and that in the cDNA being used to subtract. With the experiments performed by Kirchoff *et al.* (1990) or in the regional specific gene experiments outlined above, there is high homology between common genes thus making it possible to use high stringency conditions for hybridization thus minimizing false positive results. However, homology is probably much lower for the same gene from different species and hence lower stringency must be used. This procedure would produce increased background and lower resolution making it more difficult to identify proteins that were species specific. Thus this approach is best suited to issues of tissue or regional specificity of gene expression.

Proteome technology

Proteome technology is a molecular approach that does not rely on DNA/RNA technology. Proteome is defined as the set of PROTEins expressed by a genOME or tissue (Wilkins *et al.*, 1997). The proteome, unlike the genome, is not a fixed feature of an organism. Rather it differs from tissue to tissue, within a tissue it alters with stage of development and it can vary with tissue environment (for example endocrine status). The technique is most effectively used to study proteins in tissue. In eukaryotes there are many more proteins in a proteome than genes in a genome. This is due to alternate splicing of the mRNA and also to the complex post-translational modifications, such as glycosylation, that many proteins undergo.

Steps involved in proteome analysis are relatively straightforward and are increasingly facilitated by the ability to buy many of the components pre-made. Initially, the proteins present are separated by two-dimensional gel electrophoresis. The physical conditions of the electrophoretic separation can be varied so that over a series of gels all proteins present will be separated and visualized. The protein spots are cut out and the amino acid sequence obtained directly. This is then matched to databases of existing protein sequences to identify the protein.

Rapid improvements in protein sequencing technology mean smaller quantities of protein are required and longer stretches of amino acids can be sequenced. This lowers cost, increases throughput and makes sequence matching more reliable.

Dacheux and colleagues (Syntin *et al.*, 1996) have reported studies in pigs in which with this technique they identified five proteins and two apparently novel sequences (Dacheux *et al.*, this supplement). Recently, we have also used this approach to begin to map the proteins present in rabbit caudal epididymal fluid (B. Nixon, R. C. Jones and M. Holland, unpublished).

The resolution of two-dimensional electrophoresis is limited by the pH gradient used in the initial dimension. Current pH gradients poorly resolve proteins with pI values below 3.5 and above 7.5. In addition the resolution of the second dimension is limited by the acrylamide concentration and the degree of cross-linking used to form this gel. These difficulties could be minimized by using numerous gels of different pI range in the first dimension coupled with gradient gels or gels of different acrylamide content but then relating one gel to another to produce a comprehensive map of the proteins present is difficult.

An additional limitation comes from the system used to detect the proteins. There is a limit to the amount of protein that can be resolved by a gel system. Proteins of low abundance can prove difficult to detect. Some stains, such as silver based methods, that are very sensitive can assist with this but with these sensitive techniques staining intensity is not proportional to the amount of protein. Additional difficulties with some proteins, especially glycoproteins, which stain variably making detection unreliable.

Technology development is one of the limitations to the future of proteomics. Despite continuing significant effort from a number of companies, no equipment equivalent to the automated DNA sequencers that have made possible the rapid progress made over recent years in genomics is available. Undoubtedly machines that can use methods such as either capillary electrophoresis or serial liquid chromatography coupled with mass spectrophotometric detection will be developed with greatly enhanced resolution compared with that provided by two-dimensional electrophoresis coupled to post-separation techniques such as N or even C terminal protein microsequencing.

Expressed sequence tags

Expressed sequence tags (ESTs) have not yet been used in the study of epididymal function. The technique involves the generation of an epididymal cDNA library, clones from which are sequenced at random. It requires the power of high throughput automated sequencers and ability of complex data management systems to interpret the sequences obtained. Sequences can be obtained from either the 5′ or 3′ end. Sequencing from the 3′ end has the advantage that unambiguous identification of the same transcript, up to the first alternate slicing site, from libraries made from different tissues (or even different species) can be achieved. Homology searches can quickly identify whether an individual sequence resides in a previously sequenced cDNA or may be unique. Thus potential sequences that are specific to the epididymis can be readily identified.

When coupled with other technologies, such as polymerase chain reaction (PCR) and RACE (rapid amplification of cDNA ends), entire cDNAs of interest can be obtained quickly. There is also the intriguing possibility of using ESTs to generate hybridization chips. This procedure may provide a way to combine EST technology with the differential screening strategy described above and would significantly increase the power to identify sequences of interest.

We have undertaken some very limited EST experiments using our rabbit epididymal cDNA library. This approach quickly identified a clone with high homology to HE 2 identified by Kirchoff (J. Andrews and M. Holland, unpublished). It had previously been suggested that HE 2 is a human epididymal specific clone.

Clearly, the greater the number of ESTs from a particular species the greater the probability of determining the tissue or species specificity of any particular sequence. There are also limitations in the computer software used to identify epididymal specific sequences from the vast number of other sequences common to other tissues.

Epididymal Specific Gene Expression: How Does It Occur?

Selective expression of particular genes in individual tissues is the hallmark of differentiated organisms (for review see Wolpert, 1998). Our understanding of how this is achieved at the molecular level is rapidly expanding. Generally it would seem to involve orchestration of the action of a number of factors produced both locally and systemically.

For the epididymis it is anticipated that tissue-specific proteins would perform key roles in the process of sperm maturation. Not surprisingly, therefore, much research attention has been focused on identifying these proteins from the total protein complement present in epididymal fluid (Table 1). Perhaps one of the better examples of this is the acid epididymal glycoprotein (AEG)/ protein DE (Table 3). Such proteins arise from the expression of a repertoire of genes that are activated at a distinct point in development (that is, puberty). Identification of the genes remains relatively easy but identification of the *cis* and *trans* acting factors that regulate the tissue-specific and temporal expression of these genes is more difficult. Characterizing and understanding these genes and their

Table 3: Epididymal proteins related to rat DE from different species

Protein / Gene	Molecular mass(kDa)	Genetic properties	Species	Tissue	Homology / function
DE	32	Two mRNAs: 1.2 / 1.7kb (allelic genes)	rat, mouse, guinea -pig	Epididymis: caput, corpus, cauda Sperm: post-acrosomal region	DE: androgen-regulated epididymal secretory protein[1] Homology: metalloproteins[2], cysteine rich secretory protein (CRISP) superfamily[3], acidic epididymal glycoprotein (AEG)[4], protein IV[5], specific epididymal proteins (SEP)[6], 32 kDa rat epididymal protein (REP)[7], 4E9[8,9,10] Function: DE binds to sperm surface in a receptor–ligand fashion[11] and mediates gamete fusion through complementary sites on the oocyte surface[12]. Immunization of rats with DE leads to a significant, reversible reduction of fertility but has no apparent effect on sperm motility, viability or ability to undergo capacitation[13].
CRISP-1	29		mouse	Epididymis: corpus, cauda Spermatozoa: vas deferens, seminal vesicles, prostate, salivary gland	CRISP-1: cysteine rich secretory protein-1[3,14] Homology: mouse epididymal protein 7(MEP7)[15], mouse equivalent of AEG (Aeg1)[16,17], Aeg2[16], mouse testis specific gene (Tpx1)[18], DE[1], human testis specific gene (TPX1)[18], guinea-pig acrosomal autoantigen (AA1)[19]
ARP[d]	30	orf: 690bp gene: AEGL1 chromosome: 6p21.1–p21.2	human	Epididymis: caput, corpus, cauda Spermatozoa: post-acrosomal region vas deferens	ARP: AEG-related protein. Human functional equivalent of rodent AEG/DE[20,21]

Key to References is in Appendix 2.

regulatory elements provides an opportunity to use molecular approaches, such as selective gene knockout, that will assist in establishing the functions of the encoded proteins in maturation.

One approach is to study the 5′ untranslated region of genomic clones for these epididymal specific proteins for functionally important sites of DNA–protein interaction. Binding motifs for a number of transcription factors are well known and can readily be recognized. This does not eliminate the possibility that there is an epididymal specific transcription factor(s) but its identification would require much more complex manipulations linking the promoter to a reporter gene, the expression of which could be studied *in vitro* or *in vivo.* Whether such a factor exists is problematic as increasingly data from studies in areas other than the epididymis suggest that tissue-specific expression is a consequence of interactions of unique combinations of relatively ubiquitous transcription factors. The realisation that tissue architecture and extracellular matrix elements can also contribute to the regulation of tissue-specific gene expression in ways that remain poorly understood is also important. Identification of these factors, the nature and mechanism of their interaction, and their interaction with downstream target genes is the only way to understand what role these transcription factors play in inducing or maintaining expression of proteins specific to the epididymis and ultimately their role in epididymal function. However, there is evidence that the epididymis is even more subtle than this and indeed, in a similar way to the testis, produces unique transcripts encoding isoforms of proteins that are present in other tissues (Table 1) in addition to its repertoire of unique proteins. These arise usually as a consequence of alternate splicing events. The studies on glutathione peroxidase are perhaps the best example (Hinton *et al.*, this supplement).

The critical role that androgens play in the process of proliferation and probably differentiation of the epididymal epithelium has long been established as has the role of androgens in regulating expression of some epididymal specific genes (for review see Brooks, 1986). Of course androgens are not the only factors involved (Jones *et al.,* 1980; Holland *et al.,* 1992). Clearly components of testicular fluid which may even include the spermatozoa themselves have been shown to exert regulatory influences (Garrett *et al.,* 1990).

How the androgenic signal is modulated to produce the specific patterns of gene expression observed is unknown but a safe assumption is that, in addition to the androgen receptor, specific transcription factors are also involved. One set of transcription factors that have been shown to be differentially expressed within the male reproductive tract are some of those encoded by homeobox genes (Lindsey and Wilkinson, 1996). Homeobox proteins have a distinct homeodomain which is a 60 amino acid motif that forms three alpha helices. Key residues in the third helix bind directly to elements in the 5′ untranslated region of induced genes.

Wilkinson and colleagues (Maiti *et al.*, 1996) used androgen induction coupled with subtraction hybridization to isolate novel epididymal genes. One cDNA obtained encoded the homeobox gene *Pem.* Studies showed that the *Pem* gene was specifically transcribed in the adult male and female reproductive tract. Analysis of the genomic structure showed that there were two promoters used in a tissue specific manner. One of these promoters (P_p) is androgen dependent and ensures expression of *Pem* in the male tract. *Pem* transcripts are produced by at least three forms of alternate splicing: alternate exon inclusion, alternate exon skipping and alternate slice acceptor usage. This raises the issue of whether tissue-specific factors are involved in modulating the androgen effect.

It remains unclear which epididymal specific genes are regulated either directly or indirectly by *Pem.* An array of possible genes can be suggested ranging from regulatory molecules (5 alpha reductase, nerve growth factor) to structural proteins (AEG/CRISP 1/DE or BC/ESP 1). However, *Pem* expression in rats is confined to the distal corpus and proximal cauda epididymides thus reducing the number of potential *Pem* responsive genes to those expressed in this region.

Two transcription factors, *Pax* 2 and *PEA 3*, previously identified as being expressed in the epididymis do not seem to be under androgenic control. Hinton and colleagues (Lan *et al.*, 1998) have suggested that *PEA 3* may be involved in regulation of the epididymal specific form of gamma-glutamyl transpeptidase (GGT IV), a key enzyme in the metabolism of glutathione and postulated to serve important functions to protect spermatozoa against reactive oxygen species. Analysis of the promoter region of this transcript shows that there are several putative *PEA 3* binding motifs. *PEA 3* is a member of the *Ets* transcription factor family that have important roles in embryogenesis. *PEA 3* expression occurs in the rat initial segment coincident with GGT IV expression. *PEA 3* expression seems to be influenced by factors present in testicular fluid, as its concentration diminishes after efferent duct ligation (Lan *et al.*, 1998). *PEA 3* in other tissues is regulated by a number of factors including growth factors such as basic fibroblast growth factor (bFGF). bFGF has been shown to be a component of testicular fluid (Lan, *et al* 1998). Drevet *et al.* (1998) suggested that *PEA 3* also plays a role in repressing transcription of another of the enzymes of glutathione metabolism, glutathione peroxidase V (GPX V). Thus *PEA 3* may prove to be a key component in modulating gene expression of glutathione metabolizing enzymes.

A clear understanding of the factors involved in regulation of genes specifically expressed in the epididymis provides a way in which expression of these genes can be manipulated in a strategic way (that is genes could be selectively turned on or off). Coupled with gene knockout technology this provides a way to study directly the role of particular genes and their encoded proteins in the process of sperm maturation in a way not currently possible.

Species Restricted Proteins

Genetic homology of epididymal specific proteins among species seems the rule rather than the exception when sequence comparisons are made (Ivell *et al.*, 1998). Perhaps this is not surprising as the events of epididymal maturation are at least superficially similar across species despite differences in epididymal morphology, sperm morphology and the functions of different epididymal regions (Amann *et al.*, 1993). However, the question of whether homologous molecules perform the same biological role in the process of maturation has seldom been investigated. For example, a number of molecules homologous to the rat B/C gene have been identified from a range of species (Lareye *et al.*, this volume). On the basis of genetic homology, it is assumed that these proteins fill the role performed by B/C (that is, binding active retinoids) despite differences in molecular weight and other properties. The validity of this assumption remains untested. Comparative studies across species have traditionally provided important keys for understanding conserved physiological processes. Although there have been a number of studies of general epididymal function (R. C. Jones, this supplement) cross-species studies focusing on a particular aspect of maturation down to the molecular level have not been done. Such studies combined with molecular technologies would contribute to an understanding of maturation. For example, the gene encoding mouse mE-RABP could be selectively knocked out and these knockout mice bred with transgenic mice expressing rat protein BC to produce mice in which the rat BC gene had replaced the mouse mE-RABP. Would the rat protein fulfil the role of the mouse protein in maturation? Such studies are best conducted in species that are genetically highly related. We have recently started some studies to address this issue.

We have identified and partially characterized from the epididymis of the domestic rabbit a number of epididymal secretory proteins that bind to spermatozoa. These are designated as Rabbit Epididymal Protein with their putative molecular weight (for example REP 52). This characterization includes cloning the encoding genes and producing monospecific antisera (B. Nixon, C. Hardy, R. C. Jones and M. Holland, unpublished). We have asked the simple question: are similar molecules present in the epididymal fluid from four lagomorph species from North America? The four species chosen (Table 4) have various degrees of relatedness among themselves and to the domestic rabbit, *Oryctolagus cuniculus.* In all cases proteins of similar molecular weight to REP 52 were detected in both the caudal epididymal fluid (Fig. 1) and also in the caput fluid of all species except *L. californicus.* REP 52 could be extracted from the plasma membrane of caudal epididymal spermatozoa from all species again except *L. californicus* (Fig. 2). Why REP52 should be present in the caudal fluid from all the lagomorph species tested and present on the sperm plasma membrane of all species except one is unclear. In domestic rabbits REP 52 binds selectively to the tail of spermatozoa. Antisera to REP 52 do not visibly affect motility but do decrease sperm binding to oocytes in *in vitro* fertilization assays. The focus of future work will be to clone homologous genes from the other lagomorph species and conduct knockout experiments to determine whether similar phenotypes are

Table 4. Lagomorph species from which epididymal fluids and sperm were obtained and which were probed for the presence of REP 52

Species (common name)	Chromosome complement	Status	Distribution
Sylvilagus audbonii (Desert cottontail)	2n = 42	Very common	Mexico, Arizona, Utah parts of California
Sylvilagus nuttalli (Mountail cottontail)	2n = 42	Very common	Intermountain area from Arizona to Canada
Oryctolagus cuniculus (European rabbit)	2n = 44	Locally common	Europe, Australia, some South America
Lepus californicus (Black tail jackrabbit)	2n = 48	Locally common	Mexico to Oregon. East to Colorado
Lepus townsendii (White tail jackrabbit)	2n = 48	Locally common	Nevada to Ontario. East to Wisconsin

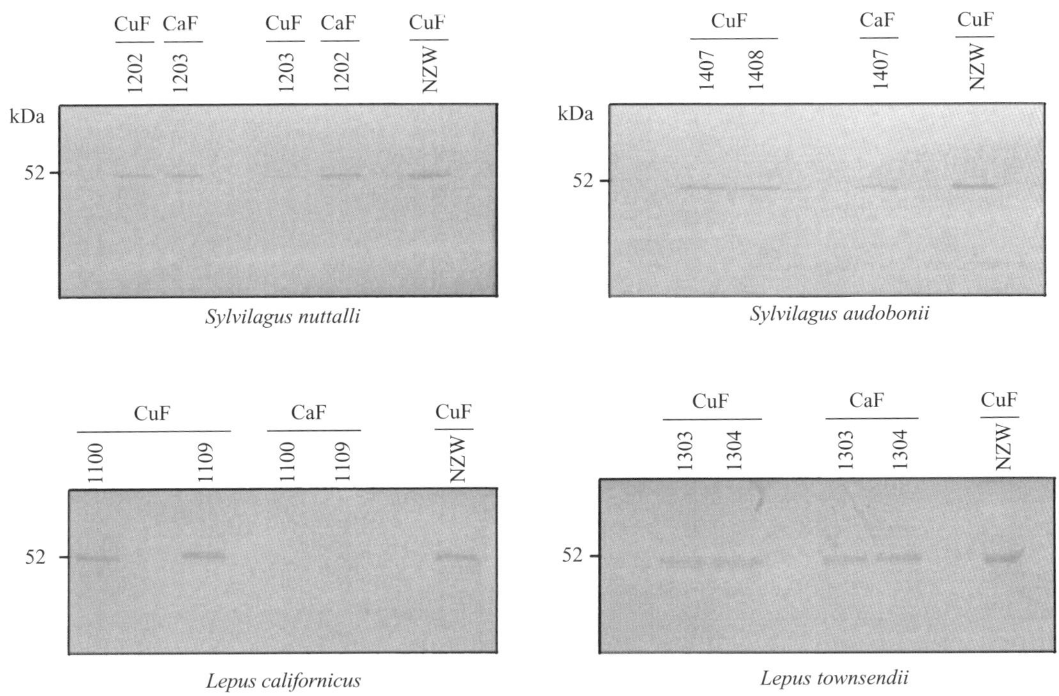

Fig. 1. Immunoreactivity, detected on western blot, to REP 52 in caput fluid (CaF) and caudal fluid (CuF) of individual animals from four lagomorph species. The vascular supply to the epididymis of all animals was perfused with saline and the epididymal fluid carefully collected from severed tubules. Spermatozoa were separated by centrifugation (800 g for 109 min at room temperature) and the supernatant harvested. Protein (20 µg) was separated using SDS-PAGE under reducing conditions and transferred to nitrocellulose membranes which were then probed with the IgG fraction of a monospecific antiserum raised to REP 52.

generated. Ultimately gene replacement studies with genes from different lagomorph species could be conducted. In the context of establishing the molecular role of REP 52 it is important to realise that immunoreactivity to REP 52 has not been detected in epididymal fluid from domestic species including dogs, cats, pigs, rams, bulls or in tammar wallabies.

Another approach that may contribute information about the species specificity of epididymal maturation will emerge from the studies of Brinster and colleagues with transplanting spermatogenic tissue between species (Clouthier *et al.*, 1996). These experiments have already shown

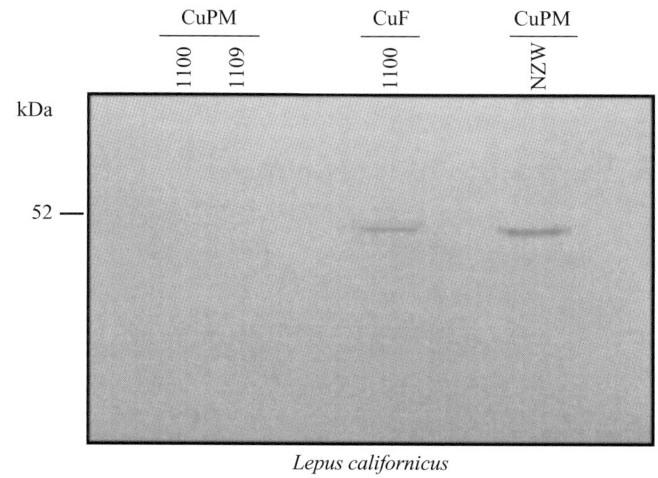

Fig. 2. Immunoreactivity to REP 52 detected in caudal plasma membrane fractions (CuPM) and cauda fluid (CuF) from *Lepus californicus.* Caudal plasma membranes were prepared using the procedure of Fayrer-Hosken *et al.* (1991). Membrane protein (20 µg) was separated using SDS-PAGE under reducing conditions and transferred to nitrocellulose membranes which were then probed with the IgG fraction of a monospecific antiserum raised to REP 52.

that rat spermatozoa can be produced successfully within a mouse testis , albeit at very small numbers. When this can be increased to larger numbers, the intriguing possibility of whether the mouse epididymis can support maturation of rat spermatozoa will be accessible for study. As we have a large number of probes for both sperm surface proteins and epididymal maturation antigens in both of these species, it will be possible to address detailed questions about the role that individual proteins play as well as a more holistic understanding of the process of maturation. Clearly, if fertile spermatozoa of both species emerge from this epididymis not only will current understanding of maturation be challenged, but also there will be new options in fields as diverse as human infertility and breeding of endangered species.

Conclusion

Molecular biology offers an array of new techniques that make possible the characterization of the repertoire of genes expressed solely by the epididymis. This characterization will permit functional roles to be directly assigned to some proteins based on homologies with genes from other tissues or species. Identification of the role of other proteins will require more difficult approaches such as gene knockout technology. The intent is that specific aspects of sperm maturation will be understood and this will lead eventually to a holistic understanding of maturation.

Appendix 1. Key to References in Table 1

[1] **Brooks DE and Higgins S** (1980) Characterisation and androgen-dependence of proteins associated with luminal fluid and spermatozoa in the rat epididymis *Journal of Reproduction and Fertility* **59** 363–375; [2] **Lea OA, Petrusz P and French F** (1978) Purification and localisation of acidic epididymal glycoprotein (AEG): a sperm coating protein secreted by the rat epididymis *International Journal of Andrology* Supplement **2** 592–607; [3] **Rankin TL, Tsuruta KJ, Holland MK, Griswold MD and Orgebin-Crist M-C** (1992) Isolation, immunolocalisation, and sperm association of three proteins of 18, 25 and 29 kilodaltons secreted by the mouse epididymis *Biology of Reproduction* **46** 747–766 ; [4] **Eberspaecher U, Roosterman D, Krätzschmar J, Haendler B, Habenicht UF, Becker A, Quensel C, Petri T, Schleuning WD and Donner P** (1995) Mouse androgen-dependent epididymal glycoprotein CRISP-1 (DE/AEG): isolation, biochemical characterization, and expression in recombinant form *Molecular Reproduction and Development* **42** 157–172; [5] **Hayashi M** (1995) Analysis of the human acidic epididymal glycoprotein-like molecule: isolation of cDNA and tissue localization *Hokkaido Igaku Zasshi* **70** 743–753; [6] **Hayashi M, Fujimoto S, Takano H, Ushiki T, Abe K, Ishikura H, Yoshida MC, Kirchhoff C, Ishibashi T and**

Kasahara M (1996) Characterization of a human glycoprotein with a potential role in sperm–egg fusion: cDNA cloning, immunohistochemical localization, and chromosomal assignment of the gene (AEGL1) *Genomics* **32** 367–374; [7] **Rankin TL, Ong DE and Orgebin-Crist MC** (1992) The 18-kDa mouse epididymal protein (MEP 10) binds retinoic acid *Biology of Reproduction* **46** 767–771; [8] **Regalado F, Pĺerez Martĺinez M, Lĺopez de Haro MS and Nieto A** (1994) Isolation and characterization of two isoforms of a retinoic acid-binding protein from rabbit epididymal secretions *Biochimica et Biophysica Acta* **1200** 235–240; [9] **Morel L, Dufaure JP and Depeiges A** (1993) LESP, an androgen-regulated lizard epididymal secretory protein family identified as a new member of the lipocalin superfamily *Journal of Biological Chemistry* **268** 10274–10281; [10] **Usselman MC and Cone RA** (1983) Rat sperm are mechanically immobilized in the caudal epididymis by "immobilin," a high molecular weight glycoprotein *Biology of Reproduction* **29** 1241–1253; [11] **Hinton BT, Palladino MA, Mattmueller DR, Bard D and Good K** (1991) Expression and activity of gamma-glutamyl transpeptidase in the rat epididymis *Molecular Reproduction and Development* **28** 40–46; [12] **Veri JP, Hermo L and Robaire B** (1993) Immunocytochemical localization of the Yf subunit of glutathione S-transferase P shows regional variation in the staining of epithelial cells of the testis, efferent ducts, and epididymis of the male rat *Journal of Andrology* **14** 23–44; [13] **Veri JP, Hermo L and Robaire B** (1994) Immunocytochemical localization of glutathione *S*-transferase Yo subunit in the rat testis and epididymis *Journal of Andrology* **15** 415–434 ; [14] **Mattmueller DR and Hinton BT** (1991) *In vivo* secretion and association of clusterin (SGP-2) in luminal fluid with spermatozoa in the rat testis and epididymis *Molecular Reproduction and Development* **30** 62–69; [15] **O'Bryan MK, Mallidis C, Murphy BF and Baker HW** (1994) Immunohistological localization of clusterin in the male genital tract in humans and marmosets *Biology of Reproduction* **50** 502–509; [16] **Syntin P, Dacheux F, Druart X, Gatti JL, Okamura N and Dacheux JL** (1996) Characterization and identification of proteins secreted in the various regions of the adult boar epididymis *Biology of Reproduction* **55** 956–974; [17] **Barber JA, Farris JA, Troedsson MHT, Crabo BG and Foster DN** (1996) Nucleotide sequence of the complementary DNA encoding equine clusterin *Animal Biotechnology* **7** 113–123; [18] **Cheng CY, Mathur PP and Grima J** (1988) Structural analysis of clusterin and its subunits in ram rete testis fluid *Biochemistry* **27** 4079–4088 [19] **Perry AC, Jones R, Niang LS, Jackson RM and Hall L** (1992) Genetic evidence for an androgen-regulated epididymal secretory glutathione peroxidase whose transcript does not contain a selenocysteine codon *Biochemical Journal* **285** 863–870; [20] **Ghyselinck NB and Dufaure JP** (1990) A mouse cDNA sequence for epididymal androgen-regulated proteins related to glutathione peroxidase *Nucleic Acids Research* **18** 7144; [21] **Ghyselinck NB, Dufaure I, Lareyre JJ, Rigaudière N, Mattéi MG and Dufaure JP** (1993) Structural organization and regulation of the gene for the androgen-dependent glutathione peroxidase-like protein specific to the mouse epididymis *Molecular Endocrinology* **7** 258–272; [22] **Okamura N, Iwaki Y, Hiramoto S, Tamba M, Bannai S, Sugita Y, Syntin P, Dacheux F and Dacheux JL** (1997) Molecular cloning and characterization of the epididymis-specific glutathione peroxidase-like protein secreted in the porcine epididymal fluid *Biochimica et Biophysica Acta* **1336** 99–109; [23] **Perry AC, Jones R and Hall L** (1993) Isolation and characterization of a rat cDNA clone encoding a secreted superoxide dismutase reveals the epididymis to be a major site of its expression *Biochemical Journal* **293** 21–25; [24] **Sosa MA, Barbieri AM and Bertini F** (1996) Purification and characterization of beta-galactosidase from rat epididymal fluid *Andrologia* **28** 217–221; [25] **Hall JC, Perez FM, Kochins JG, Pettersen CA, Li Y, Tubbs CE and LaMarche MD** (1996) Quantification and localization of *N*-acetyl-beta-D-hexosaminidase in the adult rat testis and epididymis *Biology of Reproduction* **54** 914–929; [26] **Bamberg E, Dorner F and Stöckl W** (1975) Purification of *N*-acetyl-hexosaminidase from boar epididymis by affinity chromatography *Experientia* **31** 516–518; [27] **Pokorny M and Glaudemans CP** (1975) Purification of *N*-acetyl beta-D-hexosaminidase from bull epididymis by affinity chromatography *FEBS Letter* **50** 66–69; [28] **Moore A, Hall L and Hamilton DW** (1990) An 18-kDa androgen-regulated protein that modifies galactosyltransferase activity is synthesized by the rat caput epididymidis, but has no structural similarity to rat milk alphalactalbumin *Biology of Reproduction* **43** 497–506; [29] **Harris GC, Frayne J and Nicholson HD** (1996) Epididymal oxytocin in the rat: its origin and regulation *International Journal of Andrology* **19** 278–286; [30] **Knickerbocker JJ, Sawyer HR, Amann RP, Tekpetey FR and Niswender GD** (1988) Evidence for the presence of oxytocin in the ovine epididymis *Biology of Reproduction* **39** 391–397; [31] **Kilpatrick DL and Rosenthal JL** (1986) The proenkephalin gene is widely expressed within the male and female reproductive systems of the rat and hamster *Endocrinology* **119** 370–374; [32] **Iusem ND, Pineiro L, Blaquier JA and Belocopitow E** (1989) Identification of a major secretory glycoprotein from rat epididymis: interaction with spermatozoa *Biology of Reproduction* **40** 307–316; [33] **Pryor JL, Xu W, Moore A, Ensrud KM and Hamilton DW** (1994) Putative rat sperm lipid-binding protein: isolation and partial characterisation *Molecular Reproduction and Development* **39** 289–296; [34] **Cornwall GA and Hsia N** (1997) ADAM7, a member of the ADAM (a disintegrin and metalloprotease) gene family is specifically expressed in the mouse anterior pituitary and epididymis *Endocrinology* **138** 4262–4272; [35] **Ghyselinck NB, Jimenez C, Lefrancois AM and Dufaure JP** (1990) Molecular cloning of a cDNA for androgen-regulated proteins secreted by the mouse epididymis *Journal of Molecular Endocrinology* **4** 5–12; [36] **Vernon RB** (1986) Studies of a product secreted by the mouse epididymis that associates specifically with the surface of the sperm tail *Dissertation Abstracts International, B (Sciences and Engineering)* **46** 2522; [37] **Feuchter FA, Tabet AJ and Green MF** (1988) Maturation antigen of the mouse sperm flagellum. I. Analysis of its secretion, association with sperm, and function *American Journal of Anatomy* **181** 67–76; [38] **Naz RK, Joseph A, Lee Y, Ahmad K and Bhargava MM** (1994) Expression of scatter factor/hepatocyte growth factor is regionally correlated with the initiation of sperm motility in murine male genital tract: is scatter factor/hepatocyte growth factor involved in initiation of sperm motility? *Molecular Reproduction and Development* **38** 431–439; [39] **Cornwall GA, Orgebin-Crist M-C and Hann SR** (1992) The CRES gene: a unique testis-regulated gene related to the cystatin family is highly restricted in its expression to the proximal region of the mouse epididymis *Molecular Endocrinology* **6**

1653–1664; [40] **Barksdale ZL, Caldwell SE, Aarons DJ, Young SB and Poirer GR** (1997) Characterisation of the guanidinobenzoatase in the epididymal fluids of the mouse *Molecular Reproduction and Development* **47** 204–209; [41] **Wang LF, Miao SY, Zong SD Bai Y and Koide SS** (1994) Gene encoding a mammalian epididymal protein *Biochemistry and Molecular Biology International* **34** 1131–1136; [42] **Nieto A, Gutierrez Sagal R and Perez Martinez M** (1997) Isolation and characterisation of a rabbit epididymal secretory glycoprotein that associates to the spermatozoon surface *Molecular Reproduction and Development* **46** 337–343; [43] **El Etreby MF, Beier HM, Elger W, Mahrous AT and Töpert M** (1983) Immunocytochemical localization of uteroglobin in the genital tract of male rabbits *Cell and Tissue Research* **229** 61–73; [44] **Wilson WL and Oliphant G** (1987) Isolation and biochemical characterization of the subunits of the rabbit sperm acrosome stabilizing factor *Biology of Reproduction* **37** 159–169; [45] **Nixon B, Hardy CM, Clarke HG, Jones RC and Holland MK** (1998) REP38: a rabbit epididymal secretory protein present on spermatozoa *Proceedings of The Boden Conference on The Epididymis: Cellular and Molecular Aspects* 20; [46] **Moore HD** (1981) Glycoprotein secretions of the epididymis in the rabbit and hamster: localization on epididymal spermatozoa and the effect of specific antibodies on fertilization *in vivo. Journal of Experimental Zoology* **215** 77–85; [47] **Coutu L, Des Rosiers P and Sullivan R** (1996) Purification of P26h: a hamster sperm protein *Biochemistry and Cell Biology* **74** 227–231; [48] **Boue F, Blais J and Sullivan R** (1996) Surface localization of P34H an epididymal protein during maturation capacitation and acrosome reaction of human spermatozoa *Biology of Reproduction* **54** 1009–1017; [49] **Serres C and Kann ML** (1984) Motility induction in hamster spermatozoa from caput epididymidis: effects of forward motility protein (FMP) and calmodulin inhibitor *Reproduction, Nutrition, Development* **24** 81–94; [50] **Acott TS and Hoskins DD** (1978) Bovine sperm forward motility protein. Partial purification and characterization *Journal of Biological Chemistry* **253** 6744–6750; [51] **Kirchhoff C, Osterhoff C and Young L** (1996) Molecular cloning and characterization of HE1, a major secretory protein of the human epididymis *Biology of Reproduction* **54** 847–856; [52] **Fröhlich O and Young LG** (1996) Molecular cloning and characterization of EPI-1, the major protein in chimpanzee (*Pan troglodytes*) cauda epididymal fluid *Biology of Reproduction* **54** 857–864; [53] **Perry AC, Jones R and Hall L** (1995) The monkey ESP14.6 mRNA a novel transcript expressed at high levels in the epididymis *Gene* **153** 291–292; [54] **Pera I, Ivell R and Kirchhoff C** (1994) Regional variation of specific gene expression in the dog epididymis as revealed by in-situ transcript hybridization *International Journal of Andrology* **17** 324–330; [55] **Osterhoff C, Kirchhoff C, Krull N and Ivell R** (1994) Molecular cloning and characterisation of a novel human sperm antigen (HE2) specifically expressed in the proximal epididymis *Biology of Reproduction* **50** 516–525; [56] **Kirchhoff C, Pera I, Rust W and Ivell R** (1994) Major human epididymis-specific gene product, HE3, is the first representative of a novel gene family *Molecular Reproduction and Development* **37** 130–137; [57] **Xu WD, Wang LF, Miao SY, Zhao M, Fan HY, Zong SD, Wu YW, Shi XQ and Koide SS** (1996) Identification of a rabbit epididymal protein gene *Archives of Andrology* **37** 135–141; [58] **Kirchhoff C, Habben I, Ivell R and Krull N** (1991) A major human epididymis-specific cDNA encodes a protein with sequence homology to extracellular proteinase inhibitors *Biology of Reproduction* **45** 350–357; [59] **Uhlenbruck F, Sinowatz F, Amselgruber W, Kirchhoff C and Ivell R** (1993) Tissue-specific gene expression as an indicator of epididymis-specific functional status in the boar, bull and stallion *International Journal of Andrology* **16** 53–61; [60] **Kirchhoff C, Krull N, Pera I and Ivell R** (1993) A major mRNA of the human epididymal pricipal cells, HE5, encodes the leucocyte differentiation CDw52 antigen peptide backbone *Molecular Reproduction and Development* **34** 8–15; [61] **Osterhoff C, Ivell R and Kirchhoff C** (1997) Cloning of a human epididymis-specific mRNA, HE6, encoding a novel member of the seven transmembrane-domain receptor superfamily *DNA and Cell Biology* **16** 379–389; [62] **Hutter H, Hammer A, Blaschitz A, Hartmann M, Mahnert W, Sedlmayr P, Primus G, Rosenkranz C, Gebru G, Henkel R and Dohr G** (1996) The monoclonal antibody GZS-1 detects a maturation-associated antigen of human spermatozoa that is also present on the surface of human mononuclear blood cells *Journal of Reproductive Immunology* **30** 115–132; [63] **Komori S, Kameda K, Sakata K, Hasegawa A, ToJi H, TsuJi Y, Shibahara H, Koyama K and IsoJima S** (1997) Characterization of fertilization-blocking monoclonal antibody 1G12 with human sperm-immobilizing activity *Clinical and Experimental Immunology* **109** 547–54; [64] **Poulton TA, Everard D, Baxby K and Parslow JM** (1996) Characterisation of a sperm coating auto-antigen reacting with antisperm antibodies of infertile males using monoclonal antibodies *British Journal of Obstetrics and Gynaecology* **103** 463–467; [65] **Tulsiani DR, Coleman VD and Touster O** (1988) Rat epididymal alpha-D-mannosidase: purification, carbohydrate composition, substrate specificity, and antibody production *Archives of Biochemistry and Biophysics* **267** 60–68; [66] **Beccari T, Appolloni MG, Costanzi E, Stinchi S, Stirling JL, Dellafazia MA, Servillo G, Viola MP and Orlacchio A** (1997) Lysosomal alpha-mannosidases of mouse tissues – characteristics of the isoenzymes, and cloning and expression of a full-length cDNA *Biochemical Journal* **327** 45–49; [67] **Okamura N, Tamba M, Liao HJ, Onoe S, Sugita Y, Dacheux F and Dacheux JL** (1995) Cloning of complementary DNA encoding a 135-kilodalton protein secreted from porcine corpus epididymis and its identification as an epididymis-specific alpha-mannosidase *Molecular Reproduction and Development* **42** 141–148; [68] **Dacheux F and Dacheux JL** (1988) Immunocytochemical localization of antagglutinin in the boar epididymis *Cell and Tissue Research* **252** 329–337

Appendix 2. Key to References in Table 3

[1] **Brooks DE and Higgins S** (1980) Characterisation and androgen-dependence of proteins associated with luminal fluid and spermatozoa in the rat epididymis *Journal of Reproduction and Fertility* **59** 363–375; [2] **Charest NJ, Joseph DR, Wilson EM and French FS** (1989) Molecular cloning of complementary deoxyribonucleic acid for an androgen-regulated

epididymal protein: sequence homology with metalloproteins *Molecular Endocrinology* **2** 999–1004; [3] **Kratzschmar J, Haendler B, Eberspaecher U, Roosterman D, Donner P and Schleuning WD** (1996) The human cysteine-rich secretory protein (CRISP) family. Primary structure and tissue distribution of CRISP-1, CRISP-2 and CRISP-3 *European Journal of Biochemistry* **236** 827–836; [4] **Lea OA, Petrusz P and French F** (1978) Purification and localisation of acidic epididymal glycoprotein (AEG): a sperm coating protein secreted by the rat epididymis *International Journal of Andrology* Supplement **2** 592–607; [5] **Jones R, Brown CR, von Glos KI and Parker MG** (1980) Hormonal regulation of protein synthesis in the rat epididymis: characterisation of androgen-dependent and testicular fluid-dependent proteins *Biochemical Journal* **188** 667–676; [6] **Garberi JC, Fontana JD and Blaquier JA** (1982) Carbohydrate composition of specific rat epididymal protein *International Journal of Andrology* **5** 619–626; [7] **Wong PY and Tsang AY** (1982) Studies on the binding of a 32K rat epididymal protein to rat epididymal spermatozoa *Biology of Reproduction* **27** 1239–1246; [8] **Moore A, Ensrud KM, White TW, Frethem CD and Hamilton DW** (1994) Rat epididymis-specific sperm maturation antigens. I. Evidence that the 26 kD 4E9 antigen found on rat caudal epididymal sperm tail is derived from a protein secreted by the epididymis *Molecular Reproduction and Development* **37** 181–194; [9] **Xu W and Hamilton DW** (1996) Identification of the rat epididymis-secreted 4E9 antigen as protein E: further biochemical characterisation of the highly homologous epididymal secretory proteins D and E *Molecular Reproduction and Development* **43** 347–357; [10] **Xu WH, Ensrud KM and Hamilton DW** (1997) The 26 kD protein recognised on rat cauda epididymal sperm by monoclonal antibody 4E9 has internal peptide sequence that is identical to the secreted form of epididymal protein E *Molecular Reproduction and Development* **46** 377–382; [11] **Hall JC, Tubbs CE, Li YH and Ashraf S** (1996) Characterisation of high-affinity protein D binding sites on the surface of rat epididymal spermatozoa *Biochemistry and Molecular Biology International* **40** 1003–1010; [12] **Cohen DJ, Munuce MJ and Cuasnicu PS** (1996) Mammalian sperm–egg fusion – the development of rat oolemma fusibility during oogenesis involves the appearance of binding sites for sperm protein DE *Biology of Reproduction* **27** 1239–1246; [13] **Martinez SP, Conesa D and Cuasnicu PS** (1995) Potential contraceptive use of epididymal proteins: evidence for the participation of specific antibodies against rat epididymal protein DE in male and female fertility inhibition *Journal of Reproductive Immunology* **29** 31–45; [14] **Eberspaecher U, Roosterman D, Krätzschmar J, Haendler B, Habenicht UF, Becker A, Quensel C, Petri T, Schleuning WD and Donner P** (1995) Mouse androgen-dependent epididymal glycoprotein CRISP-1 (DE/AEG): isolation, biochemical characterization, and expression in recombinant form *Molecular Reproduction and Development* **42** 157–172; [15] **Rankin TL, Tsuruta KJ, Holland MK, Griswold MD and Orgebin-Crist M-C** (1992) Isolation, immunolocalisation, and sperm association of three proteins of 18, 25 and 29 kilodaltons secreted by the mouse epididymis *Biology of Reproduction* **46** 747–766; [16] **Mizuki N and Kasahara M** (1992) Mouse submandibular glands express an androgen-regulated transcript encoding an acidic epididymal glycoprotein-like molecule *Molecular and Cellular Endocrinology* **89** 25–32; [17] **Kasahara M, Hayashi M, Yoshida MC, Nadeau JH, Fujimoto S and Ishibashi T** (1995) Mapping of acidic epididymal glycoprotein (Aeg) genes to mouse chromosome 17 *Mammalian Genome* **6** 52–54; [18] **Kasahara M, Gutknecht J, Brew K, Spurr N and Goodfellow PN** (1992) Cloning and mapping of a testis-specific gene with sequence similarity to a sperm-coating glycoprotein gene *Genomics* **5** 527–534; [19] **Foster JA and Gerton GL** (1996) Autoantigen 1 of the guinea pig sperm acrosome is the homologue of mouse Tpx-1 and human TPX1 and is a member of the cysteine-rich secretory protein (CRISP) family *Molecular Reproduction and Development* **44** 221–229; **Hardy DM, Huang TTF, Driscoll WJ, Tung KSK and Wild GC** (1988) Purification and characterisation of the primary acrosomal autoantigen of guinea pig epididymal spermatozoa *Biology of Reproduction* **38** 423–437; [20] **Hayashi M** (1995) Analysis of the human acidic epididymal glycoprotein-like molecule: isolation of cDNA and tissue localization *Hokkaido Igaku Zasshi* **70** 743–753; [21] **Hayashi M, Fujimoto S, Takano H, Ushiki T, Abe K, Ishikura H, Yoshida MC, Kirchhoff C, Ishibashi T and Kasahara M** (1996) Characterisation of a human glycoprotein with a potential role in sperm–egg fusion: cDNA cloning, immunohistochemical localisation, and chromosomal assignment of the gene (AEGL1) *Genomics* **32** 367–374

References

Amann RP, Hammerstedt RH and Veeramachaneni DN (1993) The epididymis and sperm maturation: a perspective *Reproduction Development and Fertility* **5** 361–381

Brooks DE (1981) Secretion of proteins and glycoproteins by the rat epididymis: regional differences, androgen-dependence and effects of protease inhibitors, procaine and tunicamycin *Biology of Reproduction* **25** 1099–1117

Brooks DE (1986) Androgen regulated epididymal secretory proteins associated with post testicular sperm development *Annales of the New York Academy of Science* **513** 179–194

Brooks DE and Higgins S (1980) Characterisation and hormonal dependence of proteins associated with luminal fluid and spermatozoa in the rat epididymis *Journal of Reproduction and Fertility* **59** 363–375

Clouthier DE, Avarbock MR, Maika SD, Hammer RE and Brinster RL (1996) Rat spermatogenesis in mouse testis *Nature* **381** 418–421

Cooper TG (1986) *The Epididymis, Sperm Maturation And Fertilisation* Springer-Verlag, Berlin

Dacheux J-L, Druart X, Fouchecourt S, Syntin P, Gatti J-L, Okamura N and Dacheux F (1998) Role of epididymal secretory proteins in sperm maturation *Journal of Reproduction and Fertility Supplement* **53** 99–107

Drevet JR, Lareyre J-J, Schwaab V, Vernet P and Dufaure J-P (1998) The PEA protein of the Ets oncogene family is a putative transcription modulator of the mouse epididymis-specific glutathione peroxidase gene gpx5 *Molecular Reproduction and Development* **49** 131–140

Fayrer-Hosken RA, Caudle AB and Shur BD (1991)

Galactosyltransferase activity is restricted to the plasma membranes of equine and bovine sperm *Molecular Reproduction and Development* **28** 74–78

Garrett JE Garrett SH and Douglass J (1990) A spermatozoa associated factor regulates proenkephalin gene expression in the rat epididymis *Molecular Endocrinology* **4** 108–118

Hegde UC (1997) Epididymal sperm maturation proteins *Indian Journal of Biochemistry & Biophysics* **33** 103–110

Hinton BT, Lan Z-J, Rudolph DB and Labus J C (1998) Testicular regulation of epididymal gene expression *Journal of Reproduction and Fertility Supplement* **53** 47–57

Holland MK and Orgebin-Crist M-C (1988) Characterisation and hormonal regulation of protein synthesis by the murine epididymis *Biology of Reproduction* **38** 487–496

Holland MK Vreeburg JTM and Orgebin-Crist M-C (1992) Testicular regulation of epididymal protein secretion *Journal of Andrology* **13** 266–273

Huang HFS and Johnson AD (1975) Amino acid composition of epididymal plasma of mouse, rat, rabbit and sheep *Comparative Biochemistry and Physiology* **50B** 359–362

Ivell R, Pera I, Ellerbrock K, Beiglbock A, Gebhardt K, Osterhoff C and Kirchhoff C (1998) The dog as a model system to study epididymal gene expression *Journal of Reproduction and Fertility Supplement* **53** 33–45

Jones R, von Glos KI and Brown CR (1980) The synthesis of a sperm coating protein in the initial segment of the rat epididymis is stimulated by factors in testicular fluid *ICRS Medical Science* **8** 56

Jones RC (1987) Changes in protein composition of luminal fluids along the epididymis of the tammar wallaby, *Macropus eugenii. Journal of Reproduction and Fertility* **80** 193–199

Kirchhoff C, Osterhoff C, Habben I and Ivell R (1990) Cloning and analysis of mRNAs expressed specifically in the human epididymis *International Journal of Andrology* **13** 155–167

Klinefelter GR and Hamilton DW (1984) Organ culture of rabbit epididymal tubules in a perifusion chamber *Journal of Andrology* **5** 243–258

Koskimies AI and Kormano M (1975) Proteins in fluid from different segments of the rat epididymis *Journal of Reproduction and Fertility* **43** 345–348

Lan Z-J, Labus JC and Hinton BT (1998) Regulation of gamma-glutamyl transpeptidase catalytic and protein level in the initial segment of the rat epididymis by testicular factors; role of basic fibroblast growth factor *Biology of Reproduction* **58** 197–206

Layre J-L, Marie-Genevieve M, Kasper S, Newcomer ME, Ong DE, Matusik J and Orgebin-Crist M-C (1998) Structure and putative function of a murine epididymal retinoic acid-binding protein (mE-RABP) *Journal of Reproduction and Fertility Supplement* **53** 59–65

Lindsey S and Wilkinson MF (1996) Homeobox genes and male reproductive development *Journal of Assisted Reproduction and Genetics* **13** 182–192

Maiti S, Doskow J, Li S, Nhim RP, Lawlor DA, Levan K, Lindsey JS and Wilkinson MF (1996) The *Pem* homeobox gene: androgen dependent and independent promotors and tissue-specific alternative RNA splicing *Journal of Biological Chemistry* **271** 17536–17546

Olson GE and Hinton BT (1985) Regional differences in luminal fluid polypeptides of the rat testis and epididymis revealed by two dimensional gel electrophoresis *Journal of Andrology* **6** 20–34

Orgebin-Crist M-C (1998) The epididymis across 24 centuries *Journal of Reproduction and Fertilty Supplement* **53** 285–292

Syntin P, Dacheux F, Druart X, Gatti, JL, Okamura N and Dacheux JL (1996) Characterisation and identification of proteins secreted in the various regions of the adult boar epididymis *Biology of Reproduction* **55** 956–974

Vreeburg JTM, Holland MK, Cornwall GA and Orgebin-Crist M-C (1990) Secretion and transport of mouse epididymal proteins after injection of ^{35}S-methionine *Biology of Reproduction* **43** 113–120

Vreeburg JTM, Holland MK and Orgebin-Crist M-C (1992) Binding of epididymal proteins to rat spermatozoa *in vivo. Biology of Reproduction* **47** 588–597

Wilkins MR, Williams KL Appel RD and Hochstrasser DF (1997) *Proteome Research: New Frontiers In Functional Genomics.* Springer-Verlag, Berlin

Wolpert L, Beddington R, Brockes J, Jessell T, Lawerence P and Meyerowitz E (1998) *Principles of Development* Oxford University Press, Oxford

Journal of Reproduction and Fertility Supplement **53**, 211–214

Regulation of apoptotic cell death in the rat epididymis

B. Robaire and X. Fan

Department of Pharmacology and Therapeutics, McGill University, 3655 Drummond Street, Montréal, Québec, Canada, H3Y 3H7

The rat epididymis decreases markedly in weight after orchidectomy. In these studies, we demonstrate that a time-dependent wave of apoptotic cell death occurs in some principal cells after orchidectomy. This wave moves coincidentally with the luminal content of the epididymis. Androgen treatment at the time of orchidectomy can prevent apoptotic death in all regions of the epididymis except the initial segment (Robaire and Hermo, 1988, similar to zone 1a defined by Reid and Cleland, 1957). After unilateral efferent duct ligation, apoptotic cell death in the initial segment of the epididymis is similar to that seen after orchidectomy, reduced in the caput (zones 1b,c, 2 and 3 as defined by Reid and Cleland, 1957) and absent from the corpus (defined as zones 4, by Reid and Cleland, 1957) and cauda epididymidis (defined as zones 5 and 6 by Reid and Cleland, 1957). Together, these results indicate that principal cells differ in their responses to androgens and other testicular factors both in any given cross-section and with respect to their position along the epididymis.

Introduction

Pioneering studies on the mammalian excurrent duct system by Benoit have established that the epididymis is dependent on the presence of testicular androgens (Benoit, 1926). Androgen withdrawal by orchidectomy results in a time-dependent marked weight loss of the tissue. This weight loss is in part (about 50%) due to the loss of spermatozoa and fluid from the lumen of the epididymis and in part (about 50%) due to changes in the epithelium of the tissue (Robaire *et al.*, 1977). From histological observations, it is clear that, after orchidectomy, epithelial cells become smaller and less well developed (Benoit, 1926; Robaire *et al.*, 1977), and that there is increased endocytosis by principal cells (Moore and Bedford, 1979). The content of large apical vacuoles in principal cells decreases abruptly, and there is a concomitant rise in the number of distinct dense granules and intra-epithelial lymphocytes. Ultrastructurally, orchidectomy causes the disappearance of vesicles from the cell apex, a reduction in smooth and rough endoplasmic reticulum, a drop in the volume of Golgi cisternae and an increase in lysosome content. These observations suggest a reduction in both absorption and secretion by principal cells. In contrast to the regressive response of principal cells, the ultrastructure of clear cells in the cauda epididymidis and of apical cells in the caput epididymidis appear unchanged up to 14 days after orchidectomy (Moore and Bedford, 1979).

Apoptosis is a ‘physiological’ or active cell death that is characterized by cell shrinkage, nuclear condensation, membrane blebbing, and membrane changes that lead to phagocytosis of the affected cell by its neighbours or by macrophages (Cohen, 1994). It is an active process that requires protein and RNA synthesis and the induction of a number of genes (Guenette *et al.*, 1994). DNA fragmentation by an endonuclease into nucleosomal-sized fragments (180–200 bases) is a hallmark of apoptosis. Apoptosis can be detected by *in situ* staining using the TUNEL method (labelling of 3′OH breaks in DNA) or by the presence of a DNA ladder on gel electrophoresis (Tenniswood *et al.*, 1994).

The questions addressed in the present studies are whether apoptotic cell death is involved in the androgen dependent weight loss found in the rat epididymis after orchidectomy, and if so, whether this response is dependent on androgens, testicular factors or both.

Materials and Methods

Three complementary experiments, using adult male Sprague–Dawley rats (375–400 g), were undertaken to address the above questions. In the first experiment, nine groups of adult male Sprague–Dawley rats were orchidectomized; an additional group was sham operated and served as control. One epididymis was perfused-fixed after 0.5, 0.75, 1, 2, 3, 4, 5, 6, or 7 days and the localization of apoptotic cells was determined in the initial segment, caput, corpus and cauda epididymidis by detection with the *in situ* TUNEL assay (Gavrieli, 1992). The presence of a DNA ladder was assessed in DNA isolated from the other epididymis by using agarose gel electrophoresis.

In the second experiment, rats were either left intact or orchidectomized and given either corn oil (0.2 ml day^{-1}) or treated with testosterone (0.5 or 5.0 mg per rat per day) or 5α-dihydrotestosterone (DHT, 5 mg per rat per day) to determine the effect of androgens on the presence of apoptosis. Animals were killed on days 1, 2, 3 and 7 after surgery and the epididymides were fixed with Bouin's fixative by perfusion.

In the third experiment, rats were either left intact or had their efferent ducts ligated unilaterally. Animals were killed 0.5, 0.75, 1, 2, 3, 4, 5, 6, 7, 8 and 9 days after surgery. Both epididymides were fixed as described above and the effects of withdrawal of the luminal contents on apoptosis in the various regions of the epididymis were determined.

Results

No apoptotic cells were seen in any segment of the control epididymis. After orchidectomy, apoptotic cell death was localized specifically to principal cells throughout the rat epididymis. The presence of apoptosis was confirmed with the observation of a ladder of nucleosomal sized DNA fragmentation (Fan and Robaire, 1998).

Apoptotic cells first appeared in the epithelium of the initial segment of the epididymis 18 h after orchidectomy, reached a maximum on day 2, and disappeared by day 5 after orchidectomy (Fig. 1). In the caput epididymidis, apoptosis was first found after 24 h, reached a maximum by day 3, and was detectable until day 5. In the corpus epididymidis, apoptosis was first seen on day 4, reached a peak on day 5, and was undetectable by day 6 after orchidectomy. In the cauda epididymidis, apoptosis was first seen on day 5, reached a peak on day 6, and was occasionally detected on day 7 (Fig. 1). A similar wave-like pattern was obtained whether data were expressed as the number of apoptotic cells per 100 tubules or as the percentage of tubules showing any apoptotic cells. This wave-like pattern of apoptotic cell death after orchidectomy coincided with the outward movement of the luminal content.

Even at very high doses, testosterone or DHT could not completely prevent apoptosis in the initial segment of the epididymis after orchidectomy (Fig. 2). However, apoptosis in the caput, corpus and cauda epididymidis after orchidectomy could be completely prevented by androgen treatment (Fan and Robaire, 1998). In the caput epididymidis, the rapid rise in the number of apoptotic cells between days 1 and 3 after orchidectomy was remarkably reduced by treatment with a low dose of testosterone so that no apoptotic cells per tubules were seen either 1 or 2 days after orchidectomy. The high dose of testosterone or DHT entirely prevented apoptotic cell death induced by orchidectomy in the caput epididymidis. In the corpus and cauda epididymidis, apoptosis was not seen in the control group or any of the androgen treated groups at any time. On day 7 after orchidectomy, no apoptotic cells were found in any region of the epididymis in any of the five groups.

The epithelial cells of the initial segment of the epididymis started to undergo apoptotic cell death by 18 h after efferent duct ligation. This response reached a maximum on day 2, and then was gradually reduced to zero by day 5 (data not shown). Thus, the pattern, incidence and time course of

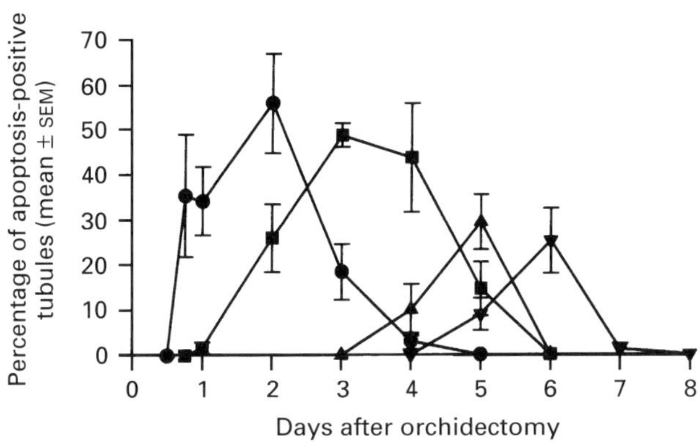

Fig. 1. Percentage of apoptosis-positive tubules in the rat epididymis after orchidectomy. Adult males were orchidectomized and, at the times indicated on the x-axis, the percentage of apoptosis-positive tubules in the initial segment (●), caput (■), corpus (▲) and cauda (▼) epididymidis were assessed using the TUNEL staining method. $n = 4$ rats per time point.

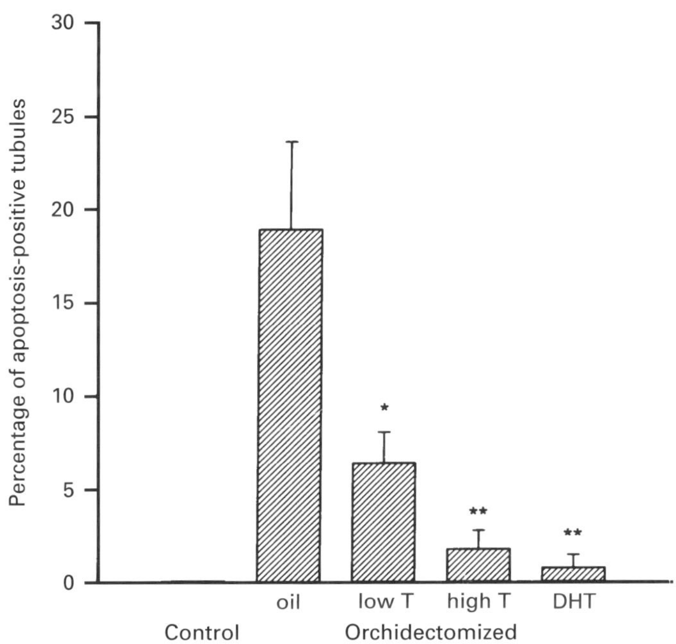

Fig. 2. Percentage of apoptosis-positive tubules in initial segment of the epididymis of control rats, or rats that had been orchidectomized and treated with oil, a low dose of testosterone (low T, 0.5 mg per rat per day), a high dose of testosterone (high T, 5 mg per rat per day) or dihydrotestosterone (DHT). $n = 8$ rats per group; values are significantly different from oil control * $P < 0.05$ and **$P < 0.01$.

apoptosis were similar in the initial segment of the epididymis in orchidectomized animals and in animals with ligated efferent ducts. After efferent duct ligation, apoptosis was first seen on day 2, reached a peak on day 4, and was detectable until day 7 in the caput epididymidis. Moreover, the incidence of apoptotic cells in the caput epididymidis after efferent duct ligation was reduced by more than one order of magnitude when compared with that found after orchidectomy. No apoptotic cells were observed in the corpus or cauda epididymidis, nor were any found in the contralateral epididymis after efferent duct ligation.

Discussion

The data presented here demonstrate that the withdrawal of androgen by orchidectomy induces a wave of apoptotic cell death in the epididymis; apoptosis in the initial segment is caused by withdrawal of androgen as well as by the removal of luminal components coming from the testis.

Ligation of efferent ductules was shown by Nicander *et al.* (1983) to result in a "...focal degeneration in the epithelium..." in the initial segment (zone 1a) by 24 h after surgery; this degeneration was reduced by 48 h after surgery. In the caput epididymidis (zones 1b,c and 2), similar degeneration was found by day 3; by days 5–7, this difference between the initial segment and the caput epididymidis had disappeared. Although these investigators described the cell degeneration as necrotic cell death, it is likely that the observed cell death was apoptosis. Sufficiently detailed morphological analyses were not done to establish whether cell death was by necrosis or apoptosis; no specific histochemical markers for apoptotic cell death were available at that time. Moreover their results are very similar to those reported by our laboratory (here, and Fan and Robaire, 1998).

These striking results raise several questions. What is the role of apoptosis in a tissue in which epithelial cells do not proliferate? What are the relative contributions of apoptosis, necrosis and cell atrophy to the weight loss after orchidectomy? What are the specific molecular events mediating apoptosis in the epididymis? Are there two distinguishable populations of principal cells in the epididymis, one more dependent on androgens than the other? If so, what is the difference between these cells? This tissue lends itself particularly well to these questions because of the time–space organization of the apoptotic wave after orchidectomy.

These studies were supported by the Medical Research Council of Canada and by NIH (AG08321).

References

Benoit J (1926) Recherches anatomiques, cytologiques et histophysiologiques sur les voies excrétrices du testicule chez les mammifères *Archives d'anatomie et d'histologie* 5 175–412

Cohen JJ (1994) Apoptosis: physiologic cell death *Journal of Laboratory and Clinical Medicine* **124** 761–765

Fan X and Robaire B (1998) Orchidectomy induces a wave of apoptotic cell death in the epididymis *Endocrinology* **139** 2128–3136

Gavrieli Y, Sherman Y and Ben-Sasson SA (1992) Identification of programmed cell death *in situ* via specific labelling of nuclear DNA fragmentation *Journal of Cell Biology* **119** 493–501

Guenette RS, Daehlin L, Mooibroek M, Wong K and Tenniswood M (1994) Thanatogen expression during involution of the rat ventral prostate after castration *Journal of Andrology* **15** 200–210

Moore HDM and Bedford JM (1979) Short-term effects of androgen withdrawal on the structure of different epithelial cells in the rat epididymis *Anatomical Record* **193** 293–312

Nicander L, Osman DI, Ploen L, Bugge HP and Kvisgaard KN (1983) Early effects of efferent ductule ligation on the proximal segment of the rat epididymis *International Journal of Andrology* **6** 91–102

Reid BL and Cleland KW (1957) The structure and function of the epididymis. I. The histology of the rat epididymis *Australian Journal of Zoology* **5** 223–246

Robaire B and Hermo L (1988) Efferent ducts, epididymis, and vas deferens: structure, functions, and their regulation. In *The Physiology of Reproduction* pp 999–1080 Eds E Knobil and J. Neill. Raven Press Ltd, New York

Robaire B, Ewing LL, Zirkin BR and Irby DC (1977) Steroid Δ^4-5α-reductase and 3α-hydroxysteroid dehydrogenase in the rat epididymis *Endocrinology* **101** 1379–1390

Tenniswood M, Taillefer D, Lakins J, Guenette R, Mooibroek M, Daehlin L and Welsh J (1994) Control of gene expression during apoptosis in hormone-dependent tissues. In *Apoptosis II: The Molecular Basis Of Cell Death* pp 283–311 Eds LD Tomei and FO Cope. Cold Spring Harbour Laboratory Press, Cold Spring Harbour

Journal of Reproduction and Fertility Supplement **53**, 215–220

HE2/EP2, an androgen-dependent protein from the epididymis of the chimpanzee, *Pan troglodytes*

L. G. Young[1]*, O. Fröhlich[1] and K. G. Gould[2]

[1]*Department of Physiology, Emory University School of Medicine, Atlanta, GA 30322, USA; and* [2]*Yerkes Regional Primate Research Center, Emory University, Atlanta, GA 30322, USA*

A cDNA clone of chimpanzee EP2 was obtained from epididymal RNA by RT–PCR and was sequenced. Chimpanzee EP2 and human HE2 cDNA were > 99% identical and the proteins were 100% identical. The derived amino acid sequence of chimpanzee EP2 showed a consensus sequence for a leader peptide typical of secreted proteins. Northern blot analysis indicated that expression of the gene encoding chimpanzee EP2 is specific to the epididymis and not to other chimpanzee tissues examined. RT–PCR and northern blot analysis of epididymides recovered from an androgen deprived adult male chimpanzee showed that the expression of EP2 is androgen dependent.

Introduction

In primates, sperm fertilizing capacity is acquired in the epididymis. Spermatozoa leaving the testis are unable to fertilize an oocyte naturally until they have interacted with epididymal secretory products (Gould and Young, 1990). During epididymal transit, the spermatozoa pass through anatomically and physiologically distinct regions: caput epididymidis, corpus epididymidis and cauda epididymidis (Smithwick and Young, 1997). In agreement with the morphological distinction, the different epididymal regions appear to have different physiological roles related to secretion and absorption of luminal contents (Hinton and Palladino, 1995).

It is hypothesized that proteins secreted by the epididymis are essential for sperm maturation (Cornwall and Hann, 1995). In the chimpanzee, spermatozoa from the caput epididymidis are immotile and do not bind to or penetrate chimpanzee ova, whereas spermatozoa from the cauda epididymidis are motile and do bind to and penetrate chimpanzee ova (Gould and Young, 1990). In humans, co-culture of spermatozoa from the caput epididymidis with epididymal tissue results in an increase in sperm motility and in sperm fertilizing capacity (Moore *et al.*, 1992). However, the identity of the epididymal components involved and the mechanisms of their interaction with spermatozoa remain unclear.

Synthesis of specific epididymal proteins is controlled by androgens which act at the nuclear DNA to regulate gene expression. Androgens induce the synthesis of five proteins in the epididymis of castrated rhesus monkeys (Arslan *et al.*, 1986) and of five proteins in cultured human epididymal tissue (Tezon *et al.*, 1987). Again, the identity of these epididymal proteins and their role in post-testicular sperm maturation remain unclear.

Recombinant DNA technology has been used to identify putative secretory proteins of primate epididymis. By differential screening of a human cDNA epididymal library, Kirchhoff *et al.* (1990) identified five clones, HE1–HE5. By RT–PCR, we demonstrated five epididymal genes in the chimpanzee, EP1–EP5, homologous to HE1–HE5. Furthermore, we demonstrated that the cDNA sequence of chimpanzee EP1 and of human HE1 are > 99% identical (Fröhlich and Young, 1996).

Epididymal specificity and androgen dependence were used as initial criteria to identify epididymal secretory proteins most likely to be involved in sperm maturation. We identified a

* Correspondence

cDNA clone, chimpanzee EP2, which codes for a protein secreted specifically by the epididymis and which is subject to androgen regulation.

Materials and Methods

Animals

Epididymal tissue from three adult male chimpanzees (*Pan troglodytes*), designated FS, LZ and BR, was analysed. These animals, aged 45 (59 kg), 20 (58 kg) and 19 (65 kg) years, respectively, were housed in facilities accredited by the American Association for Accreditation of Laboratory Animal Care. Each of these animals had sired offspring and had normal testosterone concentrations and normal semen samples immediately before the time of sampling.

Androgen deprivation

BR, the male chimpanzee used for androgen deprivation, was selected both for reproductive normality and with consideration for the genetic composition of the colony. To induce hypogonadotrophism, BR received injections of 300 mg kg^{-1} $week^{-1}$ of the GnRH agonist Antide (no. 230-13-10, Contraceptive Development Branch, Centre for Population Research, NICHHD) for a total of 6 weeks. Blood samples were obtained from BR twice a week. Serum concentrations of testosterone were determined by radioimmunoassay using kits obtained from Diagnostic Products Corp. (Los Angeles, CA).

Surgical protocols

Ketamine HCl (10–20 mg kg^{-1}) was administered by intramuscular injection and a Metofane/O_2/N_2O mixture was administered by endotracheal tube. The testes with attached epididymides were removed using standard surgical procedures with minimal tissue manipulation. After surgery, FS and LZ were euthanized for clinical reasons unrelated to reproductive function; BR was given Banamine (0.1 mg kg^{-1} four times a day; Schering-Plough, Kenilworth, NJ) to minimize post-operative discomfort during recovery.

The chimpanzee epididymides were subdivided sequentially and frozen in liquid nitrogen. Samples of other tissues were also frozen in liquid nitrogen.

Chimpanzee uterine tissue was obtained from an adult female chimpanzee euthanized for reasons unrelated to reproductive function. The uterine tissue was frozen in liquid nitrogen.

Reverse transcription–PCR analysis of tissue RNA

Total RNA was isolated by acid phenol extraction from sequential segments of chimpanzee epididymis and from chimpanzee testis, kidney and uterus. Aliquots were reverse-transcribed using the SuperScript Preamplification System (Life Technologies, Gaithersburg, MD). Reverse-transcribed samples were subjected to PCR using EP2-specific primers.

The EP2-specific PCR primers were designed on the basis of the cDNA sequence of HE2 (Kirchhoff *et al.*, 1990) (Genbank accession number A18922). The forward primer: 5′-CGGATTCCGGATGCGTTTCC-3′ corresponded to a stretch beginning at position -4 nt relative to the open reading frame. The reverse primer: 5′-GACTCATTGGCCAGATGC-3′ corresponded to a stretch ending at 88 nucleotides into the 3′-untranslated region. The PCR amplification was achieved with 30 cycles of 1 min at 92°C, 1 min at 58° or 60°C and 2 min at 72°C. Based on HE2 (Osterhoff *et al.*, 1994), the amplified PCR product was expected to be 402 bp long and to contain the entire open reading frame.

For determining the sequence of chimpanzee EP2, the PCR product was subcloned into TA

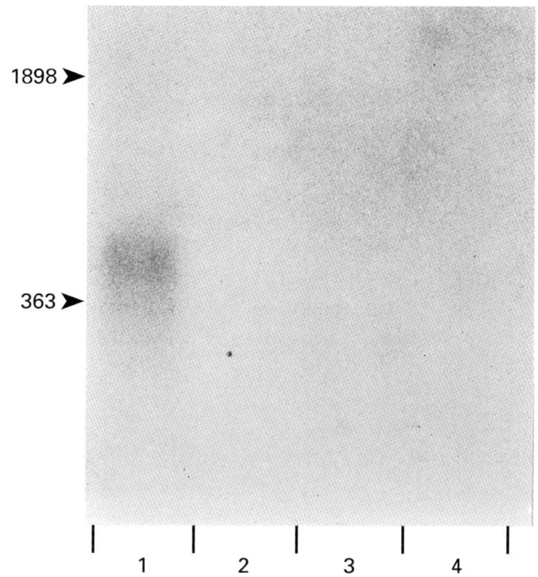

Fig. 1. Northern blot analysis of total RNA (10 μg RNA per lane) isolated from epididymis (lane 1), testis (lane 2), kidney (lane 3) and uterus (lane 4) of an androgen-normal chimpanzee (*Pan troglodytes*). Numbers on the left represent RNA molecular weight standards.

vector pGEM-T (Promega, Madison, WI) and its sequence was determined using the Sequenase 2.0 DNA sequencing kit (Amersham Life Science, Arlington Heights, IL).

Northern blot analysis

Total RNA was separated by electrophoresis on formaldehyde–agarose gels, capillary-blotted to Duralon nylon membrane (Stratagene, La Jolla, CA) and hybridized using a ^{32}P-labelled hybridization probe. This probe was prepared by random hexamer priming using Klenow fragment and the PCR product of chimpanzee EP2 as template. A cDNA probe for glyceraldehyde-3-phosphate dehydrogenase (GAPDH) served as a control (Fröhlich and Young, 1996).

Results

Sequence of EP2

Within the length of the PCR product, the DNA sequence of chimpanzee EP2 was > 99% identical to the human sequence, the only difference being two additional nucleotides (As) in the 3′-untranslated region 1 position after the stop codon. Thus, within the open reading frame, chimpanzee EP2 and human HE2 DNA and protein are identical.

Tissue specificity of EP2

Message for EP2 in chimpanzee epididymis was identified by RT–PCR. By northern blot analysis, message for EP2 (Fig. 1) is detected in chimpanzee epididymis and not in chimpanzee testis, kidney and uterus. EP2 is detected predominantly in the caput epididymidis in the chimpanzee.

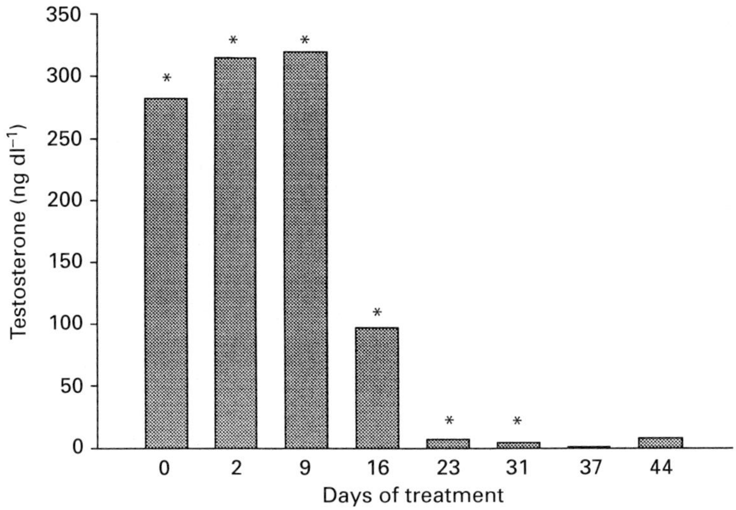

Fig. 2. Time course of androgen deprivation in a chimpanzee (*Pan troglodytes*). *Administration of the GnRH agonist antide; administration stopped at day 31.

Time course of androgen deprivation

As shown in Fig. 2, with 300 mg GnRH agonist kg^{-1} $week^{-1}$, testosterone concentrations fell to minimum values within 23 days and remained suppressed for the duration of the experiment (44 days). At day 44, the animal (BR) was castrated bilaterally.

Androgen dependence of chimpanzee EP2

Northern blot analysis comparing mRNA of EP2 in epididymides from androgen-normal and from an androgen-deprived chimpanzee showed that EP2 is absolutely androgen dependent (Fig. 3). Moreover, using RT–PCR, no signal for EP2 was detected with RNA isolated from androgen-deprived epididymides.

Discussion

The human HE2 clone was isolated by differentially screening for cDNAs present in epididymides but not testes (Kirchhoff *et al.*, 1990). Our northern blot hybridization data indicate the same tissue specificity in the chimpanzee, in that message for chimpanzee EP2 clones could be detected in the epididymis but not in the testis. The sequence identity between human and chimpanzee EP2 cDNAs suggests that the protein has the same function in the two species. However, the actual function of EP2 is not known.

The translated EP2 peptide sequence has an N-terminal leader sequence which suggests that EP2 is secreted by the epididymal epithelium into the luminal fluid. In its secreted state, it has a predicted core molecular mass of 8.5 kDa before glycosylation. There is one consensus glycosylation site close to the N-terminus of the secreted peptide, which could increase the actual molecular weight of the protein. On the basis of its small size, it is unlikely that EP2 possesses an enzymatic function. It may, however, have a signalling function which activates an as yet unknown process. Alternatively, EP2 may be a binding protein for a signalling factor.

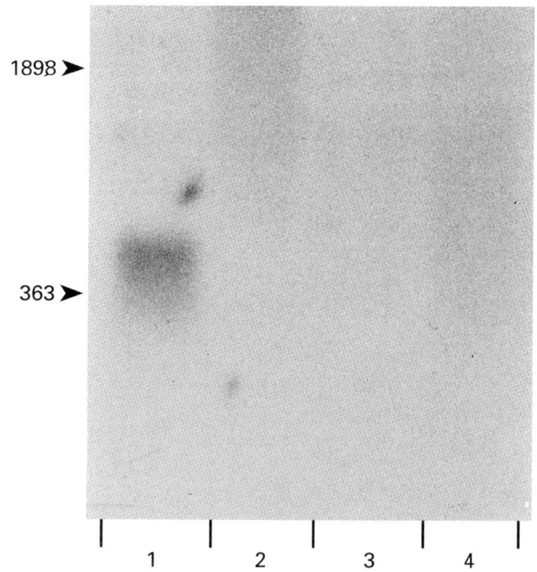

Fig. 3. Northern blot analysis of total RNA (10 μg RNA per lane) isolated from epididymis (lane 1) and testis (lane 2) of an androgen-normal chimpanzee and from epididymis (lane 3) and testis (lane 4) of an androgen-deprived chimpanzee. Numbers on the left represent RNA molecular weight standards.

Our studies with an androgen-deprived animal shows that the expression of EP2 by the epididymis depends critically on the presence of circulating androgen. Only a few of the known secretory epididymal proteins are androgen dependent (Cornwall and Hann, 1995). The androgen control of EP2 expression suggests that EP2 is important for epididymal function, and thus it may play an important role in the maturation process that spermatozoa undergo as they pass through the epididymis.

Conclusion

EP2 is an epididymis-specific, androgen-dependent secretory protein that is expressed predominantly in the caput epididymidis in the chimpanzee. The apparent identity between chimpanzee EP2 and human HE2 supports the use of the chimpanzee as a model for epididymal physiology of the human male.

This research was supported by NIH Grants RR-05994 and RR-00165.

References

Arslan M, Haider M and Qazi H (1986) Characterization and androgen dependence of specific proteins in the epididymis of the adult rhesus monkey *Archives of Andrology* **16** 67–74

Cornwall G and Hann S (1995) Specialized gene expression in the epididymis *Journal of Andrology* **16** 379–383

Fröhlich O and Young L (1996) Molecular cloning and characterization of EPI-1, the major protein in chimpanzee (*Pan troglodytes*) cauda epididymal fluid *Biology of Reproduction* **54** 857–865

Gould K and Young L (1990) Acquisition of fertilizing capacity by chimpanzee sperm *Folia Primatologia* **54** 105–108

Hinton B and Palladino M (1995) Epididymal epithelium: its contribution to the formation of a luminal fluid microenvironment *Microscopy Research and Technique* **30** 67–81

Kirchhoff C, Osterhoff C, Habben I and Ivell R (1990) Cloning and analysis of mRNAs expressed specifically in the human epididymis *International Journal of Andrology* **13** 155–167

Moore H, Curry M, Penfold L and Pryor J (1992) The culture of human epididymal epithelium and *in vitro* maturation of epididymal spermatozoa *Fertility and Sterility* **58** 776–783

Osterhoff C, Kirchhoff C, Krull N and Ivell R (1994) Molecular cloning and characterization of a novel human sperm antigen (HE2) specifically expressed in the proximal epididymis *Biology of Reproduction* **50** 516–525

Tezon J, Vazquez M, DeLarminat M, Cameo M, Pineiro L, Piazza A, Scorticati C and Blaquier J (1987) Further characterization of a model system for the study of human epididymal physiology and its relation to sperm maturation *New York Academy of Science* **513** 215–221

Smithwick E and Young L (1997) Sequential histology of the adult chimpanzee epididymis *Tissue and Cell* **29** 383–412

Journal of Reproduction and Fertility Supplement **53**, 221–226

Extratesticular sperm maturation in the brush-tail possum, *Trichosurus vulpecula*

N. J. Cooper[1], M. K. Holland[2] and W. G. Breed[1]

[1]*Department of Anatomical Sciences, University of Adelaide, SA 5005, Australia; and* [2]*Vertebrate Biocontrol Centre and CSIRO Division of Wildlife and Ecology, PO Box 84, Lyneham, ACT 2602, Australia*

The changes in distribution of protein and sugar components in, and on, the plasmalemma of the spermatozoon during epididymal transit of a marsupial, the brush-tail possum, *Trichosurus vulpecula*, are described. Freeze-fracture studies indicate a change in organization of plasmalemma intramembranous particles of both the head and midpiece of the tail as the spermatozoa pass from the caput to cauda epididymides. Staining with fluorescein isothiocyanate (FITC)-lectins shows that heads of caput spermatozoa stain with Con A, WGA, RCA_{120}, LCA and JAC, whereas those from the cauda epididymides stain only with LCA and JAC, thus suggesting that *N*-acetyl-β-D-glucosamine, α-D-glucose, or β-D-galactose may either become lost or masked during epididymal transit. A reduction of α-D-mannose is also suggested. Collectively these results show that the plasmalemma of the spermatozoon of at least this marsupial species undergoes both protein and saccharide modification during transit of the epididymis. How these findings relate to sperm maturation in preparation for sperm–egg binding has yet to be determined.

Introduction

In eutherian mammals, for fertilization to occur, spermatozoa have to undergo extratesticular maturation which takes place, in part, as they traverse the epididymis and includes both structural and functional changes in metabolism and pattern of flagellar activity (Orgebin-Crist *et al.*, 1975). Changes in the sperm plasmalemma composition and organization contribute to these modifications, which include alterations in surface charge, lectin binding, intramembranous particle (IMP) distribution, lipid and protein composition, and antibody binding (see Eddy and O'Brien, 1994; Moore and Akhondi, 1996 for reviews).

In marsupials morphological changes occur to the spermatozoon during epididymal migration (Temple-Smith and Bedford, 1976; Temple-Smith, 1994) but very little is known of the associated maturational changes of the sperm plasmalemma. However, we have extracted six proteins, not detectable in the blood plasma, from caput sperm plasma membrane from the brush-tail possum. These proteins were not evident in cauda spermatozoa, but a further eight proteins were found in detergent extracts of cauda spermatozoa that were not present in the caput spermatozoa (Lamont *et al.*, 1998).

The present study is part of a broader investigation into changes that take place to the protein and saccharide composition of the plasmalemma of the marsupial spermatozoon during epididymal transit in the brush-tail possum.

Materials and Methods

Adult male brush-tail possums (*Trichosurus vulpecula*) obtained from the Division of Animal Services, University of Adelaide, were killed with carbon dioxide, and the scrota removed. The epididymides were dissected free from the testes, divided into the caput and cauda regions, and spermatozoa extruded.

Freeze-fracture preparations of spermatozoa

Caput and cauda sperm pellets were obtained by centrifugation (13 000 *g* for 5 min) and fixed by the addition of 3% (w/v) glutaraldehyde–3% (w/v) paraformaldehyde in 0.1 mol phosphate buffer l^{-1}, pH 7.4, together with 2.5% (w/v) polyvinyl pyrrolidone, for 2–4 h at room temperature. After washing in PBS, pH 7.4, the pellets were transferred to 30% glycerol in PBS for 2 h, and samples were frozen in liquid Freon 22 at –150°C, and stored in liquid nitrogen. The specimens were fractured at 10^{-6} to 10^{-7} Torr, –115°C, replicated with platinum and carbon, cleaned by immersion in sodium hypochlorite, and examined with a Philips CM100 electron microscope.

Lectin binding of spermatozoa

Sperm suspensions from caput and cauda epididymides, 50–100 µl, were washed (700 *g* for 2 min) with 50 mmol Tris-buffered saline l^{-1} to which 0.1% (w/v) bovine serum albumin (TBS/BSA) had been added. 200 µl of the lectin-fluorescein isothiocyanate (5 µg ml^{-1}) (Sigma, St Louis) and 5 µl of propidium iodide (PI; 5 µg ml^{-1}) in PBS were added to the sperm suspension and incubations carried out in the dark at room temperature for up to 4 min. The sperm suspensions were then centrifuged at 700 *g* for 1–2 min, and resuspended in 100 µl TBS/BSA. A 5 µl drop of the sperm suspension was placed onto a slide; a coverslip was placed on top, and the slides were viewed by epifluorescence and phase contrast microscopy. FITC-lectins used were: *Concavalia ensiformis* agglutinin (Con A), *Triticum vulgaris* agglutinin (WGA), *Artocarpus integrifolia* agglutinin (JAC), *Arachis hypogea* agglutinin (PNA), *Lens culinaris* agglutinin (LCA), *Erythrina cristagalli* agglutinin (ECA), and *Ricinus communis* agglutinin (RCA_{120}).

Results

Freeze-fracture of sperm plasmalemma

Freeze-fracture replicas of caput epididymal spermatozoa showed randomly distributed 8–20 nm IMPs in the plasmalemma of the sperm head (Fig. 1a), and a similar distribution of 8–20 nm IMPs in the midpiece (Fig. 1b), although in the latter region clumping of 6–8 particles was also evident. In cauda epididymal spermatozoa only a few large IMPs were evident in the plasmalemma of the sperm head (Fig. 2a), but in the midpiece there were well-defined parallel rows of IMPs helically wound around the sperm tail (Fig. 2b). These rows were 4–5 particles wide and the particles were about 14 nm in diameter.

Lectin staining of the sperm plasmalemma

Staining with PI differentiated live from dead spermatozoa since those that were dead take up the PI into the nucleus, whereas live spermatozoa do not. Staining with FITC-lectins showed no binding of PNA or ECA to live caput or cauda epididymal spermatozoa. However, there was weak staining with Con A over the acrosomal region and WGA and RCA120 stained both the head and midpiece of caput spermatozoa. These lectins did not stain the head region of spermatozoa from the cauda epididymides but Con A stained the midpiece. Both caput and cauda spermatozoa stained positively with LCA and JAC, although the intensity of staining of the former was reduced during epididymal transit (see Table 1).

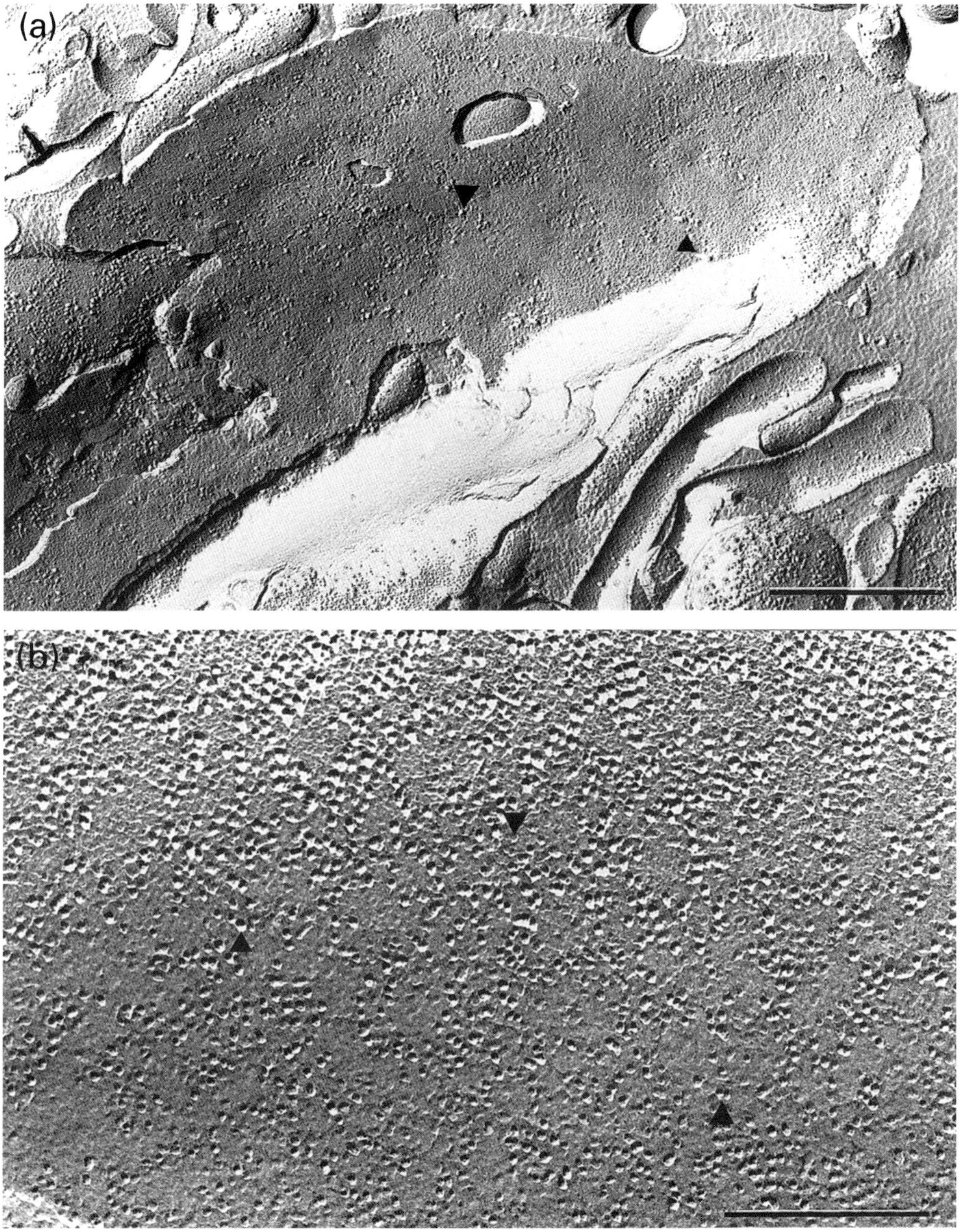

Fig. 1. Freeze fracture images of a spermatozoon from the caput epididymides of the brush-tail possum. (a) Sperm head and (b) midpiece of the sperm tail, showing randomly arranged intramembranous particles (IMPs) (arrowheads). Scale bars represent (a) 2 µm and (b) 200 nm.

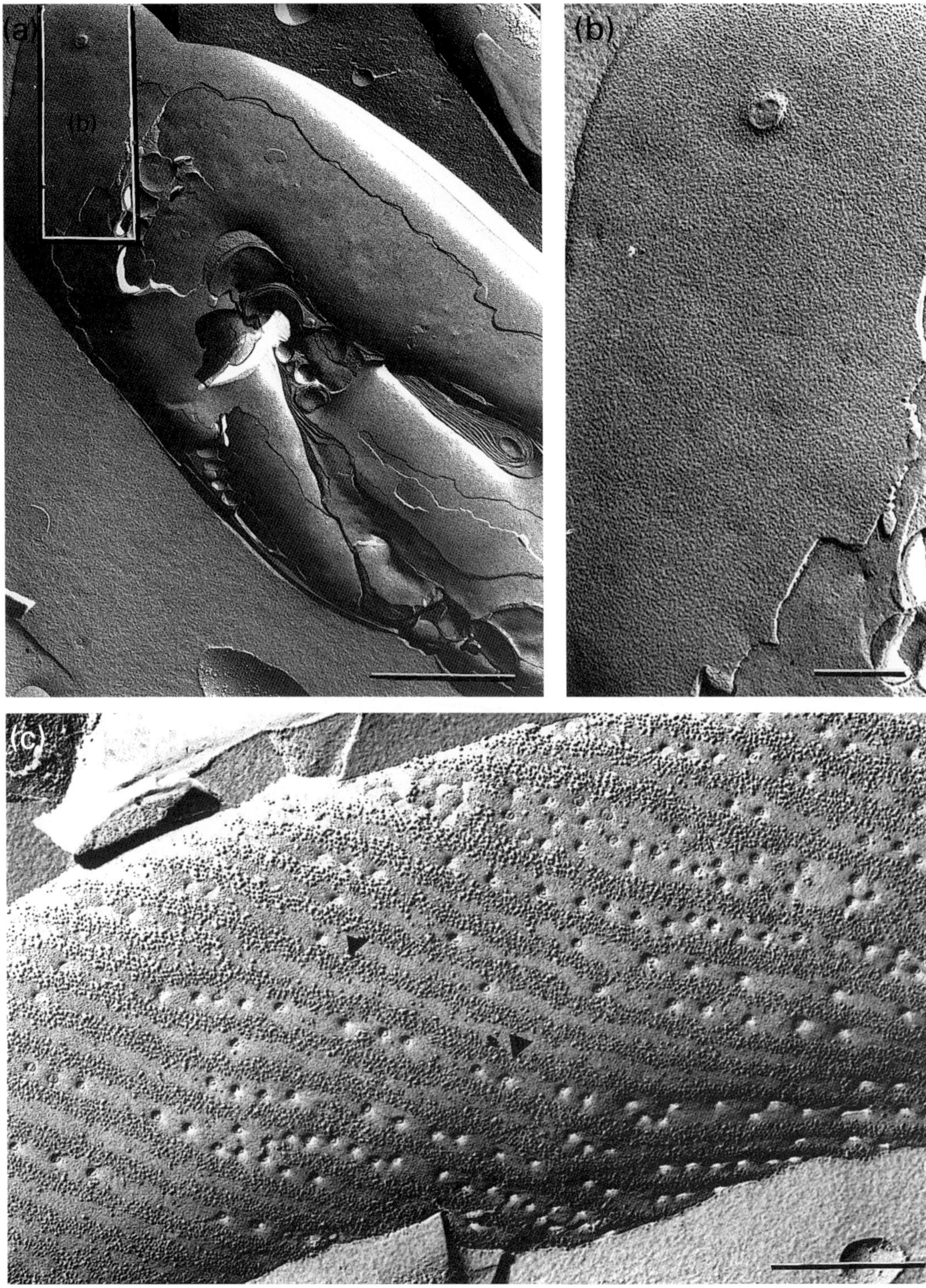

Fig. 2. Freeze fracture images of a spermatozoon from the cauda epididymides of the brush-tail possum. Sperm head (a) and (b), and midpiece of the sperm tail (c), showing virtually no large intramembranous particles (IMPs) in the sperm head, but abundant parallel rows of IMPs in the midpiece of the sperm tail (arrowheads). Scale bars represent (a) 1 µm, (b) 200 nm and (c) 2 µm.

Table 1. Distribution of sugar molecules on the plasmalemma of caput and cauda epididymal spermatozoa from brush-tail possum, *Trichosurus vulpecula*

Lectin-FITC[a]	Con A	WGA	JAC	PNA	LCA	ECA	RCA_{120}
Sugar binding specificity[b]	α-D-man α-D-glc	$(\text{D-glcNAc})_2$, NeuNAc	β-D-gal-(1-3)-D-galNAc	β-D-gal-(1-3)-D-galNAc	α-D-man	β-D-gal-(1-4)-D-glcNAc	β-D-gal
Caput spermatozoa							
Acrosomal plasmalemma[c]	+	+	+++	o	+++	o	+
Whole head plasmalemma	+	o	+++	o	+++	o	+
Midpiece plasmalemma	o	+	+++	o	+++	o	+
Caudal spermatozoa							
Acrosomal plasmalemma	o	o	+++	o	++	o	o
Whole head plasmalemma	o	o	+++	o	++	o	o
Midpiece plasmalemma	+	o	+++	o	++	o	o

Fluorescence: +++ intense; ++ moderate; + weak; o absent

[a] (FITC) lectins: Con A: *Concavalia ensiformis* agglutinin; WGA: *Triticum vulgaris* agglutinin; JAC: *Artocarpus integrifolia* agglutinin; PNA: *Arachis hypogea* agglutinin; LCA: *Lens culinaris* agglutinin; ECA: *Erythrina cristagalli* agglutinin and RCA_{120}: *Ricinus communis* agglutinin.

[b] Monosaccharide sugars expressed in an abbreviated form; data obtained from Sigma and Vector catalogues.

Discussion

In a previous one-dimensional SDS-PAGE gel electrophoretic study of sperm plasmalemma extracts we showed that, as possum spermatozoa pass along the epididymis, some proteins are lost whereas others become bound to the plasmalemma. The proteins that become bound are likely to be secreted by the epididymis and [^{35}S]methionine labelling studies indicated that the epithelium of the caput and corpus epididymides is more active in synthesizing and secreting proteins than is that of the cauda epididymidis (Lamont *et al.*, 1998).

Here we show by freeze-fracture that there is a reduction in intramembranous proteins in the plasmalemma of the sperm head during passage from the caput to cauda epididymides, whereas, by contrast, in the midpiece of the sperm tail a redistribution of proteins takes place with the result that they come to form parallel helical arrays by the time the spermatozoa reach the cauda epididymis (see also Temple-Smith, 1994).

Studies with FITC-lectins also show that the sugar components on the sperm surface change during epididymal migration. In particular WGA and RCA_{120}, which bind to the sperm plasmalemma of caput spermatozoa, did not bind to cauda spermatozoa suggesting that the sugar components *N*-acetyl-β-D-glucosamine or β-D-galactose may have either become cleaved from the sperm surface or become masked. The disappearance of staining with Con A suggest that α-D-glucose may become lost or masked and that α-D-mannose is reduced, although binding of both of these lectins to the midpiece plasmalemma is evident in cauda spermatozoa. The staining by JAC–FITC over the entire surface of the plasmalemma of both caput and cauda spermatozoa suggests that *N*-acetyl α-D-galactose-(1-3)-D-galactose may remain abundant over the whole surface of the spermatozoon during migration along the epididymis.

The authors wish to thank J. Swift of the Electron Microscopy Unit at the Institute for Medical and Veterinary Science, Adelaide for the freeze-fracture preparations, R. Harrison, Babraham Institute, Cambridge for advice on lectin staining, and the Australian Research Council for financial assistance.

References

Eddy EM and O'Brien DA (1994) The Spermatozoon. In *The Physiology of Reproduction* (2nd Edn) pp 29–44 Ed. E Knobil and JD Neill. Raven Press Ltd , New York

Lamont AE, Clark H, Cooper NJ, Holland MK and Breed WG (1998) Protein synthesis and secretion by the epididymis of the brush-tail possum, *Trichosurus vulpecula. Journal of Reproduction and Fertility* (in press)

Moore HDM and Akhondi MA (1996) *In vitro* maturation of mammalian spermatozoa *Reviews of Reproduction* **1** 54–60

Orgebin-Crist M-C, Danzo BJ and Davies J (1975) Endocrine control of the development and maintenance of sperm fertilising ability in the epididymis. In *Handbook of Physiology Section 7: Endocrinology* Vol. 5 pp 319–338. Ed. DW Hamilton and RO Greep. Waverly Press Inc., Baltimore, MD

Temple-Smith PD (1994) Comparative structure and function of marsupial spermatozoa *Reproduction, Fertility and Development* **6** 421–435

Temple-Smith PD and Bedford JM (1976) The features of spermatozoa maturation in the epididymis of a marsupial, the brush-tailed possum, *Trichosurus vulpecula. American Journal of Anatomy* **147** 471–500

Journal of Reproduction and Fertility Supplement **53**, 227–234

Chemical interference with sperm metabolic pathways

A. R. Jones

Department of Biochemistry, The University of Sydney, Sydney NSW 2006, Australia

During the 1960s, the quest for a simple non-steroidal chemical possessing male anti-fertility activity culminated with the discovery of the activity of α-chlorohydrin in 1970. Investigations into the mechanism of action of this compound revealed that it was affecting the glycolytic pathway within mature spermatozoa through its conversion to an inhibitory metabolite. Use of these and other simple chemical inhibitors has subsequently led to a clearer understanding of the metabolic pathways involved in the generation of ATP, which is necessary for sperm motility. Mature boar spermatozoa from the cauda epididymidis are almost totally reliant on the glycolytic pathway, not necessarily for the immediate generation of ATP, but for the ultimate production of lactate, which appears to be the sole substrate used for the mitochondrial production of ATP. The only exogenous substrates that support lactate production *in vitro* are fructose, glucose, glycerol and glycerol 3-phosphate and when these substrates are plentiful, there is evidence that compounds can be retained as such or as intermediates of the glycolytic pathway. When exogenous substrates are limited, the cells have the capability to mobilize endogenous compounds and to maintain the continuous synthesis of ATP.

Introduction

In the first monogragh devoted to substances affecting male fertility, Jackson (1966) described the actions of over 30 non-steroidal chemicals that were then known to cause periods of infertility, or in some cases sterility, in male laboratory animals. The majority of these compounds were biological alkylating agents and their effects were predominantly aimed at the testicular phase of spermatogenesis by inhibiting or interfering with various stages in the development of the immature spermatozoa. What was apparently obvious, however, was that an ideal male anti-fertility agent required an immediate action directed not at developing spermatozoa but at mature spermatozoa stored in the cauda epididymidis. Such a compound should be devoid of side effects, active when administered orally in low doses and have an immediate anti-fertility action, which would be abolished when administration ceased.

The Actions of α-Chlorohydrin

Several years later Coppola (1969) and then Ericsson (1970) published the results of their respective studies with low oral doses of α-chlorohydrin (3-chloropropan-1,2-diol, I, Fig. 1) on the fertility of male rats; their evidence was consistent with a type of inhibitory action directed at mature spermatozoa stored in the cauda epididymidis. Interest in determining the mechanism of this inhibitory action grew and was sustained for 15 years yielding over 250 publications (Jones, 1983). White's group eventually pin-pointed the biochemical site of action of the compound on ejaculated ram spermatozoa *in vitro* as being inhibition of the glycolytic enzyme glyceraldehyde 3-phosphate dehydrogenase resulting in the severely reduced ability to synthesize ATP from glycolysable sugars (Mohri *et al.*, 1975; Brown-Woodman *et al.*, 1978). These studies also noted that the inhibitory action

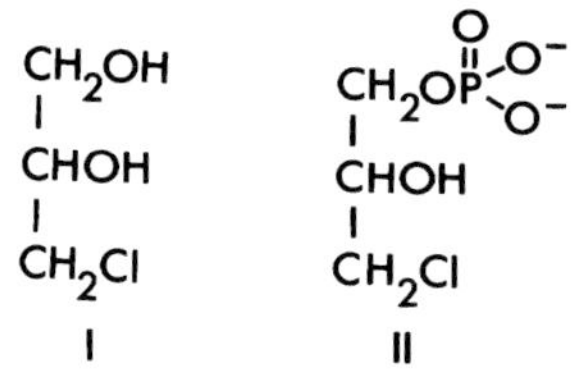

Fig. 1. α-Chlorohydrin (I) is an equimolar mixture of the (*R*)- and (*S*)-isomers; (*R, S*)-α–chlorohydrin phosphate (II) was originally suggested to be the inhibitory metabolite of α-chlorohydrin.

was not immediate but required a period of preincubation and it was suggested that because the structure of α-chlorohydrin resembled that of glycerol, glycerol kinase within mature spermatozoa was converting α-chlorohydrin to α-chlorohydrin phosphate (II, Fig. 1) which was the true inhibitory species. With the finding that caudal spermatozoa obtained from rats that had been treated with α-chlorohydrin had low motility and very low glyceraldehyde 3-phosphate dehydrogenase activity (Ford *et al.*, 1979), the mechanism of action of α-chlorohydrin as a male antifertility agent had apparently been solved.

There were many unanswered questions about α-chlorohydrin. As all cells contain glyceraldehyde 3-phosphate dehydrogenase, why was α-chlorohydrin not a general metabolic poison? Was α-chlorohydrin phosphate really the inhibitory metabolite in mature spermatozoa? Why was the inhibitory activity of α-chlorohydrin abolished *in vitro* when glycerol was the substrate? Why should inhibition of the glycolytic pathway result in low concentrations of ATP when it can be more efficiently synthesized by mitochondrial activity? In an attempt to answer these questions, we began with a detailed investigation that involved boar spermatozoa obtained from abattoir material (Hutton *et al.*, 1980) since this species was reported to be susceptible to the action of α-chlorohydrin (Johnson and Pursel, 1972). At that time it was realised that α-chlorohydrin possessed a chiral carbon atom and, therefore, existed as the (*R*)- and (*S*)-isomers with the (*S*)-isomer (III, Fig. 2) possessing the anti-fertility activity *in vivo* (Jones, 1983). We confirmed that this isomer was inhibitory towards spermatozoa *in vitro* (Stevenson and Jones, 1982) and showed that the active metabolite was (*S*)-3-chlorolactaldehyde (IV, Fig. 2) (Stevenson and Jones 1985), which possesses the same configuration as (*R*)- or (D)-glyceraldehyde 3-phosphate (V, Fig 2), the substrate for glyceraldehyde 3-phosphate dehydrogenase. Synthetic (*R, S*)-3-chlorolactaldehyde had an immediate, inhibitory activity on boar spermatozoa *in vitro* similar to that of (*S*)-chlorohydrin (Cooney and Jones, 1988), but had no activity either on the commercially available preparations of glyceraldehyde 3-phosphate dehydrogenase or the glycolytic activity of erythrocytes from eight mammalian species (Stevenson *et al.*, 1984). These results, together with the establishment that (*S*)-α-chlorohydrin is converted to (*S*)-3-chlorolactaldehyde by an $NADP^+$-dependent dehydrogenase that converts glycerol to glyceraldehyde (Stevenson and Jones, 1985), led to a more detailed proposal for its inhibitory mechanism of action within mature boar spermatozoa (Fig. 2). We also showed that α-chlorohydrin phosphate had no inhibitory activity on the oxidation of fructose (Jones and Chantrill, 1989).

Chemical Inhibition of Sperm Metabolism

During the course of these investigations it became apparent that there were some unusual aspects to the metabolic activity of boar spermatozoa and there were several dangerous precedents in the

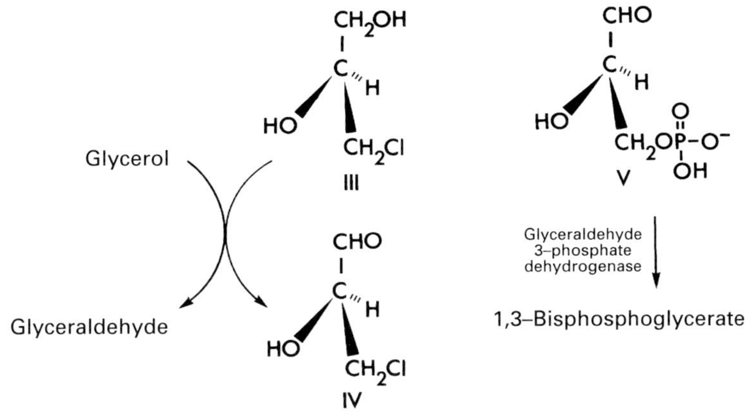

Fig. 2. (*S*)-α-chlorohydrin (III) is oxidized by a dehydrogenase, involved in the conversion of glycerol to glyceraldehyde, to (*S*)-3-chlorolactaldehyde (IV). The aldehyde inhibits glyceraldehyde 3-phosphate dehydrogenase since it has a similar structure and identical stereochemistry to (*R*)-glyceraldehyde 3-phosphate (V), the substrate for the enzyme.

literature where results obtained with spermatozoa of one species were assumed to apply to the spermatozoa of another species. In their treatise on the biochemistry of spermatozoa, Mann and Lutwak-Mann (1981) clearly recognized the diversity in metabolism between species: "Several substances other than lactic acid, such as pyruvic acid, acetic acid, glycerol and sorbitol, provide substrates for exogenous sperm respiration, but in this respect there are marked species differences. Trout spermatozoa oxidize pyruvate faster than acetate, and glucose to a small extent only. Ram and bull spermatozoa oxidize acetic acid in preference to fructose and glucose; by contrast, in human, canine and rabbit spermatozoa the reverse is true. Ram spermatozoa oxidize lower fatty acids with an even number of carbon atoms more efficiently than those with an odd number, whereas dog and cock spermatozoa oxidize acetate and propionate equally well. Ram and bull, but not boar or stallion, spermatozoa oxidize sorbitol. Glycerol markedly stimulates the respiration of bull and ram spermatozoa but has a small effect on boar, and practically none on either rabbit or stallion". With the availability of (*S*)-α-chlorohydrin and (*R, S*)-3-chlorolactaldehyde as specific metabolic inhibitors, aspects of the metabolic activity of boar spermatozoa could be investigated in detail.

It soon became apparent that the value of these inhibitors was limited. (*R, S*)-3-Chlorolactaldehyde was not particularly permeable to the cell membrane resulting in its use at quite high concentrations, which meant that toxic effects of the (*R*)-isomer were more prominent (Stevenson and Jones, 1984), whereas the onset of inhibitory activity of (*S*)-α-chlorohydrin was delayed and (*S*)-α-chlorohydrin was ineffective when glycerol was present. Spermatozoa incubated in the presence of (*S*)-α-chlorohydrin with fructose 1,6-bisphosphate as the substrate did not produce either fructose or glucose, but accumulated equilibrium quantities of fructose 6-phosphate and glucose 6-phosphate, suggesting that glycolytic intermediates can be stored within the pathway (Jones and Montague, 1991).

The only other inhibitory chemical known at that time was 6-chloro-6-deoxy-D-glucose (VI , Fig. 3), which had anti-fertility activity when administered to several species (Ford and Waites, 1981). Although it was generally assumed that spermatozoa metabolized this chlorinated sugar, 'mistaking' it for glucose 6-phosphate, to dihydroxyacetone phosphate and (*S*)-3-chlorolactaldehyde, boar spermatozoa did not metabolize it nor did it have any inhibitory activity *in vitro* (Jones and Dobbie, 1991). However, the assumption that the glycolytic enzymes of spermatozoa may not be able to distinguish between their substrates and compounds possessing a chlorine atom in place of a phosphate ester led to the synthesis of 3-chloro-1-hydroxypropanone (CHOP, VII, Fig. 3), the chloro-analogue of dihydroxyacetone phosphate. This compound was shown to be an excellent inhibitor

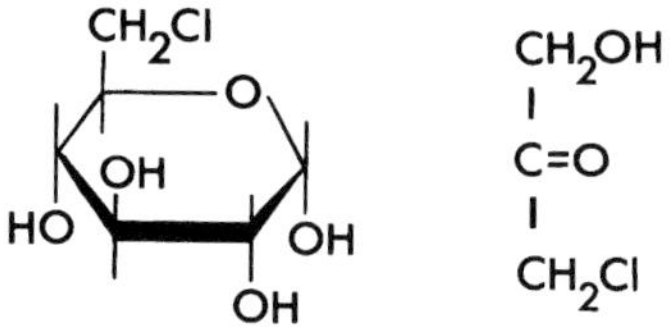

VI VII

Fig. 3. 6-Chloro-6-deoxy-D-glucose (VI) and 3-chloro-1-hydroxy-propanone (CHOP, VII) are the chlorinated analogues of D-glucose 6-phosphate and dihydroxyacetone phosphate, respectively.

of glyceraldehyde 3-phosphate dehydrogenase, presumably being converted specifically to (*S*)-3-chlorolactaldehyde by triosephosphate isomerase (Jones *et al.*, 1986). (The bromo-analogue, 3-bromo-1-hydroxypropanone, has similar inhibitory activity (Porter and Jones, 1995).) The advantage of CHOP was twofold; onset of inhibition was almost immediate and it allowed the metabolism of glycerol to be investigated.

In the presence of CHOP, boar spermatozoa metabolized fructose to fructose-1,6-bisphosphate and dihydroxyacetone phosphate, but these intermediates did not accumulate when glycerol was the substrate. This led to two findings, the first was that not only was glyceraldehyde 3-phosphate dehydrogenase inhibited but so was triosephosphate isomerase (Jones and Cooney, 1987) and a re-examination of the effects of (*R*, *S*)-3-chlorolactaldehyde and (*S*)-α-chlorohydrin on boar spermatozoa confirmed that both enzymes were inhibited (Cooney and Jones, 1988). The second finding concerned the metabolism of glycerol. The fact that fructose 1,6-bisphosphate and dihydroxyacetone phosphate did not accumulate when spermatozoa were incubated in the presence of CHOP with glycerol as the substrate enabled the metabolic pathway glycerol → glyceraldehyde → glyceraldehyde 3-phosphate to be established (Jones *et al.*, 1992), thereby explaining how these cells metabolize glycerol in the absence of glycerol kinase activity (Mohri and Masaki, 1967). Furthermore, it explained why (*S*)-α-chlorohydrin was ineffective when glycerol was the substrate (Stevenson and Jones, 1985); the same enzyme oxidized both glycerol and (*S*)-α-chlorohydrin but had a higher affinity for glycerol so that (*S*)-3-chlorolactaldehyde was not produced (Jones *et al.*, 1992).

In retrospect, the inhibitory action of CHOP, (*S*)-α-chlorohydrin and (*R*, *S*)-3-chlorolactaldehyde on the metabolic activity of boar spermatozoa should have raised questions about which substrates could be used for the generation of ATP. All three inhibitors prevented the synthesis of ATP when glucose, fructose or glycerol were substrates but could ATP be produced from other substrates? In studies involving the use of ^{14}C-labelled substrates, the only substrates oxidized to $^{14}CO_2$ were fructose, glucose, glycerol, glycerol 3-phosphate and lactate; short- and medium-chain fatty acids were not oxidized (Jones and Chantrill, 1989) nor were the ketogenic amino acids (Jones and Gillan, 1996a). The ability of lactate and the inability of pyruvate to be oxidized was surprising until it was shown that it is lactate, not pyruvate, that enters the mitochondria thus regenerating cytoplasmic NAD^+ without the requirement of a shuttle (Jones, 1997). Boar spermatozoa, therefore, are totally reliant on the glycolytic pathway for the direct production of ATP and the generation of lactate for the subsequent mitochondrial processes of the tricarboxylic acid cycle and electron transport. More particularly, boar spermatozoa generate most of their ATP by the latter process since they cannot maintain ATP production under anaerobic conditions (Jones and Chantrill, 1989).

As the cytoplasmic conversion of pyruvate to lactate regenerates NAD^+ for glyceraldehyde 3-phosphate dehydrogenase to continue functioning, our attention was focussed on the metabolism of glycerol 3-phosphate since its conversion to dihydroxyacetone phosphate would generate NADH by a glycerol 3-phosphate dehydrogenase. As there was little, if any, NAD$^+$-dependent glycerol 3-phosphate dehydrogenase activity detectable in boar spermatozoa, cells were incubated with glycerol 3-phosphate as substrate in the presence and absence of CHOP. In both cases the concentration of substrate declined rapidly and at the same rate with the ATP concentration being maintained in the absence of CHOP but declining over time in its presence (Jones and Gillan, 1996a). Use of (*R*, *S*)-α-bromohydrin phosphate, shown to inhibit the oxidation of glycerol 3-phosphate by acting as a competitive inhibitor, enabled it to be confirmed that the glycerol 3-phosphate dehydrogenase in boar spermatozoa is an FAD-linked mitochondrial enzyme (Jones and Gillan, 1996b). Consequently, boar spermatozoa use this as a *de facto* shuttle system as glycerol 3-phosphate metabolism directly produces mitochondrial $FADH_2$ and dihydroxyacetone phosphate for the production of lactate.

It became increasingly apparent that the triosephosphates occupy a pivotal role in boar sperm metabolism since they are produced by fructose, glucose, glycerol and glycerol 3-phosphate. When offered either dihydroxyacetone phosphate or glyceraldehyde 3-phosphate as substrates, boar spermatozoa rapidly interconverted them, produced fructose 1,6-bisphosphate and equilibrium amounts of fructose 6-phosphate and glucose 6-phosphate (Jones, 1998). In the presence of CHOP, however, less of these glycolytic intermediates were produced but the rates of metabolism of the triosephosphates were similar to those in its absence. This appears to indicate that there is some degree of conservation of glycolytic substrates from the triosephosphates and that there may be the formation of an as yet unknown storage metabolite. As neither glucose nor fructose were produced, futile substrate cycling, suggested to be a factor in decreasing the ATP concentrations of spermatozoa as a result of glycolytic inhibition, was not occurring (Ford and Harrison, 1987).

One problem was that the known glycolytic inhibitors affected the activity of triosephosphate isomerase and what was required was an inhibitor that did not involve this enzyme. One compound examined was 1,6-dichloro-1,6-dideoxy-D-fructose (VIII, Fig. 4), the chloro-analogue of fructose 1,6-bisphosphate. This was found to be a transient inhibitor of aldolase but was also a weak substrate for it which converted it into CHOP and (*S*)-3-chlorolactaldehyde which was inappropriate (Jones and Morin, 1995). Another chemical that we were studying was 3-bromopyruvate (IX, Fig. 4) and while this was an inhibitor of all substrates at high concentration, low concentrations were specific for stage 2 of the glycolytic pathway with specific inhibitory actions directed towards glyceraldehyde 3-phosphate dehydrogenase and 3-phosphoglycerate kinase (Jones *et al.*, 1995).

Boar spermatozoa can maintain motility and high ATP concentrations for up to 5 h at 34°C in the presence of glucose and oxygen (Kamp *et al.*, 1996), and ATP concentrations could be maintained for the same period in the absence of any exogenous substrates (Jones and Milmlow, 1997). Addition of CHOP at any time caused the ATP concentration to decline immediately and fructose 1,6-bisphosphate, dihydroxyacetone phosphate and glycerol to accumulate, indicating that endogenous compounds are being mobilized to form the triosephosphates but that these do not originate from hexoses. There appear to be two endogenous substrates that are mobilized under these conditions; one substrate generates minor amounts of glycerol 3-phosphate and the other produces glycerol suggesting that they may be diglycerides (Vazquez and Roldan 1997) or triglycerides. A more detailed NMR study has revealed that the glycerol 3-phosphate is produced from the degradation of glycerylphosphorylcholine as this decreases over the incubation period with a concomitant increase in the concentration of choline (A. R. Jones and W. A. Bubb, unpublished).

Conclusion

Selective inhibition of various metabolic pathways within boar spermatozoa has advanced our knowledge of the manner by which these cells generate the ATP which is vital for maintaining their motility within the female reproductive tract. Spermatozoa stored in the cauda epididymidis presumably generate lactate from blood glucose or use blood lactate directly and when cauda epididymides are stored at 34°C for up to 5 h after death of the animal, lactate accumulates within the spermatozoa and ATP continues to be produced (Jones and Chantrill, 1989). When ejaculated,

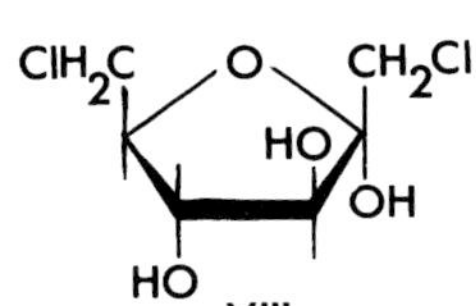

VIII

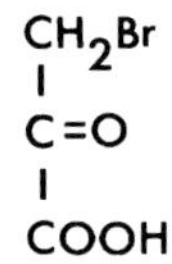

IX

Fig. 4. 1,6-Dichloro-1,6-dideoxy-D-fructose (VIII) is the chlorinated analogue of D-fructose-1,6-bisphosphate and 3-bromopyruvate (IX), an inhibitor of stage 2 of the glycolytic pathway.

they are initially supplied with fructose but what do they obtain from the female tract? Uterine washings show that the milieu is acidic, due mainly to the presence of lactate, with some glucose and only minor amounts of glycerol and glycerol 3-phosphate and no fructose (Table 1). This highlights the importance of lactate in boar sperm metabolism and, perhaps explains why an isozyme of lactate dehydrogenase not detectable in other tissues is present, as it is in the spermatozoa of several other species (Jones, 1997). One intriguing question is why boar spermatozoa metabolize glycerol since it is generally assumed that this occurs in the liver (Stryer, 1995). This may be associated with the metabolism of fructose which is converted to dihydroxyacetone phosphate and glyceraldehyde, via fructose 1-phosphate, so that glyceraldehyde, produced from either fructose or glycerol, can be converted to glyceraldehyde 3-phosphate. Whatever the reason, it is interesting to acknowledge that it is the ability of boar spermatozoa, and presumably the spermatozoa of other susceptible species, to oxidize glycerol that ultimately results in (*S*)-α-chlorohydrin having anti-glycolytic activity within these cells.

Another outcome from these studies is the metabolic 'arrangement' of the glycolytic and associated reactions which, while primarily directed towards the production of lactate, avoid the need for shuttle mechanisms to regenerate oxidized co-factors in the cytoplasm. The oxidation of glycerol 3-phosphate is essentially a *de facto* shuttle, while the reduction of pyruvate to lactate enables the regeneration of NAD^+ for glyceraldehyde 3-phosphate dehydrogenase and transfers reducing equivalents directly to the mitochondrial matrix (Fig. 5). The mechanism involved in the oxidation of glycerol to glyceraldehyde has yet to be determined.

It is possible to speculate on why sperm metabolism varies between species as Mann and Lutwak-Mann (1981) so aptly illustrated. It may be an evolutionary trait since the spermatozoa of marine worms, for example, spend hours in salt water yet they maintain constant concentrations of ATP (Kamp *et al.*, 1996) as do sea urchin spermatozoa which, in the absence of exogenous substrates,

Table 1. Substrates in uterine washings

	0.5 h after death (n = 22)	5 h after death (n = 11)
pH	5.9 ± 0.1	5.8 ± 0.1
Glucose	14 ± 5	0.5 ± 0.2
Lactate	28 ± 8	20 ± 4
Glycerol 3-phosphate	1.5 ± 0.5	0.2 ± 0.1
Glycerol	1 ± 0.3	2 ± 0.7

Uteri were removed from sows 0.5 h after death and washings taken immediately or 4.5 h after storage in saline at 34°C. Each uterine horn was flushed with 2 × 10 ml physiological saline and the washings made up to 50 ml. Values for substrates are given in μmoles per whole uterus where n = number of determinations.

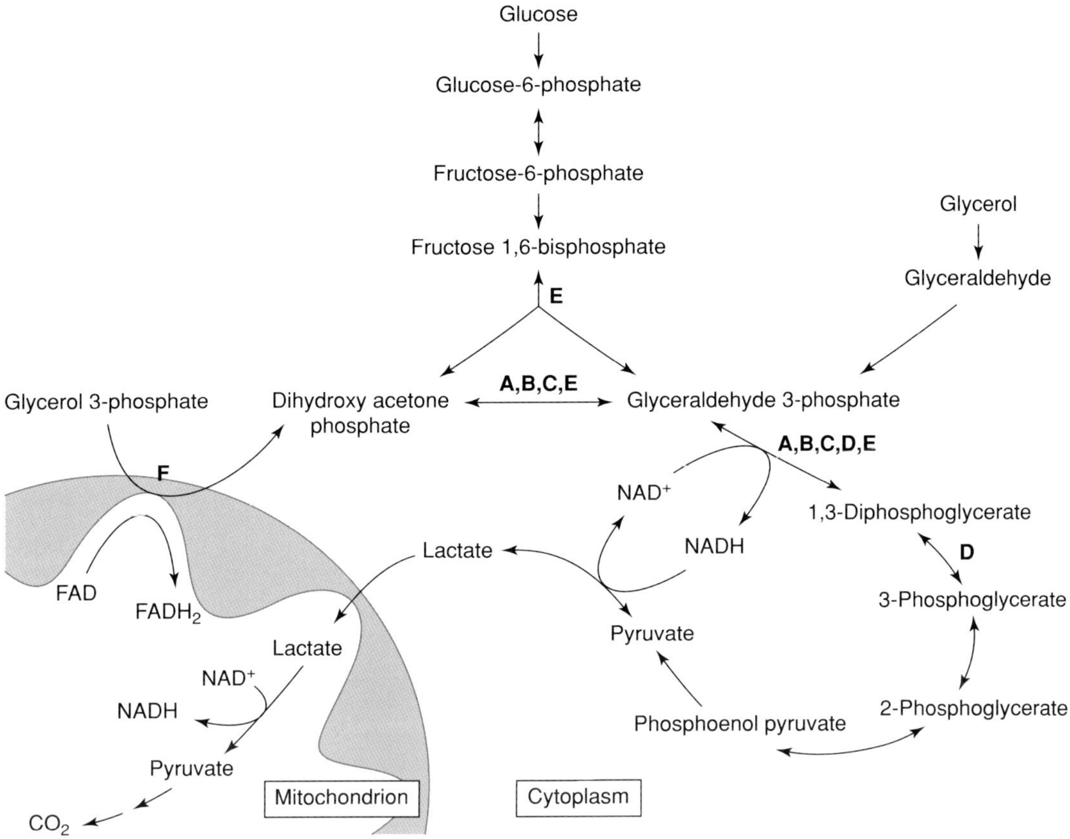

Fig. 5. The production of lactate by mature boar spermatozoa *in vitro*. Reactions susceptible to chemical inhibition are: (*S*)-α-chlorohydrin (A), (*R, S*)-3-chlorolactaldehyde (B), 3-chloro- (and bromo-)-1-hydroxypropanone (C), 3-bromo-pyruvate (D), 1,6-dichloro-1,6-dideoxy-D-fructose (E) and (*R, S*)-α-chloro- (and bromo-)-hydrin phosphate (F).

degrade stored triglycerides and generate ATP by β-oxidation of fatty acids (Mita and Nakamura, 1993). Avian spermatozoa are motile for several hours and turkey spermatozoa retain their fertilizing capacity in the female reproductive tract for several weeks (Kamp *et al.*, 1996). It may be that mammalian spermatozoa retain some of these characteristics, but have also evolved to make use of substrates available in the female reproductive tract.

References

Brown-Woodman PDC, Mohri H, Mohri T, Suter D and White IG (1978) Mode of action of α-chlorohydrin as a male antifertility agent. Inhibition of the metabolism of ram spermatozoa by α-chlorohydrin and location of block in glycolysis *Biochemical Journal* **170** 23–37

Cooney SJ and Jones AR (1988) Inhibitory effects of (*S*)-3-chlorolactaldehyde on the metabolic activity of boar spermatozoa *in vitro*. *Journal of Reproduction and Fertility* **82** 309–317

Coppola JA (1969) An extragonadal male antifertility agent *Life Sciences* **8** 43–48

Ericsson RJ (1970) Male antifertility compounds: U-5897 as a rat chemosterilant *Journal of Reproduction and Fertility* **22** 213–222

Ford WCL and Harrison A (1987) Futile substrate cycles in the glycolytic pathway of boar and rat spermatozoa and the effect of α-chlorohydrin *Journal of Reproduction and Fertility* **79** 21–32

Ford WCL and Waites GMH (1981) The effect of 6-chloro-6-deoxysugars on adenine nucleotide concentrations in and motility of rat spermatozoa *Journal of Reproduction and Fertility* **63** 75–79

Ford WCL, Harrison A, Takkar GL and Waites GMH (1979) Inhibition of glucose catabolism in rat, hamster, rhesus monkey and human spermatozoa by α-chlorohydrin *International Journal of Andrology* **2** 275–288

Hutton P, Dawson AG and Jones AR (1980) Inhibition of glycolysis in boar sperm by α-chlorohydrin *Contraception* **22** 505–512

Jackson H (1966) *Antifertility Compounds in the Male and Female* Thomas, Springfield Illinois

Johnson LA and Pursel VG (1972) Reversible infertility in male swine fed α-chlorohydrin *Journal of Animal Science* **34** 241–245

Jones AR (1983) Antifertility actions of α-chlorohydrin in the male *Australian Journal of Biological Sciences* **36** 333–350

Jones AR (1997) Metabolism of lactate by mature boar spermatozoa *Reproduction, Fertility and Development* **9** 227–232

Jones AR (1998) Triosephosphate metabolism by mature boar spermatozoa *Reproduction, Fertility and Development* **9** 557–581

Jones AR and Chantrill LA (1989) Oxidative metabolic activity of boar spermatozoa: a system for assessing anti-glycolytic activity of potential inhibitors *in vitro Reproduction, Fertility and Development* **1** 357–367

Jones AR and Cooney SJ (1987) Inhibition of triosephosphate isomerase in boar spermatozoa by (*S*)-3-chlorolactaldehyde *Biochemical and Biophysical Research Communications* **145** 1054–1058

Jones AR and Dobbie MS (1991) The male antifertility activity of 6-chloro-6-deoxyglucose *Contraception* **44** 649–655

Jones AR and Gillan L (1996a) Metabolism of glycerol 3-phosphate by mature boar spermatozoa *Journal of Reproduction and Fertility* **106** 321–327

Jones AR and Gillan L (1996b) Glycerol 3-phosphate dehydrogenase of boar spermatozoa: inhibition by α-bromohydrin phosphate *Journal of Reproduction and Fertility* **108** 95–100

Jones AR and Milmlow D (1997) Endogenous energy production by mature boar spermatozoa *Journal of Reproduction and Fertility* **111** 285–290

Jones AR and Montague MD (1991) Metabolism of fructose-1,6-bisphosphate by mature boar spermatozoa *Reproduction, Fertility and Development* **3** 609–613

Jones AR and Morin C (1995) Inhibition of glycolysis in boar spermatozoa by 1,6-dichloro-1,6-dideoxy-D-fructose *Biochimica et Biophysica Acta* **1244** 141–146

Jones AR, Bubb WA, Murdoch SR and Stevenson DA (1986) Inhibition of fructolytic enzymes in boar spermatozoa by (*S*)-α-chlorohydrin and 1-chloro-3-hydroxypropanone *Australian Journal of Biological Sciences* **39** 395–406

Jones AR, Chantrill LA and Cokinakis A (1992) Metabolism of glycerol by mature boar spermatozoa *Journal of Reproduction and Fertility* **94** 129–134

Jones AR, Gillan L and Milmlow D (1995) The anti-glycolytic activity of 3-bromopyruvate on mature boar spermatozoa *in vitro. Contraception* **52** 317–320

Kamp G, Büsselmann G and Lauterwein J (1996) Spermatozoa: models for studying regulatory aspects of energy metabolism *Experientia* **52** 487–494

Mann T and Lutwak-Mann C (1981) *Male Reproductive Function and Semen* p 199 Springer-Verlag, Berlin

Mita M and Nakamura M (1993) Lipid globules at the midpieces of *Glyptocidaris crenularis* spermatozoa and their relation to energy metabolism *Molecular Reproduction and Development* **34** 158–163

Mohri H and Masaki J (1967) Glycerokinase and its possible role in glycerol metabolism of bull spermatozoa *Journal of Reproduction and Fertility* **14** 179–194

Mohri H, Suter DAI, Brown-Woodman PDC, White IG and Ridley D (1975) Identification of the biochemical lesion produced by α-chlorohydrin in spermatozoa *Nature* **225** 75–77

Porter LM and Jones AR (1995) Inhibition of glyceraldehyde 3-phosphate dehydrogenase in boar spermatozoa by bromohydroxypropanone *Reproduction, Fertility and Development* **7** 107–111

Stevenson D and Jones AR (1982) Inhibition of fructolysis in boar spermatozoa by the male antifertility agent (*S*)-α-chlorohydrin *Australian Journal of Biological Sciences* **35** 595–605

Stevenson D and Jones AR (1984) The action of (*R*)- and (*S*)-α-chlorohydrin and their metabolites on the metabolism of boar sperm *International Journal of Andrology* **7** 79–86

Stevenson D and Jones AR (1985) Production of (*S*)-3-chlorolactaldehyde from (*S*)-α-chlorohydrin by boar spermatozoa and the inhibition of glyceraldehyde 3-phosphate dehydrogenase *in vitro. Journal of Reproduction and Fertility* **74** 157–165

Stevenson D, Ford SA, Du Toit JI and Jones AR (1984) Spermatozoal glyceraldehyde 3-phosphate dehydrogenase *Proceedings of the Australian Biochemical Society* **16** 51

Stryer L (1995) *Biochemistry* p 606 (4th Edn) Freeman, New York

Vazquez JM and Roldan ERS (1997) Phospholipid metabolism in boar spermatozoa and role of diacylglycerol species in the *de novo* formation of phosphatidylcholine *Molecular Reproduction and Development* **47** 105–112

Journal of Reproduction and Fertility Supplement **53**, 235–245

Immune responses in the epididymis : implications for immunocontraception

K. W. Beagley[1], Z. L. Wu[2], M. Pomering[2] and R. C. Jones[2]

[1]*Discipline of Pathology, Faculty of Medicine and Health Sciences and* [2]*Department of Biological Sciences, University of Newcastle, Callaghan, NSW 2308, Australia*

In recent years the need to develop vaccines against a variety of sexually transmitted diseases, the desire to treat male infertility and interest in developing alternative contraceptive methods have focused research interest on the immunology of the male reproductive tract. This paper reviews the current state of knowledge of immunity in the male tract. Both physical and immune mechanisms that operate to maintain the blood–testis barrier are discussed with regard to (i) their importance in preventing autoimmune responses against spermatozoa and (ii) how these can be overcome to induce specific immunity in the testis and efferent ducts. The role of both the systemic and mucosal arms of the humoral immune response are discussed both in terms of immune-mediated infertility and the induction of specific immunity. Finally some novel approaches to elicit immunity in the male reproductive tract are discussed.

Introduction

Although basic knowledge of the reproductive immunology of females has been established (Wira and Kaushic, 1996), males have received little attention. Nevertheless, there are important reasons to gain basic knowledge of male reproductive immunology. Sexually transmitted diseases represent a major unresolved health problem worldwide. Organisms such as human immunodeficiency virus (HIV), herpes simplex virus, human papilloma virus, *Neisseria gonorrhoeae*, *Chlamydia* species and *Treponema pallidum* are a major threat to the health of both adults and the newborn. Most of the organisms are highly contagious and are spread primarily through heterosexual contact. A second reason for understanding the immunology of the male reproductive tract is the developing interest in immunocontraception in males (Aitken *et al.*, 1993). It offers a novel approach to birth control without many of the disadvantages of current contraceptive methods used by humans, or the traditional methods of controlling reproduction in other mammals, which are becoming increasingly unacceptable on ethical grounds. A third reason is to provide a rationale for preventing or treating immunological forms of male infertility. This form of infertility is thought to account for 8% of idiopathic male infertility, and it occurs in more than 60% of men who have undergone reversal of vasectomy. This review assesses our current knowledge of the immunology of the male sperm ducts to provide a basis for solving the problems mentioned above. Although the emphasis is on the excurrent ducts of the testis, the testis is also considered for comparison and because procedures that have a primary effect on the testis may show secondary effects on the excurrent ducts.

Self Tolerance and Spermatogenesis

The major constraint on any immune response is that minimal damage is caused to self tissue. Thus the mechanisms determining the discrimination of self from non-self have been a major thrust of immunological investigation in recent times. During late fetal and early post-natal life the precursors of both T and B lymphocytes undergo random gene rearrangements within the T-cell receptor (TCR) and immunoglobulin (Ig) gene loci, respectively, such that a large repertoire of both TCR and immunoglobulin receptors are generated. Thymocytes that have undergone a productive TCR rearrangement are then selected within the thymus by processes of both negative and positive selection so that potentially self-reactive cells are eliminated (von Boehmer, 1988). Similarly antigen recognition by immature B cells within the bone marrow (of self antigen) results in clonal deletion due to apoptotic cell death (Goodnow, 1992a,b). Because self tolerance is essential to survival, the body does not rely on thymic selection alone for removal of self-reactive T cells. Clonal anergy is a state of antigen-specific suppression of a T cell resulting from activation (through the TCR) in the absence of a co-stimulatory signal provided by professional antigen-presenting cells (APCs) (Schwartz, 1997). This process is thought to have arisen to prevent autoimmune responses against self tissues not encountered in the thymus.

Sperm production does not occur until puberty, well after tolerance to self has been established and thus post-meiotic germ cells in the testis have the potential to be antigenic. The presence of anti-sperm antibodies in some infertile males and the ease with which anti-sperm antibodies are induced in experimental animals after immunization with sperm fractions in adjuvant confirm that tolerance to these antigens has not been established. In most males, however, sperm production proceeds unhindered by the immune system suggesting that there must be other mechanisms for preventing autoimmune destruction of the developing spermatozoa. Recent interest in using the immune system as a contraceptive has therefore generated considerable interest in the immune capacity and function of the male reproductive tracts.

The blood–luminal Barrier

A barrier between blood and the lumen of the seminiferous tubules was demonstrated by Setchell *et al.* (1969). It was shown to be due partly to peritubular cells which prevented the entry of peroxidase, but mainly due to specialized tight junctions between adjacent Sertoli cells which prevented the passage of most solute including lanthanum (Dym and Fawcett, 1970). The barrier in the rete testis is less efficient than that in the seminiferous tubules as judged by the exclusion of marker molecules (Kormano, 1967), and comparison of the composition of luminal fluid samples from both sites (Tuck *et al.*, 1970). There is also some entry of protein and antibody into the rete testis (Johnson, 1972; Tung and Unanue, 1970) and the concentration of immunoglobulin in rete testis fluid is about 0.2 % of that in serum (Johnson and Setchell, 1968). The peritubular capillaries around the ductuli efferentes are more permeable than testicular blood capillaries (Kormano, 1967), and in terms of the transport of fluid and solute the duct epithelium is 'leaky' to water and some inorganic ions (see Clulow *et al.*, this volume). Although there is no evidence that immunoglobulin or other protein enters the lumen from the peritubular compartment, the possibility has not been satisfactorily tested. Friend and Gilula (1972) concluded that the tight junctions between adjacent epithelial cells in the ductus epididymidis are more highly developed than elsewhere in the rat (except the seminiferous tubules) and the epithelium was shown to be impermeable to pyroentimote, lanthanum and peroxidase (Friend and Gilula, 1972). Subsequently, Suzuki and Nagano (1978) characterized the tight junctions in the initial segment of the rat using freeze fracture, and Cyr *et al.* (1995) found that tight junctions in the initial segment spanned a considerably greater length of apical plasma membrane than they did in the rest of the epididymis.

Immunological Barriers

In addition to the barriers formed as a result of tight junctions, there is also an immunological barrier to prevent leakage of sperm antigens into the systemic circulation and the subsequent induction of autoimmunity. Although the testis contains only lymphocytes in the interstitial tissues, the epithelium of the ductus epididymidis contains significant numbers of lymphocytes. These intraepithelial lymphocytes have been estimated to make up 13 % of total mucosal cells in humans (el-Demiry *et al.*, 1985), 4–5% in rats (Yeung and Cooper, 1982) and are also found in tammar wallabies (Jones *et al.*, 1984). They are therefore present in numbers similar to those found in the intestinal epithelium (Beagley and Husband, 1998) and in the female reproductive tract (Parr and Parr, 1991). The density of lymphocytes differs in various regions of the ductus epididymidis but it is agreed that $CD8^+$ cells outnumber $CD4^+$ cells in the epithelium in all regions. CD4 cells appear to be dominant in the interstitial tissues, although recent studies (M.P. Hedger, personal communication) suggest that CD8 cells also predominate in the interstitial tissues of the rat testis. It has been assumed that these cells are suppressor cells due to the expression of CD8 and that their function is to prevent the induction of immune responses to sperm antigens. However, there is little hard data to demonstrate a definite suppressor function. For example, the relative numbers of TCRγδ versus TCRαβ cells, the repertoire of cytokines secreted and the form of CD8 expressed (CD8αα versus CD8αβ) all remain to be determined. Thus while similar cells in the intestinal epithelium have been implicated in preventing immune responses against food antigens, a similar function for epididymal CD8 cells has yet to be demonstrated.

Macrophages, some containing sperm fragments, have been demonstrated in the testis in several species and it has been suggested that these cells may be involved in sequestering sperm antigen before it gains access to the systemic circulation. Staining of mouse testicular sections with antibodies for mouse macrophages and dendritic cells (Itoh *et al.*, 1995) revealed a considerable heterogeneity in staining patterns and morphology, with cells often expressing surface antigens associated with both macrophages and dendritic cells. Whether epididymal macrophages also differ in cytokine profiles and responses to inflammatory mediators is unknown.

The principal cells in the efferent ducts have been shown to express MHC class II antigen following immunization with sperm antigens in both mice and rats and injection of Freund's adjuvant alone can induce MHC class II expression and orchitis in mice. It has been assumed that these cells are acting as antigen-presenting cells as MHC class II expression precedes the development of orchitis. There is little data available, however, regarding the expression of B7 (CD80/CD86) co-stimulator molecules by these cells. It is possible therefore that if these cells are MHC class II^+ but unable to express co-stimulatory molecules such as B7, they may actually be involved in the induction of anergy (functional inactivation) in naive sperm-reactive CD4 T cells, which would occur following TCR–MHC class II interaction in the absence of signalling through the T cell CD28 molecule (Schwartz, 1997). This process may be facilitated by the binding of spermatozoa to MHC class II on principal cells by a CD4-like surface protein found on spermatozoa (Ashida and Scofield, 1987). Only one study has looked at CD80 and CD86 staining on cells in the testis of both normal BALB/c mice and autoimmune-prone non-obese diabetic (NOD) mice (Sainio-Pollanen *et al.*, 1996). Neither young (4 weeks of age) or older (17–21 weeks of age) BALB/c mice had any CD80/CD86 expressing cells in testicular sections. However, older NOD mice (14–22 weeks of age) did contain some cells expressing CD80 and CD86. These $CD80^+$ and most $CD86^+$ cells did not co-stain with CD11b/CD18 suggesting that they were not macrophages and the authors suggested that these cells may be dendritic cells; however, this was not verified by costaining with anti-CD11c, MHC class II or NLDC145. Although this study did not include examination of the epididymal tissues, the findings of lack of B7 expression in the testis support the hypothesis that antigen encounter at this site, and possibly the efferent ducts, may result in induction of anergy in potentially self-reactive T cells.

Interestingly, transplantation of allografts into the testis results in prolonged allograft survival (Head *et al.*, 1983; Kazeem, 1988; Maddocks and Setchell, 1990). One quarter of parathyroid allografts in the testis survived for >200 days compared with a normal rejection time of 7–10 days. Allografts under the rat epididymal capsule survived for only 36 days suggesting that immune privilege at this site may not be as great as for the testis. However, graft survival times in the epididymis did depend on whether the graft bed was drained by the retroperitoneal lymph nodes. Longer survival times were noted in grafts where the lymphatics drained directly into the cisterna chyli (Kazeem, 1988). These observations are consistent with a state of immunosuppression or immune privilege in this tissue.

Basal cells in the human epididymal epithelium have been shown to express macrophage antigens (Yeung *et al.*, 1994) and their ultrastructure is macrophage-like. As with CD8 cells, there is little functional data concerning the role of these cells in the induction or suppression of immune responses.

Transforming growth factor β (TGFβ) has been demonstrated in the testis and this cytokine is known to suppress a number of immune responses (Moses *et al.*, 1990). Interleukin 1 (IL-1) is present in rete testis fluid and this cytokine is involved in early activation of both B and T cells. Information regarding the expression of other cytokines in the ductus epididymidis is not available. It has been suggested that immune responses in the testis and ductus epididymidis are Th2 dominant although Th1 cells are definitely induced in rodent models of orchitis. Mechanisms that drive a dominant Th2 response at these sites have yet to be determined. No data are available on the expression of IL4 or IL12 in testis or ductus epididymidis nor have functional studies of resident APCs been carried out to determine whether these cells preferentially stimulate a Th2 (or Th1) response as has been demonstrated for dendritic cells in murine Peyer's patches (Everson *et al.*, 1996).

Epididymal and seminal plasma are known to contain significant concentrations of complement inhibitors. Epididymal spermatozoa have been shown to express clusterin, membrane cofactor protein (CD46), decay accelerating factor (CD55) and protectin (CD59). CD46, CD55 and CD59 have also been reported in seminal plasma (Bozas *et al.*, 1993; Fenichel *et al.*, 1994; Simpson and Holmes, 1994). The complement components C3 and C9 were not detected in human seminal plasma while in rabbit cauda epididymal fluids C3 is present at concentrations of 25 % of that found in serum. Thus, it appears that the activity of the complement cascade is inhibited in the testis and ductus epididymidis and presumably in the rete testis and efferent ducts. This finding is consistent with findings that complement components such as C3 and C8 are involved in the acrosome reaction (Cabot and Oliphant, 1978) and in sperm–egg interaction (Pollanen and Cooper, 1994) and the role of the epididymis in acting to decapacitate spermatozoa and stabilize the acrosome. Opinion is divided as to whether the presence of complement inhibitors can protect spermatozoa from complement-mediated lysis should antibody gain entry to the ductus epididymidis.

Entry of Immunoglobulin into the Ductus Epididymidis

In recent times efforts to develop immunocontraceptive vaccines have led to interest in how antibody gets into the epididymal lumen. This interest is based on the substantial clinical literature which demonstrates that male infertility is associated with the presence of anti-sperm antibody both bound to spermatozoa and in seminal plasma. The majority of such infertile men rarely suffer from orchitis and thus attempts to recreate this experiment of nature underpin efforts to develop a male immunocontraceptive. After intravenous (i.v.) infusion of ^{51}Cr-EDTA into rats, the concentration in serum was found to be 40 times higher than that in rete testis fluid (Setchell *et al.*, 1996). This study suggests that the barrier significantly prevents the entry of small water soluble molecules the size of EDTA (MW 292), and would thus prevent not only sperm products gaining access to the systemic immune system, but also immune products such as Ig and complement (C) from gaining entry to developing spermatozoa. Lack of Ig entry into the epididymal lumen was confirmed by a number of studies. Intravenous infusion of isotope or fluorochrome-labelled antibodies (Johnson, 1972; Pollanen and Cooper, 1995; Wong *et al.*, 1983; Yeung *et al.*, 1991) and studies of segments of ductus epididymidis incubated in solutions containing conjugated Ig all showed that Ig could penetrate extratubular interstitial tissues but did not reach the luminal compartment. A possible problem in interpretation of some of these studies is that the Ig used was not from the species being studied (i.e. sheep and rabbit IgG infused into rats). Further studies with whole Ig versus F(ab) fragments also demonstrated that there were no Fc-mediated uptake mechanisms operating in the excurrent ducts (Pollanen *et al.*, 1997). Thus despite entry into the lumen of products such as amino acids, sugars and other molecules required for sperm maturation the above studies suggest that the blood–epididymal barrier excludes Ig. Nevertheless studies in both rats and guinea-pigs immunized with isologous spermatozoa plus Freund's adjuvant and pertussis toxin demonstrated that under these conditions Ig entered the excurrent ducts. Such treatment resulted in orchitis and infertility in many animals,

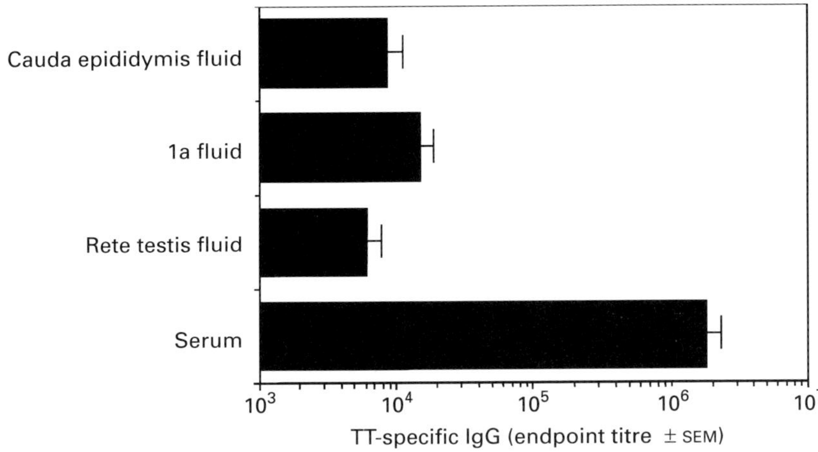

Fig. 1. Tetanus toxoid-specific IgG in serum and reproductive tract fluids. Male Wistar rats were immunized subcutaneously three times (days 0, 28 and 42) with tetanus toxoid (TT) in Freund's adjuvant. Samples were collected on day 49 and assayed for TT-specific IgG by ELISA spot assay.

and in guinea-pigs immunized with PH-20 plus adjuvant IgG was demonstrated by immunofluoresence inside the lumen of the cauda epididymidis (Tung *et al.*, 1997). In these studies, however, it is not clear whether antibody entered the lumen across the epithelium of the cauda epididymidis or as a result of inflammation upstream in the testis due to immunization with testicular antigen in adjuvant. The latter is the most likely explanation. However, in guinea-pigs injected intravenously, or directly into the testis, with anti-sperm antibodies, IgG was found bound to spermatozoa in the rete testis and caput epididymidis, but not in the seminiferous tubules, within 30 min of injection (Tung *et al.*, 1971). This antibody entry could not be attributed to inflammation.

We have used a non-reproductive tract antigen, tetanus toxoid (TT), to investigate uptake of IgG into the rete testis and excurrent ducts of male Wistar rats. Animals were immunized with TT (100 μg in Freund's complete adjuvant; CFA) on day 0 and also on days 28 and 42 with 50 μg TT in IFA. One week after the third immunization blood was collected by cardiac bleed, luminal fluids were collected by micropuncture and TT-specific IgG in all samples was measured by ELISA-spot assay. The mean endpoint titre (± SEM) of TT-specific IgG in serum was $1.825 \times 10^6 (4.78 \times 10^5)$ while that of rete testis fluid was 6.08×10^3 (1.6×10^3), 1a fluid entering the ductus epididymidis $1.49 \times 10^4 (3.8 \times 10^3)$ and cauda epididymal fluid 8.56×10^3 (2.48×10^3). Thus the percentage of TT-specific IgG found in luminal fluids as a percentage of that found in serum was 0.33 % for rete testis fluid, 0.81 % for 1a fluid entering the ductus epididymidis and 0.47 % for cauda epididymidis fluid (Fig. 1).

Mucosal Immunity and the Male Reproductive Tract

Mucosal surfaces represent the interface between the external and internal environments and are constituted in most cases by an epithelial layer one cell thick. Sampling of antibodies in mucosal secretions has shown that IgA is the dominant isotype. Because maintenance of the integrity of the mucosal epithelia is an important host defence mechanism, a unique transport mechanism has evolved to transport IgA, produced by plasma cells in subepithelial tissues, across the epithelial barrier into mucosal secretions. This mechanism involves the binding of IgA (and IgM) by secretory component (SC) (Brandtzaeg, 1985; Mostov *et al.*, 1984) expressed at the basolateral surface of mucosal epithelial cells. Only polymeric IgA and IgM is bound by SC, with monomeric forms of either isotype and IgG not able to be bound. The SC–Ig complex is then taken up by endocytosis and the endosome transcytosed across the epithelial cell. At the luminal surface the IgA (or IgM) is

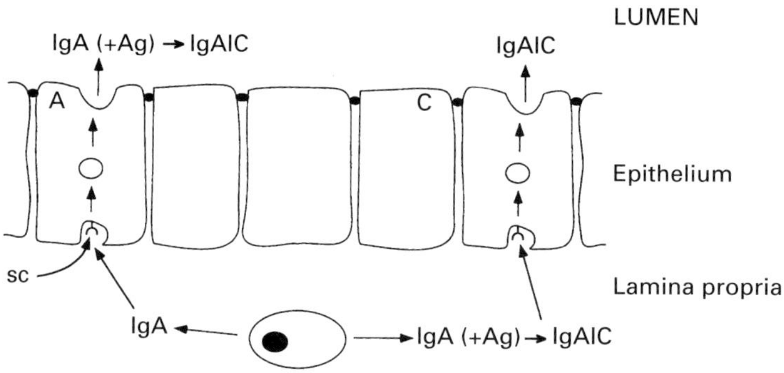

Fig. 2. Transepithelial transport of IgA. IgA produced by subepithelial plasma cells, or IgA + Ag immune complexes (AIC) are bound by secretory component (SC) on the basolateral surface of epithelial cells. IgA or IgA immune complexes are then transcytosed across the epithelial barrier and released at the luminal surface.

released into the mucosal secretions together with a small portion of the SC molecule which remains attached to the Ig molecule (Fig. 2). In this way IgA is transported into secretions while the epithelial integrity is maintained. IgA–immune complexes can also be transported across the epithelium so that antigen that has breached the epithelial barrier can be transported back into the lumen.

Another feature of mucosal responses is that the antigenic experience of one mucosal site is shared amongst other mucosal sites. Immunization into the gut, for example, gives rise to IgA antibodies not only in intestinal secretions but also in the respiratory tract, female reproductive tract, saliva and lachrymal glands. These findings have led to the definition of the common mucosal immune system (CMIS) (reviewed in Brandtzaeg *et al.* (1989) and McGhee *et al.* (1989). An important feature of the CMIS is the presence of specialised lymphoid tissues that play a major role in the induction of mucosal immunity. The best studied of these are the Peyer's patches (PP) of the mouse small intestine. PP can be divided into three distinct areas, a dome epithelium consisting of specialised antigen sampling microfold (M) cells, sometimes called follicle-associated epithelial (FAE) cells, a follicular B-cell zone and a parafollicular T-cell zone (Fig. 3). In PP, luminal antigen is sampled by M cells found on the luminal surface of the PP (Bockman and Cooper, 1973; Owen and Jones, 1974). Antigens such as bacteria, viruses, some proteins and various particulate antigens are transported into the PP by M cells (Table 2) and presented to APCs within the subluminal area. Some reports have identified MHC class II expression on M cells suggesting that they may have an antigen-presentation function; however, this is disputed by other investigators and remains to be determined. The mechanism for selective antigen uptake by M cells is unknown; however, it is thought that this occurs to prevent immune responses against food-derived antigens which make up the bulk of luminal contents. Antigen is carried to the B-cell areas where naive B cells become activated and, under the influence of T-cell cytokines, undergo isotype switching from IgD/IgM expression to cells expressing only surface IgA. During this process B cells (and T cells) acquire specific homing receptors (for example the $\alpha4/\beta7$ integrin). IgA B cells then leave the PP by the intestinal lymphatics, enter the blood circulation via the thoracic duct and home to mucosal sites such as the lamina propria of the small intestine. This tissue-specific homing is achieved by binding of the $\alpha4/\beta7$ integrin to its specific ligand (MAdCAM-1) which is found only on vascular endothelial cells in mucosal tissues such as the gastrointestinal tract, the respiratory tract and the urogenital tract (Butcher and Picker, 1996). In this way the CMIS can be divided into inductive sites, such as PP, where cells become activated by mucosal antigen and undergo isotype switching to IgA, and effector sites such as the intestinal lamina propria and subepithelial tissues associated with various mucosal surfaces where IgA is secreted and transported into mucosal secretions. The entire process is extremely dynamic as 1 metre of human small intestine contains 10^{10} IgA plasma cells (Mestecky,

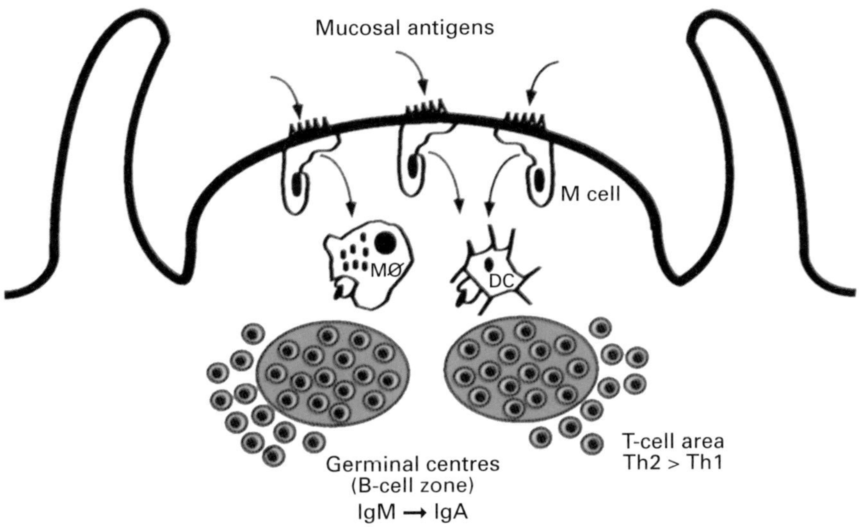

Fig. 3. Induction of mucosal immunity in Peyer's patches (PP). Luminal antigen is endocytosed by PP microfold (M) cells and transferred to macrophages (MØ) or dendritic cells (DC) in the dome region. Germinal centre B cells are activated by antigen carrying antigen-presenting cells (APCs) and under the influence of T-cell-derived cytokines undergo isotype switching to IgA. IgA B cells then acquire homing receptors that allow them to home to other mucosal sites.

1987) that have a half life of 3–5 days and must therefore be continually replaced. IgA is secreted at a rate of 3–4 g per day into the human GI tract (Mestecky, 1987). Structures similar to PP occur in the tonsils and adenoids (nasal-associated lymphoid tissues, NALT), near bronchial bifurcations (bronchus-associated lymphoid tissues, BALT) and in the appendix, colon and rectum which together with the PP in the small intestine make up the gut-associated lymphoid tissues (GALT). Immunization at any of these sites with antigen in an appropriate form results in the appearance of specific IgA in multiple mucosal secretions.

The finding of IgA antisperm antibodies in semen and reproductive tracts of infertile males (Bronson, 1985; Bronson *et al.*, 1982) and interest in the development of immunocontraceptive vaccines and vaccines against sexually transmitted diseases has prompted studies of the role of mucosal immunity in the reproductive tract of both males and females. While a considerable body of data relating to the female reproductive tract is available (Wira and Kaushic, 1996), the male reproductive tract remains largely unexplored. The presence of secretory component (SC) in the rat male reproductive tract has been demonstrated by immunolabelling. SC was found in the ejaculatory ducts, excretory ducts of several accessory glands and urethral glands, with expression being greatest in the prostate (Parr and Parr, 1989; Stern *et al.*, 1992) and 50 % of prostatic fluid IgA was associated with SC. IgA plasma cells are found in the human prostate and in the rat urethral glands (Ablin *et al.*, 1972; Doble *et al.*, 1990; Parr and Parr, 1989) and IgA was detected in organ homogenates of prostate, epididymis, ductus deferens and testis (Stern *et al.*, 1992). These findings suggest that SIgA is transported into the male reproductive tract from the prostate and sites distal to the production of spermatozoa and seminal fluids.

Wang *et al.* (1996) infused mice with radiolabelled polymeric IgA, monomeric IgA and IgG (monomeric) and investigated uptake, from serum, of antibody into various parts of the reproductive tracts of male mice. Polymeric IgA was detectable in secretions from seminal vesicles, prostate, coagulating gland and epididymis (at low concentrations), whereas monomeric IgA and IgG were not transported. Thus in mice SIgA may be transported into the excurrent ducts more widely than it is in rats.

Table 1. Components of the blood–testis barrier

Physical components
Tight junctions between Sertoli cells
Peritubular cells
Immunological components
T-cell suppression (CD8 >> CD4 in reproductive tract)
Macrophages
intraluminal phagocytosis of spermatozoa
reduced responsiveness to stimulation by inflammatory mediators
different cytokine secretion patterns
(compared with peritoneal macrophages)
T-cell anergy induction by testicular APCs?
reduced/lack of B7 expression by reproductive tract APCs
Production of suppressive cytokines eg. TGFβ
Presence of complement inhibitors eg. CD46, CD55, CD59 and clusterin on spermatozoa and in seminal plasma
Suppressive components in seminal plasma
inhibition of T-cell mitogenesis, phagocytosis and ADCC

APCs antigen-presenting cells; ADCC: antibody-dependent cell-mediated cytotoxicity

Table 2. Antigens taken up by M cells

Particles/macromolecules	Bacteria
Ferritin	*Vibrio cholerae*
Horseradish peroxidase	*Salmonella typhi*
Wheat germ agglutinin	*Mycobacterium paratuberculosis*
Cholera toxin	*Brucella abortus*
Latex particles	*Shigella flexneri*
	Escherichia coli
Viruses	Parasites
Reovirus	*Cryptosporidium*
Poliovirus	
Human immunodeficiency virus (HIV)	

These findings have been used to support the hypothesis that the reproductive tract is part of the CMIS, although it is apparent that both serum-derived and mucosal antibodies play a role in both female and male reproductive tracts. Oral and nasal immunization (Kozlowski *et al.*, 1997; Kubota *et al.*,1997; Muster *et al.*, 1995; Staats *et al.*, 1996) have been shown to induce SIgA antibody in vaginal, cervical and uterine fluids. Concentrations of antibody in female reproductive tract fluids are regulated by sex hormones and fluctuate throughout the cycle. Lymphoid aggregates are found in female reproductive tracts (Yeaman *et al.*, 1997), although their size and frequency varies with the stage of the cycle (Wira and Kaushic, 1996). Whether these aggregates serve a similar immune inductive function as PP is unclear. The situation in the male tract is less clear, however, as the area has not been studied. Mucosal lymphoid aggregates are rare in human, mouse and male rat genital tracts (el-Demiry and James, 1988; Parr and Parr, 1989).

Clifton *et al.* (1992) showed that intestinal immunization with ovalbumin (OVA) followed by intratesticular immunization resulted in OVA-specific IgA cells in testis, caput epididymidis, cauda epididymidis, ductus deferens, prostate, and bulbo-urethral gland and OVA-specific IgA in testicular homogenate. Neither intestinal immunization alone nor testicular immunization alone resulted in IgA secreting cells in the reproductive tract or IgA in testicular homogenates. While this study suggests that mucosal antibody may reach the epididymis, the authors did not look for

Table 3. Methods for targeting immune responses to the male reproductive tract

Routes of immunization (activation of mucosal immunity)
intranasal
oral
rectal
Use of replicating delivery systems
attenuated *Salmonella* sp.
vaccinia virus, poliovirus, ectromelia virus
Lactobacillus sp.
Lactococcus sp.
Adjuvants and delivery systems that target mucosal immunity
liposomes
microcarrier beads
cholera toxin and cholera toxin β subunit
E. coli heat labile toxin
DNA vaccination

orchitis in the immunized animals. As immunization involved injection into the testis of OVA emulsified in Freund's complete adjuvant, it is possible that inflammation may have affected the blood–testis barrier.

Immunization of the Male Reproductive Tract: Future Directions

While there are many obvious reasons to induce immunity in the male reproductive tract (see Introduction) this has not been attempted (with the exception of the studies of Primakoff *et al.*, 1997) despite many review articles outlining the need for such vaccination. As both mucosal and systemic immunity play a role in the male tract, lessons may be learned from attempts to induce immunity in females. Oral, uterine and vaginal immunization with attenuated polio virus induces specific antibodies in uterine and vaginal secretions (Ogra and Ogra, 1973). Oral immunization should be explored as a means of inducing immunity in the male reproductive tract. These studies also highlight the potential value of replicating delivery systems, both viral and bacterial. Immune-mediated infertility in female mice has been induced by infection with a recombinant Ectromelia virus expressing the mouse ZP3 glycoprotein (Jackson *et al.*, 1998). Attenuated *Salmonella* vectors have been shown to induce mucosal antibodies and their use to immunize feral foxes with sperm antigens is being investigated (Bradley *et al.*, 1997; Jackson *et al.*, 1994; Zhang *et al.*, 1997). The use of replicating vectors to induce immunity in males has yet to be attempted. Similarly intranasal immunization induces specific antibodies in vaginal secretions (Muster *et al.*, 1995; Staats *et al.*, 1996), but the effect on the male reproductive tract is unknown. Local immunization of the female reproductive tract also induces antibody in vaginal secretions; however, notwithstanding the studies of Clifton *et al.* (1992), this is unlikely to be a viable route in males. Studies of systemic immunization in animals almost invariably uses Freund's adjuvant. This poses obvious problems in man where to date alum remains the only accepted adjuvant. The potential of other carrier or adjuvant systems such as liposomes, immunostimulatory complexes (ISCOMs) and microcarrier particles needs to be explored. Thus as the need for vaccines targeting the male reproductive tract has been identified much work remains to fulfil the potential promised by animal studies and review articles.

This work was supported in part by a grant from the Australian Research Council and the Vertebrate Biocontrol Cooperative Research Centre.

References

Ablin RJ, Soanes WA and Gonder MJ (1972) *In vivo* bound immunoglobulins in the human prostate – their identification and possible significance *Zeitschrift fur Immunitatsforschung, Experimentelle und Klinische Immunologie* **144** 233–241

Aitken RJ, Paterson M and Koothan PT (1993) Contraceptive vaccines *British Medical Bulletin* **49** 88–99

Ashida ER and Scofield VL (1987) Lymphocyte major histocompatibility complex-encoded class II structures may act as sperm receptors *Proceedings of the National Academy of Sciences USA* **84** 3395–3399

Beagley K and Husband A (1998) Intraepithelial lymphocytes: origins, distribution and function *Critical Reviews in Immunology* (in press)

Bockman DE and Cooper MD (1973) Pinocytosis by epithelium associated with lymphoid follicles in the bursa of Fabricius, appendix, and Peyer's patches: an electron microscopic study *American Journal of Anatomy* **136** 455–477

Bozas SE, Kirszbaum L Sparrow RL and Walker ID (1993) Several vascular complement inhibitors are present on human sperm *Biology of Reproduction* **48** 503–511

Bradley MP, Hinds LA and Bird PH (1997) A bait-delivered immunocontraceptive vaccine for the European red fox (*Vulpes vulpes*) by the year 2002? *Reproduction, Fertility and Development* **9** 111–116

Brandtzaeg P (1985) Role of J chain and secretory component in receptor-mediated glandular and hepatic transport of immunoglobulins in man *Scandinavian Journal of Immunology* **22** 111–146

Brandtzaeg P (1989) Overview of the mucosal immune system *Current Topics in Microbiology and Immunology* **146** 13–25

Bronson RA (1985) The immunoglobulin class of antisperm antibodies *American Journal of Reproductive Immunology and Microbiology* **9** 142 (letter)

Bronson RA, Cooper GW and Rosenfeld DL (1982) Sperm-specific isoantibodies and autoantibodies inhibit the binding of human sperm to the human zona pellucida *Fertility and Sterility* **38** 724–729

Butcher EC and Picker L J (1996) Lymphocyte homing and homeostasis *Science* **272** 60–66

Cabot CL and Oliphant G (1978) The possible role of immunological complement in induction of rabbit sperm acrosome reaction *Biology of Reproduction* **19** 666–672

Clifton VL, Husband AJ and Kay DJ (1992) Local immunity in the male reproductive tract *Immunology and Cell Biology* **70** 301–307

Cyr DG , Robaire B and Hermo L (1995) Structure and turnover of junctional complexes between principal cells of the rat epididymis *Microscopy Research and Technique* **30** 54–66

Doble A , Walker MM, Harris JR, Taylor-Robinson D and Witherow RO (1990) Intraprostatic antibody deposition in chronic abacterial prostatitis *British Journal of Urology* **65** 598–605

Dym M and Fawcett DW (1970) The blood–testis barrier in the rat and the physiological compartmentation of the seminiferous epithelium *Biology of Reproduction* **3** 308–326

el-Demiry M and James K (1988) Lymphocyte subsets and macrophages in the male genital tract in health and disease: a monoclonal antibody-based study *European Urology* **14** 226–235

el-Demiry MI, Hargreave TB, Busuttil A, James K, Ritchie AW and Chisholm GD (1985) Lymphocyte sub-populations in the male genital tract *British Journal of Urology* **57** 769–774

Everson MP , McDuffie DS, Lemak DG, Koopman WJ, McGhee JR and Beagley KW (1996) Dendritic cells from different tissues induce production of different T cell cytokine profiles *Journal of Leukocyte Biology* **59** 494–498

Fenichel P , Cervoni F, Hofmann P, Deckert M, Emiliozzi C, Hsi BL and Rossi B (1994) Expression of the complement regulatory protein CD59 on human spermatozoa: characterization and role in gametic interaction *Molecular Reproduction and Development* **38** 338–346

Friend DS and Gilula NB (1972) Variations in tight and gap junctions in mammalian tissues *Journal of Cell Biology* **53** 758–776

Goodnow CC (1992a) B-cell tolerance *Current Opinion in Immunology* **4** 703–710

Goodnow CC (1992b) Transgenic mice and analysis of B-cell tolerance *Annual Review of Immunology* **10** 489–518

Head JR, Neaves WB and Billingham RE (1983) Immune privilege in the testis I. Basic parameters of allograft survival *Transplantation* **36** 423–431

Itoh M, De Rooij DG, Jansen A and Drexhage HA (1995) Phenotypical heterogeneity of testicular macrophages/ dendritic cells in normal adult mice: an immuno-histochemical study *Journal of Reproductive Immunology* **28** 217–232

Jackson R, Maguire D, Hinds L and Ramshaw I (1998) Infertility in mice induced by a recombinant Ectromelia virus expressing mouse zona pellucida glycoprotein 3 *Biology of Reproduction* **58** 152–159

Jackson RJ, Staats HF, Xu-Amano J, Takahashi I, Kiyono H, Hudson ME, Gilley RM, Chatfield SN and McGhee JR (1994) Oral vaccine models: multiple delivery systems employing tetanus toxoid *Annals of the New York Academy of Sciences* **730** 217–234

Johnson MH (1972) The distribution of immunoglobulin and spermatozoal autoantigen in the genital tract of the male guinea pig: its relationship to autoallergic orchitis *Fertility and Sterility* **23** 383–392

Johnson MH and Setchell BP (1968) Protein and immunoglobulin content of rete testis fluid of rams *Journal of Reproduction and Fertility* **17** 403–406

Jones RC, Hinds LA and Tyndale-Biscoe CH (1984) Ultrastructure of the epididymis of the tammar, *Macropus eugenii*, and its relationship to sperm maturation *Cell and Tissue Research* **237** 525–535

Kazeem AA (1988) A critical consideration of the rat epididymis as an immunologically privileged site *Scandinavian Journal of Immunology* **27** 149–156

Kormano M (1967) Dye permeability and alkaline phosphatase activity of testicular capillaries in the postnatal rat *Histochemie* **9** 327–338

Kozlowski PA , Cu-Uvin S, Neutra MR and Flanigan TP (1997) Comparison of the oral, rectal, and vaginal immunization routes for induction of antibodies in rectal and genital tract secretions of women *Infection and Immunity* **65** 1387–1394

Kubota M, Miller CJ, Imaoka K, Kawabata S, Fujihashi K, McGhee JR and Kiyono H (1997) Oral immunization with simian immunodeficiency virus p55gag and cholera toxin elicits both mucosal IgA and systemic IgG immune responses in nonhuman primates *Journal of Immunology* **158** 5321–5329

Maddocks S and Setchell BP (1990) Recent evidence for immune privilege in the testis *Journal of Reproductive Immunology* **18** 9–18

McGhee JR, Mestecky J, Elson CO and Kiyono H (1989) Regulation of IgA synthesis and immune response by T cells and interleukins *Journal of Clinical Immunology* **9** 175–199

Mestecky (1987) The common mucosal immune system and current strategies for induction of immune responses in external secretions *Journal of Clinical Immunology* **7** 265–276

Moses HL, Yang EY and Pietenpol JA (1990) TGF-beta stimulation and inhibition of cell proliferation: new mechanistic insights *Cell* **63** 245–247

Mostov KE, Friedlander M and Blobel G (1984) The receptor for transepithelial transport of IgA and IgM contains multiple immunoglobulin-like domains *Nature* **308** 37–43

Muster T, Ferko B, Klima A *et al.* (1995) Mucosal model of immunization against human immunodeficiency virus type 1 with a chimeric influenza virus *Journal of Virology* **69** 6678–6686

Ogra PL and Ogra SS (1973) Local antibody response to poliovaccine in the human female genital tract *Journal of Immunology* **110** 1307–1311

Owen RL and Jones AL (1974) Epithelial cell specialization within human Peyer's patches: an ultrastructural study of intestinal lymphoid follicles *Gastroenterology* **66** 189–203

Parr MB and Parr EL (1989) Immunohistochemical localization of secretory component and immunoglobulin A in the urogenital tract of the male rodent *Journal of Reproduction and Fertility* **85** 115–124

Parr MB and Parr EL (1991) Langerhans cells and T lymphocyte subsets in the murine vagina and cervix *Biology of Reproduction* **44** 491–498

Pollanen P and Cooper TG (1994) Immunology of the testicular excurrent ducts *Journal of Reproductive Immunology* **26** 167–216

Pollanen P and Cooper TG (1995) Vascular permeability to effectors of the immune system in the male rat reproductive tract at puberty *Journal of Reproductive Immunology* **28** 85–109

Pollanen P, Cooper TG, Kokk K, Saari T and Setchell BP (1997) Microvascular permeability to the F(ab')2 fragment of IgG in the male rat reproductive tract at puberty *Journal of Reproductive Immunology* **32** 221–240

Primakoff P, Woolman-Gamer L, Tung KS and Myles DG (1997) Reversible contraceptive effect of PH-20 immunization in male guinea pigs *Biology of Reproduction* **56** 1142–1146

Sainio-Pollanen S, Saari T, Simell O and Pollanen P (1996) CD28–CD80/CD86 interactions in testicular immunoregulation *Journal of Reproductive Immunology* **31** 145–163

Schwartz R H (1997) T cell clonal anergy *Current Opinion in Immunology* **9** 351–357

Setchell BP, Voglmayr JK and Waites GM (1969) A blood–testis barrier restricting passage from blood into rete testis fluid but not into lymph *Journal of Physiology* **200** 73–85

Setchell BP, Tao L and Zupp JL (1996) The penetration of chromium-EDTA from blood plasma into various compartments of rat testes as an indicator of function of the blood–testis barrier after exposure of the testes to heat *Journal of Reproduction and Fertility* **106** 125–133

Simpson KL and Holmes CH (1994) Differential expression of complement regulatory proteins decay-accelerating factor (CD55), membrane cofactor protein (CD46) and CD59 during human spermatogenesis *Immunology* **81** 452–461

Staats HF, Nichols WG and Palker TJ (1996) Mucosal immunity to HIV-1: systemic and vaginal antibody responses after intranasal immunization with the HIV-1 C4/V3 peptide T1SP10 MN(A) *Journal of Immunology* **157** 462–472

Stern JE, Gardner S, Quirk D and Wira CR (1992) Secretory immune system of the male reproductive tract: effects of dihydrotestosterone and estradiol on IgA and secretory component levels *Journal of Reproductive Immunology* **22** 73–85

Suzuki F and Nagano T (1978) Regional differentiation of cell junctions in the excurrent duct epithelium of the rat testis as revealed by freeze–fracture *Anatomical Record* **191** 503–519

Tuck RR, Setchell BP, Waites GM and Young JA (1970) The composition of fluid collected by micropuncture and catheterization from the seminiferous tubules and rete testis of rats *Pflugers Archiv – European Journal of Physiology* **318** 225–243

Tung K and Unanue E (1970) Pathogenesis of allergic orchitis *Proceedings of the Federation of the American Societies of Experimental Biology* **29** 287

Tung KS, Unanue ER and Dixon FJ (1971) Pathogenesis of experimental allergic orchitis: II The role of antibody *Journal of Immunology* **106** 1463–1472

Tung KS, Primakoff P, Woolman-Gamer L and Myles DG (1997) Mechanism of infertility in male guinea pigs immunized with sperm PH-20 *Biology of Reproduction* **56** 1133–1141

von Boehmer H (1988) The developmental biology of T lymphocytes *Annual Review of Immunology* **6** 309–326

Wang Y, Ben K, Cao X and Wang Y (1996) Transport of anti-sperm monoclonal IgA and IgG into murine male and female genital tracts from blood: effect of sex hormones *Journal of Immunology* **156** 1014–1019

Wira C and Kaushic C (1996) Mucosal immunity in the female reproductive tract: effect of sex hormones on immune recognition and responses. In *Mucosal Vaccines: New Trends in Immunization* pp 375–388 Eds H Kiyono, PL Ogra and JR McGhee. Academic Press, New York

Wong PY, Tsang AY, Fu WO and Lau HK (1983) Restricted entry of an anti-rat epididymal protein IgG into the rat epididymis *International Journal of Andrology* **6** 275–282

Yeaman GR, Guyre PM, Fanger MW, Collins JE, White HD, Rathbun W, Orndorff KA, Gonzalez J, Stern JE and Wira CR (1997) Unique CD8[+] T cell-rich lymphoid aggregates in human uterine endometrium *Journal of Leukocyte Biology* **61** 427–435

Yeung CH and Cooper TG (1982) Ultrastructure of the perfused rat epididymis: effect of luminal sodium ion concentration *Cell and Tissue Research* **226** 407–425

Yeung CH, Bergmann M and Cooper TG (1991) Non-specific uptake of IgG by rat epididymal tubules *in vitro*. *International Journal of Andrology* **14** 364–373

Yeung CH, Nashan D, Sorg C, Oberpenning F, Schulze H, Nieschlag E and Cooper TG (1994) Basal cells of the human epididymis – antigenic and ultrastructural similarities to tissue-fixed macrophages *Biology of Reproduction* **50** 917–926

Zhang X, Lou YH, Koopman M, Doggett T, Tung KS and Curtiss RR (1997) Antibody responses and infertility in mice following oral immunization with attenuated *Salmonella typhimurium* expressing recombinant murine ZP3 [published erratum appears in *Biology of Reproduction* 1997 **56** 1069] *Biology of Reproduction* **56** 33–41

Journal of Reproduction and Fertility Supplement **53**, 247–259

Effects of environmental toxicants on the efferent ducts, epididymis and fertility

Rex A. Hess

Department of Veterinary Biosciences, College of Veterinary Medicine, S. Lincoln, University of Illinois, Urbana, IL 61802, USA

Many of the reproductive toxicants have primary effects on the testis, which potentially overshadow effects downstream on the efferent ducts and epididymis. The specific target of these effects depends upon the dosage and time response. It is often necessary to design experiments that separate testosterone-dependent responses arising in the testis from direct effects on epididymal tissues and spermatozoa, to uncover the mechanisms of toxicity in excurrent ducts. Recent studies have confirmed that chemicals can also alter the time required for sperm transport through the epididymis. Currently there are approximately twenty chemicals that can be classified as epididymal toxicants. There are fewer toxicants reported for the efferent ducts, but a few overlap with epididymal effects. The benzimidazole carbamates, like many efferent ductal toxicants, induce occlusions and subsequent testicular atrophy. The mechanisms appear to be related to fluid reabsorption, sperm stasis, followed by leukocyte chemotaxis, sperm granulomas, fibrosis and often the formation of abnormal microcanals. Disruption of oestrogen receptor function in the efferent ducts also interferes with fluid reabsorption and results in testicular swelling and seminiferous tubular atrophy. Thus, studies in which testicular atrophy occurs after chronic or subchronic exposures should be examined for lesions in efferent ducts and head of the epididymis. Such lesions can lead to permanent infertility.

Introduction

Toxicology of the epididymis has received less attention than other regions of the male reproductive system. A search of the literature for the period 1995–1997 shows that the testis has been the major emphasis in toxicology (nearly 400 papers), while the number of manuscripts focused on toxicity associated with the epididymis is fewer than 90. One problem has been the difficulty in separating direct versus indirect effects on the excurrent ducts, because altered testicular function indirectly alters function of the ductal epithelium downstream. The epididymis is dependent upon androgen stimulation; therefore, any compound that decreases Leydig cell function will decrease androgenic concentration in blood and rete testis fluid, which will have subsequent effects on the epididymis, sperm maturation and fertility. One complication is the fact that a primary effect on the testis may become overwhelming and define the long-term effects on fertility, regardless of effects on the epididymis. If there is a decline in spermatogenesis or testicular atrophy ensues, it is of little consequence that clear cells in the epididymis also disappear. However, it is possible that short-term toxicity targets only the epididymis or the spermatozoa in transit. For example, α-chlorohydrin appears to have direct effects on epididymal spermatozoa without testicular effects, if the dosage is low and exposure time is short (Slott *et al.*, 1997).

If we are to begin separating direct versus indirect effects of toxicants on the male reproductive tract, it is important that experimental design be given top priority. Examining long-term exposures and moderate to high dosages will often provide only primary testicular effects that overshadow effects on the epididymis or spermatozoa. In this review, the ductuli efferentes (efferent ducts) and

Table 1. Pathways for direct effects of toxicants on the epididymis

1. Sperm target	3. Connective tissue target
Enzyme activity	Blood and lymphatic flow
Sperm proteins	Leukocyte chemotaxis
Sperm motility	Inflammation, granulomas
2. Epithelial target	Smooth muscle
Secretory proteins, ions, etc.	4. Mixed targets
Cellular degeneration	Leukocyte chemotaxis
Metabolism, ion flux, organelles	Inflammation
	Indirect action on spermatozoa

epididymis will be considered independently but referred to at times collectively as epididymis. Epididymal toxicants and their known mechanisms of action will be listed. However, the primary focus will be on a compound that targets the efferent ducts and seminiferous epithelium. This compound is benomyl, a benzimidazole carbamate fungicide. We have studied both this parent compound and its metabolite, carbendazim, because the metabolite is responsible for the primary effects on male reproduction (Lim and Miller, 1997). An understanding of the short-term, as well as the long-term, effects is essential if the causes of infertility and testicular atrophy are to be revealed.

Toxicants That Affect the Epididymis

Direct versus indirect effects

The use of two different experimental methods has improved the recognition of effects on epididymal epithelium or spermatozoa in transit. A good example is cyclophosphamide, which induces lethal mutations in males. Only when short-term studies were performed or experimental ligation of the efferent ducts was used did the investigators determine direct effects on epididymal spermatozoa or the epididymal epithelium (Qiu *et al.*, 1995). Methyl chloride is another example of a toxicant that acts directly on the epididymis (Chellman *et al.*, 1987). However, its mechanism of action is different, as it works through secondary damage to spermatozoa following an inflammatory response to treatment and the formation of granulomas. Thus, there are many pathways by which toxicants can affect the epididymis (Table 1) and we have only just begun to understand these mechanisms in a limited number of chemicals. There are approximately twenty chemicals that can be classified as epididymal toxicants, either as having direct or indirect effects on the epididymal epithelium or effects on epididymal spermatozoa (Table 2).

Effects independent of testosterone

Ethane dimethanesulfonate (EDS) and chloroethylmethanesulfonate (CMS) are alkylating antitumour agents that destroy Leydig cells and thus cause a reduction in testosterone (Klinefelter *et al.*, 1992, 1994a,b). However, both compounds also produce epididymal lesions. To determine whether the epididymal effects are independent of testicular effects, Klinefelter *et al.* (1992, 1994b) used testosterone implants to maintain androgen stimulation of spermatogenesis and the epididymal epithelium. Both chemicals caused specific disappearance of clear cells in the cauda epididymis, decreased cauda sperm counts and altered two-dimensional gel patterns of proteins in cauda spermatozoa, all independent of testosterone.

Direct effects on spermatozoa

To test the potential direct effects of EDS on epididymal spermatozoa, Klinefelter *et al.* (1992) treated spermatozoa or co-cultured spermatozoa and epididymal epithelium. Using this novel *in*

Table 2. Effects of toxicants on the epididymis

	Toxicants[1,2]																		
Effects	a	b	c	d	e	f	g	h	i	j	k	l	m	n	o	p	q	r	s
Granulomas; inflammation	x	x					x					x					x		
Spermatocoele; cysts	x	x	x	x													x		
Loss of clear cells												x	x						
Desquamation of epithelium			x											x					
Fibrosis	x																		
Decreases cauda spermatoza										x	x	x	x			x		x	
Increase sperm concentration															x				
Decrease sperm motility	x								x										
Decrease sperm transit time	x	x									x			x					
Increase sperm transit time								x					x			x			
Alter sperm protein profile	x				x						x	x	x						
Epididymal necrosis																			x
Post-implantation loss						x													
Seminiferous tubule dilation	x	x											x	x					
Testicular atrophy	x	x					x						x	x			x		x
Direct effects on spermatozoa	x													x					

[1] Chemicals:
a, -Chlorohydrin; b, Epichlorohydrin; c, α-Bromohydrin; d, glycidol (Cooper *et al.*, 1974; Ericsson, 1975; Slott *et al.*, 1997; Tsang *et al.*, 1981);
e, 6-Chloro-6-deoxyglucose (Tsang *et al.*, 1981; Wong *et al.*, 1980);
f, Cyclophosphamide (Qiu *et al.*, 1995);
g, Methyl chloride (Chellman *et al.*, 1986; Working *et al.*, 1985);
h, Guanethidine (Evans *et al.*, 1972);
i, Ornidizole (Oberlander *et al.*, 1994; Cooper *et al.*, 1997);
j, Methoxychlor (Linder *et al.*, 1992);
k, Anti-androgens (hydroxyflutamide (Klinefelter and Suarez, 1997), cyproterone acetate (Din-Udom *et al.*, 1985; Tsang *et al.*, 1981), vinclozolin (Kelce *et al.*, 1997));
l, Ethane dimethanesulfonate (Klinefelter *et al.*, 1990; 1994b);
m, Chloroethylmethanesulfonate (Klinefelter *et al.*, 1994a; 1997; Klinefelter and Suarez, 1997);
n, 1,2-Dibromo-3-chloropropane;
o, Reserpine (Wen and Wong, 1988);
p, 2,3,7,8-Tetrachlorodibenzo-p-dioxin (Gray *et al.*, 1997);
q, 2,3-Dihydro-2-1-naphthyl -41H-quinazolinone (Ericsson, 1971);
r, PCB169 (Gray *et al.*, 1995);
s, Cadmium (Nagy, 1985).

[2] See also review by Klinefelter and Hess (1998).

vitro method, they found that the effects of EDS on spermatozoa were mediated through the epididymal-epithelium and not directly on the spermatozoa. There are other examples of toxicants having direct effects on spermatozoa within the epididymal lumen. However, these effects are dose dependent; direct effects on spermatozoa occur only at the lower dosages, while higher doses of the same chemical can cause many pathological changes in the epididymis. In this category, α-chlorohydrin is the best example. At lower dosages, dose-dependent effects on sperm velocity and fertility were significant in the absence of epididymal granulomas (Slott *et al.*, 1997), possibly mediated by the inhibition of glycolysis in the spermatozoa. Spermatocoeles and granulomas are typical responses in both efferent ducts and the caput epididymis after treatments at higher dosages (Cooper *et al.*, 1974).

Alterations in sperm transit time

Another mechanism by which chemicals may interfere with fertility is an alteration in sperm transit time through the epididymis. Oestrogen treatment accelerates the rate of sperm transport in the epididymis (Meistrich *et al.*, 1975). Other experiments have also demonstrated that sperm transport can be altered by disruption of sympathetic or adrenergic innervation of the epididymis (Evans *et al.*, 1972), and thereby alter ion flux, particularly Cl^- secretion (Wen and Wong, 1988; Wong, 1990). More recent studies have shown that chloroethyl-methanesulphonate and hydroxyflutamide accelerate sperm transit through the epididymis (Klinefelter and Suarez, 1997), supporting the findings that castration or cyproterone acetate treatment enhance sperm transport. Interestingly, *in utero* exposure to 2,3,7,8-tetrachlorodibenzo-*p*-dioxin also results in altered sperm transport without obvious testicular effects in adult life (Gray *et al.*, 1997). In the light of these studies, future efforts should be devoted to uncover the physiological mechanisms responsible for sperm transport that are the target of exposure to environmental chemicals.

Toxicants That Affect Efferent Ducts

Reports indicate that smoking and ten reported compounds induce some type of toxic response in the efferent ducts (Table 3). Unfortunately, a clear understanding of their mechanisms of toxicity is lacking. However, for some chemicals there are biochemical data suggesting routes of induced injury. For example, α-chlorohydrin (or a metabolite) and 6-chloro-6-deoxyglucose (CDG) cause reductions in glucose transport and glucose metabolism (Hinton *et al.*, 1983), which could indirectly interfere with energy-dependent processes such as ion transport, in addition to their direct effects on spermatozoa. It is interesting that α-chlorohydrin and epi-chlorohydrin are metabolites of 1,2-dibromo-3-chloropropane (DBCP), a chemical responsible for the first well known case of infertility in humans caused by chemical exposure (Whorton *et al.*, 1979). All three compounds cause kidney dysfunction as well as epididymal lesions (Kluwe *et al.*, 1983). Although the literature does not indicate that DBCP affects the efferent ducts, Kluwe *et al.* (1983) did report 'dilatation of the seminiferous tubules' and long-term tubular atrophy, which are common responses to occlusion of these ducts and seen following exposure to α-chlorohydrin and epichlorohydrin (Cooper and Jackson, 1972; Cooper and Jackson, 1973; Jones, 1978; Kluwe *et al.*, 1983). Thus, it appears that the general mechanism of toxicity for these chemicals is an alteration of fluid reabsorption followed by sperm stasis and ductal occlusion. In general, there are at least six major responses of the efferent ducts to environmental toxins, which can lead to reduced fertility and even testicular atrophy (Table 4).

Ductal occlusions

An examination of the chemicals listed in Table 3 indicates that many toxicants of the efferent ducts induce occlusions. This would suggest an interference with fluid reabsorption, or that other factors such as granulomas or inflammation cause the luminal fluid to become stagnant. In 1943, Wakeley stated that most epididymal cysts in man arise from dysfunction of the efferent ducts. As more chemical toxicants are examined, this early prediction appears to be correct for animal models, too. Several mechanisms could be involved in the pathophysiology of ductal occlusions. One possibility is direct or indirect disruption of Cl^- secretions, which appear to be important for normal flow of spermatozoa in the proximal epididymis (Chan *et al.*, 1995). mRNA encoding cystic fibrosis

Table 3. Effects of toxicants on the efferent ducts

	Toxicants[1,2]										
Effects	a	b	c	d	e	f	g	h	i	j	k
Ciliary loss										x	x
Phagocytosis	x	x	x							x	
Desquamation			x							x	
Epithelial hyperplasia				x						x	
Recanalization	x	x		x							
Spermatocoele	x	x	x	x	x	x			x	x	
Sperm granuloma	x	x	x	x		x					
Inflammation	x	x			x						
Ductal occlusion	x	x	x	x		x	x			x	
Fibrosis	x	x	x				x				
Testicular swelling	x	x	x		x	x		x			
Seminiferous atrophy	x	x	x	x	x	x				x	

[1] a, Benomyl® (Hess *et al.*, 1991);
b, Carbendazim (Carter *et al.*, 1987; Gray *et al.*, 1990; Nakai *et al.*, 1992; Nakai *et al.*, 1993; Rehnberg *et al.*, 1989);
c, α- and epi-Chlorohydrin (Cooper *et al.*, 1974; Ford and Waites, 1981; Hoffer *et al.*, 1975; Jones 1978);
d, Ethylenedimethane sulfonate (Cooper and Jackson, 1972; Cooper and Jackson, 1973);
e, 6-Chloro-6-deoxyglucose (Ford and Waites, 1981);
f, Quinazolinone (Ericsson, 1975);
g, 1,3-Dinitrobenzene (Linder *et al.*, 1988a);
h, Uranyl nitrate (Mason and Young, 1967);
i, Glycidol (Jones and O'Brien, 1980);
j, Cadmium (Nagy, 1985);
k, Fluoride (Susheela and Kumar, 1991).
[2] See also reviews by Ilio and Hess, 1994; and Klinefelter and Hess, 1998.

transmembrane conductance regulator (CFTR) is more prevalent in the proximal regions of the male tract (Trezise *et al.*, 1993) and adult cystic fibrosis patients are infertile, often due to epididymal obstruction (Gaillard *et al.*, 1997).

Effects of Benzimidazole Carbamate Fungicides on Efferent Ducts and Fertility

Effects on fertility

Benomyl (methyl 1-(butylcarbamoyl)-2-benzimidazole carbamate) and its metabolite carbendazim (methyl 2-benzimidazole carbamate) are both highly effective fungicides and nematocides. Their fungicidal action is due to their ability to disrupt microtubule formation, an effect that is also extended to mammalian cells (see Hess *et al.*, 1991). Regulation of these chemicals by the US Environmental Protection Agency was based partially on their reproductive toxicity, which is associated with testicular degeneration (Carter and Laskey, 1982) and decreased fertility (Carter *et al.*, 1987; Gray *et al.*, 1990; Linder *et al.*, 1988b; Torchinskiy *et al.*, 1976). However, the early studies of benzimidazole compounds did not establish mechanisms of testicular atrophy. Infertility occurred in 50% of the males after the first week of exposure to a single dose of carbendazim (400 mg kg^{-1}), but histopathological examination of the testes revealed large variation in tubular atrophy (Carter, 1987). At first, atrophy was assumed to be the result of action of carbendazim as a microtubule poison, which has been shown subsequently to cause necrosis of mitotic and meiotic cells in the testis (Nakai and Hess, 1997) and the formation of abnormal spermatids (Nakai *et al.*, 1997). Other workers found effects on hormones in serum and testicular fluids and attempted to relate the long-term effects on sperm production to an inhibition of the testicular–

Table 4. Major responses of the efferent ductules to environmental toxins and experimental conditions

Suggested responses	Associated toxicants or experimental conditions	End results
Increased reabsorption of luminal fluid	Benomyl[1]; carbendazim[2]	Increased sperm concentration/ luminal stagnation/ Spermatocoeles/ductal occlusion
Decreased reabsorption of luminal fluid	Oestrogen receptor dysfunction[2]	Decreased sperm concentration/ dilution/luminal dilation
Phagocytosis of spermatozoa	Benomyl; carbendazim[1] α-chlorohydrin[3]	Epithelial hyperplasia/ recanalization
Epithelial desquamation	α-chlorohydrin[3] Cadmium[4]	Testicular swelling
Inflammation	Benomyl[1]; carbendazim[2]; α-chlorohydrin[3]	Testicular atrophy
Fibrosis	Benomyl[1]; carbendazim[2]; α-chlorohydrin[3]; 1,3-dinitrobenzene[5]	Decreased fertility

[1] (Hess *et al.*, 1991).
[2] (Nakai *et al.*, 1992).
[3] (Hoffer *et al.*, 1975).
[4] (Nagy, 1985).
[5] (Linder *et al.*, 1988).

hypothalamus–pituitary feedback loop (Goldman *et al.*, 1989; Rehnberg *et al.*, 1989). However, upon further examination of the histopathology, it was found that two sequential events, first in the testis and then in the efferent ducts, could answer many of the questions regarding hormonal changes, long-term atrophy of seminiferous tubules and why some males became irreversibly infertile.

Effects on seminiferous epithelium

Benzimidazole carbamate compounds cause premature sloughing of germ cells along with cleaved processes of Sertoli cell cytoplasm (Hess *et al.*, 1991; Nakai and Hess, 1994), necrosis of mitotic spermatogonia and meiotic spermatocytes (Nakai and Hess, 1997) and seminiferous tubular atrophy (Carter *et al.*, 1987; Hess *et al.*, 1991; Nakai *et al.*, 1992). The proposed mechanism contributing to sloughing is deformation of Sertoli cell cytoplasm due to the disruption of microtubules (Nakai and Hess, 1994; Nakai *et al.*, 1995). Recovery from massive sloughing of germ cells is possible if the efferent ducts remain intact; however, abnormal spermatids are formed several days after a single exposure to carbendazim and may affect fertility long after the initial testicular injury (Nakai *et al.*, 1997). These effects occur in testes with intact efferent ducts. Therefore, carbendazim can have direct effects on the seminiferous epithelium at lower dosages, independent of efferent duct dysfunction. On the basis of the severity of germ cell sloughing, we first hypothesized that occlusions in efferent ducts were caused by cellular debris that clogged the lumen only at ductal junctions. However, other chemicals also induce massive sloughing of germ cells without efferent ductal occlusions; therefore, an alternative explanation was required.

Effects on efferent ducts

Occlusion of the efferent ducts (Fig. 1) is common after exposure to the fungicide benomyl or its metabolite carbendazim (Hess *et al.*, 1991; Nakai *et al.*, 1992). This response is rapid, as an increase in testis weight is detected as early as 8 h after exposure (Nakai *et al.*, 1992). A single dose appears to be sufficient to induce ductal occlusions, but a comparison of 70 day, single-exposure data (Nakai *et al.*,

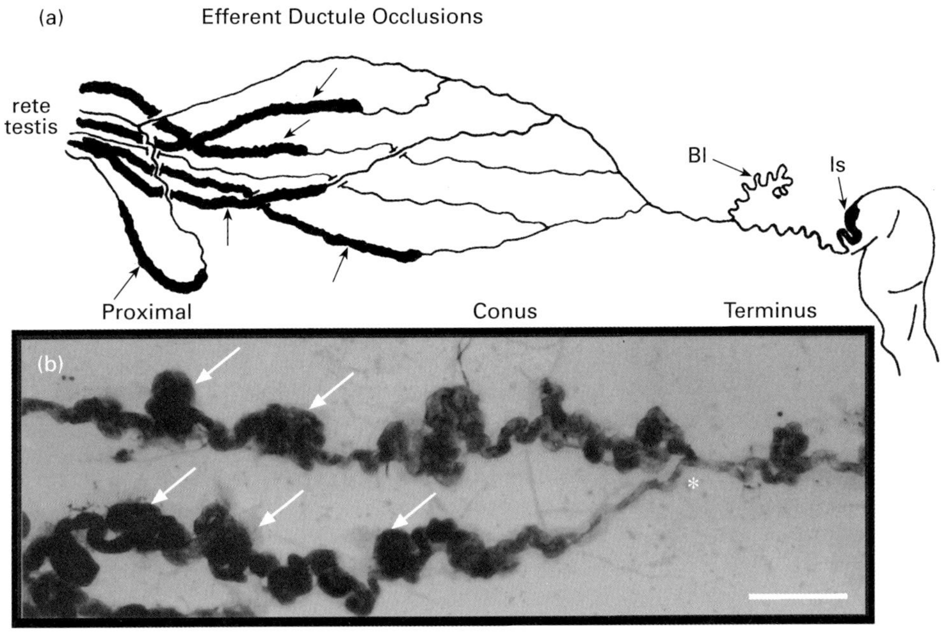

Fig. 1. (a) A drawing of microdissected efferent ducts collected from a rat 48 h after treatment with a single dose of carbendazim (400 mg kg^{-1}). This type of data was collected from photographs (similar to (b)) and tabulated in Table 5. Occlusions are noted as thick dark areas (arrows) near the rete testis. Ductal regions are identified as proximal, conus and terminus. The terminus is a single ductule that joins the initial segment epididymidis (Is), and in this case contained a small blind ending tubule (BI). (b) A photograph of microdissected efferent ducts showing occlusions (arrows). A region of normal size is noted by an asterisk near a junction. Scale bar represents 1 mm.

1992) with 245 days following exposure for 10 days (Carter *et al.*, 1987) is noteworthy because the percentage of testes with 'total seminiferous tubular atrophy' was 21% on day 70 and 50% on day 245. This suggests that either seminiferous tubular regression continues long after treatment has stopped or that the additional doses were effective in spreading damage to a greater number of efferent ducts.

Microdissection of occluded efferent ducts was performed to determine specific locations of the benzimidazole lesions (Table 5). At 12 h after treatment 75.8% of the ductules were occluded and by 24 h nearly 85% were occluded. Overall, 56% of the occlusions were located in the initial zone, 15% at junctions and 44% in the conus vasculosa. No occlusions were observed in the common efferent duct. Further measurements confirmed that the initial zone was the primary site of occlusions, as the ductules in this zone were significantly longer (41.9 mm) in treated animals compared with controls (30.7 mm). The length of the common duct did not change: 19.6 mm and 18.1 mm in control and treated, respectively.

After occlusions were formed in the efferent ducts, an inflammatory response was initiated, approximately 2–4 h later. The severity of response was dose dependent, but the onset of occlusions and time to first appearance of neutrophils in the connective tissue remained the same regardless of dosage. In controls, occlusions were not present and neutrophilic leukocytes were absent. However, 2 h after treatment, exfoliated spermatids were present in the lumen of the efferent ducts and most ductules were engorged by 4 h. Complete occlusion of the ductules occurred at 6–8 h, before the infiltration of neutrophils, which corresponded to a build-up of fluid in the testis and increased testis weight (Nakai *et al.*, 1992). Neutrophils began to appear in the connective tissue between 8–12 h after

Table 5. Carbendazim-induced occlusions of the ductuli efferentes in the adult rat[1]

Time (h) after treatment	Number of animals	Total Number of ductules	Total Number occluded	% occluded[2]	Location of occlusions[3]			
					Proximal	Junction	Conus	Terminus
12	5	33	25	75.8	13	5	12	0
24	5	32	27	84.4	16	3	11	0

[1] 400 mg kg^{-1} by single oral gavage.
[2] Overall, 80.1% of the ductules were occluded.
[3] Overall, occlusions in the proximal ductule (56%); at junctions (15%); in the conus (44%); in the terminus (0%).

treatment; therefore, it is concluded that benzimidazole carbamates have direct effects on efferent ducts rather than an indirect reaction following inflammation.

The neutrophils migrated between the junctions of endothelial cells lining small venules, producing limited haemorrhage into the connective tissue. As the leukocytes migrated between the thin smooth muscle layers of the efferent ducts, some of the muscle cells were destroyed. By 48 h, neutrophils formed between 2–5 solid layers of cells around the base of the ductules (Fig. 2a,b), where they eroded the basal lamina before penetrating between epithelial cells. Neutrophils then phagocytosed luminal debris and caused luminal contents to erupt into the lamina propria. Thus, neutrophils exhibited a specific chemotactic response toward efferent ducts containing stagnant spermatozoa and exfoliated spermatids. The leukocytes attempted to seal off the luminal contents but appeared to damage the epithelium in the process, which may have contributed to subsequent formation of fibrotic lesions and permanent infertility.

The response of efferent ductal epithelium to injury induced by occlusions appears to be dependent upon the degree of inflammation caused by the trauma. An acute inflammatory reaction may be induced by the compacted luminal contents, causing the ductal lumen to dilate (Fig. 2c). It is likely that the ductal epithelium, stretched excessively by a large bolus of testicular debris, releases a chemotactic substance, possibly a cytokine of the interleukin superfamily, which then recruits large numbers of neutrophils. Leakage of sperm antigens may draw the neutrophils toward the lumen and stimulate phagocytic activity. In other organ systems, indirect damage caused by neutrophil emigration into the interstitium and through the epithelium promotes granuloma formation and fibroblast activity (see review by Nakai *et al.*, 1993). Thus, fibrotic lesions may be an indirect result of neutrophil damage rather than direct effects of epithelial injury.

Epithelia with medium inflammatory responses often exhibited irregular epithelial growth along the edge of luminal contents and formed multiple abnormal ductules (Fig. 2d). These abnormal ductules, formed by the migration of the original epithelia and growth at the periphery of the occluded lumen, indicated that recanalization was attempted by 16 days after treatment (Nakai *et al.*, 1993). Epithelial cells of the microcanals were similar in appearance to those of blind ending tubules (Guttroff *et al.*, 1992). No evidence was found to indicate that microcanals formed patent connections between rete testis and epididymis.

Conclusions

Efferent ducts respond to toxic insult by at least two different means (Fig. 3): an increased rate of fluid reabsorption or decreased secretions (i.e. Cl^-) ; or a decreased rate of reabsorption or increased secretions. The first response leads to increased viscosity of luminal fluids, sperm stasis, ductal occlusions, granulomas and possibly fibrosis. The second response dilutes the luminal fluid, decreases sperm concentration, and leads to a decrease in sperm transit time through the epididymis. The mechanism by which benzimidazole chemicals disrupt fluid reabsorption is not

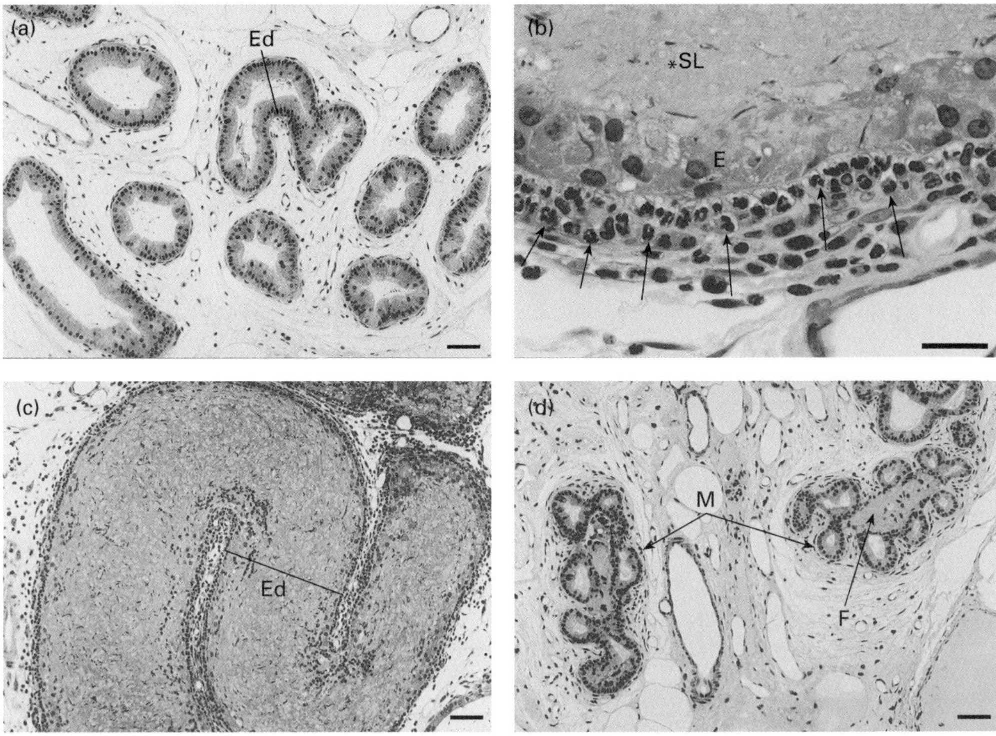

Fig. 2. (a) Efferent ducts from a control rat showing the normal diameter (Ed; bar) in the proximal conus region. (b) Occluded efferent ductule from a rat treated with a single dose of carbendazim (400 mg kg^{-1}) and fixed by vascular perfusion 48 h after treatment. The lumen is occluded with sloughed debris (Sl) from the testis. The epithelium (E) is disorganized and shows evidence of sperm phagocytosis. Neutrophilic leukocytes (arrows) completely surround the basement membrane. (c) A single occluded efferent ductule 48 h after treatment with carbendazim (400 mg kg^{-1}). The lumen is filled with debris and the diameter (Ed; bar) of the ductule has nearly doubled in size. Neutrophils line the basement membrane and are found in the lumen (dark staining nuclei). (d) Occluded efferent ducts 70 days after treatment with carbendazim (400 mg kg^{-1}) show both the fibrotic lesions (F) and abnormal microcanals (M) that have grown around the lesions. Scale bars represent: 50 μm (a,c,d) and 25 μm (b).

known. We have limited data showing a dose-dependent increase in the activity of Na^+,K^+-ATPase (Table 6), which may result from the disruption of cytoskeletal elements (Jordan *et al.*, 1995). However, effects on other pathways, such as Cl^- secretion, should also be considered. Regardless of mechanisms or the toxicant involved, once ductules become blocked, long-term results are the same, as testicular atrophy and infertility are produced. Accordingly, long-term testicular atrophy after subchronic and acute multiple exposure to any toxicant could be explained by potential efferent ductal dysfunction, a hypothesis that should be examined routinely by histopathology.

Cessation of fluid reabsorption, as seen in the oestrogen receptor knockout mouse, also leads to fluid build up within the testis and subsequent seminiferous tubular atrophy (Hess *et al.*, 1997). Thus, it appears that oestrogen may be required for normal fertility in the male. At least in the mouse, oestrogen receptor-α is required. This new role for oestrogens in the male reproductive tract raises renewed interest in the effects of xenoestrogens or environmental oestrogenic chemicals on male fertility and the decline in sperm counts. Are these effects due only to developmental anomalies, as first hypothesized (Sharpe and Skakkebaek, 1993)? Or is it possible that exposure of adults also produces oligospermia or a decline in sperm counts by the dilution of caput spermatozoa due to the inability to reabsorb fluid properly in efferent ducts (Hess *et al.*, 1997)? Increases in

Table 6. The effect of carbendazim on N^+,K^+-ATPase activity in the the ductuli efferentes of adult rats[1]

Carbendazim ($mg\ kg^{-1}$)	Number of rats	Na,K-ATPase activity[2] pmol *p*-nitrophenol mm^{-1} $tubule^{-1}$ h
0	5	7143 ± 320[a]
100	5	7767 ± 540[a,b]
200	5	8863 ± 441[b,c]
400	5	9785 ± 552[d]

[1] Single exposure by oral gavage. For details of methods, see Ilio and Hess (1992).
[2] Significant differences are indicated by different superscripts ($P < 0.05$).

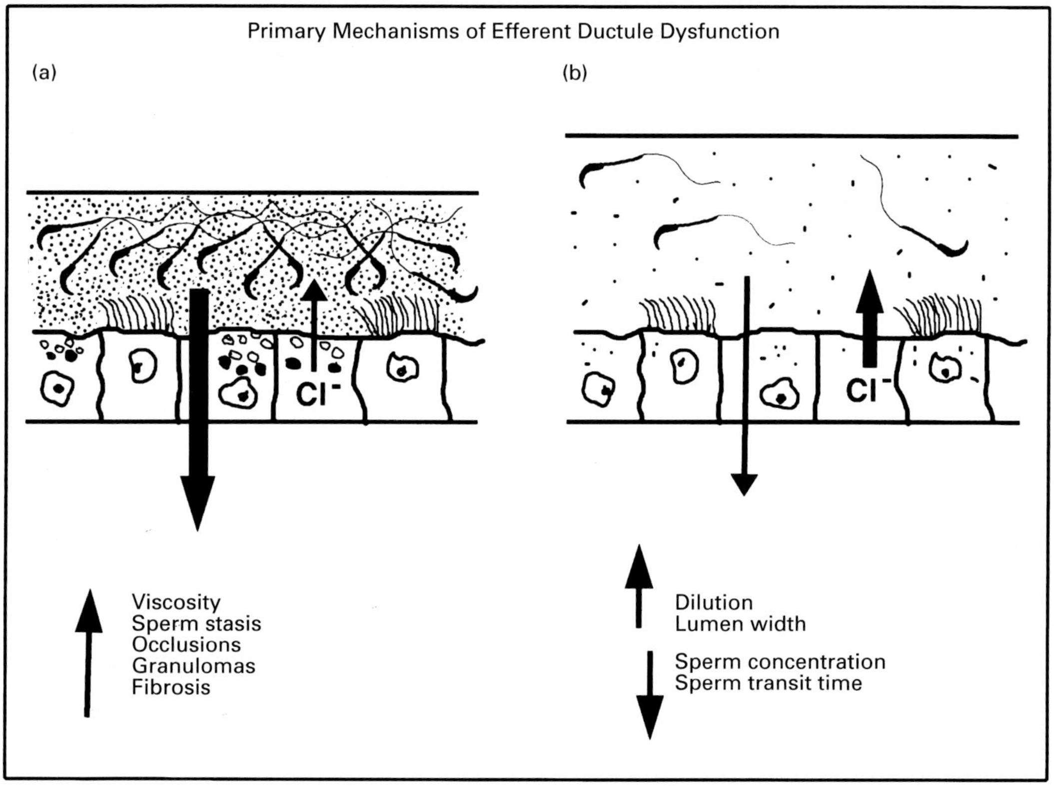

Fig. 3. (a) An illustration of toxicant effects that lead to an excessive amount of fluid reabsorption leaving behind a higher concentration of spermatozoa, protein and cellular debris in the lumen. The consequences of this effect are similar to those seen following exposure to carbendazim and lead to increases in the viscosity of luminal contents, sperm stasis, occlusions, granulomas and fibrosis. (b) An illustration of an effect leading to decreased reabsorption or increased secretions of Cl^- into the lumen. The consequences of this response are similar to those observed in the oestrogen receptor knockout mouse (Hess *et al.*, 1997), which lead to increased dilution of semen, increased luminal diameter, and decreases in sperm concentration and possibly sperm transit time.

abnormal sperm morphology could also result from abnormal fluid reabsorption, as normal spermatozoa leaving the testis would fail to mature in the epididymis if the surrounding luminal fluid did not contain the necessary concentration of factors required for sperm maturation. Thus, efferent duct dysfunction can interfere with fertility through several mechanisms and environmental chemicals have the potential to cause these effects. Future studies must address not only the pathophysiological mechanisms leading to testicular atrophy, but also the biochemical and molecular mechanisms associated with the regulation of ion and water flux across the ductal epithelium and their relationship to male infertility.

The author expresses appreciation to Dr. Ken Ilio, who as a graduate student contributed much to our understanding of Na^+,K^+-ATPase function in the efferent ducts; Dr. Masaaki Nakai, who continues to collaborate on the toxicity of benzimidazole fungicides; and Dr. Gary Klinefelter, who collaborated in writing a more comprehensive review to be published in *Reproductive and Developmental Toxicology* Ã. K. Korach (Ed) 1998. Supported by NIH grants ES05214 and ES07832.

References

Carter SD and Laskey JW (1982) Effect of benomyl on reproduction in the male rat *Toxicology Letters* **11** 87–94

Carter SD, Hess RA and Laskey JW (1987) The fungicide methyl 2-benzimidazole carbamate causes infertility in male Sprague-Dawley rats *Biology of Reproduction* **37** 709–717

Chan HC, Lai KB, Fu WO, Chung YW, Chan PS and Wong PY (1995) Regional differences in bioelectrical properties and anion secretion in cultured epithelia from rat and human male excurrent ducts *Biology of Reproduction* **52** 192–198

Chellman GJ, Morgan KT, Bus JS and Working PK (1986) Inhibition of methyl chloride toxicity in male F-344 rats by the anti-inflammatory agent BW755C *Toxicology and Applied Pharmacology* **85** 367–379

Chellman GJ, Hurtt ME, Bus JS and Working PK (1987) Role of testicular versus epididymal toxicity in the induction of cytotoxic damage in Fischer-344 rat sperm by methyl chloride *Reproductive Toxicology* **1** 25–35

Cooper ER and Jackson H (1972) The vasa efferentia in the rat and mouse *Journal of Reproduction and Fertility* **28** 317–319

Cooper ER and Jackson H (1973) Chemically induced sperm retention cysts in the rat *Journal of Reproduction and Fertility* **34** 445–449

Cooper ER, Jones AR and Jackson H (1974) Effects of alpha-chlorohydrin and related compounds on the reproductive organs and fertility of the male rat *Journal of Reproduction and Fertility* **38** 379–386

Cooper TG, Yeung CH, Skupin R and Haufe G (1997) Antifertility potential of ornidazole analogues in rats *Journal of Andrology* **18** 431–438

Din-Udom A, Sujarit S and Pholpramool C (1985) Short-term effect of androgen deprivation on intraluminal pressure and contractility of the rat epididymis *Journal of Reproduction and Fertility* **73** 405–410

Ericsson RJ (1971) Antispermatogenic properties of 2,3-dihydro-2-1-naphthyl 41H quinazolinone U-29409 *Proceedings of the Society for Experimental Biology and Medicine* **137** 532–535

Ericsson RJ (1975) Chemosterilants. In *Control of Male Fertility* pp 262–269 Ed. JJ Sciarra, C Markland and JJ Speidel. Harper & Row, New York

Evans B, Gannon BJ, Heath JW and Burnstock G (1972) Long-lasting damage to the internal male genital organs and their adrenergic innervation in rats following chronic treatment with the antihypertensive drug guanethidine *Fertility and Sterility* **23** 657–667

Ford WCL and Waites GMH (1981) The effect of high doses of 6-chloro-6-deoxyglucose on the rat *Contraception* **24** 577–588

Gaillard DA, Carre-Pigeon F and Lallemand A (1997) Normal vas deferens in fetuses with cystic fibrosis *Journal of Urology* **158** 1549–1552

Goldman JM, Rehnberg GL, Cooper RL, Gray LE, Jr, Hein JF and McElroy WK (1989) Effects of the benomyl metabolite, carbendazim, on the hypothalamic–pituitary reproductive axis in the male rat *Toxicology* **57** 173–182

Gray LE, Jr , Ostby J, Linder R, Goldman J, Rehnberg G and Cooper R (1990) Carbendazim-induced alterations of reproductive development and function in the rat and hamster *Fundamental and Applied Toxicology* **15** 281–297

Gray LE, Wolf C, Mann P and Ostby JS (1997) In utero exposure to low doses of 2,3,7,8-tetrachlorodibenzo-*p*-dioxin alters reproductive development of female Long Evans hooded rat offspring *Toxicology and Applied Pharmacology* **146** 237–244

Guttroff RF, Cooke PS and Hess RA (1992) Blind-ending tubules and branching patterns of the rat ductuli efferentes *Anatomical Record* **232** 423–431

Hess RA, Moore BJ, Forrer J, Linder RE and Abuel-Atta AA (1991) The fungicide benomyl (methyl 1-(butylcarbamoyl)-2-benzimidazolecarbamate) causes testicular dysfunction by inducing the sloughing of germ cells and occlusion of efferent ductules *Fundamental and Applied Toxicology* **17** 733–745

Hess RA, Bunick D, Lee KH, Bahr J, Taylor JA, Korach KS and Lubahn DB (1997) A role for oestrogens in the male reproductive system *Nature* **390** 509–512

Hinton BT, Hernandez H and Howards SS (1983) The male antifertility agents alpha chlorohydrin, 5-thio-D-glucose, and 6-chloro-6-deoxy-D-glucose interfere with sugar transport across the epithelium of the rat caput epididymidis *Journal of Andrology* **4** 216–221

Hoffer AP, Hamilton DW and Fawcett DW (1975) Phagocytosis of spermatozoa by the epithelial cells of the ductuli efferentes after epididymal obstruction in the rat *Journal of Reproduction and Fertility* **44** 1–9

Ilio KY and Hess RA (1992) Localization and activity of Na^+,K($^+$)-ATPase in the ductuli efferentes of the rat *Anatomical Record* **234** 190–200

Jones AR (1978) The antifertility actions of alpha-chlorohydrin in the male *Life Sciences* **23** 1625–1646

Jones AR and O'Brien RW (1980) Metabolism of three active analogues of the male antifertility agent alpha-chlorohydrin in the rat *Xenobiotica* **10** 365–370

Jordan C, Puschel B, Koob R and Drenckhahn D (1995) Identification of a binding motif for ankyrin on the alpha-subunit of Na^+,K^+-ATPase *Journal of Biological Chemistry* **270** 29971–29975

Kelce WR, Lambright CR, Gray LE, Jr and Roberts KP (1997) Vinclozolin and p,p'-DDE alter androgen-dependent gene expression: *in vivo* confirmation of an androgen receptor-mediated mechanism *Toxicology and Applied Pharmacology* **142** 192–200

Klinefelter GR and Hess RA (1998) Toxicity of the excurrent ducts and accessory organs in the male. In *Reproductive and Developmental Toxicology* Ed. KS Korach. Marcel Dekker, Inc., New York 553–591

Klinefelter GR and Suarez JD (1997) Toxicant-induced acceleration of epididymal sperm transit: androgen-dependent proteins may be involved *Reproductive Toxicology* **11** 511–519

Klinefelter GR, Laskey JW, Roberts NR, Slott V and Suarez JD (1990) Multiple effects of ethane dimethanesulfonate on the epididymis of adult rats *Toxicology and Applied Pharmacology* **105** 271–287

Klinefelter GR, Roberts NL and Suarez JD (1992) Direct effects of ethane dimethanesulphonate on epididymal function in adult rats. An *in vitro* demonstration *Journal of Andrology* **13** 409–421

Klinefelter GR, Laskey JW, Kelce WR, Ferrell J, Roberts NL, Suarez JD and Slott V (1994a) Chloroethylmethanesulfonate-induced effects on the epididymis seem unrelated to altered Leydig cell function *Biology of Reproduction* **51** 82–91

Klinefelter GR, Laskey JW, Perreault SD, Ferrell J, Jeffay S, Suarez J and Roberts N (1994b) The ethane dimethanesulfonate-induced decrease in the fertilizing ability of cauda epididymal sperm is independent of the testis *Journal of Andrology* **15** 318–327

Klinefelter GR, Laskey JW, Ferrell J, Suarez JD and Roberts NL (1997) Discriminant analysis indicates a single sperm protein (SP22) is predictive of fertility following exposure to epididymal toxicants *Journal of Andrology* **18** 139–150

Kluwe WM, Gupta BN and Lamb JC (1983) The comparative effects of 1,2-dibromo-3-chloropropane (DBCP) and its metabolites, 3-chloro-1,2-propaneoxide (epichlorohydrin), 3-chloro-1,2- propanediol (alphachlorohydrin), and oxalic acid, on the urogenital system of male rats *Toxicology and Applied Pharmacology* **70** 67–86

Lim J and Miller MG (1997) The role of the benomyl metabolite carbendazim in benomyl-induced testicular toxicity *Toxicology and Applied Pharmacology* **142** 401–410

Linder RE, Hess RA, Perreault SD, Strader LF and Barbee RR (1988a) Acute effects and long-term sequelae of 1,3-dinitrobenzene on male reproduction in the rat. I. Sperm quality, quantity, and fertilizing ability *Journal of Andrology* **9** 317–326

Linder RE, Rehnberg GL, Strader LF and Diggs JP (1988b) Evaluation of reproductive parameters in adult male Wistar rats after subchronic exposure gavage to benomyl *Journal of Toxicology and Environmental Health* **25** 285–298

Linder RE, Strader LF, Slott VL and Suarez JD (1992) Endpoints of spermatotoxicity in the rat after short duration exposures to fourteen reproductive toxicants *Reproductive Toxicology* **6** 491–505

Mason KE and Young JO (1967) Effects of cadmium upon the excurrent duct system of the rat testis *Anatomical Record* **159** 311–324

Meistrich ML, Hughes TH and Bruce WR (1975) Alteration of epididymal sperm transport and maturation in mice by oestrogen and testosterone *Nature* **258** 145–147

Nagy F (1985) Cadmium-induced alterations in the Siberian hamster epididymis *Archives of Andrology* **15** 91–104

Nakai M and Hess RA (1994) Morphological changes in the rat Sertoli cell induced by the microtubule poison carbendazim *Tissue and Cell* **26** 917–927

Nakai M and Hess RA (1997) Effects of carbendazim (methyl 2-benzimidazole carbamate; MBC) on meiotic spermatocytes and subsequent spermiogenesis in the rat testis *Anatomical Record* **247** 379–387

Nakai M, Hess RA, Moore BJ, Guttroff RF, Strader LF and Linder RE (1992) Acute and long-term effects of a single dose of the fungicide carbendazim (methyl 2-benzimidazole carbamate) on the male reproductive system in the rat *Journal of Andrology* **13** 507–518

Nakai M, Moore BJ and Hess RA (1993) Epithelial reorganization and irregular growth following carbendazim-induced injury of the efferent ductules of the rat testis *Anatomical Record* **235** 51–60

Nakai M, Hess RA, Netsu J and Nasu T (1995) Deformation of the rat Sertoli cell by oral administration of carbendazim (methyl 2-benzimidazole carbamate) *Journal of Andrology* **16** 410–416

Nakai M, Hess RA, Matsuo F, Gotoh Y and Nasu T (1997) Further observations on carbendazim-induced abnormalities of spermatid morphology in rats *Tissue and Cell* **29** 477–485

Oberlander G, Yeung CH and Cooper TG (1994) Induction of reversible infertility in male rats by oral ornidazole and its effects on sperm motility and epididymal secretions *Journal of Reproduction and Fertility* **100** 551–559

Qiu J, Hales BF and Robaire B (1995) Damage to rat spermatozoal DNA after chronic cyclophosphamide exposure *Biology of Reproduction* **53** 1465–1473

Rehnberg GL, Cooper RL, Goldman JM, Gray LE, Hein JF and McElroy WK (1989) Serum and testicular testosterone and androgen binding protein profiles following subchronic treatment with carbendazim *Toxicology and Applied Pharmacology* **101** 55–61

Sharpe RM and Skakkebaek NE (1993) Are oestrogens involved in falling sperm counts and disorders of the male reproductive tract? *Lancet* **341** 1392–1395

Slott VL, Jeffay SC, Dyer CJ, Barbee RR and Perreault SD (1997) Sperm motion predicts fertility in male hamsters treated with alpha-chlorohydrin *Journal of Andrology* **18** 708–716

Susheela AK and Kumar A (1991) A study of the effect of high concentrations of fluoride on the reproductive organs of male rabbits using light and scanning electron microscopy *Journal of Reproduction and Fertility* **92** 353–360

Torchinskiy AM, Orlova NV, Smirnova YB and Makavova LF (1976) Data on the toxicological and public health characteristics of the carbamate-group pesticide benlate *Gigiena Sanitaria* **2** 35–41

Trezise AE, Linder CC, Grieger D, Thompson EW, Meunier H, Griswold MD and Buchwald M (1993) CFTR expression is regulated during both the cycle of the seminiferous epithelium and the oestrous cycle of rodents *Nature Genetics* **3** 157–164

Tsang AY, Lee WM and Wong PY (1981) Effects of antifertility drugs on epididymal protein secretion, acquisition of sperm surface proteins and fertility in male rats *International Journal* of *Andrology* **4** 703–712

Wakeley CPG (1943) Cysts of the epididymis the so-called spermatoceles *British Journal of Surgery* **31** 165–173

Wen RQ and Wong PY (1988) Reserpine treatment increases viscosity of fluid in the epididymis of rats *Biology of Reproduction* **38** 969–974

Whorton D, Milby TH, Krauss RM and Stubbs HA (1979) Testicular function in DBCP exposed pesticide workers *Journal of Occupational Medicine* **21** 161–166

Wong PYD (1990) Abnormal fluid transport by the epididymis as a cause of obstructive azoospermia *Reproduction, Fertility and Development* **2** 115–127

Wong PY, Au CL and Ngai HK (1980) Effects of 6-chloro-6-deoxyglucose on electrolyte and water transport in the epididymis and fertility of male rats *International Journal Andrology* **3** 82–86

Working PK, Bus JS and Hamm TE, Jr (1985) Reproductive effects of inhaled methyl chloride in the male Fischer 344 rat. II. Spermatogonial toxicity and sperm quality *Toxicology and Applied Pharmacology* **77** 144–157

Journal of Reproduction and Fertility Supplement **53**, 261–270

Expression of the cystic fibrosis transmembrane conductance regulator (CFTR) mRNA in normal and pathological adult human epididymis

P. Patrizio[1] and W. A. Salameh[2]

[1]*Male Infertility Program, University of Pennsylvania Health System, Department of Obstetrics & Gynecology, Division of Human Reproduction, 3400 Spruce Street, 106 Dulles Building, Philadelphia, PA 19104– 4283, USA; and* [2]*UCLA School of Medicine, Harbor-UCLA Medical Center, Dept of Medicine, Division of Endocrinology, 1124 W Carson Street, Torrance, CA 90502, USA*

The pathogenesis of the aberrant development of the male genital tract (epididymis, vas deferens and seminal vesicles) seen in patients with congenital bilateral absence of the vas deferens (CBAVD) is still unclear. Since men with CBAVD carry mutations in the cystic fibrosis transmembrane conductance regulator gene (CFTR), it is likely that CFTR mRNA of the translated protein plays a major role in the pathogenesis of CBAVD. The aim of this study was to compare the pattern of expression of CFTR mRNA in epididymides of men with CBAVD and other types of obstruction (post-vasectomy and post-inflammatory) with that of normal non-obstructed adult epididymis. Epididymal biopsies were obtained at the time of microsurgical epididymal sperm aspiration procedures or during vaso-epididymostomy reanastomosis. A normal epididymis was obtained from an orchiectomy specimen. After standard processing for *in situ* hybridization, tissue sections were hybridized with CFTR gene-probe labelled by incorporation of digoxigenin-dUTP. After hybridization the signal was detected by an alkaline phosphatase-tagged antidigoxigenin antibody. CFTR mRNA was clearly identified in the columnar epithelium of the normal adult epididymis and vas deferens and the signal intensity was greatest in the most proximal regions of the caput epididymis. In contrast, men with genital tract obstructions due to CBAVD or post-vasectomy or post-inflammatory obstructions, had sloughing of the epithelial cells lining the lumen and as a consequence CFTR mRNA expression was lacking. In one subject (post-vasectomy obstruction), some residual caput epididymal epithelium was preserved and CFTR mRNA was detected. The abundant CFTR mRNA expression in the proximal caput of the epididymis and vas deferens under normal conditions strongly favours the hypothesis of an early obstructive process in the pathogenesis of CBAVD. The absent or severely reduced activity of CFTR protein affects the ionic exchange and fluid content within the epididymal lumen and this, in turn, can lead to excessive viscosity of the epididymal fluid, sloughing of epithelial cells expressing CFTR and further reduction in the amount of CFTR activity. As a consequence, variable segments of the epididymis and the vas deferens may be blocked and progressively obliterated. The epididymal lumen obstruction could also sustain the anatomical defects by not allowing testosterone to exert a local action on the mesonephric duct.

Background Information

Cystic fibrosis (CF) is a fatal, autosomal recessive disorder with an incidence ranging from 1 in 2000 to 1 in 2500 live births. Classic symptoms of CF are obstructive pulmonary disease, pancreatic exocrine insufficiency, gastrointestinal obstruction, failure to thrive, high concentrations of electrolytes in sweat and, in males, infertility due to absence of the vas deferens.

It is estimated that about 25% of males with obstructive azoospermia are ultimately diagnosed with bilateral congenital absence of the vas deferens (CBAVD). (In the USA, 16 000 males are infertile as a result of CBAVD.)

Anatomically, CBAVD is a disorder characterized by bilateral regression of variable portions of the epididymis, vas deferens, and in about 80% of cases, absence of the seminal vesicles. In about 10–20% of the patients, a renal anomaly is also present. These anatomical hallmarks are so strikingly similar to those observed in men with cystic fibrosis (CF) that, as early as 1971, Holsclaw *et al.* suggested that these two apparently unrelated disorders had the same genetic origin. The hypothesis was proven when mutations in the cystic fibrosis transmembrane conductance regulator (CFTR) gene (Kerem *et al.*, 1989; Riordan *et al.*, 1989; Rommens *et al.*, 1989) were found in patients with CF as well as in patients with isolated CBAVD (Dumur *et al.*, 1990; Anguiano *et al.*, 1992; Patrizio *et al.*, 1993; Zielenski *et al.*, 1995; Chillon *et al.*, 1995; Dumur *et al.*, 1996; Lissens *et al.*, 1996).

The clinical link between CF and CBAVD was also strengthened by documenting the presence of subclinical CF symptoms in the majority of men with CBAVD, including mild increases in sweat chloride concentrations, nasal polyps and chronic sinusitis.

The gene for CF was mapped to the long arm of chromosome 7 (7q31.2) (Riordan *et al.*, 1989; Kerem *et al.*, 1989); it spans approximately 230 kilobases and consists of 27 exons. The encoded protein of 1480 amino acids is a multidomain glycoprotein functioning as a low-voltage, cyclic-AMP-regulated chloride channel. This protein is present at high concentrations in the apical membranes of various epithelial cells within the organs commonly affected by CF. The presence of two transmembrane domains, each containing six hydrophobic segments and two sets of nucleotide-binding folds, led to the classification of CFTR as a member of the ATP-binding cassette (ABC) family of transporter proteins. Because CF is a recessive disease, both copies of the CFTR gene must be mutated in order to express the CF phenotype.

Currently, there are over 700 published mutations in the CFTR gene associated with the disease. In addition, there are 68 coding region and 55 non-coding region polymorphisms not associated with disease (source: CF Genetic Analysis Consortium; http://www.genet. sickkids.on.ca/).

Many patients with CBAVD, when screened for CF mutations, are found to have only one detectable mutation. Recently, by screening for mutations within the acceptor splice site of intervening sequence 8 (IVS8), more patients have been found positive. There are three variants detected in the IVS8, called 5T, 7T and 9T, consisting of five, seven and nine thymidine residues, respectively. The length of the T-tract in this site affects the splicing efficiency of exon 9; 9T is the most efficient and 5T the least. The frequency of the 5T variant among CBAVD patients is very high (Costes *et al.*, 1995; Patrizio and Zielenski, 1996) and its presence significantly reduces the amount of functional CFTR. Ultimately, it is the total amount of normal CFTR that influences the differences in phenotype between development of CF and CBAVD. When the amount of functional CFTR is less than 10%, it is reasonable to expect a full blown cystic fibrosis phenotype, wheras with concentrations of CFTR between 10 and 50%, in males, the phenotype can be of CBAVD; amounts of normal CFTR in excess of 50% are not associated with phenotypic abnormalities (Patrizio and Zielenski, 1996). With the inclusion of 5T-tract analysis, 60% of patients with CBAVD show two mutations, 25% one mutation and 15% no mutations. These data clearly support the concept that CBAVD is an incomplete phenotypic form of cystic fibrosis (Patrizio and Zielenski, 1996).

Introduction

The human epididymis is a highly differentiated organ, anatomically divided into three segments: the caput, the corpus and the cauda. From a functional standpoint, there is a dynamic exchange of fluid and proteins between the lumen and the cells lining the different portions of the epididymis. The secretory and resorptive activity of these cells is thought to be essential for the creation of an optimal microenvironment for maturation and transport of spermatozoa to occur (Wong, 1990).

The most proximal segment of the caput epididymis, also called globus major, comprises the vasa efferentia which is lined by both non-ciliated and various ciliated cells. Most of the caput is composed of vasa efferentia and at least seven types of efferent tubule connected to each other by junctions, and its embryological origin, along with the testis, is the genital ridge (Saitoh *et al.*, 1990; Yeung *et al.*, 1991). The corpus and tail of the epididymis are derived embryologically from the mesonephric or Wollfian ducts and they are lined with a variety of cells among which principal, basal, clear and halo cells are more predominant.

The development of the epididymis in men with CBAVD is highly variable. The most proximal segment of the epididymis, the caput, is always present with the same length, about 2 cm, as seen in normal men. The epididymis of the majority (65 %) of patients with CBAVD comprises the caput and the proximal portion of the corpus with a total length of 2–4 cm. The epididymis of very few (15 %) patients displays the entire caput, corpus and cauda (Patrizio *et al.*, 1994). In an attempt to explain why there should be such variability in length, a correlation with the presence of specific CFTR mutations was hypothesized. No association with any particular genotype or phenotype was found (Patrizio *et al.*, 1994).

The presence of CFTR mRNA is detectable in pancreas, lungs and male fetal reproductive tissues as early as 18 weeks (mid-trimester), when the components of the male genital tract (testes, epididymis and vas deferens) are developed (Tizzano *et al.*, 1994; Trezise *et al.*, 1993; Harris *et al.*, 1991). In postnatal life, CFTR mRNA has been localized in the epithelial cells lining the epididymal duct and the vas deferens of newborns, infants and children. The most prominent expression is in the epithelium of the caput epididymis, although it is also present in the vas deferens (Tizzano *et al.*, 1994).

The role of CFTR mRNA in the development of the epididymis and vas deferens is still unclear. In the absence of an animal model for CBAVD, two experimental approaches, one direct and the other indirect, can be formulated. A direct approach would involve the study of CFTR expression and the epididymal function in tissues of normal fetuses at different gestational ages in comparison with fetuses having known mutations in the CFTR gene. Obviously this study is not feasible. The second indirect approach is described here. We propose to compare the pattern of CFTR mRNA expression in epididymides of men with obstructions, whether due to CBAVD or post-vasectomy or post-inflammatory obstruction with that of normal non-obstructed subjects. Differences in CFTR expression could shed light on the role of CFTR in the adult epididymis and could help to formulate a hypothesis on the pathogenesis of CBAVD.

CFTR mRNA Expression in Adult Epididymis

Specimen collection

Epididymal biopsy samples were available from ten subjects. Six had a diagnosis of CBAVD, two had post-inflammatory epididymal obstruction, and the remaining two had undergone vasectomy. Epididymal biopsies were obtained at the time of microsurgical epididymal sperm aspiration (MESA), while searching for the epididymal tubule containing viable spermatozoa or at the time of vaso-epididymostomy during the identification of the epididymal tubule containing motile spermatozoa where anastomosis could be performed (Silber, 1986). In addition, an entire epididymis, obtained at the time of an orchiectomy performed for stage IV prostatic cancer, served as control. All biopsy specimens were immediately immersion fixed in 4% paraformaldehyde. The epididymis removed from the orchiectomy specimen was sectioned into small pieces and placed in Bouin's fixative immediately after collection. In all cases routine steps for embedding in paraffin wax were followed. The paraffin blocks were stored until *in situ* hybridization was performed.

Probe preparation

A human CFTR cDNA in pBluescript KS+ deposited by Tsui and co-workers was purchased from ATCC (American Type Tissue Collection catalog number 61282) (Kerem *et al.*, 1989). The plasmid was digested with EcoR I and Xba I releasing a 600 bp CFTR fragment. Negative controls

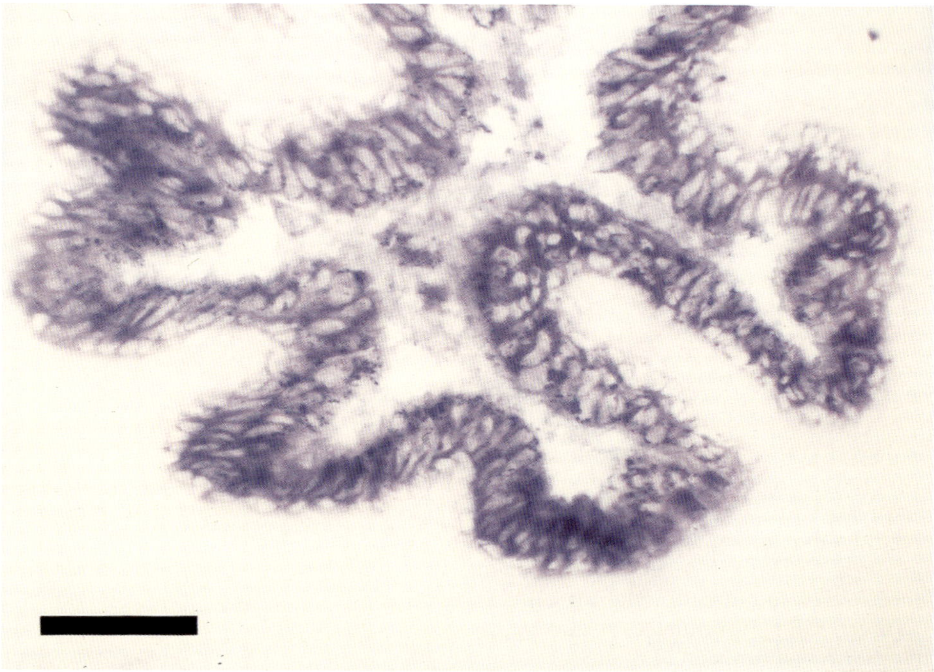

Fig. 1. Non-radioactive *in situ* hybridization of paraformaldehyde-fixed paraffin-embedded normal vas deferens using an HE-1 digoxigenin-labelled cDNA probe (positive control). Note the presence of mRNA expression in the epithelium of the vas deferens. Scale bar represents 100 μm.

consisted of using prehybridization solution without the probe or a pBR empty plasmid labelled with digoxygenin. The cDNA for HE1, a human secretory peptide abundantly expressed throughout the epididymal epithelium, was used as a positive control (Kirchoff *et al.*, 1996; Krull *et al.*, 1993). This cDNA was a gift from Kirchhoff (IHF Institute for Hormone and Fertility Research, Hamburg) and was provided in plasmid pBluescript KS+. A 450 bp HE1 fragment was generated by digestion with EcoR I and Sma I. The cDNAs were labelled by random priming with digoxygenin dUTP (Boehringer Mannheim). Efficiency of probe labelling and probe concentrations were determined by slot blotting of various labelled probe dilutions and comparing them to a prelabelled kit standard.

In situ *hybridization*

Tissues were processed for *in situ* hybridization following a modification of previously described protocols (Maggiano *et al.*,1991; Breitschopf *et al.*, 1992). Briefly, 6 μm paraffin wax sections were deparaffinized and rehydrated. Slides were treated with 0.2 mol HCl l^{-1} for 20 min and washed twice for 5 min in diethylpyrocarbonate(DEPC) treated water. Proteinase K digestion (Boehringer-Manheim) (2 μg ml^{-1}) was performed at 37 °C for 15 min. Prehybridization was done at 55 °C for 2 h in a solution containing 50% (v/v) formamide, 4×SSC, 1×Denhardt's, 125 μg salmon sperm DNA ml^{-1} and 125 μg yeast RNA ml^{-1}. Hybridization was done overnight at 55 °C in a solution containing, in addition to the above, 10% (v/v) dextran sulfate and the denatured probes at a final concentration of 5–10 ng per slide. Two consecutive 5 min post-hybridization washes were performed in 2×SSC followed by one 15 min wash at 55 °C in 0.1 × SSC.

Development of the hybridization signal was done according to Genius Kit manufacturer (Boehringer-Manheim) protocol using an alkaline phosphatase conjugated antidigoxigenin polyclonal antibody (1:500 dilution). Nitrobluetetrazolium (NBT) and X-Phosphate were used as colour substrates. Levamisole, 1 mmol l^{-1}(Sigma), was used to block any endogenous alkaline phosphatase activity. When the signal was deemed adequate, the colour reaction was stopped in Tris-Ethylenediamine tetra acetic acid (TE) pH 8.0 and slides were mounted in VectaShield aqueous mounting medium and sealed.

Results

Positive control (HE-1) expression

HE1 mRNA was abundantly expressed and localized, as previously reported, in the epithelial compartment of all sections (caput, corpus and cauda) of the normal human epididymis and vas deferens. (Figure 1 shows the expression of HE-1 mRNA in a section of normal vas deferens.)

Negative control

No hybridization signal was detected with either the pBR digoxigenin-labelled probe or with the prehybridization solution negative control, either in the normal human epididymal tissue or in areas of conserved epithelium (vasectomy). Figure 2a shows the absence of hybridization signal from the epithelial compartment of normal caput epididymis with prehybridization solution alone.

CFTR expression in epididymis and vas deferens of a normal subject

In the normal epididymis and vas deferens, CFTR mRNA was abundantly expressed in the lumen epithelium. The signal was not formally quantitated, but appears to be more intense in the most proximal segment of the caput epididymis. In addition, there was strong signal in the vas. Figure 2b shows the expression of CFTR mRNA in the proximal caput and Fig. 2c shows expression of CFTR mRNA in the vas deferens.

CFTR expression in epididymides from men with CBAVD and other obstructions

All of these samples showed post-obstructive changes or characteristic inflammatory or fibrotic changes with distortion of the epididymal anatomy. These changes included, in the majority of cases, sloughing of the epididymal epithelium and thus no detection of the CFTR mRNA signal. Patients with CBAVD showed the highest degree of microscopic anatomical alteration.

In one patient (vasectomy) a partially preserved area of epididymal epithelium was found in the caput and CFTR mRNA expression could be demonstrated (Fig. 3a). Figure 3b shows the caput epididymidis of a patient with CBAVD, positive to CFTR mutations (W-1282X/5T), with complete absence of epithelial cells and therefore absence of CFTR mRNA expression.

Pathogenesis of CBAVD

The data presented in this experiment do not provide a definitive answer for the pathogenesis of the male genital abnormalities characteristic of CBAVD.

Currently, there are two theories to explain this defect. The first theory implies a developmental, morphogenetic defect and the second an obstructive, mechanical defect. Both models rely on the notion that men with CBAVD carry mutations in the CFTR and that dysfunctions of the CFTR mRNA and its translated protein play a major role in the pathogenesis of CBAVD.

The theory favouring a developmental defect as a cause of the anatomical changes explains that the 'affected structures' have the same embryonic origin, i.e. the mesonephric duct (Trezise *et al.*, 1993). These authors and others (Harris and Coleman, 1989) claim that secretion of seminiferous tubule fluid, from which epididymal fluid 'is derived', begins post-natally (i.e. after the 'structural defects' of the epididymis and vas deferens have already occurred). As a consequence, they suggest that a primary developmental defect leads to the anatomical abnormalities seen in patients with cystic fibrosis.

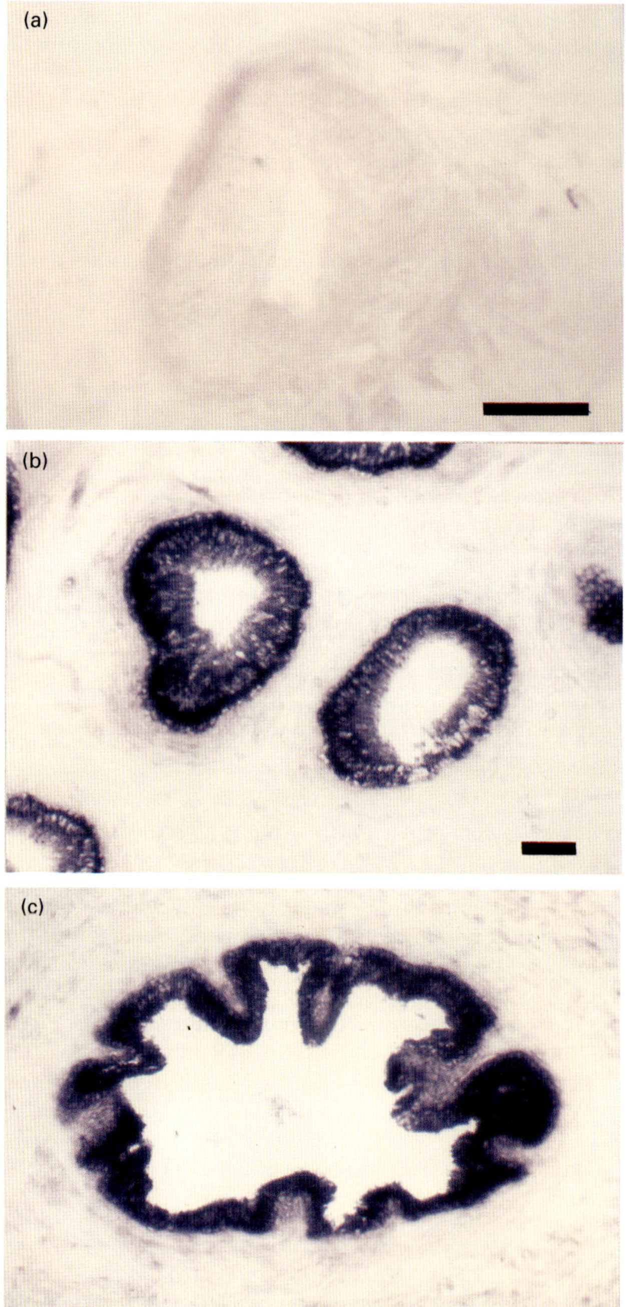

Fig. 2. Non-radioactive *in situ* hybridization of normal paraformaldehyde-fixed paraffin-embedded tissue of (a) proximal caput epididymis with prehybridization solution alone (negative control); (b) section of proximal caput epididymis and (c) vas deferens after hybridization with cystic fibrosis transmembrane conductance regulator (CFTR) digoxigenin-labelled cDNA probe. The segments with the most abundant CFTR mRNA expression are shown. (Scale bar represents 100 μm).

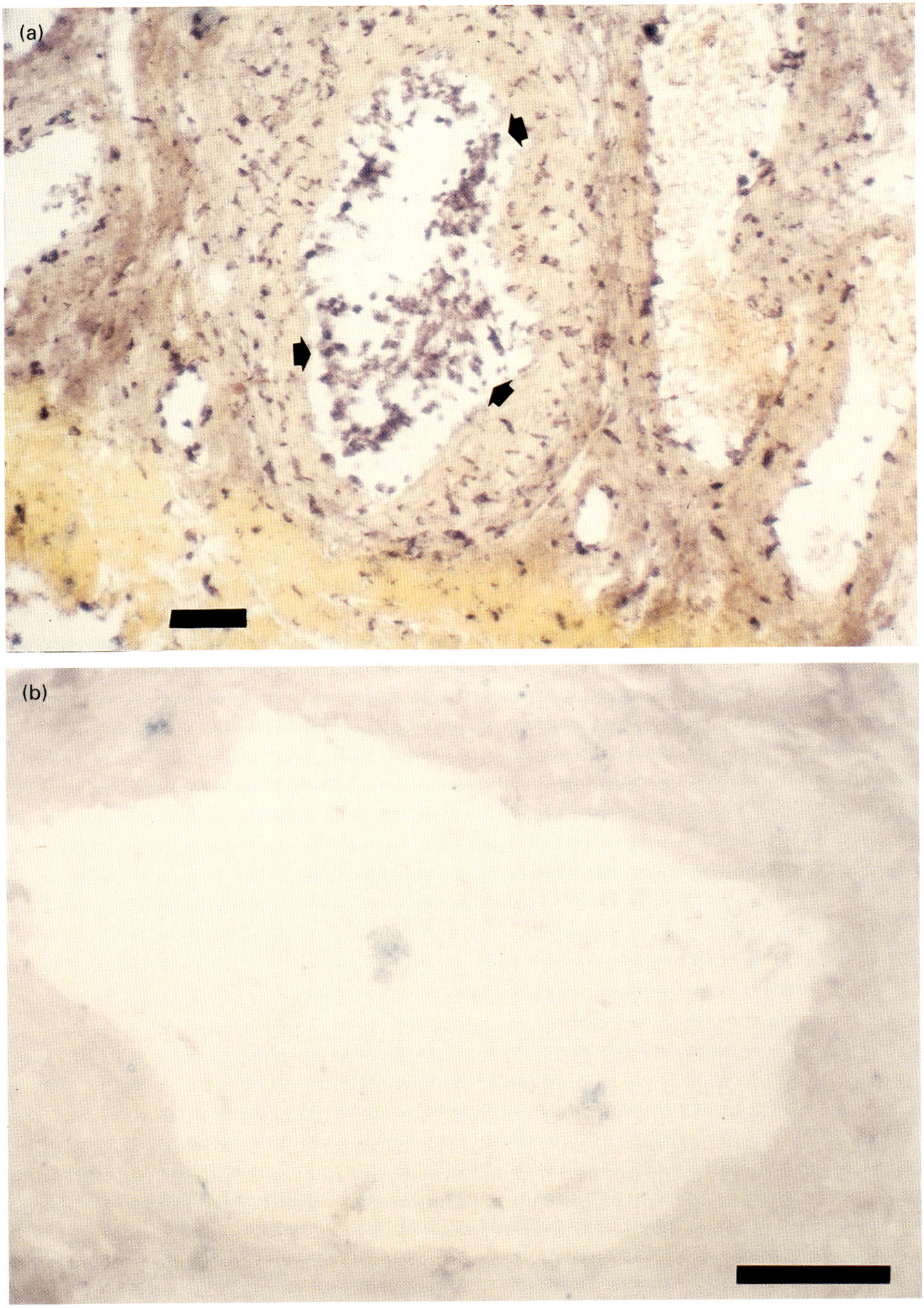

Fig. 3. Non-radioactive *in situ* hybridization of abnormal paraformaldehyde fixed paraffin-embedded biopsy specimens from (a) caput epididymis of patient post-vasectomy and (b) caput epididymis of patient with congenital absence of the vas deferens using a cystic fibrosis transmembrane conductance regulator (CFTR) digoxigenin cDNA probe. In (a) there is partial preservation (arrows) of the epididymal epithelium which shows expression of CFTR mRNA. In (b) there is complete sloughing and loss of the epididymal epithelium with absence of CFTR mRNA expression (Scale bar represents 100 μm.) Of note, the difference in diameter between the epididymal lumen of subjects with obstructions (Fig. 3a and b) and the lumen of a normal subject (Fig. 2b).

The assumption that epididymal fluid is detected only after the maldevelopment of the epididymis and the vas is problematic since there is evidence for CFTR expression in the vas of 18 week embryos and epididymal fluid secretion can be detected even in third trimester fetuses (Zondek and Zondek, 1965).

In addition, this developmental hypothesis does not explain how a dysfunctional CFTR protein would cause aberrant development. Furthermore, no data implicate CFTR in the regulation of any developmental gene expression.

An alternative hypothesis implies a progressive obstruction of the genital ducts by excessive mucus secretion as a major factor contributing to atrophy and absent portions of the epididymis and the vas deferens in men with CF and CBAVD (Wong, 1990; Tizzano *et al.*, 1994).

This hypothesis also satisfies the requirements of a previously postulated theory linking the luminal flow and content with organ damage in CF (Forstner *et al.*, 1987). It proposes that the abnormal secretions abundant in exocrine organs, such as the pancreas, predominantly affect the ducts with high protein load and low flow rate. In the epididymis and vas deferens, the abnormally concentrated protein load caused by dysfunction of the CFTR protein could produce a blockage and, consequently, progressive obliteration and disappearance of the ductal structures (Wong, 1990). In addition, the mesonephric duct must be exposed to testosterone to sustain its normal development (Siiteri and Wilson, 1974). In the absence of this local effect, epididymal fluid too viscous to allow an intraluminal flow, the development of the structures deriving from the mesonephric duct (epididymis, vas deferens and seminal vesicles) is severely impaired.

The results of our *in situ* hybridization analysis demonstrated the presence of CFTR mRNA in the columnar epithelium of normal adult human epididymis and vas deferens. The presence of CFTR mRNA in the columnar epithelium of the epididymis has been confirmed by other authors (Tizzano *et al.*, 1994). The most intense CFTR mRNA was in the most proximal portion of the epididymis (caput). The epididymides of men with CBAVD, and with post-inflammatory and with post-vasectomy obstructions do not express CFTR mRNA, because the obstructive process has created sloughing of epithelial cells. However, in a subject with post-vasectomy obstruction, an area of the caput epididymis with preserved columnar epithelium showed CFTR mRNA expression.

Areas of epithelial sloughing and absence of CFTR mRNA expression have also been reported in nasal epithelium of CF patients (Dupuit *et al.*, 1995).

A major function of the epididymis, and of CFTR gene-product, is its ability to transport electrolytes and water across the epithelial layer (Wong, 1990). In patients with CF, sodium and water reabsorption is far greater than the limited chloride secretion, and this is responsible for the blockage of exocrine outflow and for the accumulation of thick, dehydrated, mucus in the pancreas, pulmonary airways and probably in the epididymal duct remnants. In patients with CBAVD any residual CFTR function is further reduced by the sloughing of epithelial cells, thus amplifying even further the loss of CFTR activity. A recent study demonstrated that CFTR gene expression occurs also in endocervical cells throughout the menstrual cycle (Hayslip *et al.*, 1997). Therefore, the absence of CFTR gene expression due to CFTR mutations has the potential to alter female reproduction by extreme thickening of the cervical mucus.

Taken together, these data favour an early obstructive process in the pathogenesis of CBAVD. A progressive obstruction of the deferent ductal system by excessive and thick mucus secretions in the epididymal lumen is the most plausible hypothesis to explain the absence of the vas deferens and absence of variable portions of the epididymis.

Final Comments and Conclusions

In summary, in this work we tried to produce a model to explain the pathogenesis of CBAVD based on data already acquired and on new information derived from this study. CFTR mRNA is expressed in fetal male reproductive organs at 18 weeks of gestation and epididymal fluid secretion in the third trimester. CFTR mRNA is expressed in the columnar epithelial cells of adult human epididymis. CFTR mRNA, and consequently CFTR protein expression, is dependent on the integrity of the epididymal epithelium. In patients with epididymal obstruction, whether congenital (CBAVD) or acquired (post-vasectomy and post-inflammatory), there is sloughing and loss of the epithelial cells lining the epididymal lumen. As a result, there is loss of CFTR mRNA and protein expression. Mutations in the CFTR gene, as found in men with cystic fibrosis (CF) and CBAVD, are associated with lack of or decreased CFTR activity. In adults the combined presence of mutations in the CFTR gene and the sloughing of epithelial cells due to obstructive damage further reduces the amount of functional CFTR protein. CFTR plays an important role in the regulation of water and electrolyte content of the epididymal microenvironment

On the basis of these findings, we propose that the accumulation of extremely mucoid and thick epididymal fluid in ducts of narrow calibre impairs the intraluminal flow of epididymal fluid and ultimately is responsible for the atrophy and regression of variable segments of the epididymis as seen in men with CBAVD.

Several questions remain: Why are so many anatomical variations seen clinically in patients with CBAVD? Why in some patients is the epididymis fully formed but the vas is not or is replaced by a fibrous, non-patent cord, whereas in others only the caput or the corpus is present? A possible explanation is that different mutations in the CFTR gene, including the recently recognized 5T-tract variants particularly frequent in men with CBAVD, lead to differences in the amount of functional CFTR protein. The amount of functional CFTR may determine which of the variety of phenotypes is observed.

Why is the proximal segment of the caput epididymis always present? An explanation is that this segment is mainly formed by five to seven vasa efferentia that have a different embryological origin from that of the remaining part of the epididymis. Therefore, CFTR might not be involved in regulating developmental genes that are important for the canalization of the vasa efferentia. Alternatively, the efferent ducts and the most proximal region of the caput epididymis have a richer CFTR expression and, being close to the testis, receive abundant testicular fluid which keeps their patency. In more distal segments of the epididymis and in the vas deferens, the abnormally concentrated fluid caused by dysfunction of CFTR could block and obliterate these ductal structures.

What are the molecular mechanisms that underlie the observed tissue- and organ-specific differences in the response to the same defect in the CFTR gene? Are epigenetic factors responsible for the variable expression of CBAVD as illustrated by the clinical discordance in siblings with the same CFTR genotype? The variable phenotype for the same genotype in the spectrum of CF from CBAVD to complete clinical CF with pancreatic insufficiency may be caused by variability at loci other than the CFTR gene. Even though no human data support this hypothesis, it has been tested in a mouse model of CF (Rozmahel *et al.*, 1996; reviewed by Estevill, 1996). Three different phenotypes are observed in mice homozygous for CFTR gene disruption. One phenotype died by 5 weeks of age due to intestinal obstruction and rupture. The second phenotype died at weaning, and the third phenotype survived for more than six weeks. Investigation of inheritance patterns at other loci throughout the mouse genome identified an allele type at a locus on mouse chromosome 7 that was linked to the milder phenotype. The milder phenotype was associated with the presence of a calcium-activated Cl^- conductance that was not present in the mice with the severe phenotype.

Is it possible that CBAVD patients with renal agenesis and without CFTR gene mutations represent a separate disease process not related to the CFTR gene ?

Finally long-standing vasectomies are associated with loss of epithelial cells due to obstructive damage. Could the lack of CFTR activity be a significant cofactor responsible for decreasing the chances of a successful reanastomosis ?

References

Anguiano A, Oates RD, Amos JA, Dean M, Gerrard B, Stewart C, Maher TA, White MB and Milunsky A (1992) Congenital bilateral absence of the vas deferens. A primarily genital form of cystic fibrosis *Journal of the American Medical Association* **267** 1794–1797

Breitschopf H, Suchanek G, Gould RM, Colman DR and Lassmann H (1992) *In situ* hybridization with digoxigenin-labeled probes: sensitive and reliable detection method applied to myelinating rat brain *Acta Neuropathology (Berlin)* **84** 581–587

Chillon M, Casals T, Mercier B, Bassas L, Lissens W, Silber S, Romey MC, Ruiz-Romero J, Verlingue C, Claustres M, Ferec C

and Estivill X (1995) Mutations in the cystic fibrosis gene in patients with congenital absence of the vas deferens *New England Journal of Medicine* **332** 1475–1480

Costes B, Girodon E, Ghanem N, Flori E, Jardin A, Soufir JC and Goossens M (1995) Frequent occurrence of the CFTR intron 8 (TG) 5T allele in men with congenital bilateral absence of the vas deferens *European Journal of Human Genetics* **3** 285–293

Dumur V, Gervais R, Rigot JM, Lafitte JJ, Manouvriers S, Bisente J and Mazeman M (1990) Abnormal distribution of CF ΔF508 allele in azoospermic men with congenital aplasia of the epididymis and vas deferens *Lancet* **336** 512

Dumur V, Gervais R, Rigot JM, Delomel-Vinner E, Decaestecker B, Lafitte JJ and Roussel P (1996) Congenital bilateral absence of the vas deferens (CBAVD) and cystic fibrosis transmembrane regulator (CFTR): correlation between genotype and phenotype *Human Genetics* **97** 7–10

Dupuit F, Kalin N, Brezillon S Hinnrasky J, Tummler B and Puchelle E (1995) CFTR and differentiation markers expression in non-CF and delta F 508 homozygous CF nasal epithelium *Journal Clinical Investigation* **96** 1601–1611

Estivill X (1996) Complexity in a monogenic disease *Nature Genetics* **12** 348–350

Forstner G, Kopelman H, Durie P and Corey M (1987) Pancreatic and intestinal dysfunction in cystic fibrosis. In *Genetics and Epithelial Cell Dysfunction in Cystic Fibrosis* pp 7–17 Eds JR Riordan and M Buchwald. Alan R Liss, Toronto

Harris A and Coleman L (1989) Ductal epithelial cells cultured from human foetal epididymis and vas deferens: relevance to sterility in cystic fibrosis *Journal of Cell Science* **92** 687–690

Harris A, Chalkley G, Goodman S and Coleman L (1991) Expression of the cystic fibrosis gene in human development *Development* **113** 305–310

Hayslip CC, Hao E and Usala SJ (1997) The cystic fibrosis transmembrane regulator gene is expressed in the human endocervix throughout the menstrual cycle *Fertility and Sterility* **67** 636–640

Holsclaw DS, Lobel B, Jockin H and Schwachman H (1971) Genital abnormalities in male patients with cystic fibrosis *Journal of Urology* **106** 568–574

Kerem B-S, Rommens JM, Buchannan JA, Markiewicz D, Cox TK, Chakrauarti A, Buchwald M and Tsui L (1989) Identification of the cystic fibrosis gene: genetic analysis *Science* **245** 1073–1080

Kirchhoff C, Osterhoff C and Young L (1996) Molecular cloning and characterization of HE1, a major secretory protein of the human epididymis *Biology of Reproduction* **54** 847–856

Krull N, Ivell R, Osterhoff C and Kirchhoff C (1993) Region-specific variation of gene expression in the human epididymis as revealed by *in situ* hybridization with tissue-specific cDNAs *Molecular Reproduction and Development* **34** 16–24

Lissens W, Mercier B, Tournaye H, Bonduelle M, Ferec C, Seneca S, Devroey P, Silber S, Van Steirteghem A and Liebaers I (1996) Cystic fibrosis and infertility caused by congenital absence of the vas deferens and related clinical entities *Human Reproduction* **11** (Supplement 4) 55–78

Maggiano N, LaRocca LM, Piantelli M, Ranelletti FO, Lauriola L, Ricci R and Capelli A (1991) Detection of mRNA and hnRNA using a digoxigenin labelled cDNA probe by *in situ* hybridization on frozen tissue sections *Histochemistry Journal* **23** 69–74

Patrizio P and Zielenski J (1996) Congenital absence of the vas deferens: a mild form of cystic fibrosis *Molecular Medicine Today* **2** 24–31

Patrizio P, Asch RH, Handelin B and Silber SJ (1993) Aetiology of congenital absence of the vas deferens: genetic study of three generations *Human Reproduction* **8** 215–220

Patrizio P, Ord T, Silber SJ and Asch RH (1994) Correlation between epididymal length and fertilization rate in men with congenital absence of the vas deferens *Fertility and Sterility* **61** 265–268

Riordan JR, Rommens JM, Kerem B *et al.* (1989) Identification of the cystic fibrosis gene: cloning and characterization of complementary DNA *Science* **245** 1066–1073

Rommens JM, Iannuzzi MC, Kerem B, Drumm ML, Melmer G, Dean M, Rozmahel R, Cole JL, Kennedy D, Hidaka N, Zsiga M, Buchwald M, Tsui L and Collins FS (1989) Identification of the cystic fibrosis gene: chromosome walking and jumping *Science* **245** 1059–1065

Rozmahel R, Wilschanski M, Matin A, Plyte S, Oliver M, Auerbach W, Moore A, Forstner J, Durie P, Nadeau J, Bear C and Tsui LC (1996) Modulation of disease severity in cystic fibrosis transmembrane conductance regulator deficient mice by a secondary genetic factor *Nature Genetics* **12** 280–287

Saitoh K, Terada T and Hatakeyama S (1990) A morphological study of the efferent ducts of the human epididymis *International Journal of Andrology* **13** 359–375

Siiteri PK and Wilson JD (1974) Testosterone formation and metabolism during male sexual differentiation in the human embryo *Journal of Clinical Endocrinology and Metabolism* **38** 113–118

Silber SJ (1986) Diagnosis and treatment of obstructive azoospermia. In *Male Reproductive Dysfunction* pp 479– 517 Eds S Santen and R Swerdloff. Dekker publications, New York

Tizzano EF, Silver MM, Chitayat D, Benichou JC and Buchwald M (1994) Differential cellular expression of cystic fibrosis transmembrane regulator in human reproductive tissues. Clues for the infertility in patients with cystic fibrosis *American Journal of Pathology* **144** 906–914

Trezise AE, Chambers JA, Wardle CJ, Gould S and Harris A (1993) Expression of the cystic fibrosis gene in human fetal tissues *Human Molecular Genetics* **2** 213–218

Yeung CH, Cooper TG, Bergmann M and Schulze H (1991) Organization of tubules in the human caput epididymis and the ultrastructure of their epithelia *American Journal of Anatomy* **191** 261–279

Wong PYD (1990) Electrolyte and fluid transport in the epididymis. In *Epithelial Secretion of Water and Electrolytes* pp 333–347 Eds P Young and PYD Wong. Springer-Verlag, Berlin

Zielenski J, Patrizio P, Corey M, Handelin B, Markiewicz D and Tsui LC (1995) CFTR gene variant for patients with congenital absence of the vas deferens *American Journal of Human Genetics* **57** 958–960

Zondek LH and Zondek T (1965) The secretory activity of the maturing epididymis compared with maturational changes in other reproductive organs of the foetus, infant and child *Acta Paediatrice Scandinavia* **54** 295–305

Journal of Reproduction and Fertility Supplement **53**, 271–275

The role of the epididymis in human infertility

D. M. de Kretser[1], C. Huidobro[2*], G. J. Southwick[2] and P. D. Temple-Smith[2]

[1]*Institute of Reproduction and Development; and* [2]*Department of Anatomy, Monash University, Clayton, Victoria, Australia*

This review describes the role of the epididymis in human infertility, by analysing the results of epididymovasostomies which confirm that the more distal the site of obstruction the greater the chance of fertility. The use of epididymal spermatozoa for *in vitro* fertilization (IVF) yielded poor results in contrast to intracytoplasmic sperm injection using either epididymal or testicular spermatozoa. The nature of the pathology causing obstructive azoospermia is examined reviewing in particular the possible role of mercury toxicity in Young's syndrome. This review describes the results of studies that show that the level of obstruction within the epididymis is correlated with the presence of sperm antibodies and distal obstructions are associated with the presence of sperm antibodies. The demonstration that necrozoospermia decreases with increased sperm transport through the epididymis, when combined with the observation of normal testicular sperm morphology, represents the basis for the disorder termed epididymal necrozoospermia. However, to date the nature of the epididymal pathology causing this disorder remains obscure.

Introduction

The focus of attention concerning the epididymis as a cause of human infertility has been the role that it has played in obstructive azoospermia. With the increasing use of intracytoplasmic injection of spermatozoa aspirated from the epididymis or testis to achieve pregnancies, surgical correction of these obstructions is less frequent. This review explores the involvement of the epididymis as a site at which mercury toxicity may be manifested and observations indicating that specific regions of this organ may be linked to the elaboration of antisperm antibodies. The implication that the epididymis can be a hostile sperm storage site is reviewed in the condition known as epididymal necrozoospermia which is associated with infertility, severely impaired sperm motility, viability and sperm morphology.

The function of the human epididymis still remains unclear due principally to the difficulties posed in the investigation of this structure. There are considerable difficulties in obtaining tissue from normal men and hence knowledge has had to accumulate from observations on pathological materials or from the evaluation of post-mortem materials. Structural characterization of the epididymis from these sources has been possible and detailed descriptions of the cytological features and characterization of the different regions are available. However, our understanding of the function has depended on extrapolation from the results of investigations on other mammalian species.

The classical view, developed from non-human studies, that the acquisition of motility and fertilizing ability of spermatozoa are dependent on transit through the epididymis, has been challenged by the results obtained from some studies of infertile men. This review examines the results of these studies and recent data implicating the level of epididymal obstruction in antisperm antibody formation. The involvement of the epididymis in certain types of infertility is also reviewed.

* Present Address: La Clinca Las Condes, Santiago, Chile.

Is the Human Epididymis Required for the Acquisition of Fertilizing Ability by Spermatozoa?

Reviews of the results of epididymovasostomies performed to relieve obstructive azoospermia first challenged the concept that the epididymis is necessary for the acquisition of fertilizing ability by demonstrating that spermatozoa had to traverse only a very small zone of the caput epididymidis to achieve fertility *in vivo* (Schoysman and Bedford, 1986; Southwick and Temple-Smith, 1988). However, these investigators noted that the more distal the anastomotic site, the greater the chance of fertility. Subsequently, the studies of Temple-Smith *et al.* (1989) explored this possibility by undertaking a series of epididymovasostomies at different levels of the epididymis in the rabbit and assessing the fertility in these animals. They showed that some rabbits with caput anastomoses were able to achieve fertility but also noted that the percentage of fertile animals improved with the more distal anastomoses.

More recent studies confirmed the trend towards higher pregnancy rates with more distal anastomoses and also noted that the time taken for spermatozoa to appear in the ejaculate was longer (12 months) with an epididymovasostomy compared with a vasovasostomy (6 months) (Schlegel and Goldstein, 1993; Matthews *et al.*, 1995).

The use of intracytoplasmic sperm injection (ICSI) of epididymal spermatozoa into oocytes was associated with a 58% fertilization rate and a pregnancy rate of 35% per cycle (Tournaye *et al.*, 1994). These remarkable results and similar outcomes when testicular spermatozoa were used prompted suggestions that epididymal transit was not required for the acquisition of fertilizing capacity. However, caution should prevail in considering such an extrapolation since ICSI bypasses the need for penetration of the zona pellucida and sperm–oolemmal interactions. Indeed the very poor fertilization rates that were obtained when spermatozoa collected by epididymal aspiration were used for IVF support the need for epididymal maturation of spermatozoa (Temple-Smith *et al.*, 1985; Southwick and Temple-Smith, 1988). These workers found a fertilization rate of 18% and a pregnancy rate of 3% per cycle. This view is also supported by the very poor outcome in terms of fertilization after the use of epididymal spermatozoa introduced beneath the zona pellucida by microinjection. From these data it would seem reasonable to conclude that for optimal fertility *in vivo*, epididymal sperm transit, at least through the caput epididymidis, should occur. The remarkably good results achieved using testicular spermatozoa for ICSI (see McLachlan *et al.*, this supplement) are simply a reflection that this procedure bypasses several key steps in the natural process of fertilization.

The nature of the changes induced by epididymal transit that are required to facilitate fertilization still remains to be established but recent developments in this field are described in other papers in this volume (Jones, Temple-Smith, Cooper, and Ivell).

Obstructive Azoospermia due to Lesions in the Epididymis

A variety of pathological processes can result in obstruction at different levels within the epididymal duct. The molecular basis of some of these disorders has now been elucidated. One such example is the demonstration that mutations in the gene encoding the cystic fibrosis transmembrane regulator (CFTR) cause congenital absence of the vas deferens (see Patrizio *et al.*, this supplement).

Less well recognized is the condition of Young's syndrome, an association of obstructive azoospermia due to an epididymal obstruction in the region of the caput with bronchiectasis (Young, 1970; Handelsman *et al.*, 1984; Wilton *et al.*, 1990). The association of respiratory disease with infertility also occurs in Kartagener's syndrome but this defect is not epididymal in origin as it has been shown to result from disturbances in cilial beat frequency due to a genetically based absence of certain key proteins in the cilium and the axoneme of the sperm tail (Eliasson *et al.*, 1977). Examination of sperm tail and nasal cilia structure could not link Young's syndrome to the abnormalities found in the immotile cilia syndrome (Wilton *et al.*, 1990) but subtle quantitative abnormalities in a number of axonemal structures were noted. The presence of such abnormalities in a set of identical twins raised the possibility that a genetic basis may be present (Teichtahl *et al.*,

1987). In view of the linkage of congenital absence of the vas with cystic fibrosis and its respiratory disease, an examination of the CFTR gene was undertaken in patients with Young's syndrome. Mutations in the CFTR gene were not found with an increased frequency in patients with Young's syndrome (Friedman *et al.*, 1995). Hendry *et al.* (1993), and unpublished observations from our own clinic, have noted that a number of patients with Young's syndrome gave a history of Pink disease, a disorder assumed to be due to childhood mercury poisoning since that disorder disappeared after the removal of mercury from teething powders (Cheek, 1960). Pink disease disappeared in about 1960 and it is of interest that Young's syndrome has essentially disappeared from our clinical services some 25–30 years later. Formal proof of this hypothesis has yet to be established from experimental studies but the data suggest that the epididymis could be a site of action of toxic concentrations of mercury.

The applications of modern microsurgical principles to relieve epididymal duct obstruction have resulted in enhanced success rates (Silber, 1978 and 1989; Southwick and Temple-Smith, 1988). However, there is a trend for using testicular spermatozoa obtained by epididymal aspiration, or more commonly now by fine needle aspiration of the testis, for ICSI in preference to surgical correction of the epididymal lesion. However, such an approach exposes the female partner to risks of oocyte retrieval and ovarian hyperstimulation.

Links Between the Level of Epididymal Obstruction and the Formation of Antisperm Antibodies

Approximately 70% of men develop antisperm antibodies after vasectomy, but clinical observations suggest that obstruction resulting from congenital obstruction of the vas is rarely associated with the presence of antisperm antibodies. This prompted us to undertake a study to determine whether the site of epididymal obstruction correlated with the presence of antisperm antibodies in seminal plasma or in blood.

The clinical records of 180 men who underwent vasectomy reversal or epididymal microsurgery for obstructive azoospermia were evaluated to determine the presence of antibodies to spermatozoa and the level of excurrent duct obstruction. Antisperm antibodies were detected by the tray agglutination test and in some cases the indirect immunobead test was performed on seminal plasma of patients with congenital absence of the vas. A titre of 1:32 or greater was regarded as positive in the tray agglutination test (Rumke *et al.*, 1974) and in the indirect immunobead test a positive result was recorded if more than 50% of the spermatozoa showed adhering immunobeads (Clarke, 1990). The level of obstruction to spermatozoa outflow was determined at scrotal exploration and classified according to Holstein (1976). Of the 180 patients, 76 underwent epididymovasostomy and in 85 a vasovasostomy was performed. Fifteen patients had congenital absence of the vas and in four, no connection between the testis and epididymis was found. Antibodies to spermatozoa detected by the tray agglutination test were present more commonly in patients with distal obstruction particularly below epididymal level 3 (Holstein,1976) (Table 1). In those patients with a level 2 obstruction, only 14% showed antibodies, whereas this percentage rose to 68% and 74% for level 3 or vas obstructions, respectively.

A similar pattern was evident in the patients with congenital absence of the vas since the ten patients with an epididymal remnant extending to level 2a or 2b showed no detectable antisperm antibodies, whereas those with distal extensions to levels 3a and 4 demonstrated antibodies in 66–100% of cases (Table 2).

These results clearly indicate that the level of obstruction influences the likelihood of antisperm antibody formation irrespective of the aetiology. It is of note that the progression of spermatozoa to level 3 and beyond in the epididymis is associated with antisperm antibody formation in 65% or more of patients. The reasons for this association are unclear. It is recognized that maturation of spermatozoa through the epididymis is associated with changes in surface protein composition and these may elicit an antigenic response. Alternatively the more proximal epididymal epithelium may secrete substances with the capability of modulating the immune response. Neither of these suggestions explain why approximately 70% of men develop antisperm antibodies after a vasectomy.

Table 1. Patients with obstructive azoospermia

Level of obstruction*	Total number of patients	Antisperm antibodies agglutination test positive	
		n	%
Rete testis	4	0	0
Epididymis Level 1	43	6	14
Epididymis Level 2	14	2	14
Epididymis Level 3	16	11	68
Epididymis Level 4	3	2	66
Vasectomy	85	63	74

* According to classification of Holstein (1976).

Table 2. Patients with congenital absence of vas

Level of obstruction*	Total number of patients	Indirect immunobead test positive	
		n	%
Epididymis Level 2a	5	5	0
Epididymis Level 2b	5	5	0
Epididymis Level 3a	3	2	66
Epididymis Level 4b	1	1	100
Epididymis Level 4c	1	1	100

* According to classification of Holstein (1976).

Can Disordered Epididymal Function be Implicated as a Cause of Human Infertility?

Given the role attributed to the epididymis in the acquisition of sperm motility and fertilizing ability, it is not unreasonable to predict that disordered epididymal function will underlie certain disorders of sperm function. However, to date there are few examples of such disorders. One such condition is termed epididymal necrozoospermia (EN) which presents as a collection of defects that can be noted on semen analysis (Wilton *et al.*, 1988). Patients with this disorder have variable sperm concentrations linked to grossly impaired sperm motility (< 5%), markedly increased numbers of abnormally shaped spermatozoa (95%) and very poor sperm viability (< 20%). Often there are some semen analyses wherein improvements in motility, viability and morphology are linked to shortened periods of abstinence (Wilton *et al.*, 1988). Ultrastructural studies of spermatozoa showed a characteristic pattern with loss of definition of the microtubular doublets comprising the axoneme of the sperm tail. These structures take on a granular appearance and marked degeneration of the acrosome and sperm head occur. Limited studies were available on the structure of testicular spermatozoa in such patients which showed that the features of the tail, acrosome and head were normal. These data led us to the conclusion that the epididymis in such men may represent a hostile region for sperm storage.

To explore this hypothesis further, we undertook measures to decrease the time spermatozoa spent in the epididymis by asking such patients to undertake a frequent ejaculation test wherein they undertook to have an ejaculation twice a day for 5 days. By examining the first and the last samples we noted that in the patients with EN there was an improvement in sperm motility (3–7-fold increase), sperm morphology and viability in the final sample suggesting that the decreased storage time may have resulted in the improvements. Some patients show no change in their sperm concentration whereas others, probably due to limited sperm reserves, showed a significant decrease (Wilton *et al.*, 1988).

The specific epididymal pathology accounting for these features has not been established but recognition of the condition, appropriate advice regarding periods of abstinence and the use of testicular spermatozoa for ICSI have resulted in pregnancies. For our understanding of this and other human epididymal disorders to improve, there needs to be a substantial increase in our knowledge of the physiology of the epididymis. Since there is a trend to aspirate spermatozoa from the epididymis for use by ICSI and IVF, opportunities may occur for obtaining tissue samples that may facilitate studies of human epididymal pathology.

References

Cheek DB (1960) On the nature of Pink disease *Medical Journal of Australia* **1** 153–155

Clarke GN (1990) Detection of antisperm antibodies using immunobeads. In *Handbook of the Laboratory Diagnosis and Treatment of Infertility* pp 177–192 Eds BA Keel and C Webster, CRC Press, Boca Raton, Florida

Eliasson R, Mossberg B, Camner P and Afzelius B (1977) *New England Journal of Medicine* **297** 1–6

Friedman KJ, Teichtahl H, de Kretser DM, Temple-Smith PD, Southwick GJ, Silverman LM, Highsmith WE, Boucher RC and Knowles MR (1995) Screening Young's syndrome patients for CFTR mutations *American Review of Respiratory Diseases* **152** 1353–1357

Handelsman DJ, Conway AJ, Boylan LM and Turtle JR (1984) Young's syndrome: obstructive azoospermia and chronic sinopulmonary infections *New England Journal of Medicine* **310** 3–9

Hendry WF, A'hern FP and Cole PJ (1993) Was Young's syndrome caused by exposure to mercury in childhood? *British Medical Journal* **307** 1579–1582

Holstein AF (1976) Structure of the human epididymis. In *Human Semen and Fertility Regulation in Men* pp 23–30. Ese Hafez Mosby, St Louis

Matthews GJ, Schlegel PN and Goldstein M (1995) Patency following microsurgical vasoepididymostomy and vasovasotomy: temporal considerations *Journal of Urology* **154** 2070–2073

Rumke P, Van Amstel N, Messer EN and Bezemer PD (1974) Prognosis of fertility of men with sperm agglutinins in the semen *Fertility and Sterility* **25** 393–398

Schlegel PN and Goldstein M (1993) Microsurgical vasoepididymostomy: refinements and results *Journal of Urology* **150** 1165–1168

Schoysman RJ and Bedford JM (1986) The role of the human epididymis in sperm maturation and sperm storage as reflected in the consequences of epididymovasostomy *Fertility and Sterility* **46** 293–299

Silber SJ (1978) Microscopic vasoepididymostomy: specific microanastomosis to the epididymal tubule *Fertility and Sterility* **30** 565–568

Silber SJ (1989) Role of epididymis in sperm maturation *Urology* **33** 47–51

Southwick GJ and Temple-Smith PD (1988) Epididymal microsurgery and current techniques and new horizons *Microsurgery* **9** 266–277

Teichtahl H, Temple-Smith PD, Johnson JL, Southwick G and de Kretser DM (1987) Obstructive azoospermia and chronic sinobronchial disease (Young's syndrome) in identical twins *Fertility and Sterility* **47** 879–881

Temple-Smith PD, Southwick GJ, Yates CA, Trounson AO and de Kretser DM (1985) Human pregnancy by *in vitro* fertilization (IVF) using sperm aspirated from the epididymis *Journal of In Vitro Fertilisation and Embryo Transfer* **2** 119–122

Temple-Smith PD, Southwick GJ, Herrera Castaneda E, Hamer J and McClatchey M (1989) Surgical manipulation of the epididymis: an experimental approach to sperm maturation In *Perspectives in Andrology* **63** 281–290 Ed. M Serio, Serono Symposia Publications, Raven Press, New York

Tournaye H, Devroey P, Liu J, Nagy Z, Lissens W and Van Steirteghem A (1994) Microsurgical epididymal sperm aspiration and intracytoplasmic sperm injection: a new effective approach to infertility as a result of congenital bilateral absence of the vas deferens *Fertility and Sterility* **61** 1045–1051

Wilton LJ, Temple-Smith PD, Baker AGW and de Kretser DM (1988) Human male infertility caused by degeneration and death of sperm in the epididymis *Fertility and Sterility* **49** 1052–1058

Wilton LJ, Teichtahl H, Temple-Smith PD, Johnson JL, Southwick GJ, Burger HG and de Kretser DM (1990) Young's syndrome (obstructive azoospermia and chronic sinobronchial infection): a quantitative study of axonemal ultrastructure and function *Fertility and Sterility* **55** 144–151

Young D (1970) Surgical treatment of male infertility *Journal of Reproduction and Fertility* **23** 541–542

Journal of Reproduction and Fertility Supplement **53**, 277–284

The use of epididymal spermatozoa in assisted reproduction

Robert I. McLachlan

Prince Henry's Institute of Medical Research, Monash Medical Centre, Clayton, Australia 3186; and Monash IVF, 89 Bridge Road Richmond, Australia, 3121.

The use of epididymal spermatozoa in assisted reproduction (ART) permits fertility in men with surgically irremediable obstructive azoospermia. When used for conventional IVF (sperm–oocyte co-culture), epididymal spermatozoa show reduced fertilization and pregnancy rates (compared with ejaculated spermatozoa from men with a range of spermatogenic disorders) as evidence of their functional immaturity. However, when used with intracytoplasmic sperm injection (ICSI) either fresh or frozen–thawed epididymal spermatozoa produce ART success rates similar to those of ejaculated spermatozoa. The clinical place of epididymal sperm retrieval for ICSI has come under review as a result of data showing similarly good outcomes with testicular spermatozoa obtained by needle aspiration. In Australia ICSI using epididymal or testicular spermatozoa is an increasingly favoured option for vasectomy-related infertility and in other types of obstructive azoospermia for a number of reasons including better pregnancy outcomes, the less invasive nature of the procedures and less expense involved; however, this cost-benefit analysis will vary in other health systems.

Introduction

Epididymal spermatozoa have been widely used in assisted reproductive techniques (ART) whenever there is surgically irremediable congenital or acquired obstruction to sperm outflow. The task of the clinician is to counsel the couple with regard to the full range of ART options, particularly with regard to the safest, least invasive and least expensive strategy which offers a realistic prospect of pregnancy.

Conventional IVF, in which numerous motile spermatozoa are incubated with mature oocytes, demands that the spermatozoa display functions such as oocyte binding, the acrosome reaction, penetration of the zona pellucida and finally binding and penetration of the oolemmal membrane. As spermatozoa normally undergo functional maturation during epididymal passage, their premature surgical removal from the epididymis may be expected to decrease their ability to fertilize the oocyte by IVF. The first successful pregnancy obtained by IVF using epididymal spermatozoa was reported by Temple-Smith *et al.* (1985). However, success rates remained very poor (< 5% per cycle) underscoring the diminished functional capacity of these spermatozoa. These difficulties were circumvented by injecting spermatozoa under the zona pellucida; however, while offering somewhat better results than conventional IVF, clinical pregnancy rates remained poor.

The intracytoplasmic injection of a single spermatozoon (ICSI) significantly improved the prospects for normal fertilization and pregnancy using epididymal spermatozoa. Yet despite this good outcome the clinical place of epididymal surgery and sperm retrieval is under review for two reasons. First, the ICSI technique is so efficient (one spermatozoa per oocyte) and so tolerant of sperm quality (frozen–thawed epididymal spermatozoa perform as well as fresh) that numerous cycles can be undertaken from a single epididymal aspiration decreasing the need for repeat surgery. However, the greatest challenge comes from the fact that testicular spermatozoa provide equally good results and can be obtained more readily with little risk and, importantly, at a fraction of the cost.

This review will expand on these points and conclude with a view on the place of epididymal sperm retrieval in Australia and why this position may differ in other centres.

Patient Groups

Congenital bilateral absence of the vas

Congenital bilateral absence of the vas (BCAV) occurs with a prevalence of 1:2500 men and is a leading cause of obstructive azoospermia. It involves a developmental defect in the Wolffian duct structures with the seminal vesicles, vas and a variable extent of the cauda and corpus epididymides being absent. It is strongly associated with mutations of the cystic fibrosis transmembrane conductance receptor (CFTR) (see review by Lissens *et al.*, 1996; Chillon *et al.*, 1995), although the mechanism by which the CFTR mutation relates to these structural abnormalities is unclear. Only spermatozoa retrieval and ART offers any chance of fertility. Genetic screening of both partners for the commonest CFTR mutations in their ethnic group is essential before ART in order to reduce the chance of full blown CF in the offspring (see Patrizio, this volume).

Vasectomy-related infertility

Vasectomy reversal (VR) rates in Australia are now about 6% but may vary widely between countries. The prospects for pregnancy with VR are affected by a number of factors, in particular the interval between vasectomy and VR. In one large study in the USA, Belker and colleagues (1991) used microsurgical techniques for vaso-vasotomy or vaso-epididymostomy in 1469 men. Surgery provided a 76% pregnancy rate within < 3 years after vasectomy, but after 15 years of obstruction, the pregnancy rate was only 30%. Such results will not be achieved in non-specialist centres with the real success of VR in the general community clearly varying with the microsurgical skill of the surgeon and the technique of the original vasectomy. Representative figures are difficult to obtain owing to the lack of data collections and the failure to use standardized reporting criteria. A fair estimate would be that, overall, only half the VR surgeries would be expected to result in a spontaneous pregnancy within a reasonable period (for example 2 years) (McLachlan and Royce, 1996).

The failure of VR surgery relates to (i) the failure of surgery to restore patency, and (ii) poor sperm quality due to defective epididymal function, the presence of sperm antibodies and possibly to damage to seminiferous tubule epithelium (David de Kretser, personal communication). As a result failed VR is a leading cause for presentation to ART programmes in all western countries.

Post-inflammatory epididymal obstruction

Genital tract infections such as chlamydia or gonococcus can result in severe epididymal inflammation and obstruction.

Miscellaneous

Epididymal obstruction occurs in Young's syndrome where it is associated with respiratory tract disease (see deKretser, this supplement). Other causes of vas/epididymal obstruction which may result in consideration of epididymal sperm retrieval include damage to the vas during hernia surgery, anejaculation due to neurogenic problems (spinal cord injury, diabetes) or actual/functional obstruction to sperm outflow at the base of the bladder (for example after prostate surgery, congenital cysts or post-infective scarring) in which case the epididymis is the next 'upstream port of call' for sperm retrieval.

The 'Pre-ICSI' Era (1985–1993)

Temple-Smith *et al.* (1985) reported the first pregnancy using epididymal spermatozoa recovered from a vasectomized man. This approach demanded the scheduling of the epididymal sperm retrieval with oocyte collection so that fresh (and thus optimally motile) spermatozoa would be available for insemination. Such an approach is logistically difficult as the time of oocyte collection cannot be precisely predicted so that epididymal surgery may need to be rescheduled at short notice. The Monash group took the approach of treating cohorts of 10–15 patients with the aim of performing all oocyte collections and sperm retrieval during one week. Nonetheless scheduling operating theatres, oocyte collections and surgeons was indeed challenging!

Spermatozoa were recovered from the corpus or caput epididymides including, when necessary, after gentle compression of the testis to ensure the collection of fresh non-necrotic spermatozoa with optimal motility. Disappointingly the fertilization rate remained low (< 20%) and the ongoing pregnancy rate was only about 3%. The great majority of other reports showed similarly disappointing fertilization rates of 7–35% and low ongoing viable pregnancy rates (Bladou *et al.*, 1991; Patrizio *et al.*, 1994) implying that epididymal spermatozoa lacked both normal fertilizing abilities and, more importantly, that the resultant embryos did not have full developmental capabilities.

Some groups reported surprisingly good results using conventional IVF, for example Schlegel *et al.* (1994) reported a clinical pregnancy rate of 27% per cycle. In 32 IVF treatment cycles involving 28 men with BCAV, Silber *et al.* (1990) reported a fertilization rate of 26% using fresh epididymal spermatozoa, and that 21 women underwent embryo transfers with a clinical pregnancy rate of 31% per cycle. Yet later when comparing the efficacy of IVF versus ICSI using epididymal spermatozoa, it was reported that conventional IVF produced fertilization and pregnancy rates of only 19% and 4.5%, respectively and concluded that 'no programme ... using conventional IVF has > 10% pregnancy rate over the long haul' (Silber *et al.*, 1994).

These studies did provide some interesting data about the effects of the epididymal environment on the ability of the spermatozoa to fertilize with IVF. Spermatozoa from the efferent ducts or caput epididymidis tend to show the best motility (Silber 1990 *et al.*; Bladou *et al.*, 1991) and to show the least morphological evidence of degeneration (Asch *et al*, 1992). A positive correlation was reported between the length of the epididymis and the quality and fertilizing ability of spermatozoa recovered from the caput epididymidis (Patrizio *et a.*, 1994). In that study, a fertilization rate of 7% was found when the epididymal length was 0.5–1.9 cm compared with 24% when more than 4 cm was present. A similar observation was made by Schlegel *et al.* (1994). These data suggest that the more extensive and normal the interaction of spermatozoa with the epididymis, the better the functional ability of the spermatozoa. However, new spermatozoa entering an abnormal epididymal environment may suffer damage as a result and their interaction with necrotic spermatozoa within the obstructed epididymis. The basis of the obstruction (BCAV versus acquired lesions) did not appear to affect fertilization or pregnancy rates although there was a report that fertilization rates in BCAV were influenced by the CFTR mutation status (Patrizio *et al.*, 1993). Finally the presence of sperm antibodies in epididymal fluid or serum of men with BCAV did not affect the ability of epididymal spermatozoa to fertilize *in vitro* (Patrizio *et al.*, 1992).

With the development of the subzonal sperm microinjection procedure (SUZI), there was initial hope that fertilization and pregnancy rates would improve substantially. SUZI required that several motile spermatozoa be injected into the perivitelline space of each oocyte in order to achieve acceptable fertilization rates (20–40%) but as a result a high incidence of polyspermic (non-viable) fertilizations was encountered (Lacham-Kaplan and Trounson, 1994; Son *et al.*, 1996). Few comparisons of SUZI with ICSI were undertaken as SUZI was rapidly surplanted by ICSI; however, fertilization rates were clearly inferior to ICSI (Madgar *et al.*, 1996; Son *et al.*, 1996). Finally despite the transfer of normal embryos, ongoing pregnancy rates were poor, suggesting a defect in embryonic potential which remains unexplained. Pessimism continued despite the development of SUZI as did the burden and disappointment on patients and the organizational difficulties of scheduling surgeries.

Table 1. Fertilization (FR) and pregnancy rates (PR/cycle) using fresh epididymal spermatozoa and ICSI

Reference	Cycles	FR	PR/cycle	Reference	Cycles	FR	PR/cycle
Silber *et al.* (1994)	17	41%	47%	Tsirigotis *et al.* (1996)	42	48%	31%
Devroey *et al.* (1995)	7	57%	NA	Mansour *et al.* (1997)	44	60%	27%
Silber *et al.* (1995)	33	47%	60%	Rosenlund *et al.* (1997)	13	68%	43%
Nagy *et al.* (1995)	43	56%	30%	Aboulghar *et al.* (1997)	44	55%	36%
Madgar *et al.* (1996)	37	34%	19%	Fahmy *et al.* (1997)	36	60%	25%

NA = not applicable

Table 2. Results of ICSI using cryopreserved epididymal spermatozoa

No. cycles injected	No. oocytes	Fertilization rate	Pregnancies per cycle	Reference
9	106	56%	33% (3:9)	Nagy *et al.* (1995)
7	68	45%	43% (3:7)	Devroey *et al.* (1995)
97	956	48%	19% (18:97)	Holden *et al.* (1997)

The ICSI Era – Initial Impact

The dramatic success of ICSI in application to a wide range of disorders of ejaculated spermatozoa soon led to its use with epididymal spermatozoa (Silber *et al*, 1994). Results using epididymal spermatozoa were markedly better than those using any previous insemination method (Silber *et al.*, 1994; Tournaye *et al.*, 1994; Madgar *et al.*, 1996) and in many reports were similar to those reported for ejaculated spermatozoa (see Table 1). ICSI was immediately adopted as the insemination method of choice for epididymal spermatozoa.

Cryopreservation of epididymal spermatozoa

The practical difficulty of timing spermatozoa retrieval with oocyte collection, and the desire to avoid repetitive surgeries, made the consideration of freezing and thawing epididymal spermatozoa a logical extension (Devroey *et al.*, 1995). These authors reported that despite frozen–thawed epididymal spermatozoa displaying poor motility (non-progressive or only 'twitching'), fertilization and pregnancy rates were comparable to those with fresh epididymal spermatozoa, although less than those of fresh ejaculated spermatozoa. Similarly we found fertilization rates with frozen–thawed epididymal spermatozoa to be 47% which, while a satisfactory result, was less than the 73% seen with ejaculated spermatozoa (Holden *et al.*, 1997). It was also found that the results of frozen–thawed epididymal spermatozoa were poorer when spermatozoa of low vitality (< 20%) were retrieved at initial surgery. This presumably relates to the fact that poor vitality reflects stasis and subsequent necrosis of spermatozoa. Such samples would present a relatively high probability of non-viable spermatozoa (i.e. incapable of normal fertilization) being selected by chance for ICSI. Consequently we do not advise the freezing and later use of spermatozoa from samples with a < 20% vitality and advise the use of fresh testicular spermatozoa or a repeat epididymal aspiration seeking a sample from the more proximal epididymis.

In one series of 603 attempted sperm retrievals at VR, motile spermatozoa in the vasal or epididymal fluid where found only in 35% of cases leading the authors to conclude that sperm storage was not indicated in the remainder (Belker and Bergamini 1997). However, the conclusion ignores the fact that some motility may be seen after prolonged *in vitro* culture of frozen–thawed spermatozoa and that provided that vitality is maintained, the absence of motility does not indicate the absence of fertilizing ability using ICSI.

Our overall results using frozen epididymal spermatozoa and ICSI are shown in the Table 2. These results are similar to those we obtain using ejaculated spermatozoa and ICSI in an unselected population (ie. without consideration of female diagnosis or age, or cycle number).

Alternative procedures for epididymal sperm collection

Although most authors initially prefered the collection of epididymal spermatozoa at open surgery, the direct aspiration of epididymal spermatozoa for ICSI through the skin (percutaneous sperm, aspiration PESA) has been proposed as a less invasive option (Tsirigotis *et al.*, 1995). These authors later reported similar results for percutaneous aspiration versus conventional epididymal sperm retrieval, with a 53% fertilization rate, a 31% pregnancy rates per cycle and an embryo implantation rate of 14% (Tsirigotis *et al.*, 1996). PESA is now widely used under local anaesthesia and is mostly readily performed in the presence of a spermatocoele. Microsurgical puncture of the epididymis with electrical stimulation of the perivascular nerves in the spermatic cord has been proposed as a method of improving the quality of collected spermatozoa and thus of significantly enhancing fertilization and pregnancy rate (Yamamoto *et al.*, 1995, 1996). Collection of spermatozoa from the vas deferens has also been reported in anejaculation associated with diabetes, and a normal pregnancy later obtained using cryopreserved spermatozoa and ICSI (Hovatta *et al.*, 1996)

Testicular Sperm Retrieval

The failure to retrieve epididymal spermatozoa from a significant number of men with obstructive azoospermia lead to the first report that spermatozoa could be isolated directly from the testis and successfully used to produce fertilization and pregnancy (Devroey *et al.*, 1994). Numerous reports have supported the finding that testicular spermatozoa produce similar fertilization, cleavage and ongoing pregnancy rates to epididymal spermatozoa (Nagy *et al.*, 1995; Silber *et al.*, 1995; Mansour *et al.*, 1996; Fahmy *et al.*, 1997; Rosenlund *et al.*, 1997; Aboulghar *et al.*, 1997).

Recently it has been reported that testicular spermatozoa can be frozen, either as isolated spermatozoa or within seminiferous tubules, then later thawed and successfully used for ICSI (Craft and Tsirigiotis, 1995; Edirisinghe *et al.*, 1996; Cotman and Allan, 1997). This will allow the further evolution of clinical practice in which several cycles of ICSI can be undertaken from spermatozoa derived from a single biopsy. In obstructive azoospermia, very little tissue is required from the fine needle aspiration biopsy to provide enough spermatozoa for several ICSI attempts.

The Evolution of Current Clinical Practice

There are two questions to be considered: (i) When should ART be used instead of surgery? (ii) Should epididymal or testicular spermatozoa be used? In many countries, including Australia, several inter-related factors have led to a move away from VR in favour of ART, and away from the use of open epididymal sperm retrieval in favour of PESA or testicular spermatozoa in inoperable obstructive azoospermia.

Vasectomy related infertility – ART versus ICSI

Counselling couples about their prospects for initial or repeat VRs, as opposed to entry into an ART programme, is a complex issue and one frequently facing patients and ART specialists. In addition to the obstructive interval, the other critical factor is the age of the woman. Women in their late thirties face a limited time for the attainment of natural pregnancy as well as a rapidly diminishing probability of success with ART after the age of 40 years. For example, irrespective of sperm quality or origin, the probability of a live birth from an ART treatment cycle for a 42 year old woman is universally reported to be very poor (< 5%). When the prospects for successful VR are not favourable, should such couples risk their final few years of fertility in the hope that a VR will lead to a natural pregnancy or should they rather immediately enter an ART programme?

Couples must also consider issues such as the cost of surgery or ART, and the time off work associated with each treatment. One can appreciate the difficult position of a couple where the vasectomy was performed 14 years previously, the wife is 38 years and the husband is the sole income earner employed doing physical labour. The prospects of success with VR are limited and, should it fail, they have lost not only money but also invaluable time from her diminishing window of fertility. If they chose ART, there are a different set of issues to confront including the burden and risks of ovarian hyperstimulation and the as yet unproved safety of these procedures in relation to the health and fertility of the offspring.

The out-of-pocket costs of VR will depend upon the health system operating in a particular country. The Australian Federal Government provided a substantial rebate for the cost of VR until 1996 and as a result of its removal the cost of VR rose significantly. This fact, together with the greater awareness of ART options, appears to have substantially reduced the number of vasectomy reversals although the lack of a central register of VR procedures precludes quantitating this change. Indirect evidence for the reduction in VR procedures comes from data regarding sperm storage at surgery. One surrogate marker of the number of epididymal sperm retrieval procedures is the number of requests by surgeons for sperm storage during their surgeries. We have offered a sperm collection service to urologists performing VRs since 1992 in which intra-operative sperm assessment and storage of spermatozoa for later use in ART was provided. From 1992 to 1997, the number of requests for this service has progressively declined from a peak of 43 in 1995 to 24 in 1996 and to only 6 in 1997.

In several countries, including France and Australia, there is a governmental rebate for ART procedures which partially or fully covers the expenses of the couple. For example in Australia the out-of-pocket costs of a single cycle ICSI using PESA or fine needle biopsy (FNA) of the testis are about half those associated with a single VR attempt. The extent to which VR would be favoured over ART in other countries will obviously be affected by the availability of expertise in both fields, the relative costs of these treatments and perhaps cultural and religious issues.

Acceptance of testicular sperm retrieval for ICSI

In many cases epididymal spermatozoa are readily obtained by PESA and this represents a low cost and low morbidity option. For those in whom PESA is unsuccessful FAN allows sperm isolation. In the great majority of men with obstructive azoospermia, adequate numbers of spermatozoa for ICSI can be readily obtained using FNA biopsy under local anaesthesia. This procedure has been widely adopted by the ART gynaecological community, appears to have a low incidence of significant morbidity (about 1% significant haematoma), is well accepted by patients and, importantly, can be performed at little cost. With the potential for freeze–thawing of these spermatozoa, multiple attempts from a single needle biopsy can be anticipated although clear efficacy data on this approach are pending. However, as yet there is only limited, but overall reassuring, data on the safety of testicular spermatozoa in terms of birth outcomes. Finally data on the incidence of significant long-term damage to the testis, especially after repeated biopsies, are not yet available.

Conclusion

What then is the place of open epididymal sperm retrieval? If the goal is simply the provision of spermatozoa able to produce fertilization and pregnancy in ICSI, then patients and ART specialists are moving toward the use of PESA or testicular spermatozoa. Open exploratory epididymal surgery will always be more expensive, invasive and costly than FNA biopsy. Furthermore a significant number of surgeries will provide no spermatozoa (or only necrotic spermatozoa), even after the most diligent surgical exploration. Clearly if vas or epididymal surgery is to be undertaken to restore natural fertility, cryopreservation of the best fraction of spermatozoa recovered intraoperatively should be considered as 'insurance' in case of continued obstruction. Fortunately, whether epididymal or testicular spermatozoa are ultimately used for ICSI, the prospects for fertility are now good for this group of patients for whom very little hope was available only 5 years ago.

References

Aboulghar MA, Mansour RT, Serour GI, Fahmy I, Kamal A, Tawab NA and Amin YM (1997) Fertilisation and pregnancy rates after intracytoplasmic sperm injection using ejaculate semen and surgically retrieved sperm *Fertility and Sterility* **68** 108–111

Asch RH, Patrizio P and Silber S (1992) Ultrastructure of human sperm in men with congenital absence of the vas deferens: clinical implications *Fertility and Sterility* **58** 190–193

Belker A, Thomas AJ, Jr, Fuchs EF, Konnak JW and Sharlip ID (1991) Results of 1,469 microsurgical vasectomy reversal by the Vasavasostomy Study Group *Journal of Urology* **145** 505–511

Belker AM and Bergamini DA (1997) The feasibility of cryopreservation of sperm harvested intraoperatively during vasectomy reversals *Journal of Urology* **157** 1292–1294

Bladou F, Grillo JM, Rossi D, Noizet A, Gamerre M, Erny R, Luciani JM and Serment G (1991) Epididymal sperm aspiration in conjunction with *in-vitro* fertilization and embryo transfer in cases of obstructive azoospermia *Human Reproduction* **6** 1284–1287

Chillon M, Casals T, Mercier B, Bassas L, Lissens W, Silber S, Romey M-C, Ruiz-Romero J, Verlingue C, Claustres M, Nunes V, Ferec C and Estivilli X (1995) Mutations in the cystic fibrosis gene in patients with congenital absence of the vas deferens *New England Journal of Medicine* **332** 1475–1480

Cotman A and Allan JA (1997) Update on cryopreservation of seminiferous tubules *Proceedings of 16th Annual Scientific meeting of the Fertility Society of Australia, Adelaide* Abstract MP-7

Craft I and Tsirigotis M (1995) More experiences with ICSI: simplified recovery, preparation and cryopreservation of testicular spermatozoa *Human Reproduction* **10** 1623–1627

Devroey P, Liu J, Nagy Z, Tournaye H, Silber S and Van Steirteghem AC (1994) Normal fertilization of human oocytes after testicular sperm extraction and intracytoplasmic sperm injection *Fertility and Sterility* **62** 639–641

Devroey P, Silber S, Nagy Z, Liu J, Tournaye H, Joris H, Verheyen G and Van Steirteghem A (1995) Ongoing pregnancies and birth after intracytoplasmic sperm injection with frozen–thawed epididymal spermatozoa *Human Reproduction* **10** 903–906

Edirisinghe WR, Junk SM, Matson L and Yovich JL (1996) Changes in motility patterns during *in-vitro* culture of fresh and frozen/thawed testicular and epididymal spermatozoa: implications for planning treatment by intracytoplasmic sperm injection *Human Reproduction* **11** 2474–2476

Fahmy I, Mansour R, Aboulghar M, Serour G, Kamal A, Tawab NA, Ramzy AM and Amin Y (1997) Intracytoplasmic sperm injection using surgically retrieved epididymal and testicular spermatozoa in cases of obstructive and non-obstructive azoospermia *International Journal of Andrology* **20** 37–44

Holden CA, Fuscaldo GF, Jackson P, Cato A, Southwick GJ, Hauser R, Temple-Smith PD and McLachlan RI (1997) Frozen–thawed epididymal spermatozoa for intracytoplasmic sperm injection *Fertility and Sterility* **67** 81–87

Hovatta O, Reima I, Foudila T, Butzow T, Johansson K and von Smitten K (1996) Vas deferens aspiration and intracytoplasmic injection of frozen–thawed spermatozoa in a case of an ejaculation in a diabetic man *Human Reproduction* **11** 334–335

Lacham-Kaplan O and Trounson AO (1994) Micromanipulation assisted fertilisation: comparison of different techniques. In *Male Factor in Human Infertility* pp 287–304 Ed. J Tesarik, Ares Serono Symposia Publications

Lissens W, Tournaye MB, Bonduelle M, Ferec C, Seneca S, Devroey P, Silber S, Van Steirteghem A and Liebaers I (1996) Cystic fibrosis and infertility caused by congenital bilateral absence of the vas deferens and related clinical entities *Human Reproduction* **11** (Supplement 4) 55–78

McLachlan RI and Royce P (1996) The medical consequences of vasectomy *Current Obstetrics and Gynaecology* **6** 107–110

Madgar I, Siedman DS, Levran D, Yonish M, Augarten A, Yemini Z, Mashiach S and Dor J (1996) Micromanipulation improves *in-vitro* fertilization results after epididymal or testicular sperm aspiration in patients with congenital absence of the vas deferens *Human Reproduction* **11** 2151–2154

Mansour RT, Aboulghar MA, Serour GI, Fahmi I, Ramzy AM and Amin Y (1996) Intracytoplasmic sperm injection using microsurgically retrieved epididymal and testicular sperm *Fertility and Sterility* **65** 566–572

Mansour RT, Kamal A, Fahmy I, Tawab N, Serour GI and Aboulghar MA (1997) Intracytoplasmic sperm injection in obstructive and non-obstructive azoospermia *Human Reproduction* **12** 1974–1979

Nagy Z, Liu J, Cecile J, Silber S, Devroey P and Van Steirteghem A (1995) Using ejaculated, fresh, and frozen–thawed epididymal and testicular spermatozoa gives rise to comparable results after intracytoplasmic sperm injection *Fertility and Sterility* **63** 808–815

Patrizio P, Silber SJ, Ord T, Moretti-Rojas I and Asch RH (1992) Relationship of epididymal sperm antibodies to their *in vitro* fertilisation capacity in men with congenital absence of the vas deferens *Fertility and Sterility* **58** 1006–1010

Patrizio P, Ord T, Silber SJ and Asch RH (1993) Cystic fibrosis mutations impair the fertilization rate of epididymal sperm from men with congenital absence of the vas deferens *Human Reproduction* **8** 1259–1263

Patrizio P, Ord T, Silber SJ and Asch RH (1994) Correlation between epididymal length and fertilization rate in men with congenital absence of the vas deferens *Fertility and Sterility* **61** 265–268

Rosenlund B, Sjoblom P, Dimitrakopoulos A and Hillensjo T (1997) Epididymal and testicular sperm for intracytoplasmic sperm injection in the treatment of obstructive azoospermia *Acta Obstetrics Gynaecology Scandinavia* **76** 135–139

Schlegel PN, Berkeley AS, Goldstein M, Cohen J, Alikani M, Adler

A, **Gilbert BR and Rosenwaks Z** (1994) Epididymal micropuncture with *in vitro* fertilization and oocyte micromanipulation for the treatment of unreconstructable obstructive azoospermia *Fertility and Sterility* **61** 895–901

Silber SJ, Ord T, Balmaceda J, Patrizio P and Asch RH (1990) Congenital absence of the vas deferens. The fertilizing capacity of human epididymal sperm *The New England Journal of Medicine* **323** 1788–1792

Silber SJ, Nagy ZP, Liu J, Godoy H, Devroey P and Van Steirteghem AC (1994) Conventional *in-vitro* fertilization versus intracytoplasmic sperm injection for patients requiring microsurgical sperm aspiration *Human Reproduction* **9** 1705–1709

Silber SJ, Nagy Z, Liu J, Tournaye H, Lissens W, Ferec C, Liebaers I, Devroey P and Van Steirtegham AC (1995) The use of epididymal and testicular spermatozoa for intracytoplasmic sperm injection: the genetic implications for male infertility *Human Reproduction* **10** 2031–2043

Son IP, Hong JY, Lee YS, Park YS, Jun JH, Lee HJ, Kang IS and Jun JY (1996) Efficacy of microsurgical epididymal sperm aspiration (MESA) and intracytoplasmic sperm injection (ICSI) in obstructive azoospermia *Journal of Assisted Reproduction and Genetics* **13** 69–72

Temple-Smith PD, Southwick GJ, Yates CA, Trounson AO and de Kretser DM (1985) Human pregnancy by *in vitro* fertilization (IVF) using sperm aspirated from the epididymis *Journal of In Vitro Fertilization and Embryo Transfer* **2** 119–122

Tournaye H, Devroey P, Liu J, Nagy Z, Lissens W and Van Steirteghem A (1994) Microsurgical epididymal sperm aspiration and intracytoplasmic sperm injection: a new effective approach to infertility as a result of congenital bilateral absence of the vas deferens *Fertility and Sterility* **61** 1045–1051

Tsirigotis M, Pelekanos M, Yazdani N, Boulos A, Foster C and Craft IL (1995) Simplified sperm retrieval and intracytoplasmic sperm injection in patients with azoospermia *British Journal of Urology* **76** 765–768

Tsirigotis M, Pelekanos M, Beski S, Gregorakis S, Foster C and Craft IL (1996) Cumulative experience of percutaneous epididymal sperm aspiration (PESA) with intracytoplasmic sperm injection *Journal of Assistance Reproductive Genetics* **13** 315–319

Yamamoto M, Hibi H, Miyake K, Fukugaki H, Suganuma N and Tomoda Y (1995) Bulk sperm collection by epididymal micropuncture and stimulation of the spermatic nerve; a novel method for sperm retrieval for IVF for surgically irreparable vasal obstruction *International Journal of Andrology* **18** 97–102

Yamamoto M, Hibi H, Miyake K, Asada Y, Suganuma N and Tomoda Y (1996) Microsurgical epididymal sperm aspiration versus epididymal micropuncture with perivascular nerve stimulation for intracytoplasmic sperm injection to treat unreconstructable obstructive azoospermia *Archives of Andrology* **36** 217–224

Journal of Reproduction and Fertility Supplement **53**, 285–292

The epididymis across 24 centuries

Marie-Claire Orgebin-Crist

Departments of Obstetrics and Gynecology, Cell Biology, and Center for Reproductive Biology Research, Vanderbilt University, School of Medicine, Medical Center North, Room D2303, Nashville, TN 372–322633, USA

It is fitting as we are approaching the end of the 20th century to have a symposium entirely devoted to the epididymis. The first step was taken in 1992 when Dr Wong organized a one-day Symposium on 'Epididymis and Male Fertility' in Hong Kong. It became quite evident that the study of the epididymis had come of age and deserved a regular series of workshops to take stock of our knowledge and peer into the future. The series was established by holding a Boden Conference at Robertson, NSW, Australia in 1998. For this report of the conference, I have been invited to provide a historical perspective as well as some perspective for the future. Combining the two is fitting because "...the heritage of the past is the seed that brings forth the harvest of the future." (Fraser, 1934).

The first recorded description of the epididymis was made in the middle of the 4th century BC by Aristotle in his *Historia Animalium* and the first recorded description of a dissected epididymis was made by de Graaf in 1668 in his monograph *Tractatus de Virorum Organis Generationi Inservientibus*. De Graaf noted that "...the semen ... was watery and ash-like in the testis and becomes milky and thick in the epididymis" (Jocelyn and Setchell, 1972). Between 1888 and 1928 a number of scientists from the German and French schools of anatomy described the histological features of the epididymal epithelium, and from the images of secretion they were observing surmised that epididymal secretions 'nourished' the spermatozoa in the epididymal lumen. Hammar had noted in 1897 "...that in the upper part of the epididymis there is thick semen with immotile spermatozoa, whereas in the lower sections of the tail the semen is thinner and the spermatozoa are freely motile". But Tournade (1913) provided the first experimental investigation of live epididymal spermatozoa in several species. He showed that spermatozoa released from the proximal epididymis were not motile when diluted in saline, but spermatozoa released from the distal epididymis were fully motile. He wrote: "The phenomenon is general; what is its signification? Must we attribute this to an autonomous evolution, so to speak, of the spermatozoa which, still imperfect entities as they exit from the seminiferous tubules, develop into adult cells as they progress through the excurrent ducts? Or is it the result of an excitomotor action exercised by the epididymal epithelium?" Tournade favoured the second hypothesis. The implication from all these observations was that the epididymis conditioned the development of sperm motility. A number of investigators showed that the epididymis was important for sperm survival as well. Courrier (1920) observed that bat spermatozoa survived for several months in the cauda during hibernation, presumably protected by epididymal secretion. Rabbit spermatozoa survived in the epididymis for 30–60 days (Hammond and Asdell, 1926) and bull spermatozoa survived for two months (Kirillov and Mozorov, 1936) after ligation of the efferent ducts. What is remarkable in de Graff's description as well as in those of investigators 100 years ago was their intuitive acumen as they relate structure to function.

This period of intense activity culminated with the masterpiece of Jacques Benoit, who in 1926 not only provided a detailed and accurate description of epididymal histology in different species, including man, but also provided the first experimental evidence that the function of the epididymis and the survival of spermatozoa depended upon the hormones secreted by the testis. He observed that the ratio nucleus:cytoplasm in the mouse epididymis decreased after birth as the epididymis differentiated and increased markedly after castration as the epididymis dedifferentiated. He also observed that epididymal spermatozoa died quickly after bilateral castration, but not after unilateral castration. In the latter case, sperm motility remained normal on the castrated side two months after the operation. For Benoit and earlier investigators, the epididymis provided a protective environment for the survival of epididymal spermatozoa and this function depended upon a testicular hormone. Two years later, Moore showed that an injection of a testicular extract could replace this testicular hormone after castration, and in 1931 Butenandt opened the era of endocrinology by achieving the chemical synthesis of testosterone.

The consensus of these early investigations can be summarized by the last sentence of Benoit's monograph: "The role of epididymal secretions is to maintain sperm vitality, to permit the development of sperm motility, and possibly to protect them against noxious agents." Against this chorus of converging opinions, a lonely voice came from across the Atlantic. In a series of four articles published between 1929 and 1931, Young showed by artificial insemination in guinea-pigs that spermatozoa removed from the proximal epididymis were much less fertile than those removed from the distal epididymis, and concluded that during epididymal transit spermatozoa acquire not only a mature motility pattern, but also become fertile. He went on to show that immature spermatozoa isolated in the epididymis by two ligatures placed on the caput and the vas deferens became motile and fertile. He concluded "...1) that the time consumed by spermatozoa in passing through the epididymis is necessary for a completion of their development, and 2) that the changes undergone during this period represent a continuation of changes which start while the spermatozoa are still attached to the germinal epithelium and are not conditioned by some specific action of the epididymal secretion." The last part of the sentence was an over-interpretation of a flawed experiment. The ligatures did not isolate immature spermatozoa in the proximal epididymis, but rather isolated the whole epididymis. One cannot eliminate the possibility of sperm reflux from the distal to the proximal part. Even more so, since the line of division for sampling spermatozoa from the proximal and the distal part of the epididymis was at the junction of the proximal and the distal cauda, making it likely that even under normal circumstances mature spermatozoa may have been sampled with the proximal epididymis. Finally, there was only a modest increase in fertilizing ability of immature spermatozoa after 25 days of isolation (49% versus 33.3%). Nevertheless, by 1931 most of the problems and questions relating to epididymal physiology had been recognized and most of the work done since then has been to provide the experimental evidence to flesh out the insights of earlier investigators.

Surprisingly, in the ensuing 20–30 years, very few studies were published on epididymal physiology and most dealt with determination of the time necessary for spermatozoa to transit through the epididymis. Earlier studies used tracers such as India ink (Toothill and Young, 1931). After 1950, radioactive isotopes incorporated in sperm DNA were used to follow sperm transit (Ortavant, 1956; Orgebin-Crist, 1961). Surprisingly, irrespective of the species, the length of the epididymis, or the rate of sperm production, the passage of spermatozoa through the epididymis of different mammals lasts approximately 10 days.

The apparent disinterest in the epididymis during this 20–30 years span is puzzling. After the work of Benoit in 1926 and Young in 1931, there was a clear controversy that needed to be resolved. It is unlikely that investigators of that time shied away from the controversy. It is more likely that the horrendous haemorrhage of young talents in European universities caused by World War I had an impact. In addition, the forceful conclusions of Young may have appeared definitive to investigators who may not have been aware of the extensive work done by European anatomists at the turn of the century. It is also possible that, with the synthesis of steroids, the golden age of endocrinology began, favouring studies on endocrine organs such as the testis and ovary. In 1965, only 40 papers on epididymal physiology were published (Fig. 1). This contrasts with the number of publications on the testis and the ovary, which numbered 200 and 300, respectively. Whatever the reason for this disaffection, in 1964 Thaddeus Mann in his book *The Biochemistry of Semen* could refer to the epididymis as the abandoned child of the reproductive system.

A renaissance of interest in epididymal physiology occurred when detailed investigations of the motility and fertilizing ability of spermatozoa retained in discrete epididymal segments showed that the key event in sperm maturation was not the passage of time, as proposed by Young, but exposure to the luminal environment of the epididymis (Bedford, 1967; Orgebin-Crist, 1967, 1969a). The

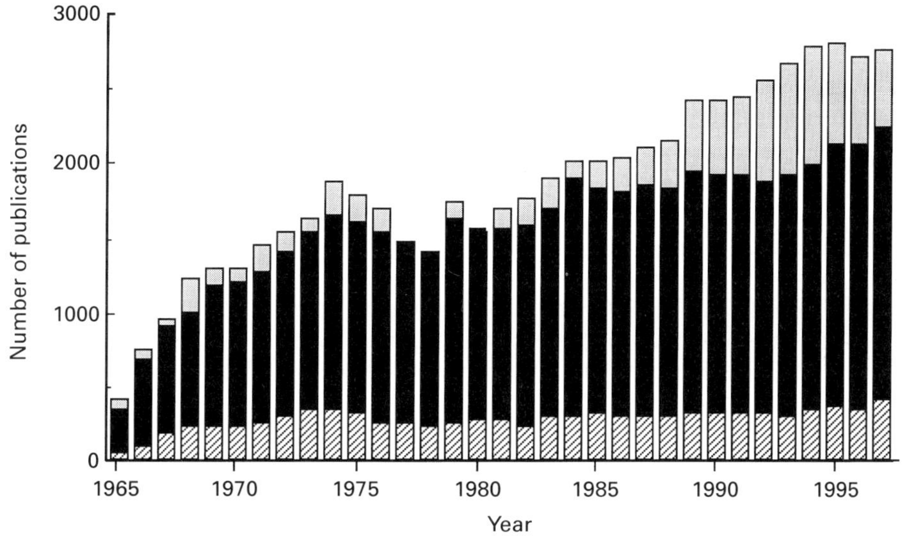

Fig. 1. Number of publications per year on the epididymis (▨), testis (■), and ovary (□) from 1965–1997.

number of publications on the epididymis per year increased from 43 in 1965 to 308 in 1975. A complete bibliography *Epididymal Physiology in Relation to Sperm Maturation* for the period 1962–1969 listed only 177 references (Orgebin-Crist, 1969b).

Studies *in vivo* done in the 1960s documented (1) that the potential for sperm motility and fertilizing ability is acquired as spermatozoa pass from the proximal to the distal epididymis; (2) that the maturation process does not end with the acquisition of fertilizing ability, since spermatozoa that have just become fertile induce a higher rate of embryonic mortality when inseminated *in vivo*; (3) that the maturation process is dependent upon an androgen-stimulated epididymis, both *in vitro* and *in vivo*; and (4) that the maturation process includes changes in sperm organelles, most prominently the plasma membrane. In 1975 I asked in a review: "What is sperm maturation? What are the specific changes that trigger the sperm fertilizing ability?" and responded: "We do not know." (Orgebin-Crist *et al.*, 1975).

This conference has given us a vantage point to see what we have learned during the past 20 years. Considerable progress has been made and, most importantly, we have come to realize that epididymal function and sperm maturation are far more complex than we could possibly imagine in the 1960s. But it is fair to say that we still do not have the response to those basic questions. It is not my intent to summarize what was presented during this meeting and forms the content of this supplement. Rather, I will highlight some areas that, in my personal, and admittedly rather biased, opinion, are ripe for further development.

There was no need to convince the participants of this symposium of the importance of the epididymis during the post-testicular lifespan of spermatozoa. During evolution, a complex system has evolved in which testicular spermatozoa are no longer able to fertilize and have to go through the processes of maturation in the male genital tract and capacitation in the female genital tract before being able to fertilize *in vivo* (R. C. Jones, this supplement).

The need for these post-testicular changes can be eliminated, since mature epididymal spermatozoa, testicular spermatozoa, round spermatids, or even secondary spermatocytes can be directly injected into the egg ooplasm with the resulting development of a viable embryo. These techniques are currently being used in the clinic. It is estimated that 5–10% of all males under age 45 suffer from infertility. The largest group of patients diagnosed with infertility suffers from idiopathic infertility. Some of these patients have subnormal semen parameters; however, the pathogenesis of their disorder, which is likely to be multifactorial, is unknown. Therefore, no rational treatment can be offered. As a result, and despite the high prevalence of male infertility in the general population, the therapeutic options for this type of male infertility are limited. Within the present state of our knowledge, the fertilization-assisted techniques offer the only hope for some infertile couples to achieve a pregnancy and these techniques are referred to by some as the ultimate treatment of male infertility. However, we should realize that we are not treating the infertile male. We are not providing a cure to the infertile male. We are exposing the normal female partner of the infertile couple to the rigors of assisted-fertilization techniques. Although assisted reproductive technology has its place in the alleviation of male infertility, the long-term goal of infertility therapy should be to promote the development of an optimum number of spermatozoa endowed with normal fertilizing ability. Although there may be practical compelling reasons for using assisted-fertilization techniques (McLachlan; de Kretser *et al.*, this supplement), their use should not overshadow other alternatives such as epididymal surgical techniques aimed at restoring the male fertility potential. Nor, in attempting to devise rational treatments for male infertility, does the advent of these techniques obviate the need to search for and understand the pathogenic mechanisms involved in male infertility and to unravel the intimate mechanisms regulating both spermatogenesis and the post-testicular maturation and storage of spermatozoa. As a corollary, a systematic approach based on a better understanding of the basic mechanisms regulating sperm maturation and survival of spermatozoa in the male genital tract will open new avenues for an effective control of male fertility.

Many studies reviewed during this meeting have confirmed that mammalian spermatozoa undergo a post-testicular maturation process, including development of fertilizing ability. In both rodents and humans, part of this maturation process can be duplicated *in vitro* by co-culture of spermatozoa and epididymal epithelium under androgen stimulation, underscoring the contribution of the epididymal epithelium to the maturation process (Moore *et al.*, this supplement). However, the elegant surgical techniques of selective regional bypasses done by Temple-Smith *et al.* (this supplement) have shown that sperm maturation may not be as regionally dependent as had been previously thought. This should be kept in mind when searching for the specific changes induced by epididymal transit that are required to promote sperm fertilizing ability.

Nevertheless, the fact that spermatozoa mature and are maintained in a viable state in the epididymis has prompted many studies on epididymal function which were amply discussed during the meeting. As spermatozoa transit through the epididymis, they are exposed to an ever-changing environment resulting from the secretory and reabsorptive properties of the epididymal epithelial cells lining the duct. A major site of fluid reabsorption is the efferent ducts. This has been known since the 1920s when Van Wagenen (1924) showed that aspermatogenesis caused by fluid accumulation occurred when ligations were placed on the efferent ducts proximally to the testis, but did not occur when the ligations were placed at the distal end of the efferent ducts. The control of fluid reabsorption by the efferent ducts is a complex process with multiple components under multi-hormonal control (Clulow *et al.*; Hess, this supplement). Likewise, the control of electrolyte and fluid transport in the epididymis involves peptide hormones and adrenergic agents (Wong, this supplement). It is likely that other epididymal functions are also under multi-hormonal control and this will be a crucial question for future study.

The recognition of the complex functional importance and regulation of the efferent ducts should prompt a re-examination of the function of another neglected part of the male reproductive tract: the vas deferens. Results of epididymovasostomy in laboratory species and in humans and of vas grafts done in rodents (Temple-Smith *et al.*, this supplement) open the possibility that the male reproductive tract may have a greater plasticity than previously considered.

Another relatively neglected area of investigation is the fate of ageing spermatozoa in the male genital tract. Under experimental conditions, luminal disintegration of spermatozoa and uptake by phagocytic cells occur from the efferent ducts to the vas deferens. But in several species, including humans, the ampullary region of the vas appears to be an important site of sperm phagocytosis. What triggers this phagocytosis or how cells are marked for destruction is not known. This is a gap in our understanding of gamete biology that needs to be filled.

The availability of molecular biology techniques has opened a new era in the study of epididymal function. This meeting has demonstrated the progress made since the first cDNA for an epididymal secretory protein was cloned by Brooks *et al.* (1986). It has illustrated that, although the duct is lined throughout its length with the same cell type, a polarized columnar principal cell, each region has a specific pattern of gene expression (Ivell *et al.*, this supplement). Furthermore, the regulation of epididymal gene expression is also region specific (Hinton *et al.*, this supplement). The regionalization of gene expression in the epididymis is striking if not unique. It is observed not only with epididymis-specific genes, but also with ubiquitously expressed somatic genes (Orgebin-Crist, 1996). It will be important to identify the regulatory factors that are responsible for region-specific expression in the epididymis. It is unlikely that these regulatory factors will be found to be specific to the epididymis. The model of combinatorial gene control proposes that regulatory proteins need not be unique. Rather, the proper combination of several factors ensures tissue-specific expression (Alberts *et al.*, 1994; Gierer, 1974). It has been estimated that the control of tissue specificity in species ranging from *Drosophila* to man may require as few as two and, at most, eight regulatory proteins (Arnone and Davidson, 1997). It is likely that the control of region-specific gene expression in the epididymis follows the same paradigm and progress is expected in the near future in deciphering the molecular mechanisms responsible for region-specific gene expression in the epididymis.

The regulation of epididymal gene expression depends on the endocrine function of the testis, but paracrine regulation is likely and is just beginning to be appreciated. The paracrine regulation may involve factors such as growth factor present in the fluid (Hinton *et al.*, this supplement), but the contribution of spermatozoa has been overlooked and may be important. Cell–cell interaction in the epididymis has until now been assumed to be unidirectional, i.e. the end products of somatic cell gene expression interacting with epididymal spermatozoa considered passive recipients. Garrett *et al.* (1990) had suggested that spermatozoa or a sperm-associated factor could regulate proenkephalin gene expression in the epididymis. The notion that cell–cell interaction in the epididymis might be bi-directional and that spermatozoa could control epididymal gene expression is intriguing and should stimulate research in the future.

Cell–cell interaction between epididymal cells and their secretory proteins and spermatozoa has received more attention. The task is far more daunting than originally envisaged. Unlike the regulatory factors controlling epididymal gene expression, which are likely to be few in number and are unlikely to be tissue-specific, epididymal gene transcripts are numerous and many are unique to the epididymis. Protein analysis by two-dimensional electrophoresis and computer image analysis has yielded a large number of proteins (Hinton *et al.*; Cooper; Dacheux *et al.*, this supplement). Even when the technique is combined with protein microsequencing, it will be difficult to determine the function of all of these epididymal proteins. Likewise, molecular biology techniques using differential cloning (Ivell *et al.*, this supplement) or analysis of Expressed-Sequence Tag (EST) (Adams *et al.*, 1991) generated from epididymal cDNA libraries yield a large number of clones. In the prostate gland, the mRNAs from most genes are of low abundance, at 0.001% of the total population. A few genes are expressed at a high abundance of 1–2% (Nelson *et al.*, 1998). The highly abundant species are often tissue specific and the majority of the low abundant transcripts are ubiquitous, shared among many tissues, implying a housekeeping function (Bishop *et al.*, 1974). This assumption, which remains to be proven for the epididymis, would narrow the number of genes to be studied, but assigning a function to these genes will be a more formidable task than determining their sequence. Many of these epididymis-specific genes encode secretory proteins. As could be expected, the first to be studied were the most abundant proteins present in epididymal fluid. A few of these secretory proteins encoded by epididymis-specific genes have been identified. They include binding proteins that may be involved in the transport of ligands between spermatozoa and epithelial cells (such as phospholipid binding protein (Araki *et al.*, 1992) and retinoic acid binding protein (Lareyre *et al.*, this supplement)) and enzymes that may either modify the composition of the plasma membrane (such as glycoprotein-modifying enzymes or proteases (Jones, Tulsiani *et al.*, this volume)), or protect the mature spermatozoa against oxidative damage during storage in the distal epididymis (such as glutathione peroxidase, γ-glutamyl transpeptidase and superoxide dismutase (Hinton *et al.*; Aitken and Vernet; Schwaab *et al.*, this supplement)). In the years to come, the list of these proteins will grow. One need not assume that each of these proteins has a definite function. Evolution has taught us that nature does not proceed in a straightforward fashion. At a molecular level, the same may apply and Jacob (1970) has used the word 'tinkering' to describe how nature uses the same building blocks in different ways to adapt to different functions. In this 'tinkering' some genes may subsist as long as they do not have a negative impact. For assessing the function of these genes, it will not be sufficient to determine homology with known proteins; their function will have to be demonstrated. In the case of a binding protein, it should be determined whether the appropriate ligand binds *in vivo* and, in the case of an enzyme, whether it is enzymatically active *in vivo*.

Despite these recent developments, it has yet to be determined how the changing composition of the epididymal fluid and the secretion of specific proteins relate to the development of sperm motility and fertilizing ability. The plasma membrane is involved in motility-related events, in the acrosome reaction, and in the fusion with the egg plasma membrane. The spermatozoon is a highly polarized cell and its plasma membrane is a mosaic of well-defined domains. Modification of the plasma membrane is a key element of the maturation process (R. Jones, this supplement). It includes binding of epididymal secretory proteins to restricted surface domains, remodelling of lipid components, and redistribution of pre-existing proteins between domains after proteolytic processing. It is likely that future studies will identify other post-translational mechanisms responsible for the remodelling of the sperm plasma membrane during maturation. However, the sperm membrane has a large array of surface proteins that can be modified during epididymal sperm maturation (Naaby-Hansen *et al.*, 1997). As discussed above, cataloguing these proteins or the epididymal secretory proteins will not be sufficient to understand the complex process of post-testicular sperm maturation. Identification of the molecular processes involved in sperm motility, sperm storage, egg recognition and fusion will help in selecting epididymal proteins that may affect these functions.

Future breakthroughs are likely to come from inactivation of the genes of interest by homologous recombination in ES cells in order to directly test their role in the context of the whole animal. This is a powerful technique that is not without surprises. Of the gene transcripts thought to mediate the fertilization process, the disruption of the ZP3 gene or the fertilin gene gave a phenotype consistent with their role in fertilization (Rankin *et al.*, 1996; Liu *et al.*, 1996; Cho *et al.*, 1998), while disruption of acrosin (Baba *et al.*, 1994) and β-galactosyltransferase (Lu and Shur, 1997) did not result in infertility. A lack of phenotype does not rule out the functional importance of a particular gene transcript. Subtle alterations, not sufficient to cause complete infertility, may occur. This appears to be the case for acrosin (Adham *et al.*, 1997) and β-galactosyltransferase (Lu and Shur, 1997). Furthermore, the lesson learned from the inactivation of the tenascin gene shows that in cases involving proteins belonging to a large family, deletion of one member of the gene family may produce no apparent phenotype, because several members of the family may have similar functions with the different members serving primarily to expand expression, while deletion of another member produces a pronounced phenotype (Erikson, 1997).

Progress will come from the disruption of genes that are thought to be important in epididymal physiology. As yet, there has been no reported gene disruption of epididymis-specific secretory proteins. Gene inactivation of the ubiquitous enzyme β-galactosidase (Matsuda *et al.*, 1997) which is highly expressed in the epididymis did not result in infertility, while inactivation of the γ-glutamyl transpeptidase gene (Harding *et al.*, 1997), which is believed to be important for sperm survival in the epididymis, resulted in infertility; but it is not clear from that study what part of the reproductive process was disrupted.

Just as importantly, progress will come from other fields, from disruption of genes that are not under investigation by epididymal physiologists. The best example is the targeted mutation of the c-ros tyrosine kinase receptor (Yeung *et al.*, this supplement). It produces a phenotype in which males are sterile. The only obvious defect is a lack of differentiation of the proximal caput epididymidis, suggesting that failure of differentiation of epithelial cells in one segment of the epididymis can affect sperm maturation and survival. Overexpression of a dominant negative RARα receptor in transgenic mice causes a disorganization of the columnar epithelium lining the cauda epididymidis followed by its transformation into a squamous-like epithelium with resulting infertility (Costa *et al.*, 1997). Other examples include male infertility caused by disruption of the apolipoprotein B gene (Huang *et al.*, 1996), the POU-homeodomain Sprm-1 (Pearse *et al.*, 1997), the protease PC4 gene (Mbikay *et al.*, 1997) the calmegin gene, a homologue of the ER chaperone calnexin (Ikawa *et al.*,

1997) and the bone morphogenic protein 8a gene (Zhao *et al.*, 1998). Both PC4 and calmegin are germ-cell specific. Gene disruption causes no obvious spermatogenic abnormality, but fertilizing ability *in vitro* is nil in the case of calmegin-null spermatozoa and severelly reduced in the case of PC4-null spermatozoa. Serine proteases are implicated in the processing of a variety of polypeptides, including cell surface proteins. Calnexin is a ubiquitous ER chaperone that plays a major role in quality control by retaining improperly folded proteins. The authors surmised that these genes may be involved in ensuring the proper maturation and processing of sperm surface molecules required for fertilization. A comparison of the sperm protein profiles between the wild-type and the mutant mice may facilitate the identification of these molecules. The apolipoprotein B gene, the Bmp8a gene and the POU-Sperm-1 gene are expressed in the testis, but also in the epididymis. Since inactivation of these genes does not affect spermatogenesis, it cannot be excluded that the infertility phenotype may have an extratesticular origin.

The new genetic technology has revolutionized the biological sciences. It has quickened the pace of research and vastly expanded the capability of the reproductive biologist to address reproductive functions and reproductive dysfunctions. Its impact has already been considerable, but with the rapid advancement of knowledge and techniques seen in recent years, we stand on the threshold of an era where one can hope that a better understanding of the molecular mechanisms involved in sperm maturation in the epididymis and the relation of epididymal maturation to the later events of sperm capacitation and sperm interaction in the female genital tract will offer rational methods of post-testicular male contraception, rational treatments of male infertility which may reduce the need to resort to invasive assisted-fertilization techniques. Despite the caveats discussed above, exciting years lie ahead. "What's past is prologue" .... (Shakespeare).

I want to thank all my past and present collaborators for their unflagging support, wealth of ideas, and unbounded enthusiasm and, in particular, Jean-Jacques Lareyre, Robert Matusik, Gary Olson, and David Ong for their helpful comments on this manuscript.

References

Adams MD, Kelley JM, Gocayne JD, Dubnick M, Polymeropoulos MH, Xiao H, Merril CR, Wu A, Olde B, Moreno RF, Kerlavage AR, McCombie WR, and Venter JC (1991) Complementary DNA sequencing: expressed sequence tags and human genome project *Science* **252** 1651–1656

Adham IM, Nayernia K and Engel W (1997) Spermatozoa lacking acrosin protein show delayed fertilization *Molecular Reproduction and Development* 370–376

Alberts B, Bray D, Lewis J, Raff M, Roberts K and Watson JD (1994) Control of gene expression. In *Molecular Biology of the Cell* pp 401–474. Garland Publishing Inc., New York & London

Araki Y, Vierula ME, Rankin TL, Tulsiani DRP and Orgebin-Crist MC (1992) Isolation and characterization of a 25 kilodalton protein from mouse testis: sequence homology with a phospholipid-binding protein *Biology of Reproduction* **47** 832–843

Aristotle (384–322 BC) *Historia Animalium*, A.L. Peck, trans., Loeb Classical Library Nos 437–438, 2 Vols., 1965, 239p. and 414p. Harvard University Press, Cambridge, MA

Arnone MI and Davidson EH (1997) The hardwiring of development: organization and function of genomic regulatory systems *Development* **124** 1851–1864

Baba T, Azuma S, Kashiwabara S and Toyoda Y (1994) Sperm from mice carrying a targeted mutation of the acrosin gene can penetrate the oocyte zona pellucida and effect fertilization *Journal of Biological Chemistry* **269** 31845–31849

Bedford JM (1967) Effect of duct ligation on the fertilizing ability of spermatozoa from different regions of the rabbit epididymis *Journal of Experimental Zoology* **166** 271–281

Benoit MJ (1926) Recherches anatomiques, cytologiques et histophysiologiques sur les voies excretrices du testicule. chez les mammiferes *Archives de Anatomie de Histologie et de Embryologie* **5** 173–412

Bishop JO, Morton JG, Rosbash M and Richardson M (1974) Three abundance classes in HeLa cell messenger RNA *Nature* **250** 199–204

Brooks DE, Means AR, Wright EJ, Singh SP and Tiver KK (1986) Molecular cloning of the cDNA for androgen-dependent sperm-coating glycoprotein secreted by the rat epididymis *European Journal of Biochemistry* **161** 13–18

Butenandt A (1931) Uber die chemisch untersuchung der sexualhormone *Zeitschrift fur Angewandte Chemie* **44** 905–908

Cho C, Bunch DO, Faure JE, Goulding EH, Eddy EM, Primakoff P and Myles DG (1998) Fertilization defects in sperm from mice lacking fertilin beta *Science* **281** 1857–1859

Costa SL, Boekelheide K, Vanderhyden BC, Seth R and McBurney NW (1997) Male infertility caused by epididymal dysfunction in transgenic mice expressing a dominant negative mutation of retinoic acid receptor alpha *Biology of Reproduction* **56** 985–990

Courrier R (1920) Sur l'existence d'une secretion epididymaire chez la Chauve-Souris hibernante et sa signification *Comptes Rendus de Societe Biologie Paris* **83** 67–69

Erickson HP (1997) A tenascin knockout with a phenotype *Nature Genetics* **17** 5–7

Fraser JE (1934) Inscription on the pedestal of a sculpture on the Constitution Avenue entrance of the National Archives Building, Washington DC. Wording devised by sculptor

James Earle Fraser, worked over by RDW Connor, First Archivist of the United States

Garrett JE, Garrett SH and Douglas J (1990) A spermatozoa-associated factor regulated proenkephalin gene expression in the rat epididymis *Molecular Endocrinology* **4** 108–118

Gierer A (1974) Molecular models and combinatorial principles in cell differentiation and morphogenesis *Cold Spring Harbor Symposia on Quantitative Biology* **38** 951–961

Hammar JA (1897) Uber secretionserscheinungen im Nebenhoden des Hundes *Archiv Anat Physiol Lpz* **Supplement** 1–42

Hammond J and Asdell SA (1926) The vitality of the spermatozoa in the male and female reproductive tracts *British Journal of Experimental Biology* **4** 155–185

Harding CO, Williams P, Wagner E, Chang DS, Wild K, Colwell RE and Wolff JA (1997) Mice with genetic γ-glutamyl transpeptidase deficiency exhibit glutathionuria, severe growth failure, reduced life spans, and infertility *The Journal of Biological Chemistry* **272** 12 560–12 567

Huang LS, Voyiaziakis E, Chen HL, Rubin EM and Gordon JW (1996) A novel functional role for apolipoprotein B in male infertility in heterozygous apolipoprotein B knockout mice *Proceedings of the National Academy of Science USA* **93** 10 903–10 907

Ikawa M, Wada I, Kominami K, Watanabe D, Toshimori K, Nishimune Y and Okabe M (1997) The putative chaperone calmegin is required for sperm fertility *Nature* **387** 607–611

Jacob F (1977) Evolution and tinkering *Science* **196** 1161–1166

Jocelyn HD and Setchell BP (1972) A treatise concerning the generative organs of men. An annotated translation of "Tractatus de Virorum Organis Generationi Inservientibus" (1968) *Journal of Reproduction and Fertility Supplement* **17** 1–76

Kirillov VS and Morozov VA (1936) Duree de conservation de la vitalité des spermatozoides de Taureau dans les épididymes isolés du testicule *Uspekhi zootekh, Nauk* **2** 19–22

Liu C, Litscher ES, Mortillo S, Sakai Y, Kinloch RA, Stewart CL and Wassarman PM (1996) Targeted disruption of the mZP3 gene results in production of eggs lacking a zona pellucida and infertility in female mice *Proceedings of the National Academy of Sciences USA* **93** 5431–5436

Lu Q and Shur BD (1997) Sperm from β1,4-galactosyltrasferase-null mice are refractory to ZP3-induced acrosome reactions and penetrate the zona pellucida poorly *Development* **124** 4121–4131

Mann T (1964) *The Biochemistry of Semen and of the Male Reproductive Tract.* Methuen, London

Matsuda J, Suzuki O, Oshima A, Ogura A, Noguchi Y, Yamamoto Y, Asano T, Takimoto K, Sukegawa K, Suzuki Y and Naiki M (1997) β-Galactosidase-deficient mouse as an animal model for G_{M1}-gangliosidosis *Glycoconjugate Journal* **14** 729–736

Mbikay M, Tadros H, Ishida N, Lerner CP, De Lamirande E, Chen A, El-Alfy M, Clermont Y, Seidah NG, Chretien M, Gagnon C and Simpson EM (1997) Impaired fertility in mice deficient for the testicular germ-cell protease PC4 *Proceedings of the National Academy of Science USA* **94** 6842–6846

Moore CR (1928) Sperm activity and testis hormone *Journal of Experimental Zoology* **50** 455–462

Naaby-Hansen S, Flickinger CJ and Herr JC (1997) Two-dimensional gel electrophoretic analysis of vectorially labeled surface proteins of human spermatozoa *Biology of Reproduction* **56** 771–787

Nelson PS, Ng WL, Schummer M, True LD, Liu AY, Bumgarner RE, Ferguson C, Dimak A and Hood L (1998) An expressed-sequence-tag database of the human prostate: sequence analysis of 1168 cNDA clones *Genomics* **47** 12–25

Orgebin MC (1961) Etude du transit épididymaire des spermatozoïdes de Taureau marqués à l'aide du ^{32}P *Annales Biologie animales Bioch Biophys* **1** 117–120

Orgebin-Crist MC (1967) Maturation of spermatozoa in the rabbit epididymis: fertilizing ability and embryonic mortality in does inseminated with epididymal spermatozoa *Annales Biologie animales Bioch Biophys* **7** 373–389

Orgebin-Crist MC (1969a) Studies on the function of the epididymis *Biology of Reproduction* **1** 155–175

Orgebin-Crist MC (1969b) Bibliography on Epididymal Physiology in Relation to Sperm Maturation *Biblphy Reprod* **14** 141–148; 289–294

Orgebin-Crist MC (1996) Androgens and epididymal function. In *Pharmacology, Biology, and Clinical Applications of Androgens* pp. 27–38 Eds S Bhasin, HL Gabelnick, JM Spieler, RS Swerdloff and C Wang Wiley-Liss Inc., New York

Orgebin-Crist MC, Danzo BJ and Davies J (1975) Endocrine control of the development and maintenance of sperm fertilizing ability in the epididymis. In *Handbook of Physiology-Endocrinology V* pp. 319–338 Eds VR Greep and DW Hamilton Williams & Wilkins, Baltimore, MD

Ortavant R (1954) Determination de la vitesse de transfert des spermatozoides dans l'epididyme de Belier a l'aide de ^{32}P *Comptes Rendus Societe Biolologie* **143** 866–871

Pearse RV 2nd, Drolet DW, Kalla KA, Hooshmand F, Bermingham JR, Jr and Rosenfeld MG (1997) Reduced fertility in mice deficient for the POU protein sperm-1 *Proceedings of the National Academy of Science USA* **94** 7555–7560

Rankin T, Familari M, Lee E, Ginsberg A, Dwyer N, Blanchette-Mackie J, Drago J, Westphal H and Dean J (1996) Mice homozygous for an insertional mutation in the Zp3 gene lack a zona pellucida and are infertile *Development* **122** 2903–2910

Shakespeare WC (1611–1613) *The Tempest* Act 2, Scene 1, line 253

Simeone FA and Young WC (1930) A study of the function of the epididymis. IV. The fate of non ejaculated spermatozoa in the genital tract of the male guinea-pig *Journal of Experimental Biology* **8** 163–175

Toothill MC and Young WC (1931) The time consumed by spermatozoa in passing through the epididymis of the guinea-pig determined by india ink injections *Anatomical Record* **50** 95–107

Tournade A (1913) Différence de motilité des spermatozoïdes prélevés dans les divers segments de l'épididyme *Comptes Rendus Societe Biologie***74** 738–739

Van Wagenen G (1924) Degeneration of germinal epithelium in the testis of the rat as a result of efferent duct ligation *Anatomical Record* **27** 189–190

Young WC (1929a) A study of the function of the epididymis I. Is the attainment of full spermatozoon maturity attributable to some specific action of the epididymal secretion *Journal of Morphology* **47** 479–495

Young WC (1929b) A study of the function of the epididymis II. The importance of an aging process in sperm for the length of the period during which fertilizing capacity is retained by sperm isolated in the epididymis of the guinea pig *Journal of Morphology* **48** 475–491

Young WC (1931) A study of the function of the epididymis. III. Functional changes undergone by spermatozoa during their passage through the epididymis and vas deferens in the guinea pig *Journal of Experimental Biology* **8** 151–162

Zhao G-Q, Liaw L and Hogan BLM (1998) Bone morphogenetic protein 8A plays a role in the maintenance of spermatogenesis and the integrity of the epididymis *Development* **125** 1103–1112

AUTHOR INDEX

SUBJECT INDEX